A Pattern-Based Approach
Atlas of Forensic Pathology

WALTER L. KEMP, MD, PhD
Montana State Chief Medical Examiner
Forensic Science Division
Department of Justice
Billings, Montana

Clinical Associate Professor
Department of Laboratory Medicine and Pathology
University of Washington School of Medicine
Seattle, Washington

RHOME L. HUGHES, MD, MS
Associate Professor
School of Engineering Medicine
Texas A&M University
College Station, Texas

JEFFREY J. BARNARD, MD
Director and Chief Medical Examiner
Dallas County
Professor
Department of Pathology
University of Texas Southwestern Medical Center
Dallas, Texas

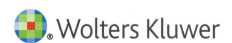

Philadelphia • Baltimore • New York • London
Buenos Aires • Hong Kong • Sydney • Tokyo

Acquisitions Editor: Nicole Dernoski
Development Editor: Ariel S. Winter
Editorial Coordinator: Varshaanaa Muralidharan
Editorial Assistant: Kristen Kardoley
Marketing Manager: Kirsten Watrud
Senior Production Project Manager: Alicia Jackson
Manager, Graphic Arts & Design: Stephen Druding
Manufacturing Coordinator: Lisa Bowling
Prepress Vendor: TNQ Technologies

Copyright © 2024 Wolters Kluwer

All rights reserved. This book is protected by copyright. No part of this book may be reproduced or transmitted in any form or by any means, including as photocopies or scanned-in or other electronic copies, or utilized by any information storage and retrieval system without written permission from the copyright owner, except for brief quotations embodied in critical articles and reviews. Materials appearing in this book prepared by individuals as part of their official duties as U.S. government employees are not covered by the above-mentioned copyright. To request permission, please contact Wolters Kluwer at Two Commerce Square, 2001 Market Street, Philadelphia, PA 19103, via email at permissions@lww.com, or via our website at shop.lww.com (products and services).

The views expressed in this work are the private views of the authors and do not purport to reflect the official policy or position of the Food and Drug Administration or any part of the US Government, nor were the materials prepared as part of official government duties.

9 8 7 6 5 4 3 2 1

Printed in Mexico

Library of Congress Cataloging-in-Publication Data

ISBN-13: 978-1-975222-50-5

Cataloging in Publication data available on request from publisher.

This work is provided "as is," and the publisher disclaims any and all warranties, express or implied, including any warranties as to accuracy, comprehensiveness, or currency of the content of this work.

This work is no substitute for individual patient assessment based upon healthcare professionals' examination of each patient and consideration of, among other things, age, weight, gender, current or prior medical conditions, medication history, laboratory data and other factors unique to the patient. The publisher does not provide medical advice or guidance and this work is merely a reference tool. Healthcare professionals, and not the publisher, are solely responsible for the use of this work including all medical judgments and for any resulting diagnosis and treatments.

Given continuous, rapid advances in medical science and health information, independent professional verification of medical diagnoses, indications, appropriate pharmaceutical selections and dosages, and treatment options should be made and healthcare professionals should consult a variety of sources. When prescribing medication, healthcare professionals are advised to consult the product information sheet (the manufacturer's package insert) accompanying each drug to verify, among other things, conditions of use, warnings and side effects and identify any changes in dosage schedule or contraindications, particularly if the medication to be administered is new, infrequently used or has a narrow therapeutic range. To the maximum extent permitted under applicable law, no responsibility is assumed by the publisher for any injury and/or damage to persons or property, as a matter of products liability, negligence law or otherwise, or from any reference to or use by any person of this work.

shop.lww.com

Walter L. Kemp:
To Dr. McKenzie Jackson, for your love of pathology and the
Forensic Files. Thank you for being my friend.

To my autopsy assistants, Kendra O'Neal and Tonya Shaffer,
for your hard work and enthusiasm and for helping me stay
sane while writing this book

To Hamo Muergerditchian, while not a physician, your assistance
in my education was invaluable and much appreciated. I miss you.

To my wife, Kelly, and her dad, Parker, thank you for your
patience, understanding, and support while
I was writing this book

To my friend, Brian Kieffer, my life was simple compared
to the challenges you have faced; with you as my friend,
I will always remember what to be thankful for

To my Aunt Lucille, for being a shining example
of kindness and generosity

Rhome L. Hughes:
To my teachers who took the time to share an extra
note of encouragement

To my students who took the time to think critically, study hard,
and marvel at all the wonders to be learned

To my family, simply for loving me

Jeffrey J. Barnard:
To my wife Terry, thank you for everything

CONTRIBUTORS

GERALD CREGO, BA
Undersheriff, Retired
Missoula County Sheriff's Office
Missoula, Montana

LYNETTE LANCON, BS
Forensic Firearm and Toolmark Examiner
Forensic Science Division
Montana Department of Justice
Missoula, Montana

ANDREW LEBRUN, D-ABMDI
Deputy Sheriff/Deputy Coroner
Carbon County Sheriff's Office
Red Lodge, Montana

SCOTT SCHLUETER, BS, D-ABFT
Forensic Toxicologist
Forensic Science Division
Montana Department of Justice
Missoula, Montana

PREFACE

While many general forensic pathology books are available, forensic pathology atlases are relatively uncommon. This atlas primarily aims to assist the reader in interpreting the patterns produced by various findings inherent to forensic pathology but also to assist the reader in learning how to look for those patterns and how to document them when they are found. Forensic pathology does not have a World Health Organization (WHO) Classification guide, and classification systems for various topics in forensic pathology (eg, gunshot wounds and asphyxia) vary from author to author. For these and other reasons, forensic pathology as a specialty sees some degree of variance in practice and determinations of the cause and manner of death between offices and between pathologists, with even experienced forensic pathologists arguing over the best practice in many areas as well as how to interpret certain autopsy findings.

To maintain consistency of style and presentation of the information throughout this book, the text was written by one author (WLK) and reviewed by the remaining two authors (JJB and RLH). The book is therefore based primarily upon the education and 20 years' experience of the lead author supplemented by the combined extensive experience of his two co-authors. The authors intend that the book will be viewed as a "user-guide" to forensic pathology, designed to assist a forensic pathologist in determining how to handle their daily cases, and not as a definitive guide to the field of forensic pathology, which in its degree of variation cannot adequately be described in an atlas or even in a textbook format. The authors hope the book will serve as a useful resource for those planning a career in forensic pathology (eg, pathology residents), or those who are early in their career in forensic pathology, and, hopefully, even offer at least a different perspective to those already well-trained in the field. If the reader wants a more in-depth review of certain topics in forensic pathology, other textbooks would better serve that purpose since based upon the relatively small amount of text space available in an atlas format, the information in this book is presented in a straight-to-the-point fashion and, hopefully, in a high-yield fashion, but as such presents the material in a different format than larger textbooks. The contributing authors are all non-forensic pathologists and were chosen for their expertise in various areas (firearms, postmortem toxicology, and death scene investigation), with the hope that readers could see how forensic pathologists can benefit from the input of such experts.

PEARLS & PITFALLS: These entries are used to address important concepts or techniques in forensic pathology that most often follow in-line with the text or images. The most common entries in the book are pearls and pitfalls and they were designed to highlight key concepts or useful points.

FAQ: These entries are commonly used to address areas in forensic pathology that are not agreed upon by all forensic pathologists, or areas that are frequently important topics in forensic pathology but might not have a clear answer. In this regard, even the three authors do not necessarily completely agree on the best answer to some of the questions. As such, each of the FAQs is written as objectively and neutrally as possible, attempting to address two sides to an argument, and to present two views to the question if more than one legitimate view was felt to exist. The reader will also see that for many FAQs, based upon information available in the literature, there is no clear answer.

CHECKLISTS: With certain types of investigations, a checklist is often provided to assist the reader in determining the steps to be taken at autopsy to identify or document the cause of death, as well as, in some situations, potential diagnoses to be considered in specific scenarios (eg, pregnancy-related deaths).

SAMPLE NOTES: In the spirit of the other books in this series, the sample notes are written to offer methods to document autopsy findings, and methods to potentially certify the cause and manner of death, given certain scenarios and autopsy findings. With the documentation of autopsy findings as well as even the certification of the cause and manner of death, there is often more than one way to do the correct thing, and the sample notes tried to address that fact.

NEAR MISSES: As with the other books in this series, the near miss section offers images and cases that have the potential to be mis-interpreted, or the potential to simply be missed. With each autopsy and investigation, there is usually always a chance to do more, and some near misses highlighted cases where an extra step brought the final answer.

ACKNOWLEDGMENTS

Completing this book was only made possible by what others have done for me through the many years. I would like to thank them for their direct and indirect contributions to my ability to write this book.

To my mom and dad, Bill and Agnes Kemp, for always supporting my love of reading and education

To Mr. Reckin, Mr. Simpson, Mr. Funk, Mrs. Roberts, Mr. Chalgren, Ms. Goyen, Mr. Cook, Ms. Gelardin, Mrs. Bland, and Mr. Hilderman for teaching me science, math, and English so that I could succeed in college

To Dr. Addis, Father Harrington, Dr. Christianson, Dr. Westwell, and Mr. Bugni, for giving me the background to succeed in medical school

To my medical school classmate Dr. Tom Nicholas, for convincing me to watch an autopsy

To Dr. Dennis Burns, for being the best mentor in autopsy pathology (and neuropathology) that a resident could ever ask for, and teaching me how to educate students

To Dr. Jeffrey J. Barnard, for being the best mentor in forensic pathology that a resident and fellow could ever ask for, for teaching me how to handle the challenges innate to this field, for always promoting a learning environment, and for helping me with this book

To Drs. Prahlow, Dolinak, Guileyardo, McClain, Spotswood, Townsend-Parchman, Urban, Salzberger, Turner, and Cohle, for teaching me forensic pathology

To Drs. Weinberg, Rogers, Timmons, and Margraf, for teaching me pediatric pathology and To Drs. White, Bigio, and Rushing, for teaching me neuropathology

To Dr. Schneider, for starting me on my teaching career and To Dr. Hesser, for asking me to teach the summer pathology course for medical students, and for giving me the motivation to develop my teaching interests

To Bev Shackelford, for the copy of Richard Lederer's *Sleeping Dogs Don't Lay*, which greatly promoted my interest in better writing

To Susan Kelly, for teaching me how to edit my own work, for teaching me how to read my own work as the reader and not as the writer, and for sticking with me as I learned the process

To Dr. Gary Dale, for teaching me how to practice forensic pathology in a rural environment and in a coroner system, and for being a great work partner

To Jerry Crego, Mickey Nelson, Dan Yonkin, and Richard Sine, for helping me write the coroner manual, for helping me fine-tune the coroner manual, and for teaching me a few things along the way

To Drs. McKeown and Skelton, for teaching me anthropology, and To Dr. Graham, for teaching me statistics and pushing my academic limits for one last time

To Dr. J. Bruce Beckwith, for teaching me pediatric pathology, and for teaching me that even the giants in medicine can still go by their first name

To Dr. Sens, for accepting my application to join the faculty at UND-SMHS, which gave me the chance to teach 2nd year medical students again and To Dr. Koponen, for being a great work partner at UND

To Dr. Rhome Hughes, for joining me at UND, for sharing our passion for teaching medical students, and for helping me with this book

To Dr. Christina Arnold, for asking me to write this book, and having faith in my abilities to produce a worthwhile forensic pathology atlas and To Drs. Elizabeth Montgomery and Dora Lam-Himlin, for agreeing with Dr. Arnold that this book would be a worthy addition to the series.

To Nicole Dernoski and Wolters-Kluwer, for accepting my proposal to write this book

To the Wolters-Kluwer team, including Varshaanaa Muralidharan, Ariel S. Winter, and Maria McAvey, for helping me submit the book, always answering my questions quickly and working with my changes, and for helping to turn the documents and photos I submitted into the final product.

To the team led by project manager, Ramkumar Soundararajan, along with Niraimathi in copyediting and Chandrasekar and Alexander in typesetting at TNQ Technologies for their work in producing the final book.

Thank you!
Willy Kemp

CONTENTS

1 PATTERN INTERPRETATION IN FORENSIC PATHOLOGY 1

2 BASICS OF AUTOPSY 5
   Introduction 6
   Hospital vs Forensic Autopsies 6
   Validity of Hospital Autopsy Permit 7
   Organ Removal at Autopsy 8
   Documentation 10

3 BASICS OF DEATH SCENE INVESTIGATION 11
   Introduction 12
   Basics of Death Investigation 12
   Importance of Scene Investigation 14
   Photography of the Scene and Body 14
   Documentation of Postmortem Changes 15
   Documentation of Discovery History and Terminal Events 17
   Near Misses 18

4 DEATH CERTIFICATION 21
   Introduction 22
   Description of Cause of Death 22
   Description of Manner of Death 23
   Description of Mechanism of Death 23
   Near Miss 26

5 IDENTIFICATION 29
   Introduction 30
   Circumstantial, Presumptive, or Tentative Identification 30
      How Formed 30
   Exclusionary Identification 30
      How Formed 30
   Positive Identification 30
      How Formed 30
   Scientific Methods to Identify a Deceased Body 33
      Introduction 33
   Fingerprints 33
      Requirements 33
      Time Frame 33
   DNA Analysis 34
      Requirements 34
      Time Frame 35
   Dental Examination 35
      Requirements 35
      Time Frame 35
   Other Forms of Scientific Identification 35
   Non-Scientific Methods of Identification 36
      Introduction 36
   Visual Identification 36
      Method 36
      Challenges 36

Physical Findings on the Body 36
   Method 36
   Challenges 36
Identification Cards 37
   Method 37
   Challenges 37
Personal Effects 38
   Method 38
Other Methods 38
Near Miss 39

6 POSTMORTEM CHANGES 41
Introduction 42
Time of Death and Early Postmortem Changes 42
   Algor Mortis 42
   Postmortem Vitreous Potassium Measurements 44
   Supravitality 44
   Rigor Mortis 44
   Livor Mortis 46
   Additional Findings Associated With Lividity 49
Decomposition 51
Important Terms Associated With Decomposition 52
   Green Discoloration of Skin 52
   Adipocere 52
   Postmortem Blisters (or Postmortem Bullae) 53
   Corneal Clouding 54
   Hemolysis 54
   Marbling 54
   Mummification and Postmortem Drying 54
   Skin Slippage 56
   Swelling/Bloating 57
   Tache Noire 59
Scene Indicators 60
Postmortem Entomology 61
   How to Collect Appropriate Specimens for Time of Death
   Determination Using Insect Activity 62
Animal Activity 63
Embalming Artifacts 65
Near Misses 67

7 NATURAL DISEASE AT AUTOPSY 71
Introduction 74
Natural Disease of the Body in General 75
   Autopsy Findings: Obesity 75
   Complications of Obesity 75
Natural Disease of the Central Nervous System 76
   Introduction 76
Intracerebral Hemorrhage 76
   Autopsy Findings 76
   Etiologies of an Intracerebral Hemorrhage 78
Cerebral Infarcts 78
   Autopsy Findings 78
Lacunar Infarct 81
   Autopsy Findings 81
Incompetent Diaphragm Sella 82
   Autopsy Findings 82
Natural Causes of Subarachnoid Hemorrhage 82
   Autopsy Findings 82

Etiologies of Subarachnoid Hemorrhage at Autopsy 82
Potential Mimics of Subarachnoid Hemorrhage 83
Meningitis 84
Autopsy Findings 84
Potential Mimics 85
Osmotic Demyelination Syndrome (Central Pontine and Extrapontine Myelinolysis) 86
Autopsy Findings 86
Association 86
Potential Mimics 86
Globus Pallidus/Basal Ganglia Necrosis 86
Autopsy Findings 86
Association of Globus Pallidus Necrosis 87
Multiple Sclerosis 88
Autopsy Findings 88
Chronic Traumatic Encephalopathy 88
Autopsy Findings 88
Seizure Disorder 89
Autopsy Findings 89
Association With Sudden Death 89
Alzheimer Disease 90
Autopsy Findings 90
Diffuse Lewy Body Disease 90
Autopsy Findings 90
Encephalitis 91
Autopsy Findings 91
Colloid Cyst 92
Autopsy Findings 92
Natural Disease of the Cardiovascular System 92
Introduction 92
Hypertensive Heart Disease 93
Autopsy Findings 93
Association With Sudden Death 93
Coronary Artery Atherosclerosis 93
Autopsy Findings 93
Association of Coronary Artery Atherosclerosis With Sudden Death 96
Gross and Microscopic Aging of an Acute Myocardial Infarct 96
Complications of Acute Myocardial Infarct 102
Aortic Dissection 105
Autopsy Findings 105
Coronary Artery Dissection 105
Autopsy Findings 105
Associations 105
Abdominal Aortic Aneurysm 106
Autopsy Findings 106
Coronary Artery Aneurysm 107
Autopsy Findings 107
Associations 107
Aortic Stenosis 108
Autopsy Findings 108
Association With Sudden Death 108
Bicuspid Aortic Valve 108
Autopsy Findings 108
Myxomatous Mitral Valve 109
Autopsy Findings 109
Association With Sudden Death 110
Potential Mimics 110

Chronic Rheumatic Mitral Valvulitis 110
    Autopsy Findings... 110
    Potential Mimic... 110
Endocarditis 111
    Autopsy Findings... 111
    Associations of Endocarditis 111
Pericarditis 113
    Autopsy Findings... 113
    Etiologies of Pericarditis 113
Myocarditis 114
    Autopsy Findings... 114
    Mimics of Myocarditis 115
Cardiomyopathies.. 116
    Autopsy Findings... 116
    Association With Sudden Death.. 117
    Mimics of Cardiomyopathy 117
Coronary Artery Anomalies Associated With Sudden Cardiac Death 118
    Autopsy Findings: Anomalous Origin of a Coronary Artery 118
    Association With Sudden Death.. 118
    Autopsy Findings: Tunneling/Bridging of Coronary Artery 119
    Association With Sudden Death.. 119
Lipomatous Hypertrophy of the Interatrial Septum 119
    Association With Sudden Death.. 120
Non-Ischemic Left Ventricular Scar... 120
    Autopsy Findings... 120
    Associated With Sudden Death 120
Lesions of the Cardiac Conduction System 120
    Introduction 120
Atrioventricular Nodal Artery Dysplasia 121
    Autopsy Findings... 121
    Association With Sudden Death.. 121
Incidental and Other Microscopic Findings in the Heart 121
    Clusters of Lymphocytes... 121
    Basophilic Degeneration 122
    Contraction Band Necrosis... 122
Natural Disease of the Respiratory System 123
    Introduction 123
Pneumonia 123
    Potential Mimics of Pneumonia 123
Aspiration Pneumonia 125
    Autopsy Findings... 125
    Mimics 126
Emphysema 126
    Autopsy Findings... 126
Asthma... 127
    Autopsy Findings... 127
Incidental Microscopic Findings in the Lung 128
    Corpora Amylacea 128
    Lentils 128
    Pulmonary Chemodectoma (Mesothelial-Like Rest).............................. 128
Natural Disease of the Hepatobiliary System... 129
    Introduction 129
Diffuse Fatty Liver 129
    Autopsy Findings... 129
    Potential Mimics 131

Cirrhosis of the Liver 132
    Autopsy Findings 132
    Potential Mimics 132
    Complications of Cirrhosis 133
Fitz-Hugh-Curtis Syndrome 135
    Autopsy Findings 135
Acute Cholecystitis 135
    Autopsy Findings 135
Acute Pancreatitis 136
    Autopsy Findings 136
    Risk Factors for Acute Pancreatitis 136
Cavernous Hemangioma 138
    Autopsy Findings 138
    Association With Sudden Death 138
Other Incidental Liver Masses 138
    Autopsy Findings 138
Natural Disease of the Genitourinary System 138
    Introduction 138
Nephrosclerosis 139
    Autopsy Findings 139
Acute Pyelonephritis 140
    Autopsy Findings 140
    Association With Sudden Death 141
Fournier Gangrene 141
    Autopsy Findings 141
Incidental Renal Masses 141
    Adenoma 141
    Renal Cell Carcinoma 141
    Adrenal Gland Rest 141
    Renomedullary Interstitial Cell Tumor 141
Natural Disease of the Endocrine System 142
    Introduction 142
Features of Diabetes Mellitus 142
    Autopsy Findings 142
Infarction of the Pituitary Gland 142
    Autopsy Findings 142
    Association 142
Hashimoto Thyroiditis 144
    Autopsy Findings 144
Pheochromocytoma 144
    Autopsy Findings 144
Incidental Findings 145
    Myelolipoma 145
    Black Thyroid 145
Natural Disease of the Gastrointestinal System 145
    Introduction 145
Esophageal Inlet Patch (Salmon Patch) 147
    Autopsy Findings 147
    Potential Mimics 148
Barrett Esophagus 148
    Autopsy Findings 148
Black Esophagus (Acute Esophageal Necrosis) 149
    Autopsy Findings 149
    Associations 149
Peptic Ulcer 150
    Autopsy Findings 150

Ischemic Colitis ... 150
   Autopsy Findings ... 150
   Potential Mimic ... 150
Intestinal Diverticula ... 150
   Autopsy Findings ... 150
Green Colon ... 152
   Autopsy Findings ... 152
   Potential Mimic ... 152
Natural Disease of the Hematolymphoid System ... 153
   Introduction ... 153
Disseminated Intravascular Coagulation ... 153
   Autopsy Findings ... 153
Thrombotic Thrombocytopenic Purpura/Hemolytic Uremic Syndrome ... 153
   Autopsy Findings ... 153
Fibrosis of the Splenic Capsule (Sugar Spleen) ... 154
   Autopsy Findings ... 154
Natural Disease of the Musculoskeletal System ... 155
   Introduction ... 152
Pregnancy-Related Deaths ... 155
   Introduction ... 155
Amniotic Fluid Embolism ... 156
   Autopsy Findings ... 156
Acute Fatty Liver of Pregnancy ... 156
   Autopsy Findings ... 156
Acute Endometritis-Myometritis ... 156
   Autopsy Findings ... 156
Placenta Accreta, Placenta Increta, Placenta Percreta ... 156
   Autopsy Findings ... 156
Peripartum Cardiomyopathy ... 156
   Autopsy Findings ... 156
Pre-Eclampsia/Eclampsia ... 157
   Autopsy Findings ... 157
HELLP Syndrome ... 157
   Autopsy Findings ... 157
Ectopic Pregnancy ... 157
   Autopsy Findings ... 157
Near Misses ... 158

8 ASPHYXIA ... 173

Introduction ... 174
Specific Forms of Asphyxia Causing Failure of Oxygen to Reach the Lung ... 178
   Introduction ... 178
   Smothering ... 178
   Choking ... 180
   Mechanical Asphyxia/Traumatic Asphyxia/Positional Asphyxia ... 181
   Vitiated Atmosphere/Suffocating Gases ... 183
   Entrapment ... 183
   Traumatic Asphyxia Combined With Smothering ... 183
Specific Forms of Asphyxia Causing External Compression of the Neck ... 184
   Hanging ... 184
   Strangulation ... 190
Other Specific Forms Of Asphyxia ... 193
   Carbon Monoxide Poisoning ... 195
   Drowning ... 195
Near Misses ... 197

9 BLUNT FORCE INJURIES 205

- Introduction 206
- Types of Blunt Force Injuries 206
  - Abrasions 206
  - Contusions 209
  - Lacerations 211
  - Fractures 214
- Pattern Interpretation of Blunt Force Injuries 214
- Blunt Force Injuries of the Head 219
- Subgaleal Hemorrhage 219
- Cranial Fractures 223
- Types of Cranial Fractures 223
  - Linear Fracture 223
  - Stellate (or Complex) Fracture 224
  - Depressed Fracture 224
  - Ring Fracture 225
  - Basilar Fracture 225
  - Comminuted Fracture 227
  - Diastatic Fracture 227
- Extra-Cerebral Hemorrhage 228
  - Epidural Hemorrhage 228
  - Subdural Hemorrhage 230
  - Subarachnoid Hemorrhage 235
- Traumatic Injuries of the Brain 239
- Type of Contusions 240
  - Coup Contusions 240
  - Contre-Coup Contusions 240
  - Fracture Contusions 242
  - Herniation Contusions 242
  - Intermediary Contusions 246
  - Gliding Contusions 246
- Blunt Force Injuries of the Neck 250
- Blunt Force Injuries of the Trunk 252
- Blunt Force Injuries of the Extremities 255
- Fractures 255
- Specific Fracture Types 257
- Extent: Incomplete vs Complete Fracture 258
  - Incomplete Fractures 258
  - Torus/Buckle Fracture 259
  - Greenstick Fracture 259
- Complete Fracture: Fracture Type Based Upon Direction 259
  - Transverse Fracture 259
  - Oblique Fracture 260
  - Longitudinal Fracture 261
  - Spiral Fracture 261
- Other Fracture Types 261
  - Comminuted Fracture 261
  - Butterfly Fracture 261
  - Segmental Fracture 262
  - Avulsion Fracture 263
- Timing of Bone Trauma 264
  - Antemortem Fractures 265
  - Postmortem Fractures 265
  - Perimortem Injuries 265
- Near Misses 268

10 SHARP FORCE INJURIES ... 273
- Introduction ... 274
- Types of Sharp Force Injuries ... 274
  - Stab Wound ... 274
  - Incised Wound ... 279
  - Chop Wound ... 281
- Sharp Force Injuries of the Bone and Cartilage ... 284
  - Introduction ... 284
  - Basic Features of Bony Defects From Sharp Force Injuries ... 284
  - Identifying Class Characteristics of Sharp Force Injuries in the Bone ... 286
  - Other Features Used to Interpret Sharp Force Wound Characteristics ... 286
- Near Misses ... 288

11 FIREARM INJURY ... 291
- Introduction ... 292
- Radiography ... 292
  - Basics of Radiography in Firearm Injuries ... 292
  - Specific Radiographic Findings Associated With Certain Types of Weapons ... 293
- External Examination ... 299
  - Overall Patterns of Injury to the Body ... 299
- Interpretation of Gunshot Wound Patterns in the Skin ... 306
  - Entrance Wounds for Handguns/Rifles ... 306
  - Exit Wounds for Handguns/Rifles ... 310
  - Features of Wound That Allow for General Determination of Range of Fire ... 316
  - Special Types of Gunshot Wounds ... 325
- Entrance and Exit Wounds for Shotguns and Relative Range of Fire ... 332
  - Features of the Shotgun Wound That Allow for Determination of Relative Range of Fire ... 333
- Internal Examination ... 337
- Mechanism of Death in Gunshot Wounds ... 340
- Composition of Projectiles ... 342
- Manner of Death Determination With Gunshot Wounds ... 344
- Near Misses ... 346

12 FIRE DEATHS ... 359
- Introduction ... 360
- Features of Thermal Injury ... 365
- Description of Flash Fire ... 367
- Autopsy Features of Fire Deaths ... 368
- Heat-Related Fractures ... 371
- Explosion-Related Deaths ... 374
- Near Misses ... 375

13 CHILD ABUSE ... 379
- Introduction ... 380
- Features of Subdural Hemorrhage ... 383
- Features of Retinal Hemorrhages ... 386
- Other Features in the Eye: Retinoschisis ... 389
- Differential Diagnosis of Subdural and Retinal Hemorrhages ... 389
- Differential Diagnoses: Glutaric Aciduria Type I and Galactosemia ... 389
- Differential Diagnosis: Congenital Heart Disease, Meningitis, and Leukemia ... 389
- Differential Diagnosis: Menkes Disease ... 390
- Differential Diagnosis: Neurosurgical Complications and

Traumatic Labor 391
Differential Diagnosis: Aneurysms 391
Differential Diagnosis: Hypernatremia 392
Differential Diagnosis: Coagulation Disorders 392
Differential Diagnosis: Accidental Injury 393
Other Important Topics With Regard to Inflicted Head Trauma
in Infants 395
    Rib Fractures 395
    Falls 401
    Apparent Life-Threatening Event 403
Alternative Theories as to the Causation of Findings Associated
With Abusive Head Trauma 403
Other Features of Child Abuse 406
    Fractures 406
    Bruising and Lacerations 408
    Burns 411
    Malnourishment and Dehydration 412
Near Misses 412

14 ENVIRONMENTAL DEATHS 423
Introduction 424
Hyperthermia 424
    Introduction 424
    Clinical Features of Heat Stroke 424
    Pattern at Autopsy 424
Hypothermia 426
    Introduction 426
    Pattern at Autopsy 426
Autopsy Findings Associated With Hypothermia 429
    Wischnewski Spots 429
    Frost Erythema 429
    Subnuclear Vacuolization of the Proximal Convoluted Tubular
    Epithelial Cells 430
    Vacuolation of Pancreatic Adenoid Cells 430
Description of Snow Immersion 430
Bodies Found in the Water 430
    Did the Decedent Drown? 430
    What Environmental and Human Factors Were Involved? 431
    Postmortem Artifacts Associated With Bodies Found in the Water ... 432
Scuba Diving-Related Deaths 432
    Causes of Death Associated With Scuba Diving 432
    How to Test for Gas Embolism and Barotrauma in
    a Scuba-Related Death 433
Electrocution 434
    Introduction 434
    Gross Appearance 434
    Microscopic Appearance 434
Dog Attacks 434
    Introduction 434
    Autopsy Findings Associated With Fatal Dog Attack 435
Snake Bite 436
    Introduction 436
    Pathologic Features of Pit Viper Injury 436
    Clinical Features of Pit Viper Injury 436
    Pathologic Features of Coral Snake Injury 436
    Clinical Features of Coral Snake Injury 436

Spider Bite 437
   Introduction 437
   Pathologic Features of Black Widow Bite 437
   Clinical Features of Black Widow Bite 437
   Pathologic Features of Recluse Bite 437
   Clinical Features of Recluse Bite 437
Other Forms of Animal Attack Encountered by Forensic Pathologists 437
High-Altitude Pulmonary Edema/High-Altitude Cerebral Edema 437
   Features of High-Altitude Cerebral Edema 437
   Features of High-Altitude Pulmonary Edema 437
   Autopsy Findings in High-Altitude Pulmonary Edema 437
Near Misses 438

15 POSTMORTEM TOXICOLOGY 443
Introduction 444
   Autopsy findings of a drug overdose 444
   Obtaining specimens for toxicologic analysis 447
   Interpretation of toxicologic results 450
   Description of postmortem redistribution and its importance 451
   Specific drugs encountered by forensic pathologists 453
Metabolites of Common Drugs 454
Ethanol 454

16 SUICIDE 463
Introduction 464
Basic Considerations When Determining That the Manner
of Death Is Suicide 464
Gunshot Wound Homicide vs Gunshot Wound Suicide 465
   Comparison of Features in Homicide vs Suicide Gunshot Wounds 465
Sharp Force Injuries Homicide vs Sharp Force Injuries Suicide 466
   Comparison of Features in Homicide vs Suicide Sharp Force Injury 466
Asphyxial Homicide vs Asphyxial Suicide 468
   Comparison of Features in Homicide vs Suicide Asphyxia 468
Near Misses 473

17 HISTOLOGY AT AUTOPSY 475
Introduction 476
Frequency of Histologic Examination at Autopsy 476
Histologic Examination of the Brain at Autopsy 478
Near Misses 479

18 EMBOLISM 483
Introduction 484
Pulmonary Thromboemboli 484
   Circumstances Under Which Pulmonary Thromboemboli Occur 484
   How to Identify 484
   Complications of a Pulmonary Thromboembolus 484
   Aging of Pulmonary Thromboemboli 486
Air Embolism 490
   Circumstance Under Which Air Emboli Occur 490
   How to Identify 490
Fat Embolism 490
   Circumstances Under Which Fat Emboli Occur 490
   Clinical Signs of Fatty Emboli 490
   How to Identify 490
Amniotic Fluid Embolism 492
   Circumstance Under Which Amniotic Fluid Emboli Occur 492
   Clinical Signs of Amniotic Fluid Emboli 492
   How to Identify 492

Bullet Embolism 493
    Circumstances Under Which a Bullet Embolism Occurs 493
    How to Identify at Autopsy 493
Septic Embolism 493
    Description of Septic Embolism 493
    Circumstances Under Which Septic Emboli Occur 493
    How to Identify at Autopsy 493
    Location of Emboli 493
Cholesterol Crystal Embolism 494
    Circumstances Under Which Cholesterol Crystal Emboli Occur 494
    How to Identify at Autopsy 494
Other Forms of Embolism 494
Near Misses 496

19 MICROBIOLOGIC ANALYSES 499
Introduction 500

20 VITREOUS ELECTROLYTE ANALYSIS 501
Introduction 502
Vitreous Electrolyte Patterns 502
Hyponatremia 503
    Causes of Fatal Hyponatremia 503
    Clinical Features of Hyponatremia 503
    How to Determine at Autopsy 503
Hyperglycemia 503
    How to Determine at Autopsy 503
Ketoacidosis 504
    How to Determine at Autopsy 504

21 SUDDEN UNEXPECTED INFANT DEATH 507
Introduction 508
Checklist for Investigation of a Sudden Unexpected Infant Death 512
Description of SUID (sudden unexplained infant death) and SIDS
(sudden infant death syndrome) 510
Identifying an overlay or other asphyxial death at autopsy 510
Microbiology Studies 512
Near Miss 513

22 IN-CUSTODY DEATHS 517
Introduction 518
Excited Delirium Syndrome 519
Restraint Asphyxia 520
Prone Restraint Cardiac Arrest 520
Conducted Electrical Weapons/Electronic Control Devices 520

23 ELDER ABUSE 525
Introduction 526
Risk Factors for Elder Abuse 526
Senile Ecchymoses 528
    Description 528
    Causes 528
Decubitus Ulcers 528
    Description 528
    Causes 528
    Risk Factors for Decubitus Ulcers 528
    Classification of Decubitus Ulcers 529
    Complications of Decubitus Ulcers 530
    Important Point 530
Near Misses 530

24 ANTHROPOLOGY ... 533
- Introduction ... 534
- Non-Human Versus Human ... 534
  - Introduction ... 534
  - Identification of Non-Human Bones ... 534
- Biological Profile ... 536
  - Introduction ... 536
- Sex ... 536
  - How Determined ... 536
  - Pelvic Features of Sex ... 538
  - Cranial Features of Sex ... 539
- Age ... 539
  - How Determined ... 539
  - Pubic Symphysis ... 540
  - Auricular Surface ... 540
  - Rib Ends ... 540
  - Cranial Suture Closure ... 540
- Ancestry ... 543
  - How Determined ... 543
  - Morphologic Analysis for Ancestry ... 543
- Stature ... 543
  - How Performed ... 543
- Variants and Natural Disease ... 546
  - Introduction ... 546
- Near Misses ... 549

25 ODONTOLOGY ... 551
- Introduction ... 552

26 MASS DISASTERS ... 555
- Introduction ... 556

27 STILLBIRTHS ... 557
- Introduction ... 558
- Basic Information Regarding Handling of a Stillborn Infant ... 558
- Basic Features of a Stillborn Fetus ... 558
- Examination of the Placenta ... 559
- Chorioamnionitis ... 559
  - Autopsy Findings ... 559
  - Potential Mimics ... 560
- Placental Abruption ... 560
  - Autopsy Findings ... 560
- Meconium Aspiration ... 561
  - Autopsy Findings ... 561
- Near Miss ... 561

28 COMMON MECHANISMS AT AUTOPSY ... 563
- Introduction ... 564
- Hypovolemic Shock ... 564
  - Mechanism ... 564
  - Causes of Hypovolemic Shock ... 564
  - Estimation of Effect of Blood Loss ... 564
  - Autopsy Findings of Blood Loss ... 564
- Cardiogenic Shock ... 564
  - Mechanism ... 564
  - Causes of Cardiogenic Shock ... 565

Septic Shock	565
Mechanism	565
Causes of Septic Shock	565
Anaphylactic Shock	565
Mechanism	565
Neurogenic Shock	565
Mechanism	565
Autopsy Findings Associated With Shock	565
Autopsy Findings of Cerebral Edema	567
Complications of Cerebral Edema	568
Autopsy Findings of Global Hypoxic Ischemic Encephalopathy	568
Near Misses	570

29 TREATMENT-RELATED AUTOPSY FINDINGS ... 573

Introduction	574
Types of Medical Devices Used	574
External Injuries Caused by Resuscitation Attempts	575
Internal Injuries Caused by Resuscitation Attempts	576
Near Misses	579

30 AUTOMOBILE ACCIDENTS ... 583

Introduction	584
Characteristic Injuries in a Motor Vehicle Accident	586
Transection of the Aorta	586
Basilar Skull Fracture	586
Flail Chest	586
Atlanto-Occipital Fracture/Dislocation (See Blunt Force Injuries Chapter)	587
Dicing	587
Stretch Abrasions/Lacerations	587
Near Misses	592

31 SPECIAL DISSECTIONS ... 595

Introduction	596
Dissection of Middle Ears	596
When Performed	596
How Performed	596
Dissection of Optic Nerves and Eyes	596
When Performed	596
How Performed	596
Dissection of Vertebral Arteries	597
When Performed	597
How Performed	597
Dissection of the Anterior and Posterior Neck	597
When Performed	597
How Performed	598
Dissection of the Cervical Vertebral Column	598
When Performed	598
How Performed	598
Examination for Pneumothorax	598
When Performed	598
How Performed	599
Examination for Air Embolus	599
When Performed	599
How Performed	599
Dissection of the Back	599
When Performed	599
How Performed	600

Dissection of the Lower Extremities 600
    When Performed 600
    How Performed 600
Dissection of the Sinoatrial and Atrioventricular Nodes 600
    When Performed 600
    How Performed 600
Dissection of the Parathyroid Glands 601
    When Performed 601
    How Performed 601
Examination of Esophagus for Varices 602
    When Performed 602
    How Performed 602
Quick Removal of the Entire Spinal Cord 603
    When Performed 603
    How Performed 603
Underwater Removal of Macerated Infant Brain 603
    When Performed 603
    How Performed 603
Maceration of the Thyroid Cartilage 604
    When Performed 604
    How Performed 604
En Bloc Removal of Female Genitalia and/or Anus (Including
the Male Anus)... 604
    When Performed 604
    How Performed 604

APPENDIX A: SELF-ASSESSMENT QUESTIONS 607

APPENDIX B: SELF-ASSESSMENT ANSWERS 633

APPENDIX C: WRITING THE AUTOPSY REPORT 641

APPENDIX D: BIAS 645

APPENDIX E: RARE BUT IMPORTANT TO CONSIDER 651

APPENDIX F: SUMMARY 661

INDEX 665

PATTERN INTERPRETATION IN FORENSIC PATHOLOGY

Rao et al described their atlas of forensic pathology as "…a guide to build one's knowledge of the variations and nuances of injury patterns encountered in actual practice today."[1] As Rao et al indicate, like other pathologists, the role of forensic pathologists is one of pattern interpretation. However, while most pathologists primarily identify patterns in histologic preparations to formulate a diagnosis, albeit with the contributions of the gross examination, immunohistochemical stains, other non-hematoxylin and eosin stains (eg, trichrome, silver stains), genetic studies, and other processes, forensic pathologists do not. Although forensic pathologists utilize light microscopy to assist in forming diagnoses from autopsy, most of their work is done primarily through gross examination and other methods.

Forensic pathologists utilize pattern interpretation in a variety of ways. First, the primary form of pattern interpretation that forensic pathologists perform is that involving gross features (ie, macroscopic autopsy findings). Forensic pathologists must make observations of gross autopsy findings to identify patterns to allow for a diagnosis. For example, forensic pathologists must observe the skin changes associated with a gunshot wound to determine whether the wound was an entrance or an exit, and, if an entrance, what was the relative distance of the body from the weapon when it was discharged. In interpreting patterns based upon gross examination, forensic pathologists must not only be able to identify the pathologic change present but also be able to separate the pathologic changes from artifacts induced by therapy, postmortem change, and any other confounding factor. In addition, pathologists must be able to distinguish natural disease from traumatic injuries, a form of pattern interpretation that is particularly important when investigating infant deaths. Second, forensic pathologists must make observations of microscopic autopsy findings to allow for a diagnosis. While forensic pathologists utilize gross examination most commonly, microscopic examination also plays an important role in their job, and the interpretation of microscopic patterns is a vital skill. For example, the finding of subnuclear vacuolation in the proximal convoluted tubular epithelial cells of the kidney is associated with ketoacidosis and hypothermia. Third, while both gross examination and microscopic examination are utilized by other pathologists in their job, albeit with a reversal of importance from that of forensic pathologists (ie, gross examination is more important than microscopic examination to forensic pathologists, while microscopic examination is more important than gross examination to surgical pathologists), these are not the only two modalities in which a forensic pathologist must interpret patterns. Forensic pathologists also utilize information from scene investigations, radiologic studies, toxicologic analysis, vitreous fluid analysis, evidence examination performed by forensic scientists (eg, firearms residue testing on clothing), forensic DNA analysis for the purpose of identification, and even genetic testing for various diseases, including inherited disorders, such as cardiomyopathies, long QT syndrome, and metabolic disorders in infants and children. As with gross and microscopic examination at autopsy, each of these modalities can present a pattern that the forensic pathologist must correctly interpret.

However, pattern interpretation in forensic pathology is not just for the purpose of making a diagnosis. In fact, in any given autopsy, a forensic pathologist may make anywhere from a few to literally hundreds of diagnoses (eg, in a decedent who is shot or stabbed many times, each injury could be technically considered its own diagnosis). Forensic pathologists must consider all of the findings (ie, diagnoses) from their autopsy (including some or all of the following: gross examination findings, radiologic findings, microscopic findings, toxicologic findings, vitreous electrolyte findings, genetic findings) and integrate that with the scene investigation findings to determine the cause and manner of death. This too is pattern interpretation—interpreting the pattern found in numerous findings to arrive at the cause and manner of death. In forensic pathology, unfortunately, a single or group of findings can be found in individuals who have died from very different causes and manners of deaths.

For example, an individual who dies as the result of a suicidal hanging can have a ligature furrow and abrasions on the neck, petechiae in the conjunctivae, and a fracture of one or both of the superior horns of the thyroid cartilage. An individual who dies as the result of a homicidal ligature strangulation can also have a ligature furrow and abrasions on the neck, petechiae in the conjunctivae, and a fracture of one or both of the superior horns of the thyroid cartilage. The distinction between the two causes and manners of death is obviously very important and involves seeing the pattern in the autopsy findings combined with other information such as the investigation. A contact gunshot wound of the back of the head may be the result of a suicide or the result of a homicide, and only correlation of the autopsy findings with the scene investigation may be able to distinguish the two situations.

Of vital importance to pattern interpretation in forensic pathology is the careful documentation of the findings that led the forensic pathologist to the final interpretation of the cause and manner of death. This careful documentation of the findings associated with the cause and manner of death also includes the documentation of any other potentially significant findings, which can include artifacts of postmortem change and negative autopsy findings (eg, no hemorrhage in a layer-by-layer neck dissection to assist in ruling out strangulation) among many others. In forensic pathology, pathologists often need to spend as much timing documenting findings that are not the cause of death as documenting those findings that were the cause of death. Although surgical pathologists, as with forensic pathologists, document their findings in a written report, surgical pathologists most frequently have a second chance to review their cases as additional slides can be cut from the tissue block. Such is not the case with an autopsy. While second autopsies (and third, and fourth…) can be performed, unless an inadequate autopsy was performed the first time, second autopsies are of questionable value, and, given that the body has been altered by the first autopsy, interpretations are impaired. Therefore, it is very important for forensic pathologists to carefully document their findings via both written report and photography. In fact, in many cases, the autopsy is not performed so much to determine the cause and manner of death as to thoroughly document the cause and manner of death for later legal proceedings (eg, a gunshot wound homicide). Thus, documentation of the autopsy findings, both in written report and photographically, is of vital importance.

Two other differences in pattern interpretation between forensic pathologists and hospital pathologists are that with a living patient, a disease process can be evaluated over time, with repeat biopsies and additional tests performed, better allowing for a final diagnosis to be made, whereas, with an autopsy, only one, albeit very extensive, examination of the body is performed and the ability to follow the progression of a disease process is not available. This difference can cause the diagnosis of some pathologic conditions at autopsy to be difficult if not impossible. The second difference, as partially described above, is that in most cases hospital pathologists can have a second look at a tumor, through additional sections made from the tissue cassettes, or from a return to the gross specimen to obtain more sections or sections from a different area. With rare exception, forensic pathologists are not able to do this. Only tissue retained at autopsy can be used in any future studies. For example, if the spinal cord was not removed at autopsy, and later in the investigation it becomes apparent that information regarding the spinal cord would be useful, this option is usually not or only very rarely available to the forensic pathologist. So, at the time of autopsy, a forensic pathologist should consider future questions about the postmortem examination, and potentially prepare for helping to answer those questions through their documentation or through the collection and preservation of tissue or blood for future testing, or evidence for future analysis (eg, in the death of a 35-year-old male with no suspicions of drug use and with no autopsy findings to indicate a cause of death, saving a purple top blood tube for future genetic testing may be useful).

Although the pattern interpretation done by forensic pathologists is frequently different than that performed by hospital pathologists, in that the pattern interpretation is not as heavily weighted toward histologic examination as most hospital pathology cases, forensic pathologists definitely interpret patterns, and actually, forensic pathologists perform pattern interpretation on at least two levels. First, the forensic pathologist must interpret gross findings, microscopic findings, toxicologic findings, radiologic findings, and other modalities to make autopsy diagnoses. Second, the pathologist must correlate the autopsy diagnoses with the scene investigation and other investigative findings to determine the cause and manner of death. In some cases, the autopsy is negative for findings and only the scene investigation, including consultation with available medical records and police reports, will identify the cause and manner of death. For example, in low-voltage electrocutions, the autopsy is often negative, but the scene investigation, if adequately performed, reveals the cause of death.

Reference

1. Rao VJ, Mittleman RE, Wetli CV. *An Atlas of Forensic Pathology*. American Society of Clinical Pathologists (ASCP); 1998.

BASICS OF AUTOPSY 2

CHAPTER OUTLINE

Introduction   6
Hospital vs Forensic Autopsies   6
Validity of Hospital Autopsy Permit   7
Organ Removal at Autopsy   8
Documentation   10

INTRODUCTION

An autopsy is a postmortem examination of the human body, which can be performed either in a hospital or forensic context and which includes both an external examination and an internal examination. In the hospital context, the autopsy can be limited by the family to only certain parts of the body; whereas in the forensic context the autopsy often cannot be limited by the family. A third situation also occurs when a family requests a pathologist, often a forensic pathologist, to perform an autopsy for a death that occurred in the hospital but most often did not have an autopsy in the hospital, or a death that occurred in a forensic context but most often did not receive a forensic autopsy. Such a situation is often termed a "private autopsy." Private autopsies can be performed for a variety of reasons: for a second autopsy, for civil purposes; for family knowledge and closure after a death; for the purpose of organ retention, most commonly the brain; or for the purpose of research and/or diagnosis, which often occurs in patients with clinically diagnosed Alzheimer disease, when the family seeks pathologic confirmation.

HOSPITAL VS FORENSIC AUTOPSIES

Hospital autopsies are generally performed to determine the mechanism of death and document the presence and extent of natural disease processes. Forensic autopsies are performed to identify the decedent; determine the cause and manner of death; and document traumatic injuries, natural disease, and postmortem changes, with collection of specimens for toxicology and evidence as dictated by the nature of the death. Requests for a hospital autopsy can come from physicians or families but must be approved by the legal next of kin. Jurisdiction for forensic autopsies is determined by state statutes governing the investigation of suspicious or undetermined deaths. While the autopsy of an individual who died under circumstances required to be reported to the coroner or medical examiner by state statutes can be performed against family wishes, as of July 2015, seven states (California, Maryland, New Jersey, New York, Ohio, Rhode Island, and Minnesota) allow families to object to the performance of an autopsy based upon their religious beliefs.[1] Statues vary by state; however, the National Association of Medical Examiners (NAME) indicates the circumstances under which a death investigation shall be performed (Table 2.1) and the circumstance under which a forensic autopsy shall be performed (Table 2.2).[2] As state statues vary fairly widely, a forensic pathologist should be aware of the specific causes under which their state's code mandates that a death investigation be performed.

At this time, most autopsies are performed in a forensic setting (eg, in a medical examiner's office). While the number of hospital autopsies performed in the United States is minimal overall, at larger teaching institutions, the number of hospital autopsies may represent a significant number. Private autopsies would require the same permission as a hospital autopsy. Private autopsy are performed in a variety of locations, including funeral homes or private medical examiner offices.

TABLE 2.1: Circumstances Under Which a Death Investigation Should Be Performed

Violent deaths
Non-natural deaths, either suspected or known
Deaths of individuals in good health
Unexpected deaths of infants and children
Deaths with unusual or suspicious circumstances
In-custody deaths
Deaths due to a disease that is a public health threat
Deaths of individuals not under physician care

TABLE 2.2: Deaths Requiring an Autopsy
Deaths due to or thought to be due to criminal violence
Unexpected death of an infant or child
Deaths associated with police action
Non-natural death in individuals in local, state, or federal institutes
Acute workplace injury
Electrocution
Drug intoxication death, unless documented
Unwitnessed drowning
Unidentified decedent
Skeletonized remains
Charred bodies
Motor vehicle accident, if required to document the injuries
Any death where forensic pathologist determines that an autopsy is necessary

VALIDITY OF HOSPITAL AUTOPSY PERMIT

The performance of a hospital autopsy specifically requires the permission of the legal next of kin, whereas a forensic autopsy does not require the permission of the legal next of kin. The order of the legal next of kin responsible for determination of whether an autopsy can be performed varies by state statutes; however, in general, the first four individuals who can grant permission for a next of kin to be performed are spouse, adult children, parents, and siblings. The first person in the list who is alive is the person who has the legal authority to determine whether an autopsy can be performed. For example, if the spouse is deceased or the spouse and decedent are divorced, the authority passes to the adult children. If several people are present within any single level of the order of next of kin (eg, there is more than one living adult child), any person in that group can give permission for the autopsy as long as none of the others in that group are known to object. As the order of permission for autopsy varies somewhat by state, and as there are potential legal repercussions if a pathologist performs an autopsy without correct permission, each pathologist performing hospital or private autopsies should know their state code governing such a determination.

Basic General CHECKLIST for a Forensic Autopsy Examination
- ☐ Obtain investigative information regarding the death, including medical records if appropriate
- ☐ Photograph the face for identification and the body overall
- ☐ Photograph injuries, using both an overall photograph for documentation of the location of the injury and a close-up photograph for documentation of the features of the injury itself
- ☐ Other useful photographs: "as-is" photograph, documenting how the body was received for autopsy
- ☐ Perform external and internal examination
- ☐ Collection of fluids for toxicology to include peripheral blood, heart blood, vitreous fluid, and urine, and can also include bile, gastric contents and liver or skeletal muscle

PEARLS & PITFALLS

Performing a forensic autopsy without some prior knowledge of the circumstances of the death is not appropriate. For example, a 33-year-old female with a known history of drug use who was found dead in her secured apartment would be handled differently than a 33-year-old female who was found dead in her car and who has a known history of type I diabetes and two myocardial infarcts, and both would be handled differently than a 33-year-old female who was found naked on the couch of her apartment with the door open, last having been known to be alive fighting with her boyfriend. The autopsy methods for evidence collection (whether obtained or not), radiography (whether performed or not), and various procedures performed at autopsy (eg, decision to perform a layer-by-layer anterior and/or posterior neck dissection) would vary between the three circumstances; however, if the only information available to the forensic pathologist is "33-year-old female," they would not know how to proceed. Also, review of the medical records may indicate a need to examine areas of the body that are not normally examined at autopsy (eg, the spinal cord).

PEARLS & PITFALLS

When documenting the body externally and internally, there are many possibilities for photographs during the course of an autopsy, which may or may not prove useful at a later time. The "as-is" photograph would document how the decedent arrived to the morgue including any clothing and medical intervention and the position of the body when it was received (eg, face-up, face-down, or on its side). Although forensic pathologists take notes during autopsies, the notes themselves can prove to be wrong (eg, transposition of left and right), and, if no photographs are available for review when the autopsy report is finalized, the errors would remain. For example, documenting an intraosseous catheter in the left leg when it was in the right leg would be easily corrected by reviewing the autopsy photographs prior to finalizing the autopsy report, and could prevent a potential problem later when the medical record and the autopsy report would differ if the error was not corrected. Routinely photographing the hands can serve as documentation of lack of injuries (or documentation of injuries present), and can be a record of blood spatter on the hands when the cause of death is a gunshot wound. Although injuries should be photographed fully cleaned, a photograph prior to cleaning may prove useful to document soot in a gunshot wound, which can be removed during the cleaning process. Routine photographs of the conjunctival surface of the eyelids and interior of the mouth can help document the presence or absence of petechiae in the conjunctivae and oral mucosa, or of injuries or lack of injuries of the oral mucosa. The liberal use of photography at the time of autopsy can provide the pathologist with a re-review of the body at the time they finalize their autopsy report and can also provide negative photographs to document their negative findings (eg, photograph of the mouth to confirm the absence of blunt force injuries).

ORGAN REMOVAL AT AUTOPSY

Two general forms of organ removal are used by offices: Leutelle (en bloc), which has also been referred to as Rokitansky, and Virchow (organ-by-organ). In the Leutelle method, the entire organ block from the tongue to the bladder is removed in one large block, which the forensic pathologist then dissects. Advantages of this method include maintaining the relationship of organs and preservation of vasculature and other interconnecting structures. In the Virchow method, organs are removed one by one and then subsequently dissected. The use of one method or the other is most often a choice by the pathologist made based upon their education and experience. Some pathologists use organ-by-organ removal for adults and en bloc removal for infants; others use organ-by-organ removal for both and others use en bloc removal for both.

PEARLS & PITFALLS

If a pulmonary thromboembolus is expected as the cause of death, removal of at least the heart and lungs en bloc may be preferable. If the thromboembolus crosses the pulmonary valve and to the branch point of the main pulmonary artery but not significantly into either the left or right pulmonary artery, organ-by-organ dissection, which would involve removing each lung by incising at the hilum, could result in the pulmonary thromboembolus possibly being missed. Another possibility to prevent such an event is opening the pulmonary artery in situ and checking for the presence or absence of a pulmonary thromboembolus at that time.

FAQ: Is a complete autopsy required to document the cause and manner of death?

Answer: NAME does recognize that limited autopsies can be performed under certain circumstances with the justification provided.[2] In all truth, essentially no autopsy is complete. In adults, the middle ears are not frequently opened. In adults and children, depending upon the nature of the death, the spinal cord is most likely not examined. The bulk of the musculoskeletal system is not examined, and, even where the skeletal system is examined (ie, the vertebral column and ribs), the periosteum is not removed, which impairs examination of the surface of the bone. While some organs may be examined grossly, they may not be examined microscopically (which often depends upon office policies and the preferences of the forensic pathologist based upon their education and experience). If the purpose of the autopsy is to determine the cause and manner of death and document the cause of death, then, if a partial autopsy can accomplish that, why is the partial autopsy not the best choice? For example, in a suicide gunshot wound of the head, the scene investigation, and not the autopsy, is the primary factor for the determination of the manner. What purpose would a complete autopsy serve if an external examination to document the entrance and exit wounds (if the gunshot perforated the head), or a limited internal examination for recovery of the projectile (if the gunshot penetrated the head) would answer the question about the cause and manner of death? While the lack of an internal examination may not allow for answering a subsequent question by the family regarding whether a brain tumor contributed to the cause of death, answering all those questions, while good if it can be done, is not the primary purpose of the forensic autopsy. Without opening the body in an otherwise natural or non-suspicious death, unexpected injuries, the identification of which would change the manner of death, would not be identified. Such is one reason why autopsies on individuals with chronic alcoholism may be performed. While chronic alcoholism itself is a cause of death, chronic alcoholics have a chance for unwitnessed trauma, and the diagnosis of a subdural hemorrhage would be missed if the head were not opened. However, the same rationale is not considered with most elderly deaths. Elderly individuals can be prone to fall and develop hip fractures. If a hip fracture is present, the manner of death is most likely accidental; however, based only upon the scene investigation and external examination, a hip fracture is likely to be missed.

If an autopsy is to be performed as a component of a death investigation, a complete autopsy (which normally includes the contents of the cranial cavity, the neck, and the contents of the trunk) is always the most thorough method, and will be the most likely to have answers to future questions that may not be identified through only a partial autopsy. The ultimate decision as to whether a partial autopsy can be performed must be based upon the forensic pathologist's experience and education and office policies.

DOCUMENTATION

While the forensic pathologist will look for patterns in the scene investigation combined with the autopsy findings to determine the cause and manner of death, they must also carefully document those findings in both their written report and autopsy photographs so that another forensic pathologist can review their work and arrive at the same interpretation. Inadequately documented autopsies will allow others to cast doubt on the determinations made by the forensic pathologist who performed the autopsy. Thus, the need for careful documentation of the autopsy findings is as vital a component of pattern interpretation as the gross examination, microscopic examination, and other testing modalities used in forensic pathology.

References

1. Grovum J. Religious freedom, states' interests clash over autopsies. *Stateline blog*. June 29, 2015. Accessed June 19, 2023. https://stateline.org/2015/06/29/religious-freedom-states-interests-clash-over-autopsies/
2. National Association of Medical Examiners Standards Committee. Forensic Autopsy Performance Standards. National Association of Medical Examiners; 2022. Approved 2005, 2010, 2015, with amendments approved 2006, 2011, 2012, 2014, 2016, and 2020; Sunset date: 2022.

BASICS OF DEATH SCENE INVESTIGATION 3

CHAPTER OUTLINE

Introduction   12

Basics of Death Investigation   12

Importance of Scene Investigation   14

Photography of the Scene and Body   14

Documentation of Postmortem Changes   15

Documentation of Discovery History and Terminal Events   17

Near Misses   18

INTRODUCTION

In the United States, two main systems of death investigation exist: coroner and medical examiner. In coroner systems, each county has an elected or appointed coroner who is charged with investigating deaths that occur in that county. The required background for a coroner varies by state, with some coroners having only a high school education and no formal training in death investigation prior to becoming coroner, whereas other coroners are physicians with some coroners even being forensic pathologists. Once an individual is elected or appointed as coroner, the continuing education required for the position varies by state. In contrast to a coroner system, in a medical examiner system, most frequently, the medical examiner is a forensic pathologist; however, in a few states, the medical examiner may be a non-forensic pathologist physician. While coroner systems are always county based, medical examiner systems can be city, county, or state based. For example, the city of St. Louis has a medical examiner, the county of Dallas has a medical examiner, and the state of Utah has a medical examiner.

In its statutes, each state has a list of scenarios that when a death occurs under that scenario, the death must be reported to the appropriate agency (either the coroner or the medical examiner, depending upon what type of system the death occurs in). While all states frequently list certain scenarios (eg, infants and deaths in custody), each state also frequently has certain scenarios listed that are specific to their state and not listed in the statutes of other states (eg, one state may require investigation into a death if the decedent was the victim of domestic abuse within the last year, whereas another state may not have this particular scenario listed in their statutes as requiring a death investigation). As the statutes are developed by politicians, quite frequently the listed scenarios under which a death must be investigated will vary depending upon their experience and preferences. Unfortunately, just because a death MUST be reported does not mean that it actually WILL BE reported. Individuals reporting deaths are most often medical providers, including physicians and nurses, and they often fail to report delayed traumatic deaths, instead attributing the death to the immediate cause of death and not the proximate cause of death.

> **PEARLS & PITFALLS**
>
> While coroners and medical examiners will most often not routinely review the death certificates for all deaths that occur in their jurisdiction, some of these non-reviewed death certificates will apply to an individual who died a non-natural death and was not referred appropriately for a death investigation. While many states require the coroner or medical examiner to approve all cremation permits for deaths in their jurisdiction, which will allow for some of these non-investigated deaths to be identified, if the decedent dies from a certified natural cause and is buried, most often the death certificate will not be reviewed by the coroner or medical examiner. Having a good relationship with funeral homes with which the coroner or medical examiner works can assist with this problem, as the funeral director can flag death certificates that they feel may be non-natural deaths, and ensure that they are referred to the coroner's or medical examiner's office.

BASICS OF DEATH INVESTIGATION

The steps performed to investigate any given death can vary from a series of phone calls to one on-site visit to the location where the body was found to multiple on-site visits to where the body was found and where the actual injury causing the death may have occurred (Figure 3.1). While each death scene is unique, if certain basic steps are followed at each scene, with some variation based upon the nature of the scene investigation, each death will be properly documented. It must be remembered that the death scene investigation, as with the autopsy, can essentially only be performed once. While second (or more) autopsies and second (or more) scene visits can be performed, the utility of each repeat attempt is greatly diminished from the original effort, and the chance to document some if

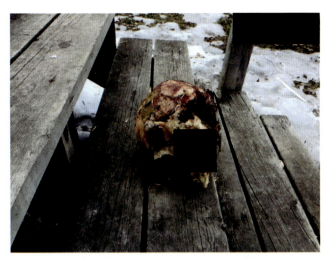

Figure 3.1. Defleshed cranium on stairs. This defleshed cranium was brought to this house by a dog. The death scene was at another location. This photo illustrates how death investigation can easily involve more than one scene investigation.

not all features of importance is gone with the repeat. That said, if the autopsy or further information obtained uncovers a finding that needs investigation at the scene, a repeat visit can easily be performed (eg, if autopsy revealed an exit site for a gunshot wound that was not identified at the scene, a return to the scene might help identify the projectile).

CHECKLIST for Death Scene Investigation[1]

The National Institute of Justice has a publication, "Every Scene, Every Time" that describes the steps each death investigation should have. These steps are divided into five categories: arriving at the scene, evaluating and documenting the scene, evaluating and documenting the body, developing decedent profile, and completing scene investigation. The steps in each of the five categories are listed below.

Arriving at the Scene
- ☐ Introduce and identify self and role
- ☐ Exercise scene safety
- ☐ Confirm or pronounce death
- ☐ Participate in scene briefing
- ☐ Conduct scene walk-through
- ☐ Establish chain of custody
- ☐ Follow laws related to evidence collection

Evaluating and Documenting the Scene
- ☐ Photograph the scene
- ☐ Record findings at scene (ie, description of scene)
- ☐ Determine probable location of injury or illness
- ☐ Collect, inventory, and ensure security of evidence
- ☐ Interview witnesses at the scene

Evaluating and Documenting the Body
- ☐ Photograph the body
- ☐ Perform external examination of body
- ☐ Collect and preserve evidence on the body
- ☐ Determine identification of the decedent

- ☐ Evaluate and record postmortem changes
- ☐ Participate in scene debriefing
- ☐ Determine next-of-kin identification procedures
- ☐ Secure remains

Developing Decedent Profile
- ☐ Record the discovery history
- ☐ Record the history of the terminal episode
- ☐ Determine decedent's medical history
- ☐ Determine decedent's psychiatric history
- ☐ Determine social history

Completing Scene Investigation
- ☐ Maintain and release jurisdiction of the body
- ☐ Perform exit procedures
- ☐ Assist family

IMPORTANCE OF SCENE INVESTIGATION

A good death scene investigation is important for a variety of reasons. First, the determination of manner of death is always contingent upon knowing at least the basics of the scene investigation. For example, an individual with the sole autopsy finding of severe coronary artery atherosclerosis may have a manner of death of homicide if the scene investigation indicated that they were being physically threatened by another person at the time of their death.[2-5] Second, while the final cause of death is most often determined at autopsy, scene investigation is important to help determine the cause of death in many cases (eg, drowning), or can be the only way to determine the cause of death in a few circumstances (eg, many cases of low-voltage electrocution, which may not leave any specific mark on the body). Third, adequate documentation of the findings at the scene can provide crucial information to support the ultimate determination of cause and manner of death and help refute future arguments against that determination. For example, a contact gunshot wound of the head could be the result of a suicide or the result of a homicide, with the scene staged to look like a suicide. The autopsy findings most likely would not be able to differentiate the two scenarios, but the scene investigation would play a critical role in that determination and the scene photographs would be important documentation to support that determination.

PHOTOGRAPHY OF THE SCENE AND BODY

For death scene photography as with autopsy photography, it is important to obtain both overall images and close-up images. An overall image is a picture that encompasses a broad range view of the scene (eg, the entire kitchen), whereas a close-up image encompasses a specific spot in the overall view (eg, the bloody knife on the kitchen floor). Overall images allow a person to see the context of the scene (eg, how different objects relate to each other) and close-up images to see the detail of different objects at the scene. Without both images, details of the scene investigation can be lost. For example, without an overall photograph, a photograph of an object may not allow for the viewer to determine where the object is or how it relates to the death scene. Also, without the overall view, the context of the close-up image is unknown. For example, if the only photograph available is of a bloody knife on the floor, the viewer would not be able to appreciate that the decedent's body was only four feet away sitting against the refrigerator. The scene can be photographed in a variety of ways; however, liberal use of photographs and attempting to record as much of the death scene as possible is best. In this regard, a video of the death scene can also help document the findings.

> **PEARLS & PITFALLS**
>
> A useful photograph is of the location where the body was found after the body has been moved. In one case, a body found only a few hundred yards from the individual's residence was decomposed. The family alleged the body had been dumped near the house sometime after the death occurred. A photograph of the ground after the body had been moved showed soil that was heavily infiltrated with decompositional fluid, which refuted the family's proposed scenario.

> **PEARLS & PITFALLS**
>
> Many potentially important findings at the scene cannot be recorded with photography, such as temperature, smells, weather conditions, or speed and flow of a water source, such as a creek or river, and should be documented in the written report so as to have a record. A photograph of the thermostat in the house, or a video of the turbulent creek or river could also be used to document such findings. One term for such findings is "ephemeral," which is defined as lasting a short time. Another related and important consideration for bodies found outdoors is that the conditions at the time the body is found may not be the same as when the person died. For example, a rockfall upon which a hiker was found dead may have actually been a waterfall at the time the hiker died.

> **FAQ:** What is the purpose of viewing a body at the hospital that has already been transported from the location where the person sustained their lethal event?
>
> **Answer:** Documentation at the hospital may help determine whether a finding was related to therapy or was present prior to the hospital course. Examining the body at the hospital will also allow the investigator to obtain hospital blood, which, depending upon the time course, may be more reliable for toxicologic analysis and interpretation of drug concentrations than autopsy blood. However, while investigation at the hospital can be performed, in most cases, investigation of the actual place where the person was transported from, especially in the case of infant deaths and some traumatic deaths, is vital to the investigation. Whether an investigation of the actual site where the decedent sustained their lethal event should be performed in addition to the hospital view is dependent upon the nature of the death, office policies, and preferences of the death investigator and forensic pathologist.

DOCUMENTATION OF POSTMORTEM CHANGES

The documentation of postmortem changes at the time of scene investigation is important. In most cases, the forensic pathologist will be performing the autopsy the day following the discovery of the decedent, or later, potentially after the body has been held in a cooler for one to several days, or after being transported in a vehicle for several hours, all of which will alter the postmortem changes, but are unrelated to the time of death (Figure 3.2A-D). In addition, one important consideration regarding evaluation of postmortem changes at the scene is whether the postmortem changes fit the body position. For example, if fixed anterior lividity is present and the body is lying on its back, then the body has been moved before the investigator arrived. However, when a body has fixed lividity that only reflects the position the body was in when the lividity fixed and not the position in which the individual died. Comparison of rigor mortis to the position that the body is found in is also important, as rigor mortis may be inappropriate for the position in which the body is found (eg, a body with rigor mortis after being killed in a chair can then be dumped in an alleyway and appear to be sitting). Another important consideration is that in children and infants, rigor mortis can develop quickly due to small muscle mass, which can lead to a misinterpretation by law enforcement that the child died earlier than what was reported and police may then incorrectly determine that the history told to them is a lie.

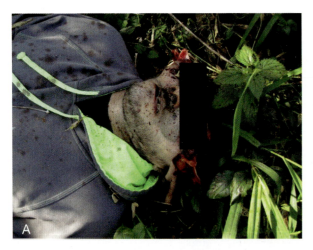
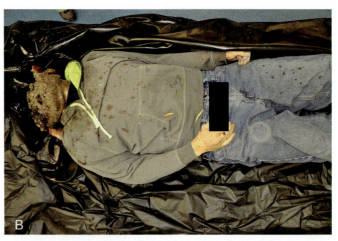
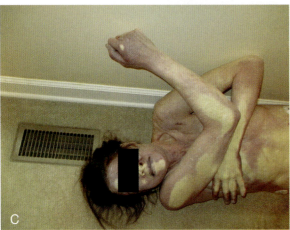
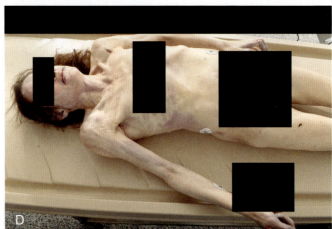

Figure 3.2. Death scene appearance versus autopsy appearance. At the scene, it is good to take photos of the body to include postmortem changes and injuries. From the time of the death scene investigation to the time of the autopsy, the appearance of both injuries and postmortem change can change, and the additional set of photographs can help the forensic pathologist interpret changes. In (**A**), at the scene, there was minimal maggot activity at the head of an individual with a self-inflicted gunshot wound; however, at the time of autopsy (**B**), there was prominent maggot activity. In (**C**), the decedent was found face-down, and when turned over, was noted to have prominent purple lividity on the anterior surface of the body; however, by the time of autopsy (**D**) the unfixed lividity had re-distributed.

FAQ: Can a postmortem temperature be taken at the scene?

Answer: While caution must be exercised using body temperature to determine time of death, it does provide an objective measurement compared to the potential subjective interpretation of blanching versus fixed lividity, or the degree of rigor mortis present. While a postmortem temperature can be obtained rectally at the death scene, usually, when the determination of time of death is most important to an investigation, the manner of death is often a homicide, and obtaining a rectal temperature at the scene would impair future collection of evidence of sexual activity. One potential method for obtaining a postmortem temperature at the scene is insertion of a thermometer into the liver. This method avoids contacting the mouth or anus and thus would not hinder future collection of evidence. The area can be photographed to show the unaltered state of the skin overlying the liver, a tiny nick in the skin made, and a thermometer, such as a standard kitchen meat thermometer, inserted and the temperature obtained. Some forensic pathologists oppose this method; however, done as above, the method should not create any significant artifacts. The track created by the thermometer can be identified in the liver parenchyma, and there will be little, if any, bleeding.

DOCUMENTATION OF DISCOVERY HISTORY AND TERMINAL EVENTS

The history regarding the terminal events is important especially if the cause of death is a condition that may produce no, minimal, or non-specific autopsy findings and require additional testing that is not normally obtained (eg, a fatal allergic reaction, and possible mast cell tryptase testing). In addition, the history regarding the terminal events may help guide the autopsy procedure. For example, if the decedent was witnessed to suddenly collapse, with little or no previous symptoms having been voiced, a cardiac condition or a pulmonary thromboembolus is a likely source and can determine how the organs are removed at autopsy and the thoroughness of the cardiac examination, such as choosing to include dissection of the sinoatrial and atrioventricular nodes. The discovery history is an important component of infant death investigation, with the determination of who placed the infant to sleep, who last knew the infant was alive, and who found the infant dead being important pieces of information; however, the discovery history can provide utility to adult death investigations as well. For example, if a boyfriend says that his girlfriend was acting fine when he left the room but that he found her dead after he returned from smoking a cigarette, suspicions of a subtle traumatic event such as a strangulation could be considered.

PEARLS & PITFALLS

If a liquid substance, such as soda pop or beer, is found adjacent to the decedent, especially if in an open container, or in a container that has had the seal broken and partially consumed, it is prudent to consider taking a sample of the liquid for potential future toxicologic testing. If the decedent is found to have died related to consumption of a drug or toxin, the family may allege that they were given the substance in the drink. Without a sample of the substance to test, this allegation could not be adequately confirmed or refuted.

PEARLS & PITFALLS

If more than one individual or pet is dead at the scene, an environmental cause (eg, carbon monoxide poisoning) or similar circumstance should be considered. If one individual and one or more pets are dead at the scene, determining whether the pets died at the same time as the decedent is important. If there is evidence the pets were alive following the individual's death (eg, scratched doors, presence of feces or urine), the likelihood of an environmental type death is less (Figure 3.3).

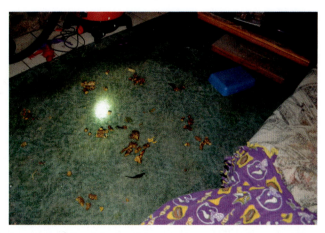

Figure 3.3. Environmental-related deaths. When there are two or more decedents and no obvious injuries that would have caused the death are apparent, an environmental hazard should be considered. If pets are found dead at the scene along with the decedent, an environmental hazard should also be considered. Determining whether the animal has been alive since the death of the individual can assist. In the photo (Figure 3.3), numerous piles of dog feces would be evidence that that dog was alive for some period of time after the decedent's death, unless the animal was known to urinate/defecate in the house.

> **PEARLS & PITFALLS**
>
> A large component of any death investigation is not actually performed at the scene, but in the form of the acquisition of appropriate records related to the death (eg, medical records, both medical and psychiatric, police reports, 9-1-1 recordings) and interviews with medical providers, law enforcement, family members, friends of the decedent, and witnesses to the terminal event. Depending upon the nature of the death, any one of these forms of records or interviews can be vital to the investigation. For example, a good social history can provide very useful information to confirm a manner of death as suicide.

> **PEARLS & PITFALLS**
>
> Death investigations frequently involve the interactions of two separate agencies: the coroner or medical examiner (depending upon what type of system the death occurs in) and law enforcement, with each agency having a different focus. Law enforcement identifies and documents crimes and coroners and medical examiners identify and document the cause and manner of death. In the case of a suspected homicide, law enforcement most likely will not let the coroner or medical examiner move the body until they have completed their investigation of the scene, and often will not even allow death investigators onto the scene itself. Unfortunately, such circumstances lend themselves to conflict between agencies, which serves no useful purpose. If the death investigators can develop a rapport with the law enforcement agencies and promote understanding and cooperation, such as by teaching law enforcement officers how the death investigator's examination of the body can assist the scene investigation through interpretation of postmortem changes, both parties will benefit.

NEAR MISSES

Near Miss #1: Natural disease presenting as motor vehicle accident. When a motor vehicle accident occurs, the first thought is that the decedent sustained injuries in the accident; however, it is very possible for an accident to occur after the decedent sustains a natural death. In Figure 3.4A, the decedent's car was found impacted against a tree; however, at autopsy, no lethal injuries are identified. The decedent had hyperinflated lungs (Figure 3.4B) and was determined to have had status asthmaticus, and died as a result.

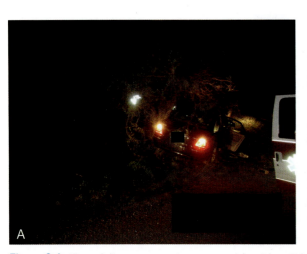
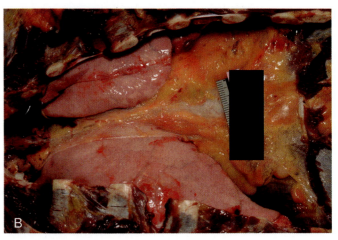

Figure 3.4. Natural disease presenting as potential accident. While the scene investigation suggested injuries sustained in a motor vehicle accident as the cause of death (**A**), autopsy identified asthma as the cause of death (**B**).

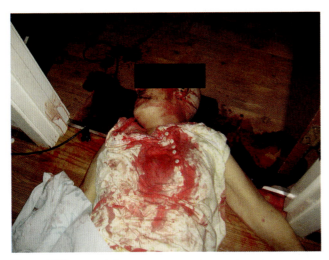

Figure 3.5. Natural disease process with prominent hemorrhage. The decedent in Figure 3.5 has lung cancer that eroded into a vessel, resulting in exsanguination.

Near Miss #2: Exsanguination due to lung cancer. While a copious amount of blood at the death scene is preliminarily concerning for a traumatic death, numerous natural disease processes can result in there being a significant amount of blood at the scene. Ruptured esophageal varices in patients with cirrhosis, a bleeding duodenal ulcer, hemorrhage from a skin neoplasm, or hemorrhage from a ruptured varicose vein can all result in a prominent amount of blood at the scene. In Figure 3.5, the decedent had lung cancer that eroded into a vessel.

Near Miss #3: Contusion at scene versus at autopsy. At scene investigation, the coroner identified a prominent bruise on the posterior surface of the right leg (Figure 3.6A); however, at autopsy, the bruise was not nearly as prominent (Figure 3.6B). The movement of unfixed lividity, decomposition, and other changes can easily alter the appearance of wounds from the time of the scene investigation until the performance of the autopsy.

Near Miss #4: Elderly homicides can be very subtle, with minimal external examination findings. For example, an older female who is being cared for by her son is found dead in her bed, with only petechial hemorrhages on the conjunctivae and face identified by external examination. Autopsy identifies hemorrhage in the neck musculature. A high degree of caution is best when investigating any death of an elderly individual, even when they were expected to die. If care is not taken, these non-natural deaths can easily be missed.

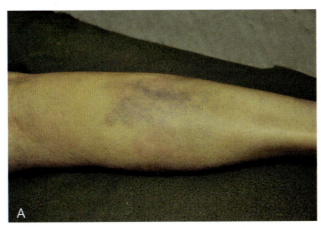 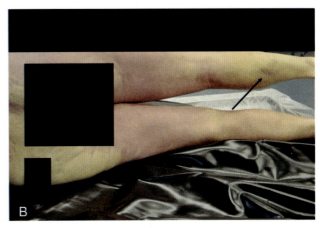

Figure 3.6. Scene photographs versus autopsy photographs of images. On the posterior surface of the right leg is a prominent contusion (**A**), which was diminished in intensity, but still visible at the time of autopsy (arrow) (**B**).

References

1. National Institute of Justice. *Death Investigation: A Guide for the Scene Investigator (Every Scene, Every Time)*. US Department of Justice; 1999.
2. Hlavaty L, Sung L. Applying the principles of homicide by heart attack. *Am J Forensic Med Pathol*. 2016;37(2):112-117.
3. De Giorgio F, Arena V, Arena E, et al. Homicide by heart attack? *Leg Med*. 2009;11(suppl 1):S531-S532.
4. Turner SA, Barnard JJ, Spotswood SD, Prahlow JA. "Homicide by heart attack" revisited. *J Forensic Sci*. 2004;49(3):598-600.
5. Davis JH. Can sudden cardiac death be murder? *J Forensic Sci*. 1978;23(2):384-387.

DEATH CERTIFICATION 4

CHAPTER OUTLINE

Introduction 22

Description of Cause of Death 22

Description of Manner of Death 23

Description of Mechanism of Death 23

Near Miss 26

INTRODUCTION

Although the forensic autopsy has many purposes, the ultimate goal of each autopsy is the accurate certification of the cause and manner of death. Many resources are available to assist medical examiners with completion of death certificates[1,2]; however, with death certification there are oftentimes many correct ways to word a cause of death based upon a series of investigative and autopsy findings (ie, the cause of death can for many if not all deaths be worded in more than one way, each of which can be considered correct). As far as the manner of death, although there are suggested guidelines for many situations,[2] honest debate regarding how to certify the manner of death in many situations often exists.[3] In short, each forensic pathologist's preferences for how to certify the cause and manner of death in any given situation will depend greatly upon their training and experience; however, each pathologist must also remember that their final determination as to the cause and manner of death must be defensible in a court of law as well as the court of public opinion. While the cause and manner of death are recorded on the death certificate, the mechanism of death is not required; however, it is important for forensic pathologists to also understand mechanism of death.

DESCRIPTION OF CAUSE OF DEATH

The cause of death is the pathologic change that initiated the sequence of events that resulted in the death of the individual. Common causes of death encountered by forensic pathologists include coronary artery atherosclerosis, blunt force injuries, drug overdose, and gunshot wounds. On the death certificate, four lines are provided for the cause of death; however, on any given case, no more than one line needs to be filled in. If more than one line is completed, the forensic pathologist needs to ensure that one condition leads to the next (ie, the most recent condition leading to death is listed on the upper line and the most remote condition that started the chain of events is listed on the lowest filled-in line). The cause of death can originate seconds to years before the time of death of the individual. For example, a gunshot wound of the head is a cause of death and can originate at or seconds before the decedent's actual time of death, whereas atherosclerotic cardiovascular disease is also a cause of death and can originate years before the actual time of death. The terms "proximate cause of death," "intermediary cause of death," and "immediate cause of death" are also used.[4] The proximate cause of death is the pathologic condition that started the chain of events in motion (ie, the most remote). The immediate cause of death is the condition that developed closest to the actual time of death of the decedent. The intermediary cause(s) of death is/are the condition(s) that developed between the proximate and immediate causes of death. For example, if the cause of death is hemopericardium due to ruptured acute myocardial infarct due to coronary artery thrombosis due to coronary artery atherosclerosis, the immediate cause of death is the hemopericardium. The proximate cause of death is the coronary artery atherosclerosis. The ruptured acute myocardial infarct and coronary artery thrombosis are intermediary conditions.

SAMPLE NOTE: WHAT IF A DECEDENT HAS MORE THAN ONE CAUSE OF DEATH?

Quite frequently, autopsy alone or autopsy combined with scene investigation and/or medical review will reveal competing causes of death, with each one potentially contributory to the cause of death. For example, if a decedent with a non-traumatic seizure disorder is found dead and at autopsy 75% stenosis of the left anterior descending coronary artery is identified, there are two possible causes of death. In such situations, the forensic pathologist must decide which condition was the more likely cause of death, and list one as the cause of death and the other potentially in "Other significant conditions" or potentially list the cause of death as Undetermined and in parentheses list the competing conditions. For example, the death certificate could be certified as "Undetermined (non-traumatic seizure disorder versus critical coronary artery atherosclerosis)." Another way to handle the situation would be to list both of the conditions as the cause of death, such as "Non-traumatic seizure disorder complicated by coronary artery atherosclerosis." If the two competing causes of death are of different manners, favoring the non-natural manner of death is most likely the better option for death certification.

DESCRIPTION OF MANNER OF DEATH

In most jurisdictions, there are only five manners of death. In a natural death, the death is entirely due to a natural disease process. In a homicide, the death is due to the volitional, intentional, and harmful actions of another person, which were directed at the decedent. The individual who caused the death did not have to intend for the death of the decedent, and could have merely been intending to hurt or scare them; however, even if the intent was not their death, if the person dies, the manner of death is best certified as homicide. In a suicide, the death is due to a self-inflicted injury with the intent of causing one's own death or causing self-harm. In an accident, a harmful event occurs; however, there was no intent for the harmful event to scare, harm, or kill another individual. In an undetermined death, there is insufficient information from the scene investigation in combination with the autopsy and other testing to determine the manner of death. For any given circumstance, different pathologists may have different criteria for using undetermined as the cause of death.

DESCRIPTION OF MECHANISM OF DEATH

A mechanism of death is the physiologic abnormality caused by the pathologic lesion(s) that constitute the cause of death. Mechanisms are very non-specific, and each mechanism can usually occur due to a wide range of underlying causes of death. For example, exsanguination is a mechanism of death that could occur secondary to traumatic causes (eg, gunshot wound or stab wound of the neck) or natural causes (eg, ruptured esophageal varices). Because they are non-specific and can be due to a variety of underlying causes, often a mixture of traumatic and non-traumatic conditions, listing a mechanism of death by itself on the death certificate is not acceptable unless perhaps with a caveat (eg, cardiac dysrhythmia of undetermined natural etiology). At the same time, listing a mechanism of death in addition to the cause of death is acceptable. For example, one pathologist may prefer to list a cause of death as hanging, whereas another pathologist may prefer to list a cause of death as asphyxia due to hanging.

PEARLS & PITFALLS

The length of time between an injury and the patient's ultimate death does not affect the determination of manner. If an individual sustains an injury that sets up their death many years later, the circumstances of the injury still determine the manner of death (Figure 4.1). For example, if an individual sustains an injury in a motor vehicle accident that causes paraplegia and then 10 years later succumbs to a urinary tract infection leading to sepsis, the injuries sustained in the accident are the underlying (ie, proximate) cause of death and the manner is accident, assuming neither the decedent or any other person intentionally caused the motor vehicle collision. This concept is often not understood by clinical physicians, who will certify a cause of death based upon the most immediate condition, often ignoring the inciting condition, and will miscertify the manner of death as natural. Careful review of the death certificate for clues as to the etiology of the final pathologic process (eg, when the cause of death is listed as pneumonia, but in other significant conditions, rib fractures are listed) will assist with identifying these non-natural deaths. In addition, considering why a young individual has paraplegia or quadriplegia or another often trauma-induced condition can also assist in identifying these situations and preventing a miscertification of manner of death.

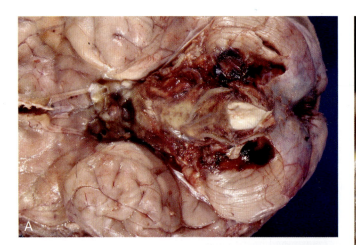
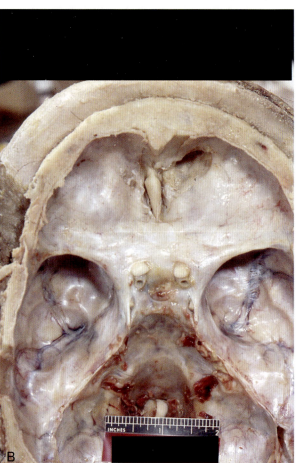
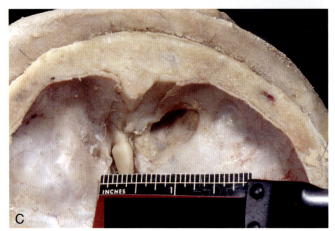

Figure 4.1. Meningitis due to remote gunshot wound. The state Bureau of Vital Statistics identified a death certificate in which the physician listed meningitis as the cause of death and a gunshot wound as a significant contributory condition, but certified the manner as natural. The body was brought for autopsy. At autopsy, meningitis was identified (**A**). In the right orbital plate was a fistula between the frontal sinus and the cranial cavity (**B** and **C**). Sinusitis led to meningitis, which caused the immediate death; however, the fistula was the result of a gunshot wound the decedent sustained over a decade before their death. As they were shot by another person, the death certificate was certified as meningitis due to remote gunshot wound of the head, and the manner of death was certified as homicide.

> **FAQ:** Can cause of death always be determined at autopsy?
>
> **Answer:** No, on occasion, autopsy in combination with scene investigation and ancillary testing cannot identify a cause of death. These situations often occur in the infant population as both sudden natural death in infants and accidental smothering (ie, overlay), which is the frequent differential diagnosis, both leave no specific findings, and the cause of death is often certified as sudden unexplained infant death (SUID), with the manner certified as undetermined, acknowledging that the underlying cause could be natural or non-natural. In the adult population, when the autopsy, scene investigation, and toxicologic analysis do not reveal a cause of death, molecular testing to identify a cardiac genetic mutation may assist; however, it will not necessarily provide a definitive answer. Also, many drugs and toxins that can cause death are not identified upon routine testing, and if scene investigation or some other aspect of the death investigation does not guide the testing, these will remain undetermined deaths, as the causative agent may not be identified during routine testing.

FAQ: How significant of an injury is required for the injury to determine the manner of death?

Answer: The answer to this question may vary somewhat based upon the training and experience of the forensic pathologist. While some forensic pathologists feel that if any injury, no matter how seemingly minor, contributed to the cause of death, that the circumstances of the injury determine the manner of death, other forensic pathologists may accept minor injuries as contributory to the cause of death but not requiring a manner of death other than natural.

PEARLS & PITFALLS

Although the exact wording used for a cause of death may vary between forensic pathologists (eg, Blunt force injuries vs Blunt force trauma), and while the determination of manner may vary between forensic pathologists, it is important for each individual pathologist to be as consistent as possible in their use of terms and their reasoning for determining a manner of death. The work of forensic pathologists is utilized by a broad range of individuals, including coroners, law enforcement, and county attorneys. When forensic pathologists are consistent in their approach, it is easier for other agencies to adapt and work with them.

FAQ: How specific does the death certificate have to be?

Answer: This question actually applies to many aspects of the death certificate, but before answering the question, it is best to remember that the purpose of the death certificate is the collection of data for public health, and the more information available to public health agencies on the death certificate, the better; however, it must also be remembered that the cause and manner of death are used for legal purposes, both criminal and civil, and that the opinion rendered by the person signing the death certificate must often be defended in court, both civil and criminal, as well as to family members who often have questions about the death. First of all, "how specific" can apply to the filling in of one of four lines on the death certificate for cause of death versus three or four lines. While filling in three to four lines versus only one line provides more information for public health agencies to use, one must be cautious to not get too specific or include conditions that are unnecessary or incorrect. For example, "Gunshot wound of the head" is an acceptable one-line cause of death. Adding another line, "Subdural hemorrhage," given that autopsy identified some subdural hemorrhage, would imply survival time. Yes, there may be subdural hemorrhage, but did it actually by itself contribute to the cause of death? Second, "how specific" can apply to what might otherwise be called "lumpers and splitters." One pathologist may word a cause of death as "Multiple gunshot wounds," whereas another pathologist may list the cause of death as "Gunshot wound of the chest" and list "Gunshot wounds of the extremities" as a contributory cause. Another example would be that one pathologist may list "Blunt force injuries" as the cause of death, whereas another pathologist may list "Flail chest due to multiple rib fractures due to blunt force injuries of the chest," and "Lacerations of the scalp and fractures of the extremities" as contributory conditions. While the approach of listing specific injuries (or natural disease) and separating between those most directly causing death and those that contributed to the death provides more information to public health agencies, the forensic pathologist should ensure that they can defend the distinction. While the public health agencies may enjoy more detailed death certificates, fewer details on a death certificate allows a forensic pathologist a little more freedom to discuss their conclusions later in court. Third, "how specific" can apply to the listing of various drugs, microorganisms, or cancer types on the death certificate. "Multi-drug overdose" is not as useful of information as "Mixed drug toxicity (methamphetamine and heroin)"; and "Metastatic carcinoma" is not as useful of information as "Metastatic squamous cell carcinoma of the lung." In addition, if cultures are performed and identify a specific organism causing an infectious disease process at autopsy, including the name of the organism in the cause of death is preferable to omitting it from the record. In those situations, more specific is better.

> **FAQ:** Can a psychiatric diagnosis be listed in "Other significant/other contributory conditions" when an individual commits suicide?
>
> **Answer:** While the argument is made that the cause of death should only be the pathologic condition that started the physiologic abnormality that led to the individual's death, Dr Petty makes a good argument that other conditions if they contributed to the circumstances of the death, even though they did not directly contribute to the physiologic mechanism of death, can and should be listed in the "Other significant/other contributory conditions."[5] If an individual commits suicide, it would be hard to argue that their on-going depression or acute ethanol intoxication, which lowers inhibitions, did not contribute to the circumstances.

> **FAQ:** What conditions can be listed in part II of the death certificate (contributory conditions)?
>
> **Answer:** While many death certificates will have no conditions listed in part II, some may have several conditions listed in part II. The forensic pathologist should just ensure that all conditions listed in part II contributed to the death and were not just listed because they were an interesting finding at autopsy. The forensic pathologist may have to defend their inclusions on the death certificate at a later time, so caution is appropriate.

Key points to completing the death certificate

- Complete the autopsy and ensure that medical records and investigative reports are available as appropriate
- Make sure the investigator obtains the information necessary to complete the death certificate, including time of death and, for non-natural deaths, the place and time of injury.

> **PEARLS & PITFALLS**
>
> Funeral directors can assist with the identification of improperly completed death certificates. As advocates for the family of the deceased, if the funeral home can identify an incorrect death certificate and contribute to a natural manner of death being appropriately changed to an accidental manner of death, that amendment may greatly assist the decedent's family financially if the deceased had accidental death insurance.

NEAR MISS

A completed death certificate was received by a funeral home. The clinical physician had certified the cause of death as natural death after comfort measures due to severe sepsis due to extensive necrotic wounds of the left buttock, hip, and perineum. The physician listed diabetes mellitus, paralysis, malnutrition, and neglect as contributory conditions. The manner was certified as natural. The funeral home called the coroner who obtained medical records. The cause of death was then re-certified as complications of remote gunshot wound and neglect. The manner was certified as homicide.

References

1. Centers for Disease Control and Prevention. *Medical Examiners' and Coroners' Handbook on Death Registration and Fetal Death Reporting, 2003 Revision*. Centers for Disease Control and Prevention; 2003.
2. Hanzlick R, Hunsaker JC, Davis GJ. *A Guide for Manner of Death Classification*. 1st ed. National Association of Medical Examiners; 2002.
3. Davis GG. Mind your manners. Part I: history of death certification and manner of death classification. *Am J Forensic Med Pathol*. 1997;18(3):219-223.
4. Prahlow J. *Forensic Pathology for Police, Death Investigators, Attorneys, and Forensic Scientists*. Springer; 2010.
5. Petty CS. Multiple causes of death: the viewpoint of a forensic pathologist. *J Forensic Sci*. 1965;10(2):167-178.

IDENTIFICATION 5

CHAPTER OUTLINE

Introduction 30

Circumstantial, Presumptive, or Tentative Identification 30
- How Formed 30

Exclusionary Identification 30
- How Formed 30

Positive Identification 30
- How Formed 30

Scientific Methods to Identify a Deceased Body 33
- Introduction 33

Fingerprints 33
- Requirements 33
- Time Frame 33

DNA Analysis 34
- Requirements 34
- Time Frame 35

Dental Examination 35
- Requirements 35
- Time Frame 35

Other Forms of Scientific Identification 35

Non-Scientific Methods of Identification 36
- Introduction 36

Visual Identification 36
- Method 36
- Challenges 36

Physical Findings on the Body 36
- Method 36
- Challenges 36

Identification Cards 37
- Method 37
- Challenges 37

Personal Effects 38
- Method 38

Other Methods 38

Near Miss 39

INTRODUCTION

Although the primary function of forensic pathologists is the performance of autopsies to determine cause and manner of death, in some cases, the forensic pathologist must also positively identify decedents. For the purpose of body handling and initial record keeping, unidentified decedents will most often initially be designated with the normal office specific case number as well as "Unknown" or "John Doe"/"Jane Doe," or another system of nomenclature that offices have for naming unidentified bodies. However, in some cases, a circumstantial, presumptive, or tentative identification for the decedent is known based upon the site of death and the subsequent scene investigation (ie, the decedent's name is known but additional confirmation is required to reach a positive identification). In this case, the decedent's body may temporarily be labeled with the possible correct name (eg, a presumptive identification) until additional methods, which can be either scientific or non-scientific or both, have been used to confirm the identification for the body. In addition, it is also important to understand that features about the unidentified body may be used as an exclusionary identification, which can be used to rule out certain missing individuals as the identity for the decedent.

CIRCUMSTANTIAL, PRESUMPTIVE, OR TENTATIVE IDENTIFICATION

HOW FORMED

A circumstantial identification is developed based upon the known situation under which the body was found (eg, a body being found in a locked apartment may circumstantially be identified as the renter of that apartment if only one person was known to reside in the apartment), whereas a presumptive or tentative identification indicates that, while an identification has been made, a more definitive method is necessary to confirm a positive identification. Each of the three terms (ie, circumstantial, presumptive, or tentative) could potentially be used relatively interchangeably because each indicates essentially the same thing: that a preliminary identification has been made; however, an additional step is required before a positive identification is made. This additional step to reach a positive identification usually involves the use of a scientific method. For example, if a burned body is found in a locked apartment that, by rental records, has a sole individual, the identification as the renter could be considered circumstantial, presumptive, or tentative, until a more definitive method for identification has been performed (eg, dental or DNA analysis).

EXCLUSIONARY IDENTIFICATION

HOW FORMED

An exclusionary identification is made when an individual has a physical characteristic or other characteristic that excludes them from being a certain missing individual. For example, if a female body is recovered from a river and is believed to be the body of a woman who was known to have gone missing 3 days earlier but the body recovered from the river has a large tattoo of a sports team's emblem on the upper back, something which the missing woman was known to not have, then the body in the river can be excluded as being the missing woman, and the search for the missing woman can continue, and the process of identifying the body found in the river can also continue.

POSITIVE IDENTIFICATION

HOW FORMED

Weedn defined a positive identification as a "legally sufficient unique identification based upon an objective comparison of pre- and postmortem information."[1] Essentially, records that were created while the individual was alive are compared to records created after the individual was found dead to determine whether they represent the same person. The records being compared can include photographs, fingerprints, dental examinations, and other items.

A positive identification must always be made before final disposition of the body as "presumptive and exclusionary identification are tentative and may be challenged."[1] Developing that positive identification requires that the criteria used to identify an individual are unique to that individual, or sufficiently unique as to exclude other possible individuals. As such identification requires the comparison of known information about a person available in pre-existing records to physical findings made through the examination of the deceased body, useful records to develop a positive identification include reports of missing persons, fingerprints, dental records, medical records, antemortem x-rays and computed tomography scans, employment records, and police records.[2]

> **PEARLS & PITFALLS**
>
> Positive identification in the living is most often accomplished through the presentation of a photo identification card to the examiner (eg, showing a passport photo to the Transportation Security Administration officer prior to boarding an airplane). The same method is employed by death scene investigators, coroners, and medical examiners to make a positive identification of a deceased body (ie, finding a wallet with a university identification card in the front pocket of the decedent's pants and then comparing the photograph on the identification card to the face of the decedent); however, traumatic injuries (eg, a shotgun wound of the head) and postmortem changes, including rigor, lividity, and other color changes associated with decomposition, can alter the appearance of an individual, complicating a visual comparison between antemortem photographs and the postmortem appearance of the body. Also, that the wallet in the pocket is not actually that of the decedent is not impossible.[3] In both the living and the dead, comparison of the face of the individual to a photo identification card would fulfill the above criteria for a positive identification; however, the idea that such an identification could not be challenged is not accurate. In fact, it could easily be argued that a deceased man with a wallet in his back pocket with a photo identification card with a photograph that appears to match the decedent is only a circumstantial identification and not a positive identification.

Ernst stated, "Whenever there is a question as to the identity of the decedent, or the possibility of confusion exists regarding the decedent's identity, the decedent should be identified scientifically, if possible."[4] Although developing a positive identification for each decedent investigated by an office through a scientific method is the ideal procedure, doing so is likely not possible for every office to do because of limited resources. However, in certain cases (eg, a homicide or when two or more decedents are at the scene, for example, in a car accident, and are of similar age and other physical features), performing a scientific identification even when presented with a strong visual identification of the decedent should be considered, as any subsequent courtroom proceedings may require a more stringent identification.

KEY FEATURES: Steps to Help Identify an Unknown Body
- Potentially establish a circumstantial or presumptive identification based upon where decedent was found (eg, a leased apartment or a vehicle registered to the decedent).
- Items located on the body may allow for at least a presumptive identification. These items could include a wallet with a driver's license, the decedent's name on dentures (Figure 5.1) or wedding ring, or personal papers or cards with the body.
- Comparison of tattoos and scars found on the body to those indicated in police records, or identified through interviews with the family, or in medical records (Figure 5.2A-C).
- If available, compare fingerprints on file to those obtained from the unidentified body.
- Identify the decedent's dentist from interviews with the family or through another source so that antemortem dental records can be obtained.
- Antemortem radiographs can be obtained for comparison to orthopedic hardware in the body.
- Medical records may contain identifying numbers for orthopedic hardware and implanted devices (eg, pacemakers) in the body.
- Obtain DNA standard from body through blood, hair, teeth, or bone and compare to known standard for decedent or known biologic relatives.

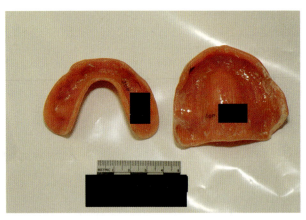

Figure 5.1. Decedent's name on the dentures. Oftentimes, the decedent's name will be found on the dentures.

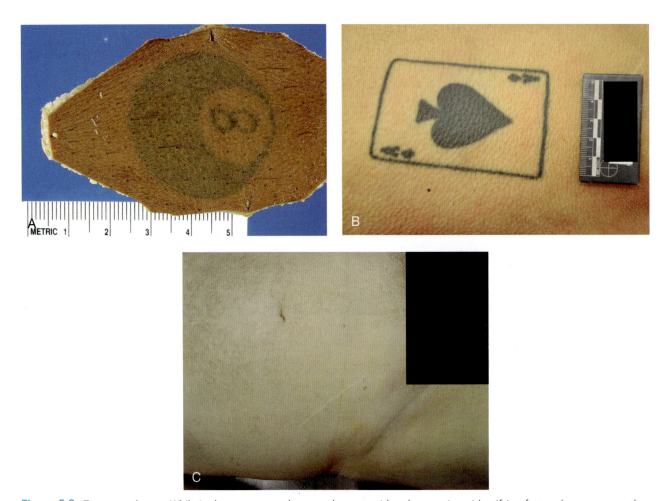

Figure 5.2. Tattoos and scars. While in the past tattoos have not been considered as a unique identifying feature because more than one individual can have the same tattoo (**A** and **B**), when combined with circumstantial factors, and given the significant number of unique tattoos that are now often present on individuals, tattoos can serve as a method of identification. Unlike tattoos, scars are probably less commonly used to develop an identification; however, under certain circumstances, when combined with other factors, scars can assist in identification (**C**).

> **PEARLS & PITFALLS**
>
> When using tattoos to identify the body, when talking with a family, ask for their knowledge of tattoos on the body first, and compare that information to what is on the body, which is probably preferable to telling the family what tattoos were found, as this may bias their answers. Other than the family, a record of tattoos for the decedent may be available through law enforcement agencies or the military. In regard to fingerprints, while latent print examiners have access to databases of fingerprints, a local fingerprint card for the decedent may not be on file, so finding out whether such a print card is available is important.

KEY FEATURES: Useful Techniques for Identification of Decedent
- Visual identification
- Personal effects and tattoos
- Fingerprint comparison
- Dental comparison
- DNA analysis
- Frontal sinuses radiographs

SCIENTIFIC METHODS TO IDENTIFY A DECEASED BODY

INTRODUCTION

The three main scientific methods used to identify a human body are fingerprint analysis, DNA analysis, and dental examination. Although these are the three most commonly employed methods, there are other methods available including frontal sinus comparison and identifying numbers on orthopedic hardware or other medical devices such as pacemakers and breast implants.

FINGERPRINTS

REQUIREMENTS

To use fingerprint analysis to identify an individual, a postmortem set of the decedent's prints is required, and the decedent must have antemortem fingerprints on file that the latent print analyst has access to. Another option is that if a body is tentatively identified, and there is a known source for that individual's fingerprints at the scene or elsewhere (eg, a water glass at their residence that they are known to use), partial fingerprints can be obtained from the object found at the scene and compared to the fingerprints obtained from the decedent at the time of autopsy to see if they match. This method, of course, depends upon whether the decedent was essentially the sole user of the object selected for developing a fingerprint from.

TIME FRAME

If a latent prints analyst is given a set of fingerprints from a decedent, and if that decedent has a set of antemortem fingerprints available for comparison purposes, a positive identification can be made in 20 minutes to 2 hours.

> **PEARLS & PITFALLS**
>
> Decomposition can affect the ability to obtain fingerprints from a body. Although mummification will cause the skin to harden, fingerprints can still be obtained through one of several methods: rehydration of the digits, removal of fingerprint pads, use of a drying gel applied to the fingertips, or photographs (Figure 5.3).[5,6] Any of these four techniques could be used to produce a fingerprint for identification in the case of mummification. In addition, application of baby powder to the fingertips to better define ridge detail or removal of the superficial tissue and transillumination are two other methods that can be employed.[7] Photographs can also work when the body is decomposed but not mummified.

DNA ANALYSIS

REQUIREMENTS

A source of nuclear DNA from the decedent (eg, blood, hair roots, buccal swab, soft tissue, or bone) is required and the decedent must have a record of their nuclear DNA on file in a system accessible by the DNA technologist (eg, CODIS). Unlike fingerprints, an antemortem record of an individual's nuclear DNA is less common. For example, in Texas, on each individual's driver's license is a thumbprint; however, most individuals do not have their nuclear DNA on file. Biologic relatives of the decedent (eg, children or parents) can easily provide a known source for DNA comparison. And, as above with the discussion of the use of fingerprints to identify an individual, if a body is tentatively identified, and there is a known source of the decedent's nuclear DNA (eg, comb with hair), a DNA sample can be obtained from the known object and the DNA technologist could compare the DNA from the known object to the DNA sample from the unidentified body to see if a match is present. Of importance, when a nuclear DNA analysis is performed, not every single base pair in the decedent's DNA is analyzed, instead, only large blocks of the DNA are compared; therefore, identical twins will have the same forensic DNA results, but will have unique fingerprints.[1] In addition to nuclear DNA, mitochondrial DNA (mtDNA) can also be obtained from samples from the decedent and used to assist in identification of the remains.

While the standard bone specimen taken for DNA analysis is a segment of the shaft from a long bone such as the femur or tibia (Figure 5.4), with increasing postmortem interval, small cancellous bones instead of a cortical segment have been shown to provide better DNA yield rates.[8] Finger and toenails can also potentially be used as a source of DNA.[9] If a sample of nuclear DNA cannot be developed, mtDNA can also serve as a source for identification.[10]

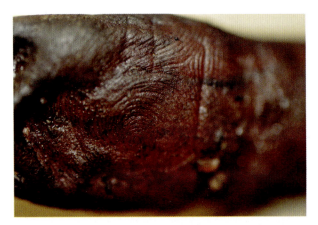

Figure 5.3. Photograph of decomposed fingerprint. While decomposition can impair the ability to obtain fingerprints, several methods, including photography, are available to develop fingerprints in such a situation.

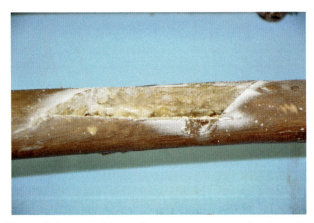

Figure 5.4. Cortical bone for DNA specimen. When sampling bone for DNA analysis, the shaft of long bones is often used as the source. When obtaining the specimen it is best to block out a segment from one side, thus not transecting the bone and allowing for the overall structure of the bone to be maintained.

TIME FRAME

From start to finish, the minimal amount of time required for analysis of nuclear DNA is around 3 days. However, given work flow and other issues, the actual time required may be weeks to months.

DENTAL EXAMINATION

REQUIREMENTS

A radiograph of the decedent's upper and lower teeth, and access to the decedent's antemortem dental records for comparison are needed. Unfortunately, at night or on weekends, access to the antemortem dental records, if they must be obtained from a dentist's office, may be challenging; also, the name of the decedent's dentist must be known. Phillips and Stuhlinger indicated, as a result of their study, that, when examined by trained personnel (including dental hygiene students), a single amalgam can be used to make a positive identification.[11] For trained forensic odontologists, the presence of amalgams is not required for identification, as comparison of features of the natural tooth (eg, the root structure) between the antemortem and postmortem radiographs can allow for identification. Even in edentulous individuals, analysis by a forensic odontologist may allow for a positive identification.[12]

TIME FRAME

As with fingerprints, dental comparison, if the antemortem records are available for review, can be performed quickly, allowing for confirmation of identification within minutes to hours.

OTHER FORMS OF SCIENTIFIC IDENTIFICATION

Other than fingerprints, DNA analysis, and dental examinations, other forms of scientific identification are available including numbers on orthopedic hardware (Figure 5.5), frontal sinus analysis, and dental features in photos of the decedent.[13-18] Orthopedic hardware, even when it has no identifying numbers, can potentially be used to identify individuals just based upon comparison of the antemortem and postmortem radiographs assessing for physical characteristics of the orthopedic hardware. Antemortem radiographs, if located, can be compared to the postmortem radiographs (Figure 5.6A and B). In addition, numbers on breast implants can also be used to potentially identify a decedent.

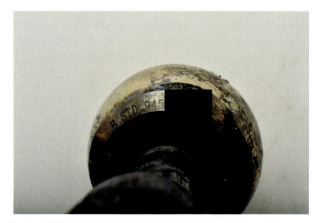

Figure 5.5. Identifying numbers on orthopedic femoral implant. This individual found in a burned building was tentatively identified by circumstances and positively identified by comparing numbers identified on the orthopedic hardware to numbers listed in the medical records.

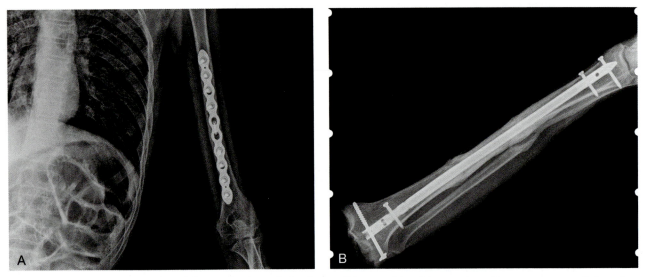

Figure 5.6. Orthopedic hardware. While not all orthopedic hardware will have an identifying number, the mere presence of the orthopedic hardware can allow for comparison of antemortem and postmortem radiographs to contribute to the identification of an individual. Examples of orthopedic hardware in a humerus (**A**) and tibia (**B**) are illustrated.

NON-SCIENTIFIC METHODS OF IDENTIFICATION

INTRODUCTION

The advantage of non-scientific methods of identification is that they can be performed by the death investigator, coroner, or medical examiner, with no special equipment or training; however, their uniqueness (ie, to be able to be matched to a specific person) is highly variable, and each as the sole method of identification of a decedent should be approached with caution.

VISUAL IDENTIFICATION

METHOD

To make a visual identification, the face of the decedent is compared to an antemortem photo of the decedent, for example, a driver's license or family photo.

CHALLENGES

Visual identification is generally viewed as the least reliable method for identification of a body, especially when performed by friends or family.[1-3,19] As described above, positive identification requires objective assessment, and family members or friends are likely to be anything but objective when viewing the body of the decedent and misidentification can occur.[19] A carefully composed photograph can help alleviate this potential difficulty.

PHYSICAL FINDINGS ON THE BODY

METHOD

Comparison of scars and tattoos on the body with those known to be on the missing individual whom the body is felt to represent.

CHALLENGES

As with visual identification, using markings on the body such as tattoos and scars to identify an individual must be done with caution. The finding of a single scar in the right lower quadrant of the abdomen is hardly unique, as many people in the population have had an appendectomy, which produces such a scar; however, a person with 50+ tattoos well-documented in past records offers a relatively unique appearance. Weedn states, "skin markings are of considerable importance for identification. Natural birthmarks, significant scars, or congenital deformities will usually provide presumptive identification, if not positive identification."[1]

> **PEARLS & PITFALLS**
>
> While color changes associated with decomposition and especially mummification can obscure tattoos, there are techniques to allow for better visualization of the skin markings. Hydrogen peroxide applied to the skin can bleach the discolored skin and allow the tattoo to be visualized (Figure 5.7A-D). Infra-red photography can also be used to highlight the tattoo in a decomposed body (Figure 5.8A and B).

IDENTIFICATION CARDS

METHOD

Identification cards offer one possible way to identify an unknown body through visual identification.

CHALLENGES

As described above, a wallet with a photo identification card is very useful in identifying a deceased individual, but the possibility of a similar-appearing person having stolen that wallet should always be considered, or, in the case of a car accident or plane crash, mixture of personal effects between bodies is also quite possible.

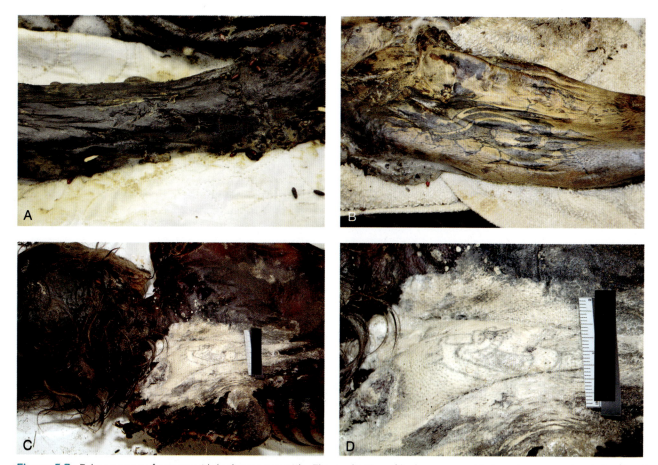

Figure 5.7. Enhancement of tattoos with hydrogen peroxide. The application of hydrogen peroxide to a decomposed and discolored area of skin with a tattoo (**A**) can allow for much better visualization of the tattoo (**B**). (**C** and **D**) are an overall and a close-up photograph of another tattoo brought out by application of hydrogen peroxide. When applying the hydrogen peroxide use some caution as prolonged exposure to the hydrogen peroxide (eg, overnight) can cause the decomposed tissue to break down.

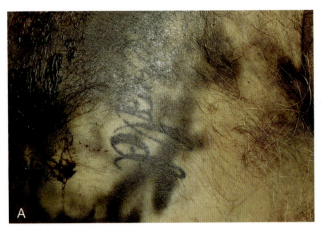 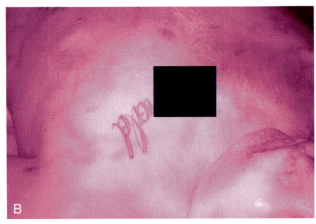

Figure 5.8. Enhancement of a tattoo with infra-red photography. Use of infra-red photography can allow for better visualization of a tattoo (**A** and **B**).

PERSONAL EFFECTS

METHOD

Items received with the body are compared to items that the missing person is known to have. For example, dentures may have a person's name and/or social security number on it. A wedding ring or pocket knife with an engraved name, a known personal item always carried by an individual, personal papers with names and signatures, and such also offer ways to identify a body.

OTHER METHODS

Other methods of identification exist and include internal findings consistent with medical records of a decedent, radiology (eg, frontal sinus and vertebral column findings), analysis of skeletal remains to determine ancestry, age, sex, and stature, facial reconstruction, and hair analysis.

> **FAQ:** What steps should be taken if a body cannot be identified at the time of autopsy or within a relatively short time frame thereafter?
>
> **Answer:** If a deceased body remains unidentified after the autopsy and disposition of the body is required, the forensic pathologist should obtain all the necessary information to allow for subsequent identification, which would include (1) photographs of the face and body, including all scars, tattoos, and any other potentially identifying features, (2) retention of hair and a bloodspot card for DNA analysis, (3) full-body radiographs, especially to document frontal sinus features, vertebral column, any orthopedic hardware, any healed fractures, and any other skeletal changes (spinal abnormalities, variation in rib structure, skeletal anomalies including deformations), and (4) documentation of the clothing and personal effects received with the body to include brand and sizes.[13] If a blood spot card cannot be obtained due to the condition of the body (eg, the body is decomposed or skeletonized), a segment of cortical bone and/or a molar tooth can be retained. Although dental radiographs of the decedent can be obtained, if the body is decomposed or skeletonized, the maxilla and mandible can also be retained for use in future identification.

NEAR MISS

An individual was found in a skeletonized condition. As part of the examination of the remains, the individual's personal effects were examined (Figure 5.9A). While wedding rings can sometimes have inscriptions that can be used for identification, none was present in this case. The decedent's glasses were present (Figure 5.9B). Analysis of the prescription of the eyeglasses could provide information that may help identify an individual.

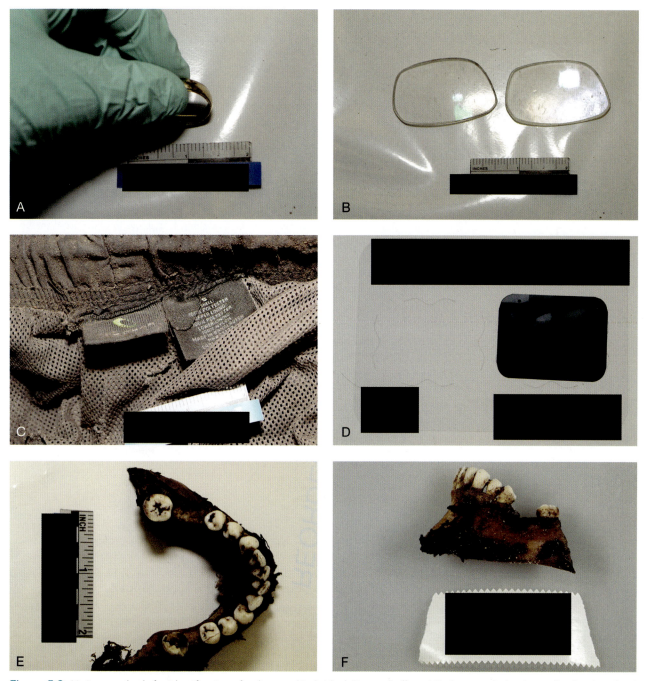

Figure 5.9. Various methods for identification of a deceased individual. Personal effects (**A**), the prescription lenses for the decedent's eyeglasses (**B**), and clothing features (**C**) can aid in the identification of a deceased individual. The presence of features in antemortem radiographs (**D**) may not be present in the skeletal remains (**E** and **F**) as teeth can be lost in the intervening period.

In addition, examination of clothing (Figure 5.9C) can provide information that may help with identification, such as clothing sizes and brands. Dental records were present; however, tooth #19 was shown to have an amalgam (Figure 5.9D). In the skeletal remains, tooth #19 was not present (Figure 5.9E and F). While a tooth can be absent in the skeletal remains but present in the antemortem records (eg, a tooth can be lost between the time the dental radiographs were obtained and the time the skeletal remains were found), a tooth that is absent in the antemortem radiographs should not be present in the skeletal remains, unless it is a dental implant or other artificial type of tooth. The absence of tooth #19 in the skeletal remains did not exclude the decedent (whose identification card was also present at the scene).

References

1. Weedn VW. Postmortem identifications of remains. *Clin Lab Med*. 1998;18(1):115-137.
2. Stahl CJ. Identification. In: Fisher RS, Petty CS, eds. *Forensic Pathology: A Handbook for Pathologists*. National Institute of Law Enforcement and Criminal Justice; 1977:64-71.
3. Brady WJ. *Medical Investigation of Deaths in Oregon*. 2nd ed; 1976.
4. Ernst MF. Medicolegal death investigation and forensic procedures. In: Froede RC, ed. *Handbook of Forensic Pathology*. 2nd ed. College of American Pathologists; 2003:1-10.
5. Haglund WD. A technique to enhance fingerprinting of mummified fingers. *J Forensic Sci*. 1988;33(5):1244-1248.
6. Fields R, Molina DK. A novel approach for fingerprinting mummified hands. *J Forensic Sci*. 2008;53(4):952-955.
7. Morgan LO, Johnson M, Cornelison J, Isaac C, deJong J, Prahlow JA. Two novel methods for enhancing postmortem fingerprint recovery from mummified remains. *J Forensic Sci*. 2019;64(2):602-606.
8. Mundorff A, Davoren JM. Examination of DNA yield rates for different skeletal elements at increasing postmortem intervals. *Forensic Sci Int Genet*. 2014;8(1):55-63.
9. Allouche M, Hamdoum M, Mangin P, Castella V. Genetic identification of decomposed cadavers using nails as DNA source. *Forensic Sci Int Genet*. 2008;3(1):46-49.
10. Lutz S, Weisser HJ, Heizmann J, Pollak S. mtDNA as a tool for identification of human remains. Identification using mtDNA. *Int J Legal Med*. 1996;109(4):205-209.
11. Phillips VM, Stuhlinger M. The discrimination potential of amalgam restorations for identification: part 1. *J Forensic Odontostomatol*. 2009;27(1):17-22.
12. Nuzzolese E, Torreggianti M. The need for a complete dental autopsy of unidentified edentulous human remains. *Forensic Sci Res*. 2022;7(2):319-322.
13. Schmidt G, Kallieris D. Use of radiographs in the forensic autopsy. *Forensic Sci Int*. 1982;19(3):263-270.
14. Takeshita H, Nagai T, Sagi M, et al. Forensic identification using multiple lot numbers of an implanted device. *Med Sci Law*. 2014;54(1):51-53.
15. Blessing MM, Lin PT. Identification of bodies by unique serial numbers on implanted medical devices. *J Forensic Sci*. 2018;63(3):740-744.
16. Bukhamseen AH, Aldhameen AA, Alzayyat NT, et al. The use of orthopedic surgical devices for forensic identification: a systematic review. *Acta Biomed*. 2022;93(3):e2022082.
17. Kanchan T, Krishan K, Menezes RG, Suresh Kumar Shetty B, Lobo SW. Frontal sinus radiographs-A useful means of identification. *J Forensic Leg Med*. 2010;17(4):223-224.
18. Silva RF, Pereira SD, Prado FB, Daruge EII, Daruge E. Forensic odontology identification using smile photograph analysis-case reports. *J Forensic Odontostomatol*. 2008;26(1):12-17.
19. Uzun I, Daregenli O, Sirin G, Müslümanoğlu O. Identification procedures as a part of death investigation in Turkey. *Am J Forensic Med Pathol*. 2012;33(1):1-3.

POSTMORTEM CHANGES 6

CHAPTER OUTLINE

Introduction 42

Time of Death and Early Postmortem Changes 42
- Algor Mortis 42
- Postmortem Vitreous Potassium Measurements 44
- Supravitality 44
- Rigor Mortis 44
- Livor Mortis 46
- Additional Findings Associated With Lividity 49
  - Tardieu Spots 49

Decomposition 51

Important Terms Associated With Decomposition 52
- Green Discoloration of Skin 52
- Adipocere 52
- Postmortem Blisters (or Postmortem Bullae) 53
- Corneal Clouding 54
- Hemolysis 54
- Marbling 54
- Mummification and Postmortem Drying 54
- Skin Slippage 56
- Swelling/Bloating 57
- Tache Noire 59

Scene Indicators 60

Postmortem Entomology 61
- How to Collect Appropriate Specimens for Time of Death Determination Using Insect Activity 62

Animal Activity 63

Embalming Artifacts 65

Near Misses 67

INTRODUCTION

Unless a body is well embalmed, it undergoes a series of changes after death that lead to skeletonization. The first three of these changes occurring in the early postmortem period are algor mortis, which is cooling of the body; livor mortis, which is discoloration of the skin and internal organs due to pooling of blood; and rigor mortis, which is stiffening of muscles. Following the development of these first three changes, decomposition (a combination of putrefaction, autolysis, and insect and animal activity) occurs. With insect activity, the soft tissue of the body will be degraded entirely leaving only the skeletal elements.

> **FAQ:** What is the utility of the identification of postmortem changes?
>
> **Answer:** The most important aspect of the accurate identification of postmortem changes is to not confuse them with antemortem injuries or a natural disease process. Knowledge of the general types of postmortem changes and their spectrum of appearances can prevent this from occurring. Postmortem changes can also be used in (1) confirming historical information (eg, Do the postmortem changes present conform to the position in which the body is found, or do they indicate that the body has been moved?) and (2) the potential determination of time since death.

TIME OF DEATH AND EARLY POSTMORTEM CHANGES

Introduction: The determination of time of death, which involves estimating how much time has passed since death occurred, can be based upon an objective measurement (eg, body temperature or vitreous potassium concentration), or a subjective interpretation (eg, supravital reactions of muscle, interpretation of rigor or livor mortis, or degree of putrefaction). The condition of gastric contents may assist in the determination of length of time between the decedent's last meal and their time of death. In addition to changes of the body itself, scene indicators (eg, date on the last mail received at the house) and entomology can be used to help determine the time of death.

> **PEARLS & PITFALLS**
>
> The accurate determination of time elapsed since death is problematic. As said by Brady, "Never express an opinion on the time of death without first inquiring when the deceased person was last known alive. It is embarrassing to state that death probably occurred at a given time, only to discover that the person was known to be alive several hours or days later"; and "Since postmortem changes vary widely, depending upon the temperature, clothing, and other factors, extreme caution on specific estimates is important. The coroner's physician who places the time of death in the television murder at 7:14 AM yesterday is an unreal fantasy"; and "Time of death estimation should ideally be made from the examination of the body at the scene of death as soon as possible after it is found. Moving to surroundings of different temperatures may affect the criteria used in time estimation." All three quotes highlight important features regarding time since death determination, being the marked variability that changing conditions, or that variable initial conditions, can have on such a determination, and the effects that a wrong determination can have on credibility of the forensic pathologist who does so.[1]

ALGOR MORTIS

Algor mortis is postmortem cooling of the body. The postmortem temperature of the body can most easily be determined via rectal thermometer or insertion of a thermometer into the liver through a small incision in the abdominal wall.

> **PEARLS & PITFALLS**
>
> After being found unresponsive, almost all infants are transported to the hospital, with the hope that they can be resuscitated, as opposed to adults who, under the same circumstances, are more likely to be pronounced dead at the scene. With infant deaths (and with adult deaths), the hospital can obtain a rectal temperature for investigators. While a temperature is not an absolute indicator as to the time since death, a distinct difference between the expected temperature of the body and the actual temperature of the body can be useful (eg, if the parents say they last knew the baby was alive 2 hours ago, a postmortem rectal temperature of 80 °C can be significant).

Using algor mortis to determine the time since death: Forensic pathology textbooks list generalized formulas to determine the time since death based upon the body temperature (Table 6.1). However, when using the cooling of the body, Lew and Matshes indicate that no single formula is applicable to all cases.[7]

TABLE 6.1: Published General Time Frames for the Development of Algor Mortis

Author	Time Frame
DiMaio and DiMaio[2]	Time since death = 37 °C − rectal temperature °C + 3 h
	Time since death = (98.6 °F − rectal temperature °F)/1.5 h
Clark et al[3]	Decrease of 1.5 °F per hour after death
Spitz and Fisher[4]	Decrease of 2.0 °F-2.5 °F per hour for first few hours after death, with average loss of 1.5 °F-2 °F for first 12 h and 1 °F per hour for the next 12-18 h
Spitz and Fisher[5]	Decrease of 1 °F-1.5 °F per hour after death
Semple[6]	15-20 h for a body to cool

> **FAQ:** What is the most reliable method to determine the interval since death using postmortem body changes?
>
> **Answer:** The nomogram method, which was developed by Henssge, has received the most investigation and is described as the most precise and most reliable.[8]
> The nomogram designed by Henssge is available to assist in determination of time since death (https://www.rechtsmedizin.uni-bonn.de/dienstleistungen/for_Med/todeszeit/). To use this nomogram, several data points are needed: knowledge of the features of the death scene (eg, clothing, bedding, sunlight exposure), ambient temperatures at the death scene, rectal temperature, body weight, and knowledge of corrective factors.[8] Madea lists corrective factors based upon the clothing, air (still or moving), whether body and clothing are wet, and bedding present or not.[8] The corrective factors are needed as the nomogram is for a naked body on a dry surface in still air. It assumes no radiation (eg, sun or heater), no antemortem abnormality in body temperature (eg, no fever or hypothermia); that the place of death is the same as the place where the body was found; that there are no changes in cooling; that there is no significant thermal conductivity of the surface that the body is on; and that there is no extended period between injuries and death.

POSTMORTEM VITREOUS POTASSIUM MEASUREMENTS

While the electrolytes in the postmortem blood are not useful in establishing the time since death, vitreous electrolytes, specifically potassium, have been used because of the relatively protected environment of the vitreous fluid, with loss of selective membrane permeability occurring at around 120 hours after death in the vitreous fluid, but within only a few hours after death in the blood.[8] Numerous authors have developed formulas to use the potassium concentration of the vitreous fluid to determine the time since death. Madea summarizes the various equations proposed by each author and offers comments regarding the development or use of the formulas.[8] For example, Sturner's formula requires the body to have been refrigerated following the death.

SUPRAVITALITY

Supravitality is the postmortem electrical or mechanical excitation of tissues, often skeletal muscle, which is due to the fact that tissue metabolism (creatine kinase activity and anaerobic glycolysis) continues after death for some period. Mechanical excitability is tested by hitting the muscle with a scalpel or other similar object and electrical excitability is determined through the use of electrodes.[8] Some form of mechanically induced excitability can be elicited for upward of 24 hours after death, and some form of electrical excitability can be elicited for upward of 16 hours after death. In addition to electrical and mechanical excitability, chemical excitability of the iris to various compounds (eg, atropine, acetylcholine) can be tested, with postmortem excitability for atropine remaining for 3 to 10 hours after death.

RIGOR MORTIS

Skeletal muscle cells do not die immediately when a person dies, as muscle has a glycogen store that it can continue to use for the production of energy. Rigor mortis is not contraction of the muscle, it is a hardening or stiffening of the muscle fibers that occurs after death due to chemical changes, including, most importantly, loss of adenosine triphosphate (ATP) but also decreased cellular pH due to production of lactic acid and dehydration.[2,7,9,10] ATP is produced during anaerobic glycolysis, which is why rigor mortis is delayed after death, until the ATP concentration falls to <85% of its normal value.[8] When muscles are alkaline, they are flexible, but with accumulation of lactic acid, the muscles becomes acidic and rigor mortis progresses; later, when the muscles become alkaline again, they become flexible[11] as the increased ammonia contributes to breakdown of the protein.[8] As rigor mortis does not represent contraction of the muscle, it does not cause postmortem movement of the body, or flexion or extension at the joints.[12] The onset of rigor mortis is hastened by infection, increased body temperature, terminal seizure or hyperactivity, electrocution, or increased environmental temperature.[1,2,7] Rigor mortis manifests as stiffening of the muscles that opposes gravity (Figures 6.1 and 6.2).

SAMPLE NOTES: KEY FEATURES THAT CAN BE USED TO DESCRIBE RIGOR MORTIS IN AN AUTOPSY REPORT

The strength of rigor mortis can subjectively be determined by an examiner, in how much pressure is required to break rigor mortis. If rigor mortis is easily broken with gentle palpation, either the rigor mortis is just beginning to form, or it is passing. Other features of the examination should help determine which is the correct scenario (eg, is the associated lividity blanching or fixed, with blanching lividity expected when rigor mortis is forming, and fixed lividity expected when rigor mortis is passing). Assessment of more than one joint is also useful as rigor mortis, while it affects all muscles equally, manifests itself in the smaller muscles first followed by the larger muscles (eg, smaller muscles of the hands and face first, followed by larger muscles of the proximal extremities).

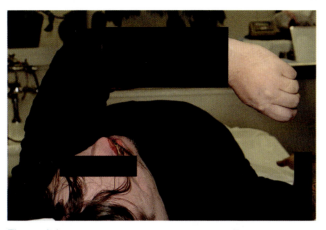 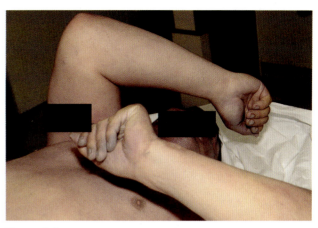

Figure 6.1. Rigor mortis. Due to postmortem stiffening of the muscles, the upper extremity remains raised against gravity.

Figure 6.2. Rigor mortis. Due to postmortem stiffening of the muscles, the upper extremities remain raised against gravity.

PEARLS & PITFALLS

Stiffening of the body due to cold temperatures can occur and can mimic rigor mortis. When rigor mortis is present, livor mortis will also be present.

Using rigor mortis to determine the time since death: Table 6.2 indicates various authors' interpretations of the time course of rigor mortis.

Findings associated with rigor mortis: Through its actions on the muscle, rigor mortis can cause specific changes. Cutis anserina is when "goose bumps" form due to rigor of the erector pili muscle, which is attached to the hair shaft (Figure 6.3). Postmortem ejaculation after death, which is expulsion of semen from the penis after death, is due to rigor mortis affecting the tunica dartos muscles (Figure 6.4).

PEARLS & PITFALLS

The presence of seminal fluid at the tip of the urethra in a male should not be misinterpreted as a sign of sexual activity just prior to death.

TABLE 6.2: General Times Frames for the Appearance of Rigor Mortis

Author	First Appears	Fully Developed	Dissipates (Passes)
Madea[8]	3 ± 2 h	8 ± 1 h	Duration: 57 ± 14 h
			Complete resolution: 76 ± 32 h
Lew and Matshes[7]		8-12 h	
Nashelsky and McFeeley[13]	1-6 h	6-24 h	12-36 h
McLemore and Zumwalt[14]	Develops in first 1-12 h	Stays full fixed for 12 h	Dissipates in 12 h
DiMaio and DiMaio[2]	2-4 h	6-12 h	36 h to 6 d
Clark et al[3]	Jaw: 2-3 h	24 h after death	48 h after death
Brady[1]	2-4 h	Remains for 24-48 h	
Spitz and Fisher[5]	1-4 h	12 h	
Smith and Fiddes[10]	4-5 h (in jaw, at 3 h)	8-12 h	10 h to 3 d
Semple[6]	2 h	Lasts for 16-20 h	

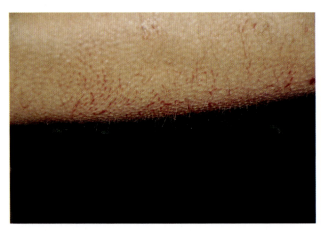

Figure 6.3. Cutis anserina. The dimpling of the skin combined with the erect hair simulates "goose bumps" and is due to postmortem stiffening of erector pili muscles.

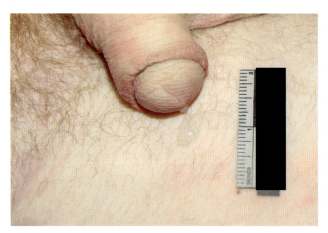

Figure 6.4. Seminal fluid at tip of urethra of the penis.

LIVOR MORTIS

Livor mortis represents postmortem pooling of the blood due to cessation of circulation and gravity's subsequent effects on the blood and manifests as a red-purple discoloration of the skin. At first, after initial formation, lividity is still capable of redistribution with changing of the position of the body (eg, if a person died face-down, and the body lies that way for 1-2 hours, they will have lividity on the anterior surface of their body, and then, if they are flipped face-up and the body is allowed to lie that way for 1-2 more hours, they will have lividity on the posterior surface of the body). When lividity is present, any pale area of skin within that lividity indicates a point of compression (eg, if an individual dies and is face-down with their forearm underneath them, they will have a pale band of skin in the lividity where the forearm was compressing the skin of the torso and not allowing lividity to form) (Figures 6.5 and 6.6).

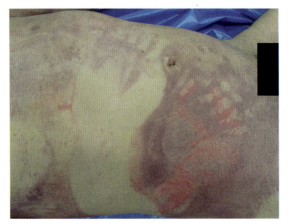

Figure 6.5. Anterior lividity. The red-purple discoloration of the skin is broken in areas by pallor. The pallor corresponds to the hands and forearm, which the body was lying on.

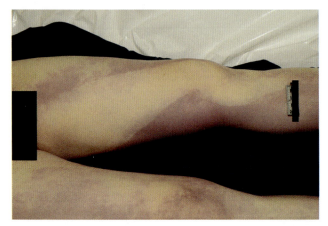

Figure 6.6. Anterior lividity. The left lower extremity manifests a red-purple discoloration, which is lividity. The strip of pallor extending along the lividity was produced by something pressing against the anterior surface of the left lower extremity as the lividity formed (ie, the left lower extremity was pressed against something on the ground beneath it).

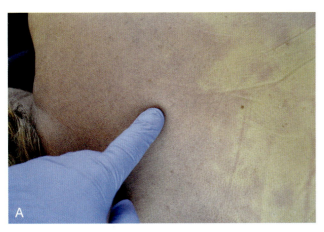

Figure 6.7A. Blanching lividity. Pressure is applied to lividity on the posterior surface of the body.

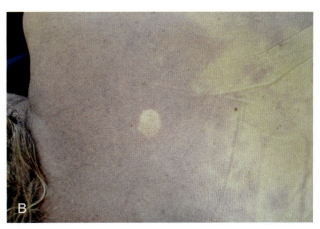

Figure 6.7B. Blanching lividity. When the pressure is released, a pale area appears where the finger pressure was applied, because the blood is still mobile in the vessels, and pressure causes it to be displaced.

SAMPLE NOTE: FEATURES ABOUT LIVOR MORTIS THAT ARE USEFUL TO DOCUMENT IN AN AUTOPSY REPORT

The location of lividity and whether or not the lividity is blanching or fixed is useful, in that it can potentially help narrow the time frame since death. This is accomplished via visual examination and palpation, looking at the body and identifying where lividity is present (eg, anterior or posterior surface of the body, or both, and if both, potentially left or right side) and pushing on the skin with the fingertips. If the skin becomes pale, the lividity is blanchable. If the skin remains red-purple, after compression the lividity is fixed (Figures 6.7A, 6.7B, 6.8A, and 6.8B). The color of the lividity is useful to document. In most situations, the lividity will be a red-purple, or purple color, such as in Figures 6.5 to 6.8A, 6.8B. A light red or cherry red appearance to the lividity can occur in individuals exposed to carbon monoxide, cyanide, or when the body was refrigerated after death (or if the death occurred in a cold environment) (Figures 6.9-6.11).

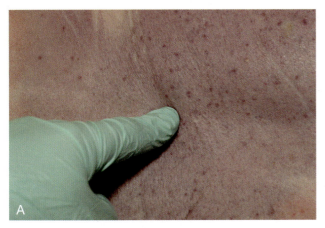

Figure 6.8A. Fixed lividity. Pressure is applied to lividity on the posterior surface of the body.

Figure 6.8B. Fixed lividity. When the pressure is released, essentially no pale area appears where the finger pressure was applied, because the blood is not mobile in the vessels, and pressure does not cause it to be displaced.

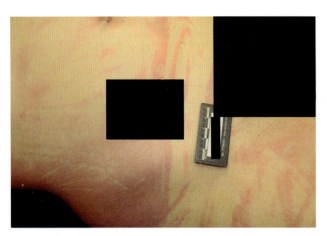

Figure 6.9. Anterior cherry red lividity. Compare the coloration of the lividity to Figures 6.5 to 6.8. This individual died as the result of carbon monoxide poisoning.

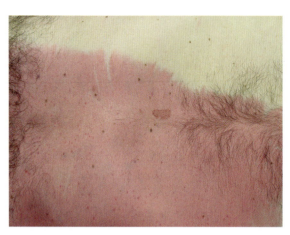

Figure 6.10. Cherry red lividity. Note the sharp line of difference between the lividity and the normal skin (this image just provides a marked contrast between skin with lividity and that without lividity). The lividity is cherry red and this individual also died from carbon monoxide poisoning.

Process of formation of livor mortis: Livor mortis (ie, lividity or hypostasis) is due to pooling of blood in blood vessels. Without the heart pumping blood through the vessels, it will pool (ie, stagnate). Since the heart stops pumping at death, lividity should start forming immediately; however, enough must form for it to be visible in the skin. Once it starts forming, lividity does not just go from blanching to fixed all at once. In other words, during the process of fixation, in some areas, the lividity will be fixed, and in other areas it will blanch. For example, if a body is left face-down long enough for lividity to form, but not completely fix, and then it is turned on its back, the body can have fixed lividity on both the anterior and posterior surfaces of the body. Fixation itself is caused by congealing of blood within vessels and diffusion into the extravascular tissue.[4] Lividity can occur in a living person. If the heart is so weak that it does not pump blood well, stasis can occur (eg, the lower extremities of a patient with congestive heart failure).

Using livor mortis to determine the time since death: General time frames for the appearance of livor mortis, as described by various authors, are listed in Table 6.3.

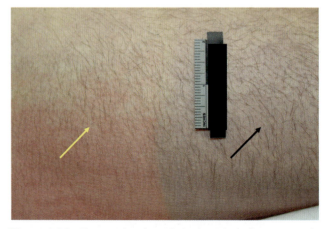

Figure 6.11. Cherry red and purple lividity. The yellow arrow indicates cherry red lividity and the black arrow indicates red-purple lividity. When the skin is uncovered, the lividity tends to appear cherry red; however, if the skin is covered (eg, by clothing or even an EKG pad), it tends to appear more red-purple. This can help distinguish cherry red lividity that is due to refrigeration from that due to carbon monoxide exposure.

TABLE 6.3: General Time Frames for the Appearance and Fixation of Livor Mortis

Author	Appearance After Death	Fixation
Madea[8]	15 min to 3 h	Incomplete: 6-12 h Complete: >12 h
Lew and Matshes[7]	3-4 h	10-12 h
Nashelsky and McFeeley[13]	2-4 h	8-12 h
DiMaio and DiMaio[2]	30 min to 2 h	8-12 h
Clark et al[3]	15 min to 2 h after death	Fixation begins 2-4 h after death
Brady[12]	First appearance: 20 min	Fixed at 6 h, but blanching can remain for 24 h
Spitz and Fisher[5]	Begins immediately Perceptible: 2 h Well-developed: 4 h	8-12 h
Smith and Fiddes[10]	Shortly after death	6-12 h
Gonzales et al[11]	Appears 20 min to 1 h in plethoric; and 1-4 h in anemic	Complete in 12 h

ADDITIONAL FINDINGS ASSOCIATED WITH LIVIDITY

Tardieu Spots

In areas of intense lividity, engorgement of vessels can cause vessels to rupture, causing punctate areas of hemorrhage (Figures 6.12-6.14).

> **PEARLS & PITFALLS**
>
> Lividity can be confused with bruising. Two methods to distinguish lividity and bruising, if observation and context are not enough, are (1) if necessary, incision into the skin at a site of a bruise will reveal hemorrhage in the soft tissue (eg, fat), and not at the sites of lividity and (2) lividity, if not fixed, will blanch to pressure, while a bruise will not. Tardieu spots can be confused with petechiae. Tardieu spots only occur in areas with lividity, whereas petechial hemorrhages can involve otherwise normal skin (ie, no lividity).

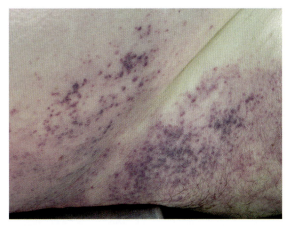

Figure 6.12. Tardieu spots. All of the red-purple spots are Tardieu spots, and occur in areas of intense lividity, where blood vessels have ruptured. Note that the adjacent area of pale skin (ie, without lividity in the flexural region in the right upper corner) does not have Tardieu spots. If the spots were present in this pale skin, then they are not from lividity, and another mechanism must be considered.

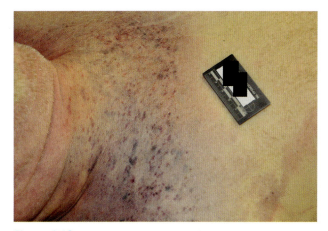

Figure 6.13. Tardieu spots. The skin of the chin, neck and upper chest has lividity. The punctate hemorrhages are Tardieu spots. The paler skin at the right of the image (ie, no lividity) does not have such hemorrhages. When the hemorrhages are associated only with areas of lividity, they are most likely a postmortem phenomenon.

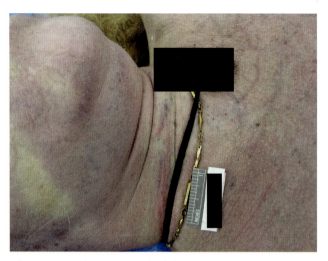

Figure 6.14. Tardieu spots. In the image to the left associated with anterior lividity are numerous punctate red hemorrhages. Because of their distribution, they could mimic changes due to strangulation; however, other than these hemorrhages, neither scene investigation nor autopsy identified any findings to suggest strangulation as a cause of death.

Other uses of lividity: The color of the lividity can provide important clues as to the cause of death. Normal lividity is a red-purple color, which is appropriate as it is deoxygenated blood. Exposure to carbon monoxide, freezing temperatures, and cyanide can cause a brighter red coloration.[7]

PEARLS & PITFALLS

In refrigerated bodies, it is not uncommon to see both red and purple lividity, and, with increasing periods of refrigeration, the amount of red lividity will increase, and can mimic carbon monoxide poisoning. However, in a covered region, such as underneath an electrocardiography patch, the skin with lividity will most often maintain the purple coloration even with prolonged refrigeration and can help separate the two etiologies for the color of the lividity.

PEARLS & PITFALLS

If a time after death determination is necessary, using only one method is not the preferred choice, and instead, using multiple methods is more reliable. Madea provides a chart to be used by forensic pathologists or other death investigators which lists various characteristics to be combined in determining a time since death (eg, features of lividity, muscle contraction).[8] When using the chart, lividity and rigor mortis "maximum" would indicate the time at which no additional lividity or rigor mortis developed either during the investigation or during the autopsy. Thumb pressure indicates that light thumb pressure causes blanching of the lividity. In addition to interpretation of lividity and rigor mortis, the chart does incorporate use of supravital methods, including electrical and chemical stimulation of muscles.

Use of gastric contents to determine time since death: Evaluation of gastric contents does not allow for a determination of time since death, but it could allow for a determination of time from the individual's last meal to their time of death. General times given for gastric emptying are 1 to 3 hours for a light volume meal, 3 to 5 hours for a medium volume meal, and 5 to 8 hours for a large volume meal[8]; however, several general mechanisms can affect the emptying time of the stomach including transient delayed gastric emptying (eg, acute viral gastroenteritis), chronic gastric stasis (eg, diabetes mellitus, gastroesophageal reflux), and rapid gastric emptying (eg, after gastric surgery, duodenal ulcer disease).

DECOMPOSITION

Decomposition is the breakdown of the body occurring after death, due to autodigestion (ie, the body's own enzymes destroying tissue, termed autolysis), putrefaction resulting from bacterial proliferation, and insect and animal activity. Three general stages are early decomposition (characterized by bloating), moderate decomposition (characterized by release of gases with tissue decay), and advanced decomposition (characterized by skeletonization).[7]

Factors affecting decomposition: The rate of decomposition is affected by many different factors including ambient temperature; outdoor vs indoor location; submersion in water or burial in ground (both have slower decomposition rates than on land); insect and animal activity; mummification and adipocere formation (both impair further decomposition); amount of blood in body (ie, individuals who have bled out before death will decompose more slowly because bacterial growth is impaired); obese vs thin (decomposition is faster in obese people as they tend to retain heat); heavy clothing; tight clothing (delays decomposition); and sepsis, which would speed decomposition.[2,3,7]

> **FAQ:** What is the purpose of performing an autopsy on a decomposed individual, given the condition of the body?
>
> **Answer:** The purpose of an autopsy is always, first and foremost, to determine the cause and manner of death. Although decomposition affects the appearance of the body, it does not invalidate the purpose of the autopsy. In some cases, decomposition and associated changes may obscure or even erase the cause of death; however, in most cases, the cause and manner of death can still be determined. That the autopsy is unpleasant for some or that the findings may be difficult to identify should not discourage the performance of an autopsy in a decomposed individual, as much information can still be discovered. Toxicology can be performed on decomposed tissue, with skeletal muscle or liver commonly being submitted for analysis.

SAMPLE NOTES: WORDING OF CAUSE OF DEATH IN DECOMPOSED INDIVIDUALS

If an autopsy is performed on a decomposed individual and no cause of death is identified, as long as the scene investigation did not reveal any suspicious circumstances and the toxicologic analysis does not provide a cause of death, the cause of death can be based upon the individual's known medical history as appropriate (eg, non-traumatic seizure disorder as the cause of death in a decomposed body, where the person had a history of a seizure disorder and autopsy, toxicology, and scene investigation revealed no suspicious findings). Alternatively, the cause of death could be worded in a generalized fashion, such as "Undetermined natural disease." If the autopsy is negative but some aspect of the scene investigation was suspicious (eg, young female found dead in her apartment with the whereabouts of her known boyfriend being unknown), both the cause and manner of death can be certified as undetermined.

IMPORTANT TERMS ASSOCIATED WITH DECOMPOSITION

GREEN DISCOLORATION OF SKIN

Description: Green discoloration of the skin most often begins in the right lower quadrant of the abdomen (Figure 6.15), presumably due to the closeness of the underlying cecum and large intestines (containing proliferating bacteria) to the skin. While this green discoloration most often begins in the right lower quadrant of the abdomen in relation to the cecum, it then becomes more diffuse with time (Table 6.4; Figures 6.16 and 6.17).

Time frame of occurrence: The appearance of the green discoloration of the abdomen is reported as around 24 to 48 hours by most authors. For example, the reported times include 24 hours,[15] 24 to 48 hours,[3,11,13] and 24 to 36 hours.[2]

ADIPOCERE

Description: A waxy, hard, or brittle change occurring in warm and moist conditions (Figure 6.18A-C), in which neutral fats are converted to oleic, palmitic, and stearic acids.[2] Adipocere formation can occur in bodies immersed or partially immersed in relatively warm water for an extended period of time.

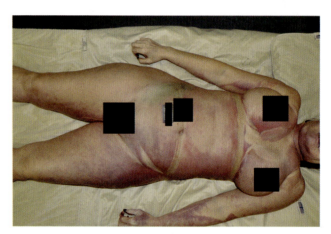

Figure 6.15. Green discoloration of skin of right lower quadrant of the abdomen.

TABLE 6.4: General Timing of Putrefactive Changes (Figures 6.15-6.17)

Time	Changes
>1-2 d	Green discoloration of some of abdominal wall (eg, right lower quadrant)
	Early collapse of eye globes
>3-5 d	Green discoloration of most of abdominal wall
	Green discoloration of skin of other regions of body
	Purge (ie, leakage of body fluid from mouth and nose)
>8-12 d	Entire body green
	Bloating of abdomen, scrotum, soft tissue of face
	Hair begins to peel
>14-20 d	Entire body green
	Decompositional bullae (or decompositional blisters)
	Fingernails peel

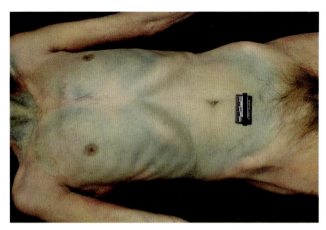

Figure 6.16. Green discoloration of trunk and neck.

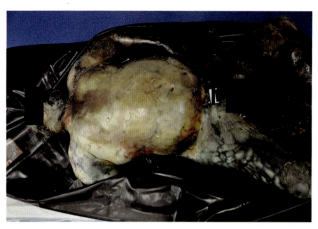

Figure 6.17. Green discoloration of entire body as well as bloating of the abdomen, scrotum, and face (eyelids and lips).

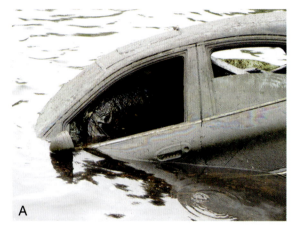

Figure 6.18A. Body in vehicle. The vehicle was found in a shallow body of water just off a highway. Visible through the driver's window is the body.

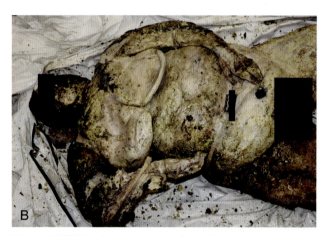

Figure 6.18B. Body at autopsy. On the surface of the decomposed body is a friable green-yellow substance, which is the adipocere.

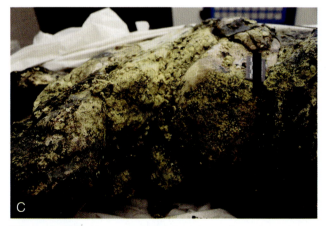

Figure 6.18C. Close-up of trunk. On the surface of the decomposed body is a friable green-yellow substance, which is the adipocere.

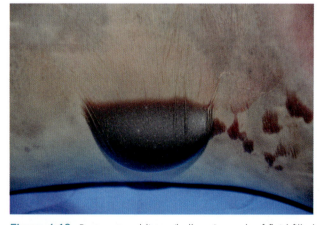

Figure 6.19. Postmortem blisters/bullae. A pouch of fluid-filled decompositional fluid has formed on the side of the trunk. The postmortem blisters rupture very easily, and can release the fluid within.

POSTMORTEM BLISTERS (OR POSTMORTEM BULLAE)

Description: Fluid-filled sacs in the skin (Figure 6.19), formed by exudation of fluid into the space created when the epidermis sloughs from the dermis. Rupture will release a watery, discolored, pungent fluid.

> **PEARLS & PITFALLS**
>
> Decomposition can occur rapidly in individuals dying of sepsis associated with various species of *Clostridium*. Culture of the fluid in a decompositional blister can identify the bacteria. Caution is appropriate as overgrowth of clostridial species from the gastrointestinal tract (ie, not related to the cause of death) is very common after death.

CORNEAL CLOUDING

Description: The cornea appears cloudy (Figure 6.20), instead of clear.

Timing of corneal clouding: If eyes are exposed to the air (eg, eyelids are open), corneal clouding can occur within a few hours,[11] and if eyes are closed, within 24 hours.[2,3]

HEMOLYSIS

Description: Rupture of red blood cells. With hemolysis during the postmortem period, ultimately a red staining of the vascular intima occurs.

MARBLING

Description: Dark green, green-red, red, or red-brown branching pattern (Figures 6.21 and 6.22) on the skin due to intravascular hemolysis and reaction of hemoglobin from red blood cells with hydrogen sulfide produced by bacteria.[2]

Time frame of occurrence: Marbling is reported as beginning at 3 to 4 days.[15]

MUMMIFICATION AND POSTMORTEM DRYING

Description: Mummification is when the skin becomes firm and yellow to yellow-black to red-black to black discolored (the colors do not progress in this order necessarily; it merely shows the range of color changes associated with mummification). This change most commonly occurs in a warm but dry environment and often affects the fingers and hands first but can ultimately involve the entire body (Figures 6.23 and 6.24). Mummification of the body is a process brought about by the effects of environment on the decomposing body; it is not the same as the procedure used on the dead in ancient Egypt.

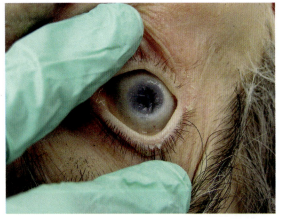

Figure 6.20. Corneal clouding. The cornea is cloudy and not as clear as normal. This change can occur quickly if the eyelids are open and the cornea exposed, and more delayed if the eyelids are closed.

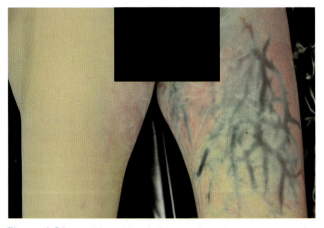

Figure 6.21. Marbling. The dark green branching pattern on the left thigh is marbling.

CHAPTER 6 POSTMORTEM CHANGES 55

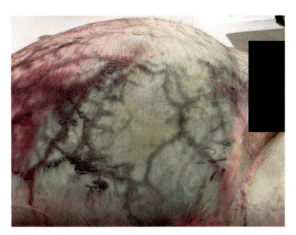

Figure 6.22. Marbling. The dark green branching pattern on the skin of the abdomen is marbling. The abdomen is also distended from the accumulation of gas in the abdominal cavity which is formed as the result of decomposition.

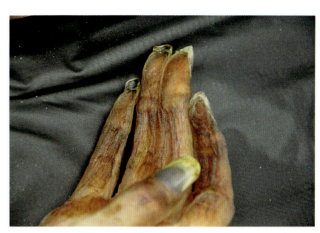

Figure 6.23. Mummification of the hands. The skin of the fingers is yellow-brown discolored and semi-translucent. The texture of the involved skin is firm (ie, dried). Mummification commonly involves the fingers and toes first.

PEARLS & PITFALLS

Postmortem drying can produce a dark red, or dark red-brown or dark red-black discoloration of the lips or of the male or female genitalia (Figures 6.25 and 6.26). These changes should not be confused with trauma.

PEARLS & PITFALLS

While mummification of the hands can impair the ability to obtain fingerprints, there are several methods which can be used. Re-hydration of the tissue, whether from soaking or injection into the tissue, can allow for fingerprints to be obtained. Dental hardening gel (also used by firearms and toolmark examiners) can make a very nice cast of the fingerprint, which can be used for identification. Also, just a macro photograph, if a wide depth of field is obtainable, can also serve to produce a fingerprint that can be used for identification.

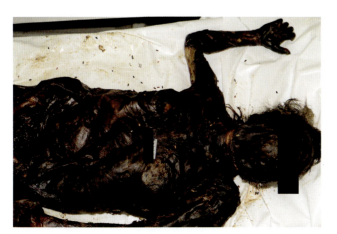

Figure 6.24. Mummification of the body. The skin of the entire body has a generalized dark red-brown discoloration. The texture of the skin is firm (ie, dried.).

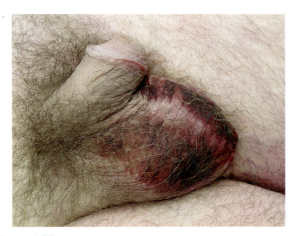

Figure 6.25. Postmortem drying of the scrotum. The red black discoloration of the scrotum can mimic inflicted injury.

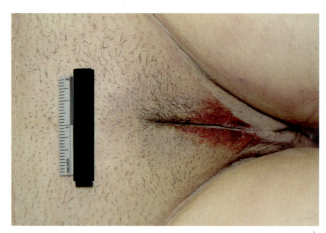

Figure 6.26. Postmortem drying of the labia. The dark red discoloration along the medial aspect of the labia majora is postmortem drying, which can mimic injury.

SKIN SLIPPAGE

Description: Sloughing of the epidermis (not the entire skin, which is composed of both epidermis and dermis), which can peel away from the body under pressure early, such as when a body is moved, or, later in the process of decomposition can be present when the body is first examined (Figures 6.27 and 6.28).

Time frame of occurrence: The range in the literature is broad: 96 hours,[3] within a few hours in a warm environment,[7] or within 5 to 6 days.[15]

> **PEARLS & PITFALLS**
> After skin slippage has occurred, the underlying dermis often becomes dried and discolored. This discoloration can have a variety of colors and can be misinterpreted as antemortem injuries, such as an abrasion (Figure 6.29A and B).

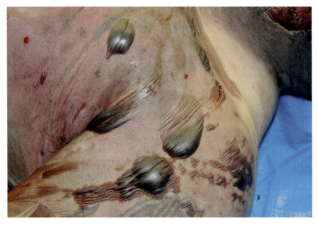

Figure 6.27. Skin slippage and blister formation. Often when skin slippage occurs, decompositional fluid will accumulate in the pocket that is formed.

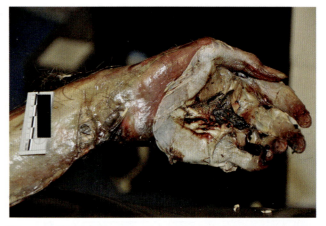

Figure 6.28. Skin slippage. The epidermis of the hands and feet can slough off. When this occurs fingerprints can potentially be obtained by placing the sloughed epidermis over a gloved finger, which can then be used to make a fingerprint.

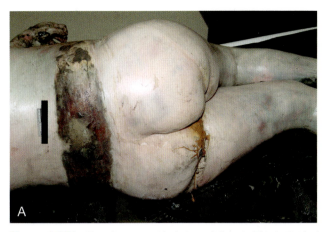

Figure 6.29A. Skin slippage with drying of dermis. This individual was found in the water, clothed. The epidermis of essentially the entire body had sloughed off. The individual was in clothes, which prevented exposure to the air, except the lower back, since the clothes had bunched upward to expose this area. The expulsion of fecal contents is due to increased intra-abdominal pressure from build-up of postmortem gas.

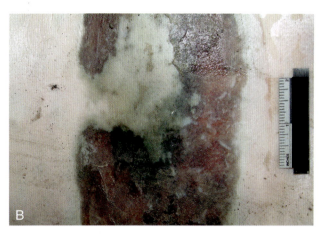

Figure 6.29B. Close-up of the dried dermis on the lower back after sloughing of the epidermis.

SWELLING/BLOATING

Description: Due to postmortem gas formation by bacterial organisms that are proliferating after death, tissue that is normally loose (ie, little substance and much space to expand) will swell. Swelling of the body is due to increased pressure because of gas formation. This increased pressure can cause purging of fluid from the mouth (Figure 6.30) and other orifices.

Locations: Bloating of the abdomen is common (Figure 6.31A-C). The gases formed by decomposition are manifested on a radiograph as streaks of radiolucency in the skeletal muscle (Figure 6.32). Other areas distended by gas formation include the eyelids, lips, tongue, breasts (Figure 6.33), external genitalia (Figure 6.34), and anus.

Time frame of occurrence: The listed time course varies from begins at 2 to 3 days[13] to beginning to end of bloating in 3 to 6 days[3] to begins at 2 to 3 days, with marked swelling by 14 days[15] to generalized bloating of body by 60 to 72 hours.[2]

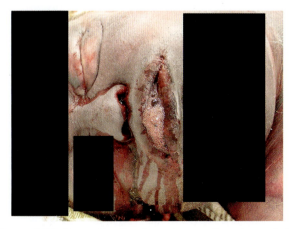

Figure 6.30. Purge. Exuding from the nostrils and mouth is a foamy, watery, hemorrhagic fluid. This can mimic a gastrointestinal hemorrhage. The eyelids and lips are also swollen.

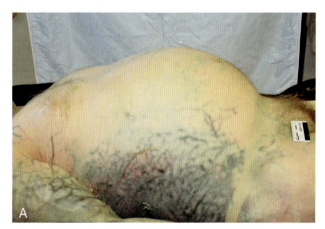

Figure 6.31A. Postmortem distension of abdomen, pre-incision. The abdomen is bulged and tense, due to postmortem gas formation associated with overgrowth of gastrointestinal bacteria.

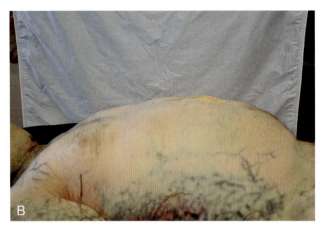

Figure 6.31B. Postmortem distension of abdomen, post incision. Incision into the abdominal wall causes a release of gases and shrinks the abdomen more toward its normal size.

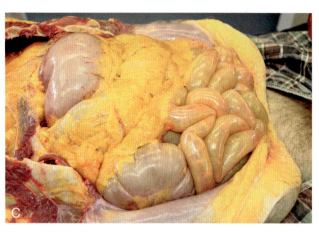

Figure 6.31C. Opening of the abdominal cavity reveals distension of the stomach and small and large intestine due to postmortem gas formation, which partly contributes to the appearance in Figure 6.31A.

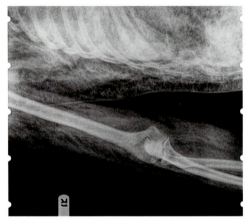

Figure 6.32. Postmortem gas formation in musculature. An x-ray of a decomposed body reveals gas formation throughout the musculature (ie, the streaked radiolucencies).

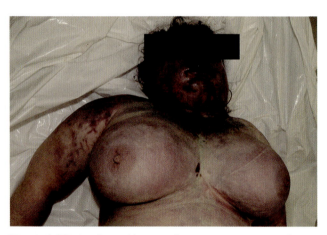

Figure 6.33. Swelling of breasts due to postmortem gas formation. Parts of the body with more loose connective tissue swell with postmortem gas formation, as gas moves into those areas. Breasts are one example.

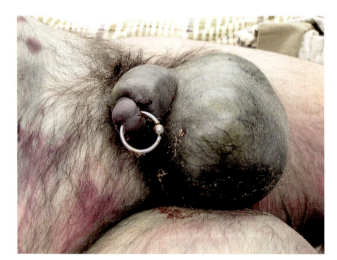

Figure 6.34. Postmortem swelling of scrotum due to postmortem gas formation. Due to the significant amount of gas the scrotum can accommodate, swelling of the scrotum in a decomposed body can be quite marked.

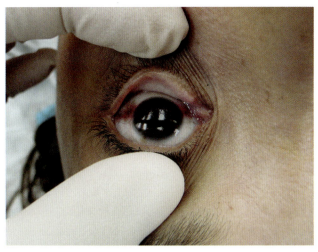 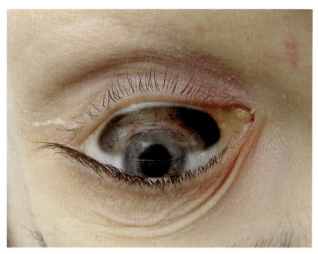

Figure 6.35. Tache noire. The red discoloration of the sclera medial and lateral to the iris.

Figure 6.36. Tache noire. The discoloration of the sclerae in this case was interpreted by the coroner as trauma.

TACHE NOIRE

Description

The lesion is postmortem drying of the sclera (Figures 6.35 and 6.36), which produces a triangular discoloration of the sclera medial and lateral to the cornea in a horizontal plane, with the base of the triangle at the cornea, or a broad or thin band of discoloration. The coloration can be red, red-yellow, red-brown, brown, or black. Tache noire is due to exposure of the sclerae to the air and is indicative that the eyelids were at least partially open before the body was discovered.

> **PEARLS & PITFALLS**
>
> Postmortem purge should not be mistaken for a gastrointestinal hemorrhage or evidence of trauma. Tache noire can also potentially be misinterpreted as trauma.

Using decomposition to determine the time since death: While the rate of decomposition depends upon many factors (eg, a body in a car in Alaska in the winter will not follow the same time frame for decomposition as a body in a car in Arizona in the summer), a general time frame and course for decomposition is listed in Table 6.5 (Figure 6.37A and B).

TABLE 6.5: Stages of Decomposition

Stages of Decomposition (Clark et al)[3]
Each Occurs at Roughly 24 h Intervals, Assuming 70 °F and 30% Humidity, With the Exception of Stages VIII-X

Stage	Features (*Were Explained Above)
I (putrid)	Early putrid odor, lividity fixed, rigor passing, tissues tacky
II (putrid)	Green discoloration of abdomen,* hemolysis,* intense livor, no rigor, early skin slippage,* drying of nose, lips and fingers*
III (putrid)	Tissue gas on x-ray, prominent hemolysis, tissues soft and slick, skin slips easily
IV (bloating)	Early body swelling, discoloration of the head, no discolorations of the trunk, gas in heart, marbling,* bullae/blisters*
V (bloating)	Moderate swelling,* discoloration of head and trunk
VI (bloating)	Maximal body swelling
VII (destruction)	Release of gases, exhausted putrefied soft tissues; total destruction of blood
VIII (destruction)	Partially skeletonized; adipocere* (Figure 6.37A and B)
IX (skeleton)	Skeleton with ligaments
X (skeleton)	Skeleton with no soft tissue

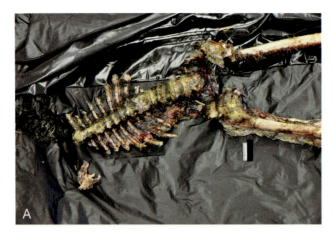

Figure 6.37A. Partially skeletonized body. The upper three-fourths of the body would fit for stage IX above (skeleton with ligaments).

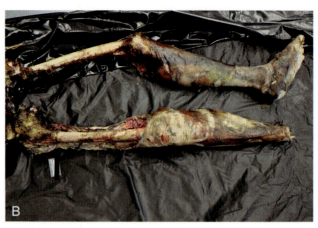

Figure 6.37B. Partially skeletonized body. Given the soft tissue present on the legs and feet, although the upper three-fourths of the body matches more with stage IX, the body in its entirety is more compatible with stage VIII.

SCENE INDICATORS

The use of scene indicators can be very helpful in establishing a time of death (Figures 6.38 and 6.39). Scene indicators include weekly medication containers, receipts, newspapers and other mail, and routines reported by witnesses. For example, one man was known to close his curtains every night at 8:00 pm, he was last known alive at 4:00 pm and found dead the next day with his curtains still open. The coroner opined that the cause of death was between 4:00 pm and 8:00 pm. The use of scene indicators to help determine the time of death is supported by numerous authors. "This last method of attempting to determine when an individual died, although unscientific, is often more accurate than determinations made by scientific means."[2] "Circumstances and evidence about the body will generally furnish more useful information than an examination of the body. Undelivered newspapers or mail, dated prescriptions, etc."[1] "The witness may relate information that can be helpful in more accurately determining the interval since death, for example, that the discoverer had been unsuccessfully phoning the decedent for 12 hours prior to coming to the residence to check on their welfare."[16]

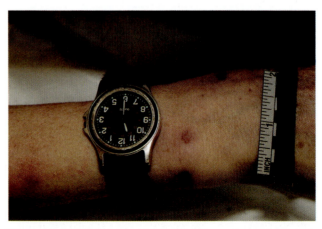

Figure 6.38. Watch as scene indicator. This watch worn by an individual who died during a motor vehicle accident was broken during the accident and displays the time of the accident, which was the time of death.

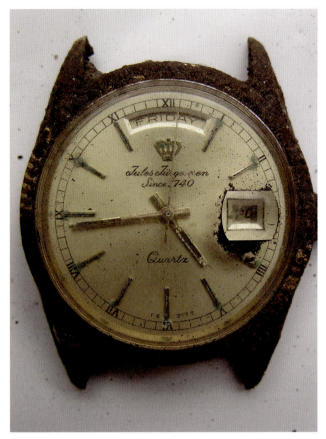

Figure 6.39. Watch found with skeletal remains. Given the watch is wind-up device, this watch, which was found with skeletal remains, and with a history of the decedent's last known time being alive, provided a date of death after over 20 years.

POSTMORTEM ENTOMOLOGY

> **FAQ:** What is the utility of insects to help determine a time of death?
>
> **Answer:** In deaths where insect activity is present, which can occur in a large number of cases potentially as flies will deposit eggs very soon after death (Figure 6.40A and B), analysis of the maggots (Figure 6.41), pupae (Figure 6.42), and other insects present, such as beetles, by a trained examiner can help narrow the possible time of death significantly.

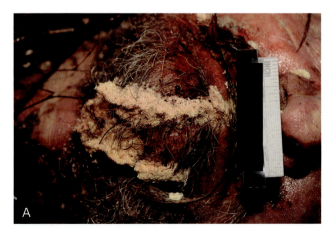

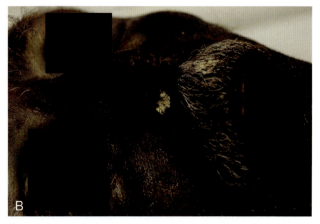

Figure 6.40A. Fly eggs. A large aggregate of fly eggs is present within the beard of this deceased individual (ie, just adjacent to and including the mouth).

Figure 6.40B. Fly eggs. In the right nasal orifice of this decomposed individual is an aggregate of fly eggs.

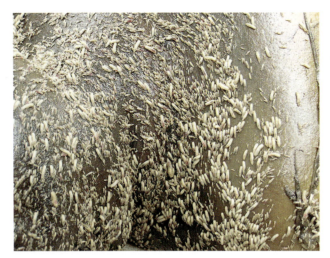
Figure 6.41. Maggots. From fly egg to fly, the insect proceeds through several stages. Using the maggots to determine time of death involves collecting numerous maggots of each size present, and submitting both living and dead maggots to the entomologist for evaluation.

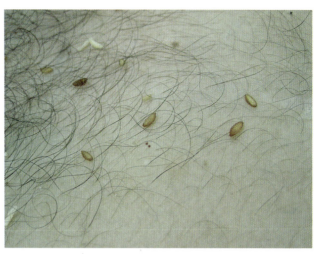
Figure 6.42. Pupa casings. With each stage, prior to finally emerging as a fly, a pupae casing is produced.

HOW TO COLLECT APPROPRIATE SPECIMENS FOR TIME OF DEATH DETERMINATION USING INSECT ACTIVITY

To best utilize insect activity to determine a time of death, entomologists will need a variety of materials and data: (1) multiple (if possible) examples of all adult insects present as well as all stages of larvae present, including both on the body and underneath the body; (2) both living and dead samples of larvae. Living larvae must be placed in an appropriate container (to allow for the entry of air) and with available food (eg, a fragment of liver). Dead larvae can be obtained by placing living larvae into formalin; however, they must be heat-killed—if the larvae are not heat killed, bacteria in the larvae will cause decomposition of the larvae from the inside; and (3) as much information about the environmental temperature, both current and past, as possible. All specimens should be sent to the consulting forensic entomologist as soon as possible. A forensic pathologist who wishes to consult with a forensic entomologist would be best served by prior communication with that forensic entomologist to learn collection protocols and other important information, so as, when the consult is needed, the case is handled in the most complete manner possible.

> **PEARLS & PITFALLS**
>
> Postmortem insect activity is often most concentrated at natural orifices (eg, eyes, ears, mouth, anus) and at unnatural orifices (eg, gunshot wounds, stab wounds). Understanding this concept can aid in the evaluation of a decomposing body for injuries, as an unusual amount of insect activity at an area where a natural orifice is not found can clue an examiner to more closely examine this area for injuries; however, failure to appreciate this concept can cause an examiner to miss an injury that is otherwise obscured by the insect activity (Figure 6.43A and B).

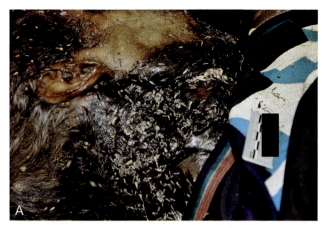

Figure 6.43A. Insect activity masking injury. When the body was received, maggot activity was noted. The amount of insect activity on the right side of the neck was out of proportion to that in other areas of the body where no natural orifice was present.

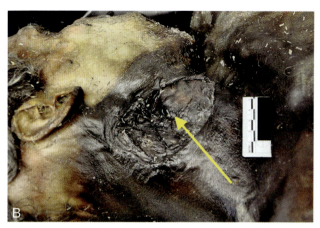

Figure 6.43B. Insect activity masking injury. After removal of the maggots from the neck, a superficial incised wound (yellow arrow) of the right side of the neck was identified.

ANIMAL ACTIVITY

FAQ: What is the importance of postmortem animal activity in death investigation?

Answer: Everything from insects to grizzly bears can feed on the body or be found on the body after death, with some being present prior to death (Figures 6.44-6.50). Changes produced by these creatures must not be interpreted as antemortem trauma. In addition to wild animals, household pets, such as dogs and cats, will also feed on the body. One key feature in helping to distinguish antemortem injury from postmortem change introduced by animals feeding on the body is evidence of reaction. When animals feed on the body postmortem, the edges of the wound will have no or minimal reactive changes (eg, hemorrhage into the soft tissue). Microscopic examination would reveal no hemorrhage (although, if a person dies immediately after sustaining injuries, they also will not manifest an inflammatory reaction at the site of the injury).

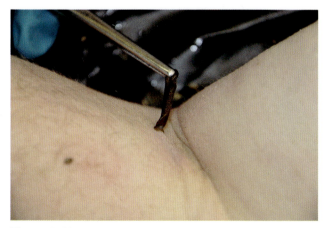

Figure 6.44. Leech. In this body removed from a lake, several leeches were found attached to the body.

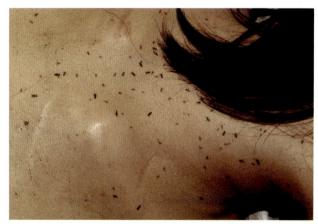

Figure 6.45. Lice on the body. In this case, the lice were present prior to death; however, insect activity on the body after death, such as ants or cockroaches, can result in postmortem injuries of the skin that can mimic antemortem injuries.

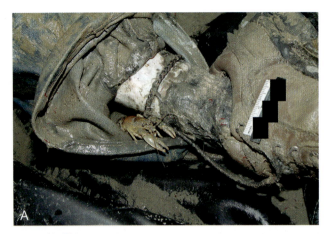

Figure 6.46A. Crayfish. In the pants leg of this body recovered from a river, live crayfish were identified.

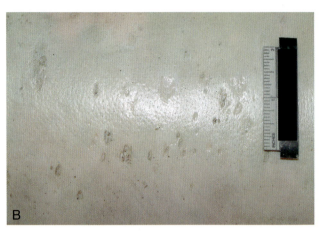

Figure 6.46B. Back of individual in Figure 6.46A. On the back were numerous superficial defects in the dermis. These changes are consistent with postmortem predation.

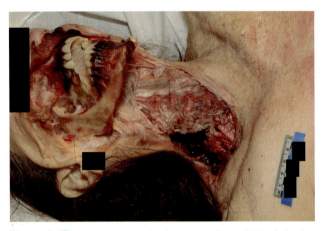

Figure 6.47. Postmortem animal activity. This individual died in her house, and her dog ate her remains. A large portion of skin and soft tissue are absent from the face and neck, but note how essentially little hemorrhage there is, which indicates the postmortem nature of the defect.

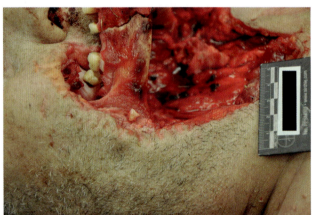

Figure 6.48. Postmortem animal activity. Along the edge of a defect created by postmortem animal predation, note the numerous linear defects in the skin and underlying dermis, which is consistent with chewing and subsequent teeth marks.

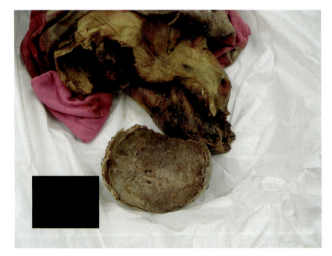

Figure 6.49. Postmortem animal (dog) activity. This individual died in her house of natural disease. After her death, her dogs consumed most of her head and upper body. At the top level of the shirt that the body is clothed in is the level of the diaphragm (ie, the dogs ate most of the head and all of the neck and chest).

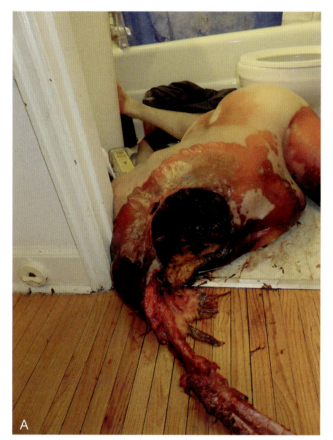

Figure 6.50A. Postmortem animal activity. This individual died of natural disease at their residence. The extent of postmortem predation by domesticated animals can be significant.

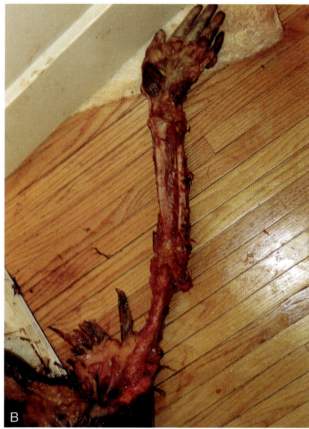

Figure 6.50B. Postmortem animal activity. Close-up of essentially skeletonized upper extremity after postmortem predation by a domestic animal.

EMBALMING ARTIFACTS

FAQ: Do forensic pathologists ever autopsy bodies that have already been embalmed?

Answer: Not uncommonly, forensic pathologists will need to perform an autopsy on an embalmed body. For example, if a medical examiner releases jurisdiction on a death in their area for an individual who died from a presumed natural death, and later evidence comes forward suggesting the cause of death may have been traumatic, a body might be brought to the medical examiner's office after it has already been embalmed.

FAQ: What are the challenges associated with autopsying previously embalmed bodies?

Answer: As with other categories of postmortem changes, correctly identifying the etiology of embalming artifacts as associated with the embalming procedure and not as an antemortem injury or natural disease process is most important.

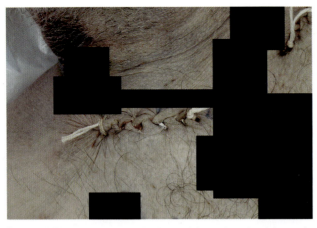 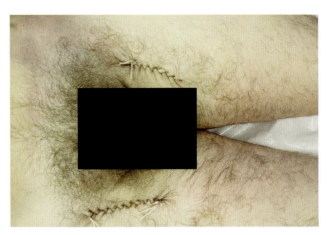

Figure 6.51. An incision at the base of the right side of the neck. Vascular access was obtained at this site, and then sutured closed.

Figure 6.52. Bilateral incisions in the femoral regions.

With the embalming procedure, the funeral director will cut down to the vasculature, often at one point (eg, the right subclavian or carotid artery), but sometimes numerous points, and use the vascular access point to cycle embalming fluid through the vasculature (Figures 6.51 and 6.52). In addition, incisions are made in the abdomen and trochars inserted to embalm the internal organs. After the incision is made, the incision is either sutured or an embalming button is placed in the incision (Figure 6.53). The use of trochars to introduce embalming fluid into the organs most often produces numerous slitlike defects in the organ parenchyma (ie, artifactual stab wounds). Other than embalming, other procedures performed can include placing a tan or colorless cap on the globes of the eye (Figure 6.54), wiring of the maxilla and mandible together (Figure 6.55), and placement of cream on areas that tend to desiccate (eg, eyelids and lips).

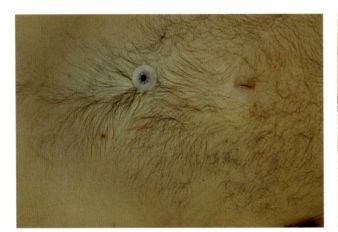 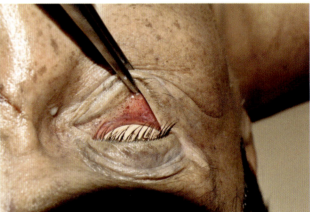

Figure 6.53. Embalming button. Superior to the umbilicus is a white plastic button that was placed by the funeral director after embalming the abdomen. With the device not in place, the defect in the skin could mimic an injury.

Figure 6.54. Tan plastic cap on eye. A tan cap covers the eye globe. The lower eyelid has florid petechiae also.

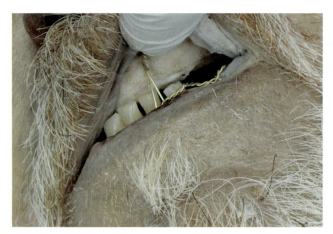

Figure 6.55. Wired jaw.

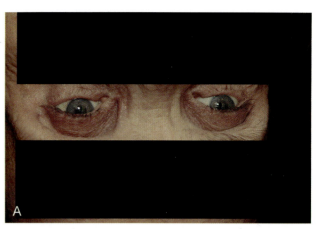

Figure 6.56A. Clear cornea. In a body with clear cornea, the time since death, if the eyelids were closed at the time the body was found, is often cited as 24 hours or less.

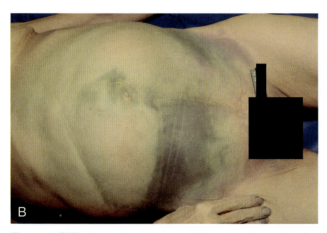

Figure 6.56B. Green discoloration of abdomen. Green discoloration of the abdomen often appears in the right lower quadrant around 24 hours after death. This abdominal wall reveals green discoloration of over half the area, indicating a time frame of greater than 1 day, and possibly 2 to 3 days or more. The body in Figure 6.56A is the same as the body in Figure 6.56B. This body could provide two different times since death based upon which area is examined.

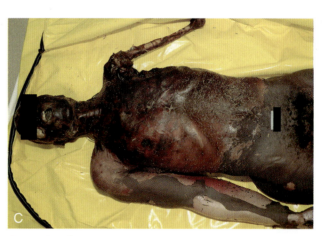

Figure 6.56C. Partial skeletonization. The body to the left has skeletonization of the left upper extremity and the right upper extremity has skin and soft tissue in place. Considered separately, each represents a different time since death; however, given that they are both present in the same body, the time since death was the same for both. The individual was found in the woods and had a jacket on. The sleeve covering the left upper extremity was bundled around the shoulder, thus exposing the soft tissue of the left upper extremity to predators, whereas for the right upper extremity, the sleeve was down, protecting the soft tissue from predators.

NEAR MISSES

Near Miss #1: Although postmortem changes of the body can be used to estimate time since death, these changes must be interpreted with caution as a significant number of factors can either speed up or slow down the rate of decomposition. Established equations for determining time since death involve using data based upon a set number of parameters and changes in these parameters can significantly change the results, and, for any given death, those parameters may not be known. Figure 6.56A-C represents how one body can, depending upon the area that is examined, show changes consistent with two different times since death.

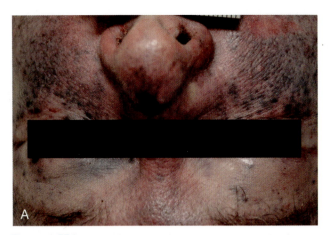

Figure 6.57A. Face of a woman found unresponsive in her house. Note the numerous periorbital petechial hemorrhages.

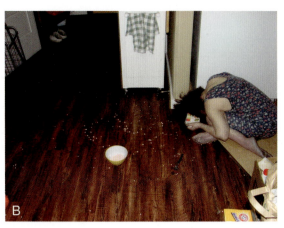

Figure 6.57B. Scene photograph corresponding to Figure 6.57A. The body was found face down. Due to the face-down position, there can be congestion of the face, often intense, which can potentially mimic a strangulation.

Near Miss #2: While petechiae are not specific for asphyxia, when petechiae are identified, the possibility of strangulation is often considered. When an individual is face down, petechiae can form in the conjunctivae postmortem. Congestion of the vessels in the eye due to gravity dependent pooling of blood followed by bursting of capillaries (such as the formation of Tardieu spots in the skin) can lead to conjunctival petechiae, conjunctival hemorrhages, and periorbital petechiae, and can mimic the findings of a strangulation (Figure 6.57A and B).

KEY FEATURES of Postmortem Changes

- Determination of time since death from postmortem changes must be approached very cautiously, as too many factors affect the timing. A safe determination of time of death is the date and time the body is found, followed by either "(found)" or "(pronounced)," as both of these dates and times are well established for any given death. An investigator should not feel the need to be more specific just because the death certificate asks for a date and time of death. For most deaths, the date and time of death is easy to determine as the person is pronounced dead by a doctor in the hospital, but for forensic cases, this is not so easy, and death investigators must not feel required to provide information that they cannot accurately provide. Misrepresentation, even when based upon honest and good intentions, of the date and time of death can have detrimental effects on later prosecution or civil court action.
- Recording of postmortem changes is best made at the scene, as transport of the body and subsequent cooling (or warming) make future determinations less useful.
- Postmortem changes, even though they may not allow for a good determination of time of death, must always be recorded as part of the investigation. These changes may be used to refute or corroborate subsequent witness accounts regarding the death, and can provide other useful information.
- Do not assume that a decomposed body will not yield useful information. Although decomposition impairs in some cases the determination of cause and manner of death, it does not preclude it.
- Be aware that numerous postmortem changes can produce findings that mimic antemortem trauma or natural disease.

References

1. Brady WJ. *Medical Investigation of Death in Oregon*. 2nd ed. 1976.
2. DiMaio VJ, DiMaio D. *Forensic Pathology*. 2nd ed. CRC Press; 2001.
3. Clark MA, Worrell MB, Pless JE. Postmortem changes in soft tissues. In: Haglund WD, Sorg MH, eds. *Forensic Taphonomy: The Postmortem Fate of Human Remains*. CRC Press; 1997.
4. Spitz WU, Fisher RS. *Medicolegal Investigation of Death*. 3rd ed. Charles C. Thomas; 1993.
5. Spitz WU, Fisher RS. *Medicolegal Investigation of Death*. 1st ed. Charles C. Thomas; 1973.
6. Semple A. *Essentials of Pathology and Morbid Anatomy*. W.B. Saunders; 1890.
7. Lew E, Matshes E. In: Dolinak D, Matshes E, Lew E, eds. *Postmortem Changes in Forensic Pathology: Principles and Practice*. Elsevier Academic Press; 2005.
8. Madea B. Methods for determining time of death. *Forensic Sci Med Pathol*. 2016;12(4):451-485.
9. Bate-Smith EC, Bendall JR. Rigor mortis and adenosinetriphosphate. *J Physiol*. 1947;106(2):177-185.
10. Smith S, Fiddes FS. *Forensic Medicine: A Textbook for Students and Practitioners*. 10th ed. J & A Churchill, Ltd.; 1955.
11. Gonzales TA, Vance M, Helpern M, Umberger CJ. *Legal Medicine: Pathology and Toxicology*. Appleton-Century-Crofts, Inc.; 1954.
12. Norris R. On the nature of rigor mortis. *J Anat Physio*. 1867;1(1):114-119.
13. Nashelsky M, McFeeley P. Time of death. In: Froede RC, ed. *Handbook of Forensic Pathology*. 2nd ed. College of American Pathologists; 2003.
14. McLemore J, Zumwalt RE. Postmortem changes. In: Froede RC, ed. *Handbook of Forensic Pathology*. 2nd ed. College of American Pathologists; 2003.
15. Rutty GN. Post-mortem changes and artefacts. In: Rutty GN, ed. *Essentials of Autopsy Practice*. Vol. 1. Springer; 2001.
16. Ernst MF. Medicolegal death investigation and forensic procedures. In: Froede RC, ed. *Handbook of Forensic Pathology*. 2nd ed. College of American Pathologists; 2003.

NATURAL DISEASE AT AUTOPSY

CHAPTER OUTLINE

Introduction 74

Natural Disease of the Body in General 75
- Autopsy Findings: Obesity 75
- Complications of Obesity 75

Natural Disease of the Central Nervous System 76
- Introduction 76

Intracerebral Hemorrhage 76
- Autopsy Findings 76
- Etiologies of an Intracerebral Hemorrhage 78

Cerebral Infarcts 78
- Autopsy Findings 78

Lacunar Infarct 81
- Autopsy Findings 81

Incompetent Diaphragm Sella 82
- Autopsy Findings 82

Natural Causes of Subarachnoid Hemorrhage 82
- Autopsy Findings 82
- Etiologies of Subarachnoid Hemorrhage at Autopsy 82
- Potential Mimics of Subarachnoid Hemorrhage 83

Meningitis 84
- Autopsy Findings 84
- Potential Mimics 85

Osmotic Demyelination Syndrome (Central Pontine and Extrapontine Myelinolysis) 86
- Autopsy Findings 86
- Association 86
- Potential Mimics 86

Globus Pallidus/Basal Ganglia Necrosis 86
- Autopsy Findings 86
- Association of Globus Pallidus Necrosis 87

Multiple Sclerosis 88
- Autopsy Findings 88

Chronic Traumatic Encephalopathy 88
- Autopsy Findings 88

Seizure Disorder 89
- Autopsy Findings 89
- Association With Sudden Death 89

Alzheimer Disease 90
- Autopsy Findings 90

Diffuse Lewy Body Disease 90
- Autopsy Findings 90

Encephalitis 91
- Autopsy Findings 91

Colloid Cyst 92
- Autopsy Findings 92

Natural Disease of the Cardiovascular System 92
- Introduction 92

Hypertensive Heart Disease 93
- Autopsy Findings 93
- Association With Sudden Death 93

Coronary Artery Atherosclerosis 93
- Autopsy Findings 93
- Association of Coronary Artery Atherosclerosis With Sudden Death 96
- Gross and Microscopic Aging of an Acute Myocardial Infarct 96
- Complications of Acute Myocardial Infarct 102

Aortic Dissection 105
- Autopsy Findings 105

Coronary Artery Dissection 105
- Autopsy Findings 105
- Associations 105

Abdominal Aortic Aneurysm 106
- Autopsy Findings 106

Coronary Artery Aneurysm 107
- Autopsy Findings 107
- Associations 107

Aortic Stenosis 108
- Autopsy Findings 108
- Association With Sudden Death 108

Bicuspid Aortic Valve 108
- Autopsy Findings 108

Myxomatous Mitral Valve 109
- Autopsy Findings 109
- Association With Sudden Death 110
- Potential Mimics 110

Chronic Rheumatic Mitral Valvulitis 110
- Autopsy Findings 110
- Potential Mimic 110

Endocarditis 111
- Autopsy Findings 111
- Associations of Endocarditis 111

Pericarditis 113
- Autopsy Findings 113
- Etiologies of Pericarditis 113

Myocarditis 114
- Autopsy Findings 114
- Mimics of Myocarditis 115

Cardiomyopathies 116
- Autopsy Findings 116
- Association With Sudden Death 117
- Mimics of Cardiomyopathy 117

Coronary Artery Anomalies Associated With Sudden Cardiac Death 118
- Autopsy Findings: Anomalous Origin of a Coronary Artery 118
- Association With Sudden Death 118
- Autopsy Findings: Tunneling/Bridging of Coronary Artery 119
- Association With Sudden Death 119

Lipomatous Hypertrophy of the Interatrial Septum 119
- Autopsy Findings 119
- Association With Sudden Death 120

Non-Ischemic Left Ventricular Scar 120
- Autopsy Findings 120
- Associated With Sudden Death 120

Lesions of the Cardiac Conduction System 120
- Introduction 120

Atrioventricular Nodal Artery Dysplasia 121
- Autopsy Findings 121
- Association With Sudden Death 121

Incidental and Other Microscopic Findings in the Heart 121
- Clusters of Lymphocytes 121
- Basophilic Degeneration 122
- Contraction Band Necrosis 122

Natural Disease of the Respiratory System 123
- Introduction 123

Pneumonia 123
- Autopsy Findings 123
- Potential Mimics of Pneumonia 123

Aspiration Pneumonia 125
- Autopsy Findings 125
- Mimics 126

Emphysema 126
- Autopsy Findings 126

Asthma 127
- Autopsy Findings 127

Incidental Microscopic Findings in the Lung 128
- Corpora Amylacea 128
- Lentils 128
- Pulmonary Chemodectoma (Mesothelial-Like Rest) 128

Natural Disease of the Hepatobiliary System 129
- Introduction 129

Diffuse Fatty Liver 129
- Autopsy Findings 129
- Potential Mimics 131

Cirrhosis of the Liver 132
- Autopsy Findings 132
- Potential Mimics 132
- Complications of Cirrhosis 133

Fitz-Hugh-Curtis Syndrome 135
- Autopsy Findings 135

Acute Cholecystitis 135
- Autopsy Findings 135

Acute Pancreatitis 136
- Autopsy Findings 136
- Risk Factors for Acute Pancreatitis 136

Cavernous Hemangioma 138
- Autopsy Findings 138
- Association With Sudden Death 138

Other Incidental Liver Masses   138
- Autopsy Findings   138

Natural Disease of the Genitourinary System   138
- Introduction   138

Nephrosclerosis   139
- Autopsy Findings   139

Acute Pyelonephritis   140
- Autopsy Findings   140
- Association With Sudden Death   141

Fournier Gangrene   141
- Autopsy Findings   141

Incidental Renal Masses   141
- Adenoma   141
- Renal Cell Carcinoma   141
- Adrenal Gland Rest   141
- Renomedullary Interstitial Cell Tumor   141

Natural Disease of the Endocrine System   142
- Introduction   142

Features of Diabetes Mellitus   142
- Autopsy Findings   142

Infarction of the Pituitary Gland   142
- Autopsy Findings   142
- Association   142

Hashimoto Thyroiditis   144
- Autopsy Findings   144

Pheochromocytoma   144
- Autopsy Findings   144

Incidental Findings   145
- Myelolipoma   145
- Black Thyroid   145

Natural Disease of the Gastrointestinal System   145
- Introduction   145

Esophageal Inlet Patch (Salmon Patch)   147
- Autopsy Findings   147
- Potential Mimics   148

Barrett Esophagus   148
- Autopsy Findings   148

Black Esophagus (Acute Esophageal Necrosis)   149
- Autopsy Findings   149
- Associations   149

Peptic Ulcer   150
- Autopsy Findings   150

Ischemic Colitis   150
- Autopsy Findings   150
- Potential Mimic   150

Intestinal Diverticula   150
- Autopsy Findings   150

Green Colon   152
- Autopsy Findings   152
- Potential Mimic   152

Natural Disease of the Hematolymphoid System   153
- Introduction   153

Disseminated Intravascular Coagulation   153
- Autopsy Findings   153

Thrombotic Thrombocytopenic Purpura/Hemolytic Uremic Syndrome   153
- Autopsy Findings   153

Fibrosis of the Splenic Capsule (Sugar Spleen)   154
- Autopsy Findings   154

Natural Disease of the Musculoskeletal System   155
- Introduction   155

Pregnancy-Related Deaths   155
- Introduction   155

Amniotic Fluid Embolism   156
- Autopsy Findings   156

Acute Fatty Liver of Pregnancy   156
- Autopsy Findings   156

Acute Endometritis-Myometritis   156
- Autopsy Findings   156

Placenta Accreta, Placenta Increta, Placenta Percreta   156
- Autopsy Findings   156

Peripartum Cardiomyopathy   156
- Autopsy Findings   156

Pre-Eclampsia/Eclampsia   157
- Autopsy Findings   157

Hellp Syndrome   157
- Autopsy Findings   157

Ectopic Pregnancy   157
- Autopsy Findings   157

Near Misses   158

INTRODUCTION

A large number of deaths investigated by a medical examiner's or coroner's office will be due to natural causes. In the National Association of Medical Examiner's (NAME) "Forensic Autopsy Performance Standards, Standard B3 Selecting Deaths Requiring Forensic Autopsies," which reads, "The forensic pathologist shall perform an autopsy when:" although some scenarios would cover some natural deaths (eg, autopsies on infants and children and deaths in custody), none of the scenarios specifically address when a forensic pathologist shall perform an autopsy in the event of an apparent natural death.[1] Thus, whether an autopsy is performed on a presumed natural death is most often based upon forensic pathologist's preference and office policies, which can vary from essentially no autopsies performed on suspected natural deaths to autopsies performed on a large number of suspected natural deaths; however, even if no autopsy is performed, a cause and manner of death must still be assigned if the death falls within the jurisdiction of the coroner or medical examiner. Based upon their study population, Nashelsky and Lawrence determined that when no autopsy is performed, the cause of death determination is incorrect in about 30% of cases, and in a small number of deaths in which no autopsy is performed (<5%), a non-natural death will be missed.[2] In their study population, Gill and Scordi-Bello found less of a difference in the cause of death determination (around 10%) than Nashelsky and Lawrence, but a similar number of non-natural deaths were missed when no autopsy was performed (<5%).[3] Based upon the results of these two studies, the only way to identify all non-natural deaths would essentially be to autopsy all deaths that fall within a coroner's or medical examiner's purview, which would not be possible in most if not all jurisdictions in the United States.

Whether the actual cause of death is a natural condition, forensic pathologists will frequently encounter natural disease processes at autopsy and must be able to identify them. When a natural disease process is discovered in a decedent who has died a traumatic death, the forensic pathologist must be able to determine whether the natural disease is an incidental finding in an otherwise traumatic death (eg, a renal mass in a person who died in a motor vehicle accident) or whether the natural disease may have played a role in the death (eg, a coronary artery thrombus in a person who died in a motor vehicle accident). In addition to determining whether a natural disease played a role in a decedent's death, forensic pathologists must also be able to distinguish natural disease from traumatic injuries, postmortem changes, and therapeutic injuries, which can all mimic natural disease. The reverse is also true.

The range of natural disease conditions and the range of findings within any one natural disease process that can be encountered by a forensic pathologist are broad, and one chapter in an atlas cannot adequately cover the spectrum. The conditions listed below are based upon common conditions encountered by a forensic pathologist, important mimics, and conditions that have a high likelihood of being the cause of death or having contributed to the cause of death.

FAQ: Why should an autopsy be performed in an otherwise traumatic death, when lethal injuries can be documented either radiographically or via external examination?

Answer: While the cause of death may be known through clinical procedures already performed (eg, a computed tomography (CT) scan), documentation of the pathologic changes by a forensic pathologist may be important for future court proceedings, remembering that clinical physicians are not the best at identifying the specifics of traumatic injuries (eg, entrance vs exit gunshot wounds). Also, autopsies are frequently requested by attorneys to rule out natural disease as a competing cause of death for situations in which criminal charges will be filed, especially drug overdoses. If no autopsy is performed, a defense attorney may try to implicate natural disease as the actual cause of death, even in circumstances such as a motor vehicle accident when the decedent was not the driver, and thereby seek to confuse the jury as to the guilt or innocence of the defendant. An autopsy would provide the information to refute such claims. In addition, in civil claims, the autopsy findings will be used to help determine life span, which can affect the monetary outcome.

> **FAQ:** A tumor is identified during an autopsy. How far must the forensic pathologist go to identify the tumor type?
>
> **Answer:** Unfortunately, most if not all medical examiner's offices do not have the financial resources to study every tumor encountered at autopsy with the range of immunohistochemical stains, genetic testing, and other testing modalities that are often required in the clinical setting. How far a forensic pathologist goes to study any given tumor will depend upon the nature of the case, office policies, and preferences of the pathologist. Having hospital surgical pathologists with whom to regularly consult regarding the diagnosis of incidental tumors identified at autopsy is a valuable asset for a forensic pathologist.

NATURAL DISEASE OF THE BODY IN GENERAL

AUTOPSY FINDINGS: OBESITY

Obesity is a common disease process encountered at autopsy, wherein the overall weight of the body is increased. While a subjective interpretation of obesity can be made based upon a visual inspection of the body, using body mass index (BMI) calculators (https://www.cdc.gov/healthyweight/assessing/bmi/adult_bmi/english_bmi_calculator/bmi_calculator.html) can provide an objective determination.

COMPLICATIONS OF OBESITY

Obesity is a risk factor for cardiomegaly, including massive cardiomegaly (heart weight of >1000 g); steatosis and steatohepatitis of the liver (ie, non-alcoholic fatty liver disease [NAFLD]); pulmonary thromboembolism; diabetes mellitus; pulmonary hypertension and systemic hypertension; obstructive sleep apnea; dyslipidemia; cholelithiasis; cancers (including endometrial, prostatic, colonic, and renal); osteoarthritis; menstrual irregularities and pregnancy difficulties; and buried penis, which is due to envelopment of the shaft of the penis with adipose tissue.[4-10]

> **FAQ:** Is obesity itself a risk factor for coronary artery atherosclerosis?
>
> **Answer:** Some authors have described that obesity is not necessarily a risk factor for coronary artery atherosclerosis, and a higher BMI may actually be protective against coronary artery atherosclerosis.[11,12] However, other authors have identified an association between obesity and coronary artery disease.[13-15] Obesity is a known risk factor for sudden cardiac death[16,17]; however, with sudden cardiac death in obese individuals with a BMI > 50, the underlying pathologic cause of sudden death may be cardiac hypertrophy rather than coronary artery atherosclerosis.[17]

> **PEARLS & PITFALLS**
>
> Obesity is a risk factor for asphyxiation after motor vehicle accidents specifically when inversion of the body occurs.[18] In such a situation, listing obesity as a contributory condition on the death certificate would be acceptable.

> **PEARLS & PITFALLS**
>
> Obesity will speed decomposition, especially if there are other factors affecting the rate, such as heavy clothing or bedding, or nearness of the body to a heat source.[19] Because of this increased rate of decomposition, the time of death of an obese individual can be misinterpreted as having occurred a greater length of time before they were found dead than the actual length of time between death and discovery.

> **PEARLS & PITFALLS**
>
> Obstructive sleep apnea, which can be a complication of obesity, is a risk factor for sudden cardiac death.[20-24] In a review of 25 individuals with obstructive sleep apnea who died suddenly, Zhang et al found different cardiac findings among the decedents including non-specific cardiomyopathy (including left ventricular hypertrophy without or without dilation), hearts without a morphologic cause of death but which frequently had right ventricular dilatation, and other cardiac conditions.[24]

NATURAL DISEASE OF THE CENTRAL NERVOUS SYSTEM

INTRODUCTION

The natural diseases of the central nervous system that are most commonly encountered during a forensic autopsy include strokes (both cerebral infarcts and intracerebral hemorrhage), ruptured berry aneurysms, meningitis, multiple sclerosis, seizure disorders, and tumors (most commonly meningiomas). While the identification of neurodegenerative diseases is normally outside the scope of a forensic pathologist's expertise, who most often lack additional formal training in neuropathology, the basic diagnosis of Alzheimer disease and diffuse Lewy body disease for the purpose of a standard forensic autopsy can potentially be made with additional stains (eg, Bielschowsky silver stain of selected regions of the cortex in the case of Alzheimer disease, and α-synuclein immunohistochemical stain of selected regions of the cortex in diffuse Lewy body disease).[25]

> **FAQ:** When should the brain be fixed in formalin for future dissection?
>
> **Answer:** While fixation of the brain allows for a better examination and the opportunity to send the brain to a neuropathologist if necessary, organ retention has been a legal and ethical issue for medical examiner's offices. The decision to retain a brain for formalin fixation and future examination is based upon office policies and the preference of the forensic pathologist performing the autopsy.

INTRACEREBRAL HEMORRHAGE

AUTOPSY FINDINGS

Gross examination will reveal a large mass of blood within the cerebral parenchyma (Figure 7.1A and B). While not necessary to make the diagnosis, microscopic examination will reveal disruptions of the cerebral parenchyma that are filled with extravasated red blood cells. Microscopic examination may potentially assist in the determination of the etiology of the hemorrhage if the etiology is not otherwise apparent from the clinical history or other autopsy findings (eg, microscopic examination would allow for the identification of cerebral amyloid angiopathy).

> **PEARLS & PITFALLS**
>
> If the intracerebral hemorrhage ruptures through the cortical surface of the cerebral hemisphere, a subdural hemorrhage can result. With a brainstem hemorrhage, a basilar subarachnoid and subdural hemorrhage can also result (Figure 7.2A-C). In these situations, the subdural hemorrhage would represent one feature of an otherwise natural manner of death, and should not be mistaken for a traumatic cause of death. If the intracerebral hemorrhage ruptures into the ventricular system (Figure 7.3A and B), or if blood from a bleeding arteriovenous malformation or a vascular tumor enters the ventricular system (Figure 7.4), the ventricular system will expand, pushing on the brain from the inside and causing a flattening of the gyri and effacement of the sulci, mimicking cerebral edema.

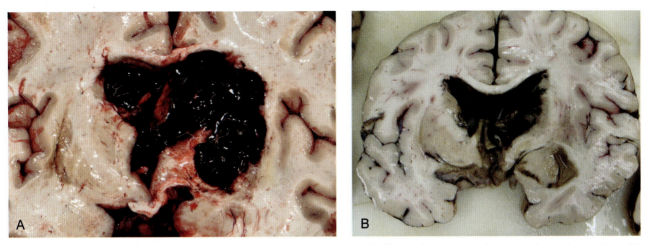

Figure 7.1. Intracerebral hemorrhage. In both (**A** and **B**), there is an intracerebral hemorrhage centered on the right caudate nucleus. (**A**) is an unfixed brain and (**B**) is a fixed brain.

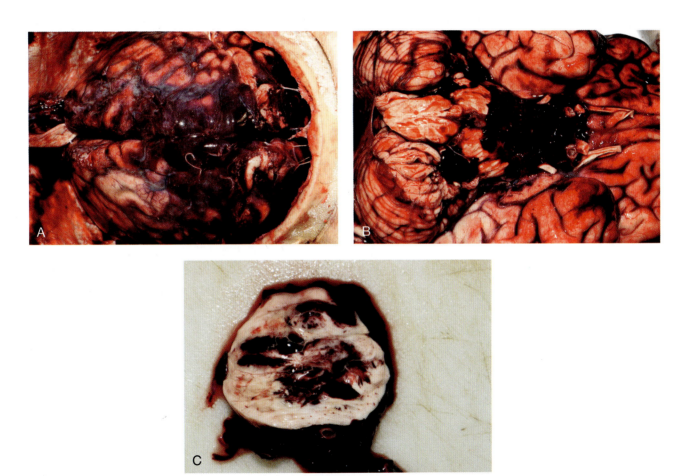

Figure 7.2. Brainstem hemorrhage. Upon opening the brain, a subarachnoid hemorrhage was identified (**A**). The gyri were still relatively rounded and the sulci open, especially anterior. At the base of the brain was subarachnoid hemorrhage (**B**). Note that there is space between the right cerebellar tonsil and the brainstem (ie, there was no tonsillar molding). There was a diffuse large patchy hemorrhage in the pons and midbrain (**C**). Given that the decedent was witnessed to fall and had no significant injuries, and given the lack of well-developed cerebral edema, the hemorrhage in the brainstem was determined to be a natural event and not a Duret hemorrhage secondary to edema. The basal ganglia, cerebellum, and brainstem are common locations for hypertension-associated intracerebral hemorrhage.

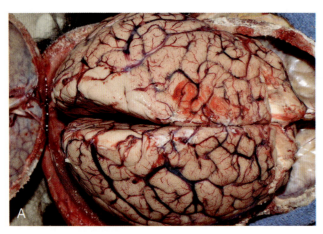
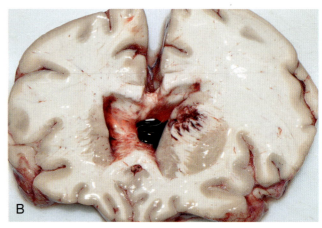

Figure 7.3. Intracerebral hemorrhage mimicking edema. From the outer surface, the brain appears to be markedly edematous, with flattening of the gyri and effacement of the sulci (**A**). The decedent sustained an intracerebral hemorrhage centered on the right basal ganglia (**B**); however, instead of dissecting into the parenchyma, the hemorrhage entered the ventricular system, filling the ventricles and distending the brain, creating the appearance of edema.

ETIOLOGIES OF AN INTRACEREBRAL HEMORRHAGE

When the underlying cause of an intracerebral hemorrhage is systemic hypertension, the hemorrhage is usually centered on the basal ganglia, the cerebellum, or the brainstem. When an intracerebral hemorrhage occurs in a location that is not typical for a hypertensive-type hemorrhage (ie, a lobar hemorrhage), two important conditions to consider are expansion of a cerebral contusion and cerebral amyloid angiopathy (Figure 7.5). Vascular malformations, neoplasms, and bleeding disorders are other possibilities.[26]

CEREBRAL INFARCTS

AUTOPSY FINDINGS

The gross and microscopic findings allow for a relative determination of the age of the infarct because, depending upon the length of time since the infarct occurred, the affected portion of the brain will have different findings that correlate with the time frame. Early

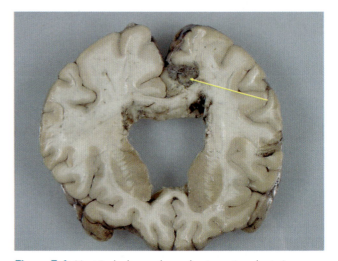

Figure 7.4. Ventricular hemorrhage due to ruptured arteriovenous malformation that mimics cerebral edema. From the external surface of the brain, this individual appeared to have edema, with flattening of the gyri and effacement of the sulci; however, the source was an arteriovenous malformation (arrow), that ruptured into the right lateral ventricle, distending the ventricular system and mimicking cerebral edema.

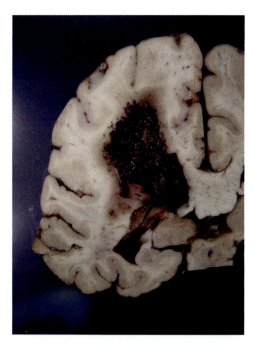

Figure 7.5. Lobar hemorrhage. This individual crashed their vehicle and was subsequently hospitalized and died shortly thereafter. Sectioning of the brain revealed a hemorrhage centered posterior to the left basal ganglia. While expansion of a contusion was a possible cause, no contusions were identified. Microscopic examination did not disclose amyloid angiopathy or another potential cause. The etiology of the lobar hemorrhage was not satisfactorily determined.

in the course, microscopic examination will reveal red neurons within 12 hours and the gray matter will be dusky around 2 days (Figure 7.6A-C).[27] With the infiltration of macrophages, the tissue will begin to break down and have a more friable appearance (Figure 7.6D and E), which will be around 2 weeks.[27] Ultimately, the affected region will be cystlike (Figure 7.6F and G) in weeks to months.[27] The distribution of the infarct will help determine the vessel involved (eg, if the infarct is along the greater longitudinal fissure on the right side of the anterior portion of the right cerebral hemisphere, the lesion causing the infarct affected the right anterior cerebral artery) (Figure 7.7).

> **PEARLS & PITFALLS**
>
> While an intracerebral hemorrhage can rapidly cause death and present as a sudden unexpected death, the death from a cerebral infarct is most often delayed, with the decedent having associated complications such as malnutrition and pneumonia. While a large cerebral infarct could potentially cause sudden death, unless the inciting thrombus or embolus is discovered in a cerebral artery, this cause of death would most likely not be identified at autopsy because some time (up to hours to a day) must pass before the brain manifests identifiable pathologic changes of a cerebral infarct.

> **PEARLS & PITFALLS**
>
> A remote cortical contusion and a remote cerebral infarct can appear similar. On gross examination, remote cortical contusions are found at the crest of gyri and have a wedge shape, with the apex pointed inward, whereas remote infarcts are found at the depths of sulci and have a flasklike shape. On microscopic examination, a remote cerebral infarct will have an intact sub-pial layer of parenchyma, which gets its nutrients and oxygen from the meningeal vessels (Figure 7.8), whereas a remote cortical contusion will not have this intact sub-pial layer. However, caution is advised in interpretation of the microscopic findings, as adjacent to a remote cortical contusion can be a region of infarction.

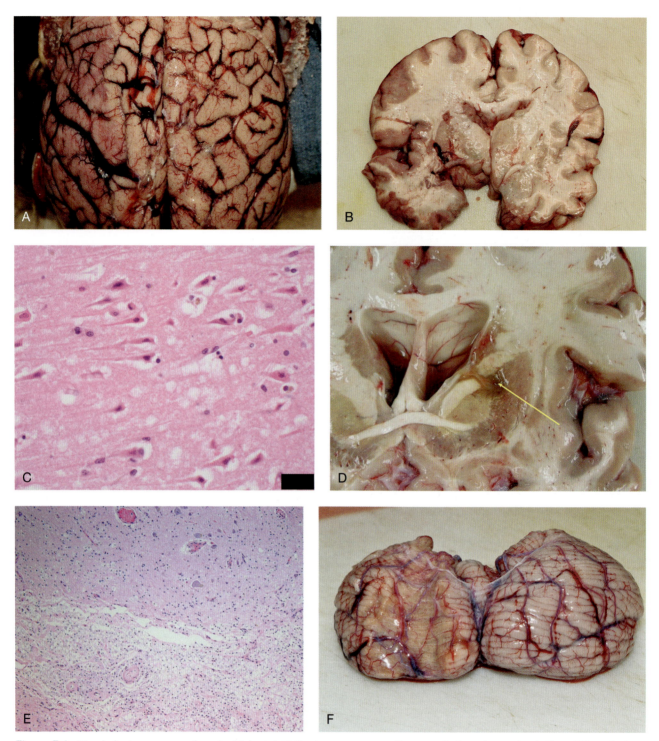

Figure 7.6. Morphologic sequence of cerebral infarct. Initially, the gray matter will appear dusky or hemorrhagic (**A** and **B**), and microscopic examination can reveal red neurons (**C**). The infarcted region will then become soft and friable (arrow, **D**), which corresponds to the removal of dead neurons and debris by macrophages (**E**, low power). At this point, microscopically, the infarct will have a very well-defined junction from the surrounding viable tissue. Ultimately, a cystic region will be present (**F** and **G**). Microscopic examination would reveal gliosis at the edge of the infarcted region.

CHAPTER 7 NATURAL DISEASE AT AUTOPSY

Figure 7.6g (continued)

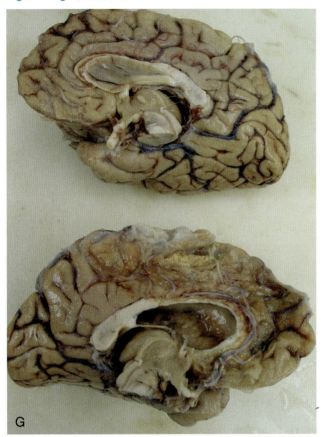

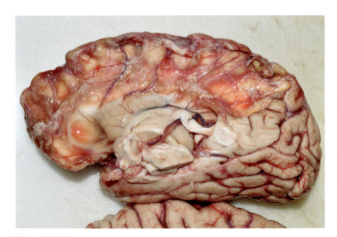

Figure 7.7. Infarct in the distribution of the right anterior cerebral artery. This individual sustained an infarct of the right frontal and parietal lobes along the greater longitudinal fissure, which is the distribution of the right anterior cerebral artery.

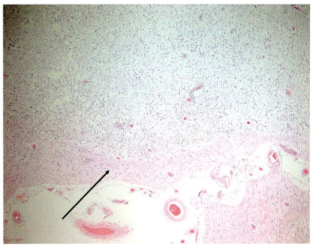

Figure 7.8. Subpial sparing. Just underlying the pia mater is a thin strip of histologically preserved cerebral parenchyma (arrow), which survived the underlying infarct as illustrated by the sheets of foamy histiocytes, because of the ability to get oxygen and nutrients from meningeal vessels (low power). In a contusion, this thin surviving strip of subpial parenchyma would not be present.

LACUNAR INFARCT

AUTOPSY FINDINGS

Lacunar infarcts are small (around a few millimeters) cavitary defects often located in the basal ganglia region or the brainstem. Lacunar infarcts are commonly associated with a history of systemic hypertension.

INCOMPETENT DIAPHRAGM SELLA

AUTOPSY FINDINGS

The dural opening through which the pituitary stalk passes is markedly widened (Figure 7.9), which allows the arachnoid mater to prolapse into the sella turcica, pushing on the pituitary gland. This finding is very common at autopsy, and, while it can potentially lead to pituitary gland atrophy and empty sella syndrome, in almost all cases, the pituitary gland is just flattened on the floor of the sella turcica.

NATURAL CAUSES OF SUBARACHNOID HEMORRHAGE

AUTOPSY FINDINGS

With a subarachnoid hemorrhage, blood underlying the arachnoid mater will be present at autopsy, which can be identified grossly or microscopically (Figure 7.10). The subarachnoid hemorrhage should be centered on the underlying condition leading to its formation. For example, subarachnoid hemorrhage due to a ruptured berry aneurysm is most commonly found at the base of the brain, centered on the circle of Willis.

ETIOLOGIES OF SUBARACHNOID HEMORRHAGE AT AUTOPSY

Common causes of subarachnoid hemorrhage include trauma, ruptured berry aneurysms (Figure 7.11A-C), and ruptured arteriovenous malformations. A ruptured berry aneurysm represents the etiology for about 85% of subarachnoid hemorrhages that have occurred due to a natural cause.[28] The most common location for a berry aneurysm is the middle cerebral artery.[29] Alcohol intoxication, sexual activity, and stimulant use (eg, cocaine and methamphetamine) have been associated with berry aneurysm rupture.[30-33] Smoking, hypertension, and cerebral amyloid angiopathy are also risk factors for subarachnoid hemorrhage.[33,34]

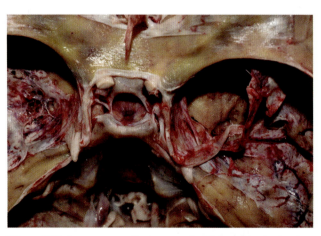

Figure 7.9. Incompetent diaphragm sella. The opening in the dura through which the pituitary stalk passes is markedly widened.

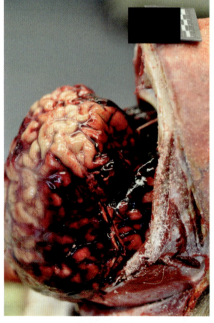

Figure 7.10. Subarachnoid hemorrhage. Underlying the arachnoid are extravasated red blood cells. While a subdural hemorrhage, unless organized, will fall away from or can be wiped away from the surface of the brain, a subarachnoid hemorrhage cannot.

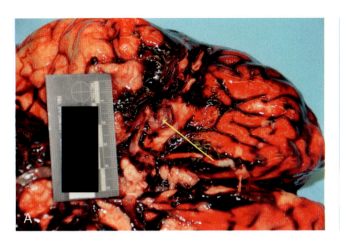
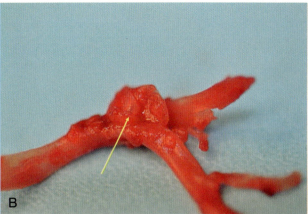
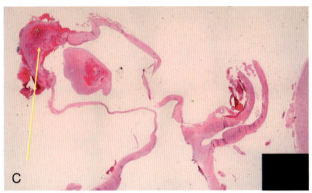

Figure 7.11. Berry aneurysm. In (**A**), the berry aneurysm arises from the right middle cerebral artery (arrow). Berry aneurysms commonly arise at branch points in the circle of Willis (arrow, **B**). Microscopic examination of a ruptured berry aneurysm can reveal fibrin and neutrophils at the rupture site (arrow, **C**, low power). The presence of hemosiderin at the location of the aneurysm could represent a past bleed (ie, a sentinel leak) or a delayed period over which the rupture occurred.

POTENTIAL MIMICS OF SUBARACHNOID HEMORRHAGE

When the head is in a prone position (or, potentially supine) for an extended period of time, some degree of subarachnoid hemorrhage may form associated with congestion and decomposition (Figure 7.12). In addition, when the cranium is opened, venous channels are often cut and some amount of blood can leak onto the cerebral surface. In a photograph, this displaced blood could mimic a subarachnoid or subdural hemorrhage, since it forms a very thin layer; however, it is easily removed with a towel at the time of autopsy. If the photographs are to be potentially reviewed by another forensic pathologist, such removal may be prudent to prevent future disagreement as to the nature of the blood on the surface of the brain.

PEARLS & PITFALLS

When a subarachnoid hemorrhage is encountered at autopsy, especially if the cause of the hemorrhage is not obvious (eg, trauma in a motor vehicle accident), the etiology of the subarachnoid hemorrhage must be identified. If the hemorrhage is centered at the base of the brain, the etiology is most likely a ruptured berry aneurysm. The aneurysm should be identified at the time of the autopsy, using water to rinse away the subarachnoid blood. If the brain is instead fixed in formalin, identification of the berry aneurysm is much more difficult, as dissecting away the fixed hemorrhage is likely to damage the delicate aneurysm. If no aneurysm is identified, other etiologies must be considered such as vertebral artery dissection, arteriovenous malformations, bleeding disorders, hemorrhage from the cervical region of the vertebral column, basilar artery dissections, tumors, pregnancy-induced hypertension, and even neurodegenerative diseases, such as multi-system atrophy.[35-39] Despite all efforts to determine the etiology of a subarachnoid hemorrhage, it is possible that in some cases, no underlying condition will be identified. In the context of the remainder of the autopsy and the scene investigation, if trauma can be ruled out, the underlying etiology of the subarachnoid hemorrhage may be presumed natural in origin.

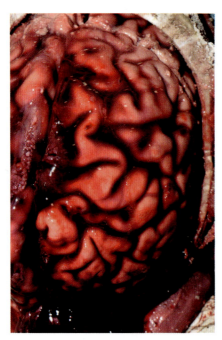

Figure 7.12. Congestion mimicking subarachnoid hemorrhage. This individual died as the result of sepsis and was in a prone position for 2 days before autopsy. At autopsy, despite refrigeration, there was some degree of decomposition of the head and neck region.

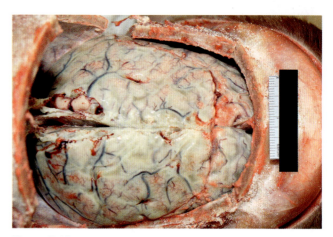

Figure 7.13. Bacterial meningitis. This individual had *Streptococcus pneumoniae* meningitis.

PEARLS & PITFALLS

Pseudo-subarachnoid hemorrhage is a radiologic entity where certain conditions can mimic subarachnoid hemorrhage on imaging and thus be misinterpreted as subarachnoid hemorrhage by the radiologist. Such misinterpretation could impact the determination of whether an autopsy is necessary in any given case, and could bias a forensic pathologist's interpretation of autopsy findings, and thus is an important condition for them to be aware of. Pseudo-subarachnoid hemorrhage is commonly due to cerebral edema, which can appear on CT scan as a subarachnoid hemorrhage.[40] Other conditions that have been reported to cause pseudo-subarachnoid hemorrhage include infections, subdural hemorrhage, diabetic ketoacidosis, hyponatremia, hyperhemoglobinemia, valproate toxicity, sudden infant death syndrome (SIDS), and cerebellar infarction.[41]

MENINGITIS

AUTOPSY FINDINGS

The classic appearance of the brain in bacterial meningitis will be pus-covered, which is most frequently due to *Streptococcus pneumoniae* (Figure 7.13); however, this appearance does not apply to all forms of bacterial meningitis. With *Neisseria meningitidis*, the meninges will actually appear fairly normal; however, the skin will often have a splotchy rash and the adrenal glands will be hemorrhagic (ie, Waterhouse-Friderichsen syndrome)[42] (Figure 7.14A and B). If the meningitis is basal in location, tuberculosis or a dimorphic fungus (ie, *Blastomyces*, *Coccidioides*, and *Histoplasma*) should be considered (Figure 7.15).

PEARLS & PITFALLS

It is important to consider that trauma may have played a role in the development of meningitis. Identification of the possible source of the bacteria (eg, a sinusitis or otitis media), and determination of whether trauma was involved (eg, through history or identification of some form of cranial trauma) is important, as the manner of death may be non-natural.

CHAPTER 7 NATURAL DISEASE AT AUTOPSY

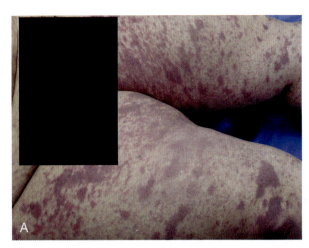
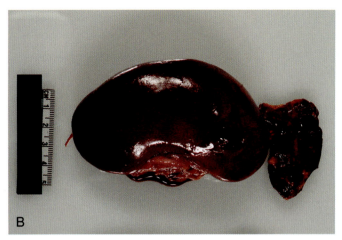

Figure 7.14. Meningitis due to *Neisseria meningitidis*. This individual died as the result of meningitis due to *Neisseria meningitidis*. While the meninges usually appear normal, other features of the disease include a splotchy skin rash (**A**) and bilateral adrenal gland hemorrhage, that is, Waterhouse-Friderichsen syndrome (**B**). This pattern is important to identify as individuals with *Neisseria meningitidis* are highly contagious and exposed individuals are often treated with antibiotics prophylactically.

PEARLS & PITFALLS

Waterhouse-Friderichsen syndrome is also associated with *S. pneumoniae* infections in individual who are post-splenectomy.[43]

POTENTIAL MIMICS

With increased age of decedents, the arachnoid granulations can develop a fair amount of fibrosis (Figure 7.16), which could mimic pus on the surface of the brain; however, this change would essentially only be present along the greater longitudinal fissure, and, if necessary, microscopic examination, revealing the absence of a neutrophilic infiltrate, would easily distinguish the two conditions.

PEARLS & PITFALLS

In a severe infection, the bone marrow can release large number of immature granulocytes, which can be the dominant cell type present in the exudate if the meningitis is examined microscopically. These immature cells can, especially with some degree of postmortem change or other cellular breakdown, can easily mimic lymphocytes.

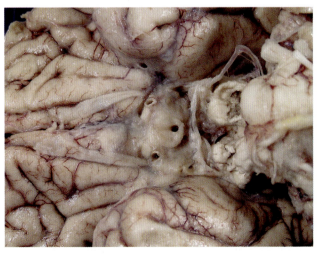

Figure 7.15. *Coccidioides immitis* meningitis. This individual died from *Coccidioides immitis* meningitis, which, like tuberculosis, produces a basilar meningitis.

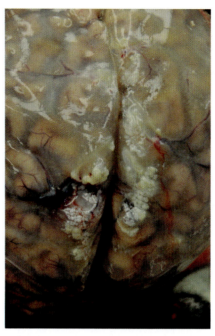

Figure 7.16. Fibrosis of arachnoid granulations. Fibrosis of the arachnoid granulations in older individuals can potentially mimic pus, and appear as a meningitis.

OSMOTIC DEMYELINATION SYNDROME (CENTRAL PONTINE AND EXTRAPONTINE MYELINOLYSIS)

AUTOPSY FINDINGS

In central pontine myelinolysis, the center of the pons will have a gray discoloration or friable defect (Figure 7.17A and B). Microscopic examination will reveal foamy macrophages but preservation of neurons (Figure 7.17C). Extrapontine myelinolysis commonly involves the basal ganglia.[44]

ASSOCIATION

While central pontine and extrapontine myelinolysis have most frequently been associated with the clinical rapid correction of hyponatremia, in forensic autopsies, the condition does occur in non-treated patients and has been associated with excessive consumption of water, vomiting, complications of thermal burns, and chronic alcoholism,[45-47] all of which are associated with potential significant electrolyte abnormalities.

POTENTIAL MIMICS

An infarct of the brainstem can mimic central pontine myelinolysis; however, with an infarct, no histologically viable neurons will be present in the area of damage; whereas in central pontine myelinolysis, the foamy macrophages will be found among histologically viable neurons.

GLOBUS PALLIDUS/BASAL GANGLIA NECROSIS

AUTOPSY FINDINGS

The basal ganglia nuclei, often the globus pallidus, are necrotic, which can vary from small foci within the nucleus to the entire nucleus being affected. The gross changes are the same as those of a cerebral infarct (Figure 7.18A and B). Microscopic examination can reveal the variety of appearances associated with variable timing of an infarct (eg, from red neurons to a cystic space in the gray matter).

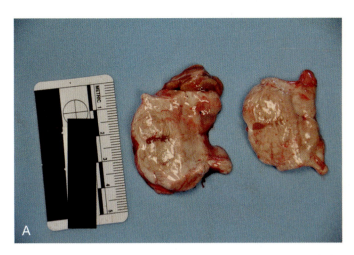
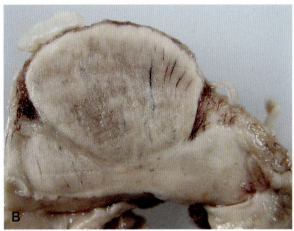
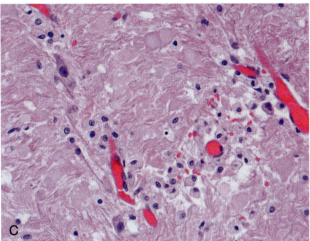

Figure 7.17. Central pontine myelinolysis. In the center of the pons will be a gray discoloration or friable region (**A** and **B**). On longitudinal section, the lesion can resemble a football. Microscopic examination (**C**, high power) will reveal macrophages with scattered histologically viable neurons, whereas, with an infarct, which is in the differential diagnosis, histologically viable neurons would not be present. In (**C**), spheroids are also present.

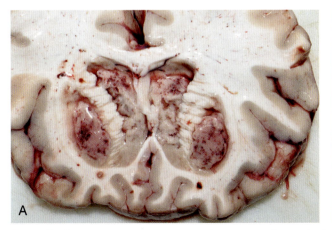
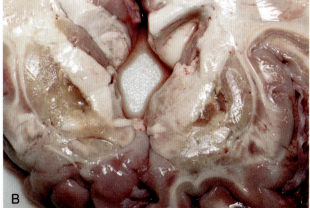

Figure 7.18. Globus pallidus necrosis. Both images are from individuals who had a delayed death associated with a drug overdose. In (**A**), the basal ganglia nuclei are necrotic. Each nucleus actually completely shelled out from its respective position. (**B**) is from an overdose that occurred several weeks prior to death, with the necrotic region having the appearance of an organizing cerebral infarct.

ASSOCIATION OF GLOBUS PALLIDUS NECROSIS

While globus pallidus necrosis has been historically associated with carbon monoxide exposure, in their review of the condition, Yarid and Harruff found that in 27 cases, globus pallidus necrosis was associated with drug overdose most commonly, but also heart disease and asphyxia, as well as a few cases associated with chronic ethanolism, Huntingtonlike disorder, remote trauma, rheumatic heart disease, and cerebral artery gas embolism.[48] Of the cases of carbon monoxide poisoning in their office records, Yarid and Haruff found that none were associated with globus pallidus or basal ganglia necrosis.[48] In agreement, Alquist et al described globus pallidus necrosis in opiate addicts.[49] However, in comparison to Yarid and Haruff, Chen et al described globus pallidus necrosis in nearly two-thirds of patients who attempted suicide via exposure to burning charcoal, but the mortality rate had only been 3%.[48,50] Therefore, globus pallidus/basal ganglia necrosis is most likely a change that occurs over time and not in the relatively acute time frame that carbon monoxide poisoning causes death as most frequently seen by a forensic pathologist at autopsy.

MULTIPLE SCLEROSIS

AUTOPSY FINDINGS

Multiple sclerosis is a disorder of demyelination characterized by plaques in the white matter (Figure 7.19A and B). One good region to search for plaques is at the junction of the corpus callosum with the adjacent cerebral parenchyma. If the diagnosis of multiple sclerosis is known, or identified upon dissection of the brain, removal of the spinal cord would best help determine the extent of the disease process.

> **PEARLS & PITFALLS**
>
> A past history of head trauma has been described as a risk factor for the development of multiple sclerosis.[51] If a decedent is determined to have died from the complications of multiple sclerosis, determining whether or not they have a past history of head trauma would be prudent. If the multiple sclerosis can be linked timewise to the head trauma, the manner of death may be related to the traumatic event.

CHRONIC TRAUMATIC ENCEPHALOPATHY

AUTOPSY FINDINGS

Chronic traumatic encephalopathy (CTE), a neurodegenerative disease associated with repetitive head trauma, is characterized by an abnormal accumulation of hyperphosphorylated tau in neurons and astrocytes, which are found in an irregular pattern around small blood vessels at the depth of the cortical sulci.[52] Early in the disease, the hyperphosphorylated tau is confined to the cortical gray matter, but with progression of the disease,

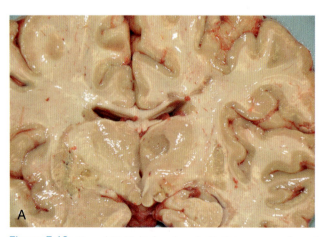
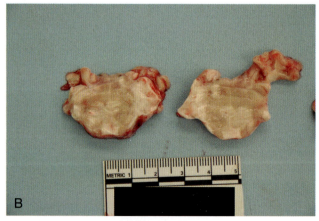

Figure 7.19. (**A** and **B**) Multiple sclerosis. Both images are from the same patient, and illustrate the patchy nature of the disease, with plaques at the angles of the lateral ventricles and both in the cerebral hemispheres and the brainstem.

> **PEARLS & PITFALLS**
>
> While chronic traumatic encephalopathy has been described in individuals with repetitive head trauma (eg, boxers and football players), Iverson et al discussed the pathologic findings of CTE in individuals with substance abuse, temporal lobe epilepsy, and neurodegenerative diseases, including amyotrophic lateral sclerosis (ALS) and multiple system atrophy.[53]

> **PEARLS & PITFALLS**
>
> As chronic traumatic encephalopathy has been associated with suicide, and as families are potentially aware of the diagnosis of CTE given its portrayal in the media, when autopsying individuals who have committed suicide and have in their past a history of repetitive head injuries, it would be useful to save sections of the brain that will allow for the future diagnosis of CTE should the family request it.

hyperphosphorylated tau can be identified in the diencephalon, the brainstem, and medial temporal lobe structures, such as the hippocampus, entorhinal cortex, and the amygdala.[52]

SEIZURE DISORDER

AUTOPSY FINDINGS

Upon gross examination of the brain in individuals with a seizure disorder, most frequently, no mass or other specific lesion will be identified, unless the decedent's seizures are due to trauma, and even if the seizures are trauma-related, gross examination of the brain may still reveal no pathologic changes as the pathologic changes from previous head injury can be subtle to non-existent on gross examination of the brain. Microscopic examination of the hippocampus in individuals with a seizure disorder can reveal mesial temporal sclerosis (Figure 7.20A-C), which is neuronal loss in Ammon's horn associated with gliosis.[54-56] While not a specific neuropathologic finding, contusions of the tongue can be found in people with seizure disorders. In fact, the identification of contusions of the tongue in a decedent with little or no available history at the time of autopsy may clue a forensic pathologist as to the possible mechanism of death as a seizure, albeit with the understanding that decedents with a contusion of the tongue may not have sustained a seizure.

ASSOCIATION WITH SUDDEN DEATH

SUDEP (sudden unexpected death in epilepsy) causes the death of 1 in 1000 individuals with epilepsy each year.[57,58] One important risk factor for SUDEP is whether or not the decedent had generalized tonic-clonic seizures and how often they had those seizures.[57] Determining that the seizure disorder itself is the cause of death is a diagnosis of exclusion and requires ruling out other causes of death. In addition to being a cause of sudden death, a seizure disorder can contribute to death from another mechanism (eg, choking on food triggered by the seizure, or blunt force injuries of the head occurring after a seizure-induced fall). If the seizure is non-traumatic in origin, the manner of death for SUDEP is natural; however, if the decedent dies as a result of a traumatic situation induced by the seizure (eg, choking on food), the manner is accident.

> **PEARLS & PITFALLS**
>
> When the cause of death is a seizure disorder, the etiology of the seizure disorder must be determined. If the seizure disorder is traumatic in origin, the nature of the trauma determines the manner of death. For example, if the individual developed a seizure disorder after an assault by another person and the seizure disorder was determined to be the cause of death, the manner of death could be certified as homicide.

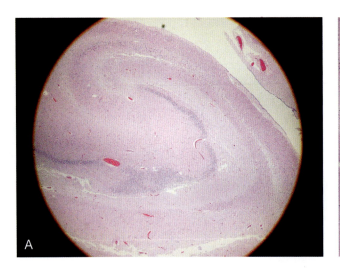
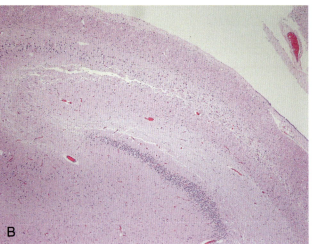
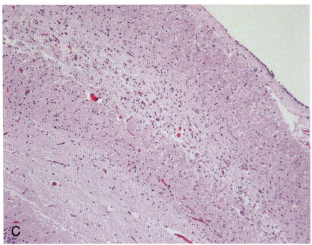

Figure 7.20. (**A-C**) Mesial temporal sclerosis. In the CA1 sector of the hippocampus is complete loss of neurons associated with some gliosis (low, medium, and high power, respectively).

> **PEARLS & PITFALLS**
>
> If an individual has a seizure and as a result ends up in a face-down position or other position that impairs their breathing, a positional asphyxial death can occur as in the post-ictal state, the decedent may not be able to move.

ALZHEIMER DISEASE

AUTOPSY FINDINGS

Gross examination of the brain can reveal atrophy (Figure 7.21A). Microscopic examination of the cerebral parenchyma will reveal neurofibrillary tangles, senile plaques, granulovacuolar degeneration, and Hirano bodies (Figure 7.21B-D). The plaque distribution in correlation with the age and symptomatology of the patient will determine the likelihood of Alzheimer disease as the diagnosis.[25]

DIFFUSE LEWY BODY DISEASE

AUTOPSY FINDINGS

Microscopic examination of the cerebral parenchyma, including specifically the entorhinal cortex and cingulate gyrus, will reveal cortical Lewy bodies; however, these Lewy bodies

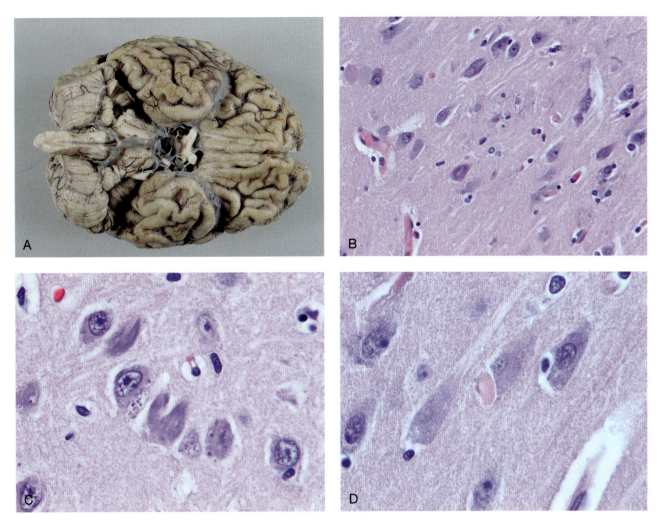

Figure 7.21. Alzheimer disease. Gross examination of the brain can reveal atrophy, with widening of the sulci (**A**). Microscopic examination can reveal plaques (**B**, high power), neurofibrillary tangles (**C**, high power), and Hirano bodies (**D**, high power). Hematoxylin and eosin are not the best method to assess for the changes, with thioflavin-S, or Bielschowsky silver stains being much better methods that can be used, and the changes must always be correlated with the symptoms of the decedent as the pathologic changes of Alzheimer disease also occur with increasing age.

are difficult to identify on hematoxylin and eosin (H&E) stain and require α-synuclein immunohistochemical staining to best differentiate them. Diffuse Lewy body disease is the second most common cause of dementia, and often, individuals diagnosed with Alzheimer disease in actuality have diffuse Lewy body disease.

ENCEPHALITIS

AUTOPSY FINDINGS

While the necrotizing feature of herpes simplex virus encephalitis provides gross evidence of the underlying disease process,[59] other forms of encephalitis may only present with cerebral edema, or no gross pathologic findings at all. The microscopic diagnosis of encephalitis is based upon the findings of microglial nodules, inflammatory cells in the Virchow-Robin spaces, and neuronophagia (Figure 7.22A and B).

PEARLS & PITFALLS

Microglial nodules and/or perivascular cuffing of the vessels, particularly of the nucleus and/or the spinal tract of the fifth cranial nerve, can be an incidental finding at autopsy and is not necessarily indicative of a significant disease process.[60]

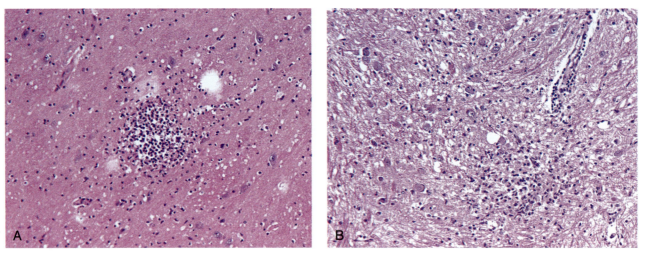

Figure 7.22. Encephalitis. The microscopic features of encephalitis are microglial nodules (**A** and **B**, medium power), lymphocytic cuffing in the Virchow-Robin spaces of vessels (**B**, medium power), and neuronophagia.

COLLOID CYST

AUTOPSY FINDINGS

A colloid cyst is composed of a fibrous capsule with an inner layer of mucin-producing or ciliated epithelium and with the cyst containing periodic acid-Schiff (PAS)–positive mucoid material.[61] Colloid cysts are a rare congenital cyst of the brain, most often found in the third ventricle and can cause sudden death, with the cyst obstructing the flow of cerebrospinal fluid and leading to hydrocephalus.[62] Lagman et al indicate that of 107 individuals who died as the result of a colloid cyst, the mean diameter of the cyst was 2.0 cm, with a range of 0.5 to 7.9 cm.[63]

NATURAL DISEASE OF THE CARDIOVASCULAR SYSTEM

INTRODUCTION

At autopsy, the most commonly encountered natural diseases of the cardiovascular system include coronary artery atherosclerosis and its complications, cardiomegaly (most often associated with underlying hypertension but also alcohol-induced dilated cardiomyopathies), and some valvular disorders (bicuspid aortic valve and myxomatous mitral valve); however, the range of diseases which the forensic pathologist might encounter in the heart is broad, including also pericarditis, myocarditis, endocarditis, coronary artery dissections, other valvular heart disease, cardiomyopathies, coronary artery anomalies, and conduction system abnormalities.

PEARLS & PITFALLS

If a decedent with an implanted cardiac device sustains a sudden death, with no identifiable cause at autopsy, the medical device representative may be able to do a postmortem interrogation of the device and determine whether or not the decedent sustained a lethal cardiac dysrhythmia at the time of their collapse, which can help determine the cause of death and time of death.[64,65] If the implanted device is an implantable cardioverter-defibrillator, care must be taken during removal at autopsy to prevent electrical shock.[66] A magnet placed on the device or the use of certain types of gloves reportedly can prevent shock.[67]

HYPERTENSIVE HEART DISEASE

AUTOPSY FINDINGS

Associated with systemic hypertension, the heart will be enlarged. When measuring the weight of the heart, it is best to include as little of the great vessels as possible and ensure that the chambers are cleared of postmortem clots, both of which can significantly increase the measured weight of the heart. The thickness of the chamber walls can also be measured; however, it is important to not include the trabecular muscle in the measurement. Microscopic examination can reveal hypertrophied cardiac myocytes, identified by enlarged and rectangular nuclei. Some increased interstitial and perivascular fibrosis may also be present.

ASSOCIATION WITH SUDDEN DEATH

Many authors report that cardiac hypertrophy, which is a feature of hypertensive heart disease, is well associated with sudden cardiac death.[68-71] As such, individuals with hypertensive heart disease have an increased risk for sudden cardiac death. Individuals who sustain a sudden cardiac death related to hypertensive heart disease are often asymptomatic prior to their death and frequently do not have an antemortem diagnosis of hypertension.[68]

> **FAQ:** What weight of the heart can be accepted as representing a cause of death?
>
> **Answer:** Various sources are available to compare the weight of the heart at autopsy to reference ranges developed by authors based upon their analysis of large numbers of autopsy heart weights.[72-77] Kumar et al describe the normal heart weight for a 60 to 70 kg person as 320 to 360 g, but do not distinguish based upon the sex of the individual.[27] In addition, Schoppen et al provide an online calculator to determine the threshold for cardiomegaly for decedents after sudden cardiac death at an age less than 40 years (https://labs.feinberg.northwestern.edu/webster/heart_weight).[78]
>
> Instead of comparing the autopsy weight to weight reference ranges developed by other authors, some forensic pathologists use absolute cutoffs, such as 400 g or 500 g, as a guide to whether or not the cardiomegaly is a cause of death. Basso et al indicate that a 500 g heart weight in an adult male and a 400 g heart weight in adult female are acceptable as a cutoff for a measure of a significant and potentially lethal increase in heart weight if no other comparison is available.[79] While it would seem to be the best method of the two described above, comparing heart weight at autopsy to available reference ranges will not always work, such as if the population upon which the author's reference ranges are developed do not match those of the decedent. For example, based upon a Japanese population, Kakimoto et al found cutoff values for hypertrophy as 407 g in males and 327 g in females, which varies from Basso et al's values mentioned above.[79,80] In conclusion, the determination of a sudden cardiac death due to a cardiac dysrhythmia induced by an enlarged heart is a diagnosis of exclusion and requires ruling out other possible causes of death. How each pathologist approaches the answer to this question is based upon their education and preferences, but consistency is important.

> **PEARLS & PITFALLS**
>
> While hypertension is a risk factor for the development of atherosclerosis and is a cause of cardiac hypertrophy, an enlarged heart by itself, regardless of the cause of cardiac enlargement, is also a risk factor for the development of coronary artery atherosclerosis.[81]

CORONARY ARTERY ATHEROSCLEROSIS

AUTOPSY FINDINGS

Serial sections of the coronary arteries will reveal variable degrees of stenosis due to atherosclerotic plaque. Plaques can be stable or unstable, with unstable plaques having an acute change, such as hemorrhage (Figure 7.23A and B). Thrombi, which can be

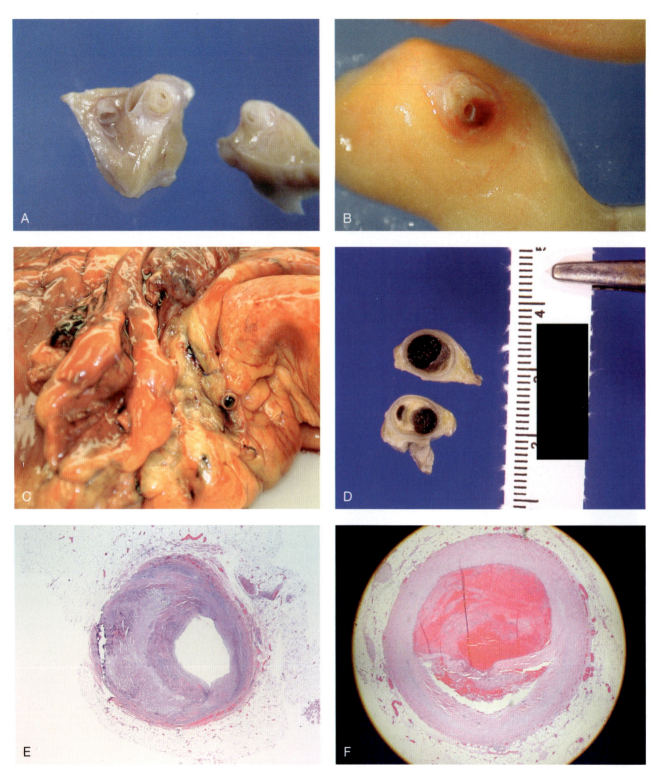

Figure 7.23. Coronary artery atherosclerosis and complications. (**A**) is a significantly stenotic plaque, with only a tiny residual lumen; however, the plaque is stable, with no evidence of an acute change, which is in contrast to (**B**), which is a plaque with focal hemorrhage. (**C** and **D**) are examples of coronary artery thrombi. Care must be taken to not confuse postmortem clots with antemortem thrombi. Postmortem clots often do not distend the lumen and appear more gelatinous in texture. (**E**) illustrates the fibrous cap and atheromatous core of a stable plaque, although there is a small focus of extravasated red blood cells (low power). (**F** and **G**) (low and high power) illustrate a ruptured plaque with resultant occlusive thrombosis. The thrombogenic atheromatous material can be seen at the rupture point of the fibrous cap in (**G**) (high power). (**H**) (low power) illustrates an intraplaque hemorrhage, which has expanded the size of the plaque, but not ruptured the fibrous cap. The lumen is patent. (**I**) (low power) is a non-occlusive thrombus. Thrombi can form secondary to rupture of the plaque and exposure of the atheromatous core, but also due to fissuring or erosion of the plaque. (**J**) is an occluded coronary artery. The cross section reveals areas of yellow discoloration, which represents the atheromatous material, and a gray peri-central region, which, upon gross inspection, could be a thrombus but could also be an atheromatous core. Microscopic examination would allow for a more definitive determination of the nature of the coronary artery lesion.

Figure 7.23 (continued)

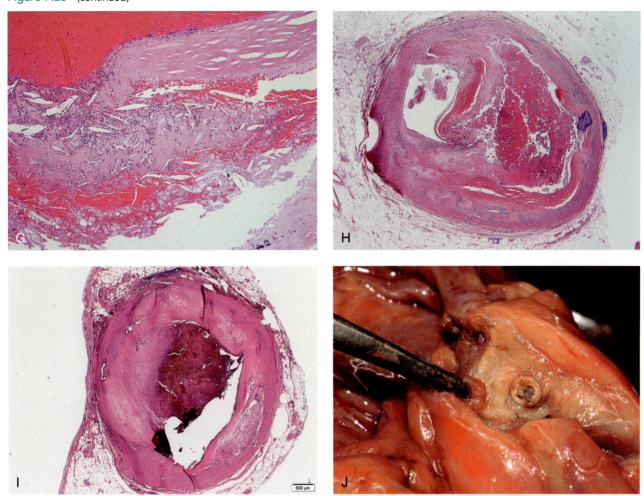

associated with an acute change in the plaque that leads to rupture, can also be identified during sectioning of the coronary arteries (Figure 7.23C and D). The section intervals, ideally, should be close enough together so that each segment of the coronary artery produced can be seen completely through to the other side, which will ensure that the entire length of the coronary artery is examined for areas of stenosis or obstruction. Thrombi and significant sites of stenosis can be very short (eg, a few millimeters in length) and if long segments of coronary artery are produced during the sectioning process, which do not allow for visualization of the entire length of the vessel, a significant lesion can easily be missed. While the coronary arteries can be opened longitudinally, this method would essentially preclude determination of the degree of stenosis as the degree of stenosis is based upon the cross-sectional appearance. Also, the tip of the scissors could dislodge or disrupt thrombi. Microscopic examination of a coronary artery lesion can help identify the features of the plaque such as the thickness of the fibrous cap and any acute changes in the plaque that might not have been visible grossly, and can confirm that a gross finding of a suspected thrombus is in actuality a thrombus, as a plaque composed of a prominent atheromatous core can easily mimic an acute thrombus on gross inspection (Figure 7.23E-J).

SAMPLE NOTES: DOCUMENTATION OF CORONARY ARTERY ATHEROSCLEROSIS AT AUTOPSY

Ideally, the location of each atherosclerotic plaque (eg, proximal, mid, or distal) in each of the major epicardial coronary arteries and the degree of stenosis caused by each plaque would be documented. Using a diagram of the heart can facilitate the recording of such data. While the degree of stenosis can be assessed in subjective terms (eg, mild, moderate, and severe), this method does not give the reader as clear of an indication of the degree of stenosis as a percentage number would (eg, 65%). The degree of stenosis can be expressed as a single estimate (eg, 75%) or as a range (eg, 65%-75%). Having a series of images available for comparison such as either actual gross and microscopic images of coronary artery atherosclerosis or a simple diagram can assist in the determination of the degree of stenosis[82] (Tables 7.1 and 7.2). Using Image J (https://imagej.nih.gov/ij/download.html), the percentage of stenosis can be directly calculated from a digital image.

FAQ: Does the degree of stenosis identified at autopsy correlate with the degree of stenosis caused by the coronary artery lesion in the living person?

Answer: Autopsy cannot accurately determine how much dilation a particular vessel is capable of to compensate for the atherosclerosis. Perfusion of the coronary arteries provides tension against the wall, whereas, this pressure is not present at autopsy. Sheppard and Davies have interesting photographs of perfusion fixed coronary arteries with atherosclerotic plaque that demonstrate how a lesion that is deemed to be of significance at autopsy may not actually be as stenotic in the living person.[83]

ASSOCIATION OF CORONARY ARTERY ATHEROSCLEROSIS WITH SUDDEN DEATH

Markwerth et al indicate that coronary artery stenosis (of any degree) associated with a normal myocardium or with fibrosis of the myocardium is not clearly consistent with sudden death; however, plaques associated with contraction band necrosis or complicated plaques associated with normal myocardium or with fibrosis are consistent with sudden death.[84] However, Basso et al indicate that an atherosclerotic plaque with coronary luminal stenosis >75% is highly probable as the cause of sudden cardiac death.[85] In their study of 5869 cases of sudden death, 600 of which had histologic study of the coronary arteries, Holmström et al found that only around 50% of the individuals had an acute plaque change (intraplaque hemorrhage, or a plaque rupture or erosion), with the other around 50% of the group just having a stable plaque.[86]

PEARLS & PITFALLS

Cocaine and amphetamine use have been associated with intimal hyperplasia in the coronary artery[87-89] (Figure 7.24). This intimal hyperplasia can lead to significant sites of stenosis, but the lesions can have minimal to none of the typical atheromatous component found in most plaques.

GROSS AND MICROSCOPIC AGING OF AN ACUTE MYOCARDIAL INFARCT

Grossly, pallor of the myocardium or red discoloration, which occurs with reperfusion, occurs around several hours to 1 day after the inciting event, with variable degrees of

TABLE 7.1: Representative Degrees of Stenosis (Gross Appearance)

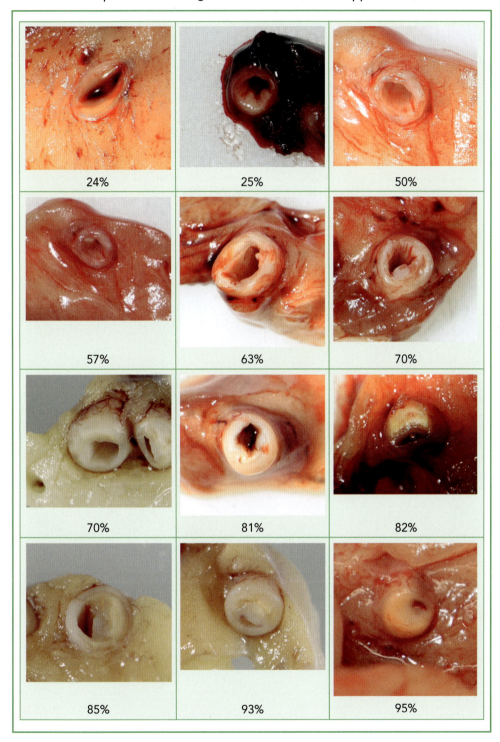

coagulative necrosis, contraction band necrosis, and some neutrophilic infiltrate present upon microscopic examination (Figure 7.25A-C).[27] Ill-defined fibrous scarring can easily mimic a recent acute myocardial infarct, causing pallor of the section of the heart (Figure 7.25D). Lividity can mimic a reperfused acute myocardial infarct.

Grossly, yellow discoloration with variable amounts of contraction of the myocardium occurs from one to 10 days after the inciting event.[27] The associated microscopic changes will be coagulative necrosis and neutrophilic infiltrate centered at 1 to 3 days, with subsequent macrophage infiltration centered around 3 to 7 days, and early granulation tissue

TABLE 7.2: Representative Degrees of Stenosis (Microscopic Appearance)

25%	40%	46%
49%	60%	62%
67%	71%	84%
85%	90%	99%

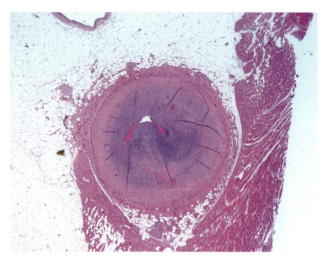

Figure 7.24. Intimal hyperplasia in cocaine user. The coronary artery is significantly stenotic; however, essentially all of the stenosis is produced by intimal hyperplasia, with essentially no atheromatous change present in the lesion (low power).

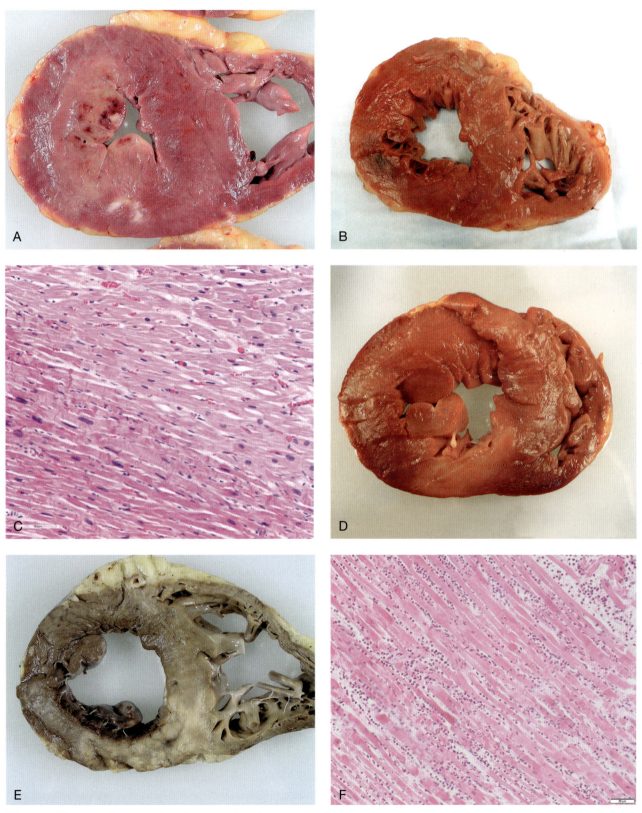

Figure 7.25. Aging of a myocardial infarct, grossly and microscopically. (**A**) is an acute myocardial infarct with pallor and focal hemorrhage of the myocardium. With reperfusion, hemorrhagic discoloration of the infarct can occur (**B**). Early changes can include coagulative necrosis and contraction band necrosis with minimal neutrophilic infiltrate (**C**; high power). In the inferior wall of the left ventricle in (**D**) is an area of pallor, which could mimic an acute myocardial infarct. Close inspection reveals some white fibrous scar and microscopic examination revealed only a remote infarct. The yellow discoloration in the inferior-septal wall of the left ventricle in (**E**) is an acute infarct, with the corresponding microscopic examination revealing coagulative necrosis and neutrophils (**F**, medium power).

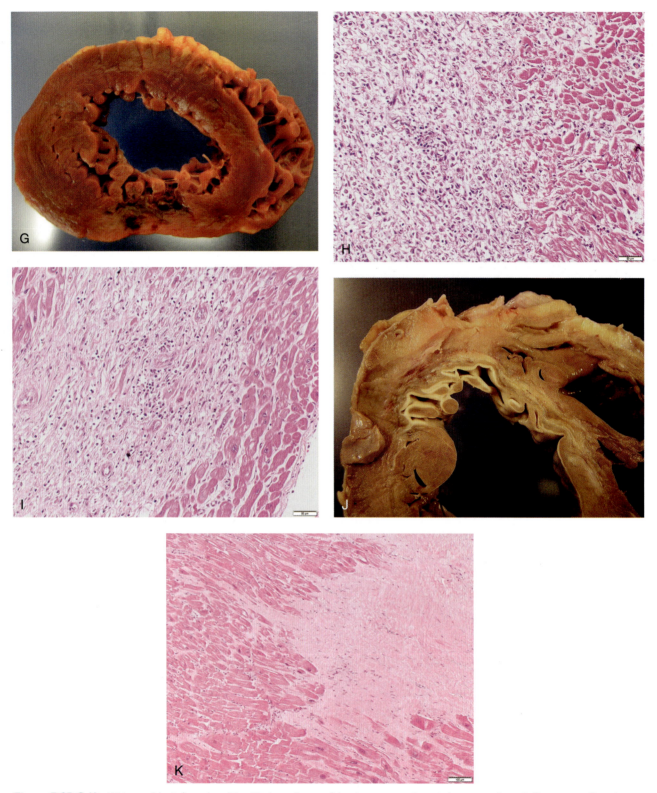

Figure 7.25 G-K (**G**) is an older infarct than (**E**), with the collapse of the tissue secondary to the macrophage infiltrate engulfing the dead cells and debris (**H**, medium power). (**I**) is fibrotic but still cellular (medium power). (**J** and **K**) are a remote infarct, with thinning of the anterior wall of the left ventricle associated with fibrous scar, and the myocardium replaced by a dense acellular region of fibrosis microscopically (**K**, low power).

centered around 7 to 10 days[27] (Figure 7.25E-H). In addition, hemosiderin would be present about 2 to 3 days following the infarct, assuming hemorrhage was a component. The microscopic findings are easier to interpret and less subjective than the gross appearance.

Grossly, gray discoloration/translucent tissue occurs from 2 weeks to 2 months post infarct as granulation tissue forms and develops into a scar.[27] The myocardium can have

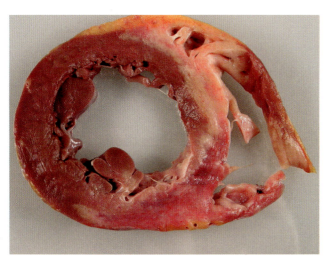

Figure 7.26. Sarcoidosis of the heart. Although the gross appearance is similar to a remote myocardial infarct, the coronary arteries had no significant sites of stenosis, and microscopic examination revealed granulomas associated with fibrosis.

a variety of appearances microscopically. Macrophages will remove the neutrophils and dead myocytes. Granulation tissue with collagen and new blood vessel formation will develop, and gradually become a dense acellular scar (Figure 7.25I-K), which takes about 2 months.[27]

With a dense fibrous scar, the myocardium will have a well-defined area of firm white discoloration, which on microscopic examination is fibrosis with little to no cellularity. While a white fibrous scar in the myocardium is most consistent with remote ischemic injury, other conditions can produce a similar finding. If no significant degree of atherosclerosis is present in the coronary arteries, microscopic examination of the scar may reveal another etiology such as sarcoidosis (Figure 7.26).

PEARLS & PITFALLS

When an individual sustains a sudden death and is found to have a remote myocardial infarct, close examination of the edges of the infarct is useful, as is microscopic examination of those regions. As the remote myocardial infarct indicates past ischemic injury, current ischemic injury (ie, the cause of the decedent's death) may be found at the rim of the past injury, as that area has proven itself sensitive to ischemic injury before (Figure 7.27A and B).

PEARLS & PITFALLS

Following an acute myocardial infarct, the individual must survive for some period of time if gross and microscopic changes in the heart are to be appreciated at autopsy. Some microscopic changes can occur within an hour or so though (eg, wavy fiber changes) (Figure 7.28). Available clinical history and testing (eg, electrocardiographic (ECG) changes and/or cardiac troponin concentrations) may provide additional information.

PEARLS & PITFALLS

If a decedent has been resuscitated and/or if catecholamines have been given to the decedent, interpretation of contraction band necrosis as a sign of ischemic injury must be done carefully, as both of these situations (ie, resuscitation and catecholamines) are associated with contraction band necrosis as well.[84]

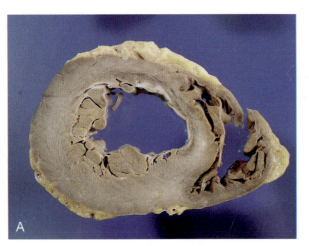 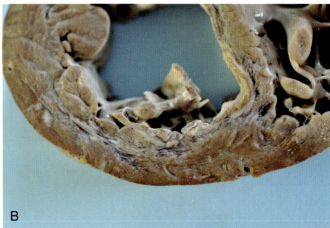

Figure 7.27. (**A** and **B**) Remote myocardial infarcts with hemorrhagic discoloration of the rim. At the rim of both remote myocardial infarcts is a hemorrhagic discoloration. This discoloration may be recent ischemic injury or it may just be congestion associated with the scar. Microscopic examination is necessary to definitively distinguish between the two possibilities.

COMPLICATIONS OF ACUTE MYOCARDIAL INFARCT

At autopsy, individuals who have survived the initial period after the development of an acute myocardial infarct can die from subsequent complications. If the infarct involves >40% of the myocardium, heart failure can develop (Figure 7.29A).[27] With a transmural infarct, rupture of the myocardium can occur. Following free wall rupture, a hemopericardium occurs, which can rapidly lead to death (Figure 7.29B-D). Rupture of the interventricular septum or papillary muscle of the mitral valve can also occur after an acute myocardial infarct; however, symptomatology and a delay before death may allow those individuals to seek medical care, and not present as a sudden death in a forensic context. Kumar et al describe that rupture occurs 3 to 7 days following the infarct; however, Buja and Butany describe that ruptures occur in two peaks, one at <24 hours and the other at 3 to 5 days following the infarct.[27,90] Acute mitral insufficiency does not require rupture of the papillary muscle as just infarction can affect its function (Figure 7.29E).

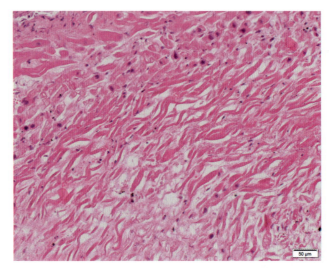

Figure 7.28. Wavy fibers. Wavy fibers are the earliest histologic change of an acute myocardial infarct. As in the image, coagulative necrosis can accompany the change. Just wavy fibers without accompanying coagulative necrosis or contraction band necrosis should be interpreted cautiously to prevent miscalling artifact as early ischemic injury (high power).

Mural thrombi, with potential resultant emboli, could present as a sudden death following embolization to a coronary or cerebral artery (Figure 7.29F). While post-myocardial infarct–related pericarditis is not a likely cause of death, the finding of pericarditis necessitates a search for the etiology, of which an acute myocardial infarct is one possibility (Figure 7.29G).

> **PEARLS & PITFALLS**
>
> Both calcification of the coronary arteries and previous stent placement can impair the examination of the coronary arteries at the time of autopsy. If a detailed examination of the coronary arteries is necessary, the entire coronary artery length can be dissected from the surface of the heart and placed in a decalcifying solution to allow for close examination of calcified vessels. Methods to examine coronary arteries with stents in place are also available.[91,92]

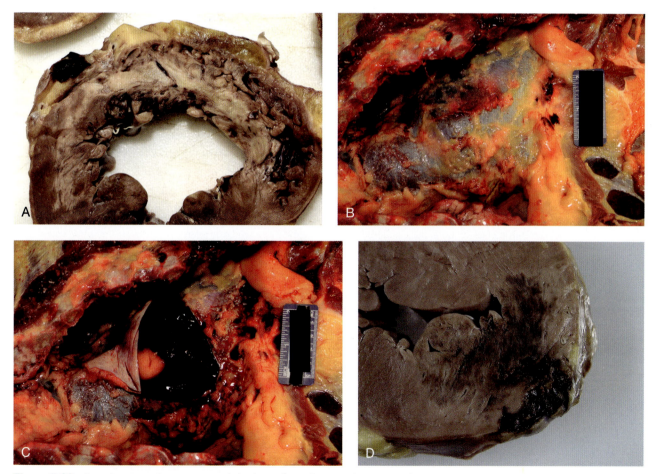

Figure 7.29. Complications of acute myocardial infarct. If an infarct involves >40% of the myocardium, heart failure can develop. (**A**) is a large infarct in the distribution of the left anterior descending coronary artery and involves about 40% of the myocardium in the section. (**B-D**) illustrate a hemopericardium due to a ruptured acute myocardial infarct. The blue discoloration of the unopened pericardial sac indicates blood around the heart (**B**). Upon opening the pericardial sac, the amount of blood should be measured (**C**). The rupture site can be identified in situ within the left or potentially right ventricle wall. If the infarct involves the right ventricle it is most likely due to extension from an inferior left ventricular wall infarct. The rupture site can be quite obvious with a wide gap in the myocardium, or more serpiginous and difficult to identify (**D**).

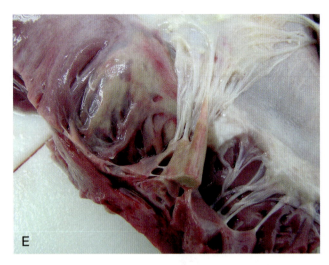
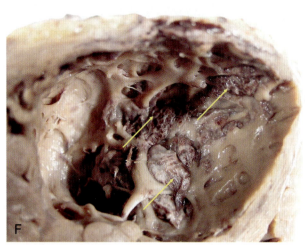
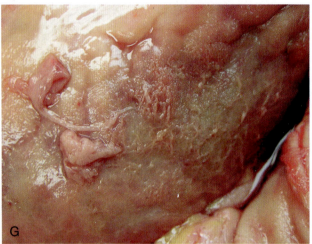

Figure 7.29 E-G Infarction of the papillary muscle with or without rupture can lead to mitral insufficiency. In (**E**), the papillary muscle is infarcted, but not ruptured. Mural thrombi (arrows) can form on the endocardial surface of the ventricle at the site of the infarct (**F**). These mural thrombi can stay in place, or potentially embolize. Focal pericarditis can overlie an infarct, when the infarct is transmural (**G**). Dressler syndrome is more diffuse and occurs weeks after the infarct.

SAMPLE NOTE: POTENTIAL WORDINGS FOR THE DEATH CERTIFICATE WHEN CORONARY ARTERY ATHEROSCLEROSIS IS THE KNOWN OR SUSPECTED UNDERLYING ETIOLOGY

If an individual dies suddenly under non-suspicious circumstances and is thought to have coronary artery disease because of their age, sex, family history, and other risk factors (history of smoking, diabetes mellitus, high cholesterol, and hypertension) but no autopsy is performed, the cause of death may be worded as "Arteriosclerotic cardiovascular disease" or "Atherosclerotic cardiovascular disease." Of the two wordings, arteriosclerotic cardiovascular disease is the more broad choice and covers more possible specific entities. If the individual has a history of hypertension, this diagnosis can be incorporated into the cause of death statement, such as "Hypertensive and arteriosclerotic cardiovascular disease" or "Hypertensive and atherosclerotic cardiovascular disease."

If an individual dies suddenly and an autopsy identifies significant stenosis of a coronary artery by atherosclerotic plaque (eg, around 75%), the cause of death may be worded in one of several ways, "Coronary artery atherosclerosis." "Severe coronary artery atherosclerosis," and "Critical coronary artery atherosclerosis," among others. If the certifier so wishes, a mechanism could be added. For example, "Cardiac dysrhythmia due to severe coronary artery atherosclerosis" is acceptable.

If clinical history (eg, history of ECG changes or elevated troponin I) and/or autopsy findings identify an acute myocardial infarct associated with an acute coronary artery change such as acute thrombosis, the death certificate can be worded as "Acute myocardial infarct due to Thrombosis of the coronary artery due to Coronary artery atherosclerosis." If an individual is found unresponsive, with no subsequent clinical evaluation, and an autopsy identifies severe coronary artery atherosclerosis, but no acute changes in the myocardium, it is best not to include "acute myocardial infarct" in the cause of death statement, as there is no evidence of such a pathologic process.

AORTIC DISSECTION

AUTOPSY FINDINGS

A tear in the intima of the aorta occurs, leading to blood tracking through the media in the outer two-thirds (Figure 7.30A), and eventually rupturing back in to the lumen of the aorta, or out through the adventitia, with a resultant hemopericardium (Figure 7.30B) or hemothorax most likely, but with retroperitoneal hemorrhage also possible. Within the wall of the aorta can be a variable amount of blood, varying from a thick hematoma to just separation of the wall with minimal hemorrhage in the cleavage plane (Figure 7.30C-E). Microscopic examination of the aorta can be performed to identify any pathologic process that may be related to the dissection, including inflammation or cystic medial degeneration (Figure 7.30F), which is found in both systemic hypertension and Marfan syndrome.

SAMPLE NOTES: DOCUMENTATION OF AORTIC DISSECTION AT AUTOPSY

The originating tear in the intima can be described by size and location, such as distance from the aortic valve. The tear in the intima may not be reflective of the subsequent tear in the outer adventitia. Filling the aorta with water will allow for an appreciation of the size of the defect through which blood was escaping from the aorta into the surrounding tissue or into the adjacent cavity (Figure 7.31A and B).

CORONARY ARTERY DISSECTION

AUTOPSY FINDINGS

In the wall of the coronary artery will be hemorrhage, which is visible grossly (Figure 7.32A). Microscopic examination could confirm the hemorrhage (Figure 7.32B). Like in aortic dissection, the hemorrhage is most often in the outer two-thirds of the media.

ASSOCIATIONS

Coronary artery dissection is a rare cause of ischemic cardiac disease and is commonly associated with pregnancy but can occur in males as well.

> **PEARLS & PITFALLS**
>
> Examination of a coronary artery dissection, if close attention is not paid to the appearance, can lead to misinterpretation of the lesion as a thrombus in the coronary artery lumen.

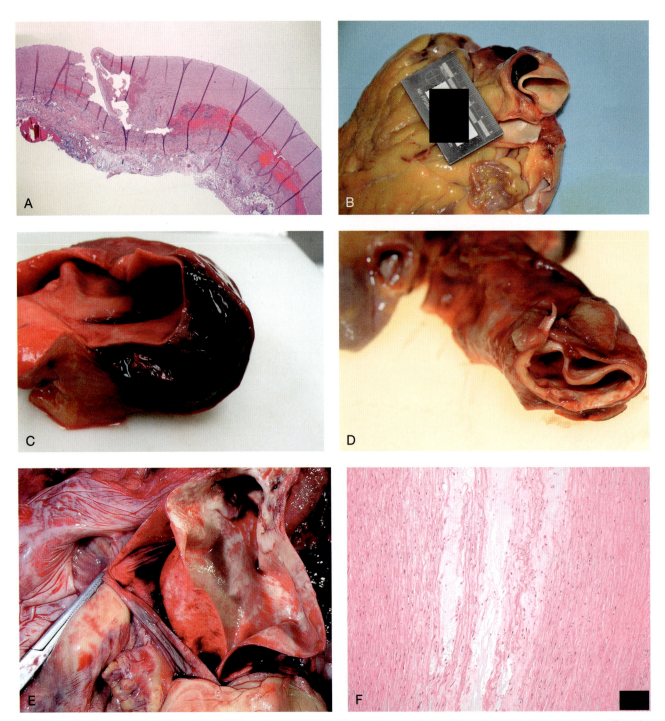

Figure 7.30. Features of aortic dissection. The dissection causes a tear in the intima, which then dissects through the media, normally in the outer two-thirds of the wall (**A**, low power). The dissection can continue to the aortic valve, leading to aortic insufficiency, but can also tear out of the adventitial surface near the aortic valve, and within the pericardial sac, leading to a hemopericardium (**B**). The amount of blood in the wall can be prominent (**C**) or minimal, with essentially just a separation of the aortic wall present (**D** and **E**). Cystic medial degeneration is found in patients with hypertension and Marfan syndrome, appearing as myxoid acellular areas with the media (**F**, medium power).

ABDOMINAL AORTIC ANEURYSM

AUTOPSY FINDINGS

In the abdominal aorta, the most common form of an aneurysm is a saccular out-pouching from the wall of the aorta that ruptures into the retroperitoneum, and the hemorrhage can extend into the peritoneal cavity. While ruptured abdominal aortic aneurysms can be found

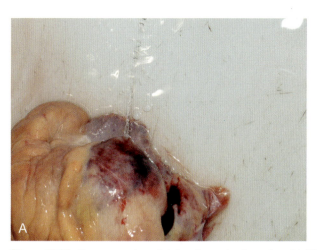 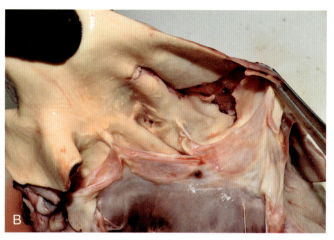

Figure 7.31. Demonstration of defect in aortic dissection. By filling the aorta with water, the size of the defect in the adventitia can be appreciated. While the water flowing from the aorta is in a thin stream, implying a pinhole defect in the adventitia (**A**), the corresponding tear in the intimal surface is much more extensive (**B**).

as the cause of death at forensic autopsy, the identification of an unruptured abdominal aortic aneurysm is potentially of importance to surviving relatives, as there is a familial component to some abdominal aortic aneurysms.[93]

CORONARY ARTERY ANEURYSM

AUTOPSY FINDINGS

The coronary artery will be dilated, which can be associated with thrombosis and/or rupture (Figure 7.33).

ASSOCIATIONS

Coronary artery aneurysms are most commonly associated with Kawasaki disease; however, they have been associated with other conditions as well, including COVID-19 (coronavirus disease 2019), idiopathic hypereosinophilic syndrome, polyarteritis nodosa, and Behçet syndrome.[94-98]

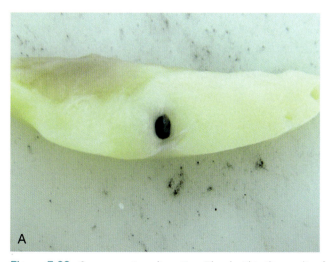 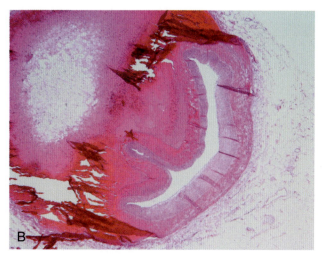

Figure 7.32. Coronary artery dissection. Blood within the media of the vessel, visible both grossly (**A**) and microscopically (**B**). The decedent in (**A**) was a male.

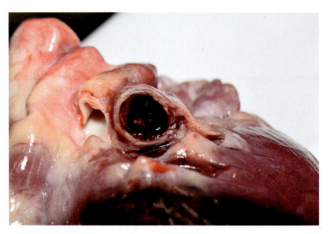

Figure 7.33. Coronary artery aneurysm. The proximal distribution of both the left anterior descending and right coronary arteries were markedly dilated. No evidence of an on-going vasculitis was identified upon microscopic examination.

AORTIC STENOSIS

AUTOPSY FINDINGS

Aortic stenosis is caused by fibrosis and calcification of the aortic valve cusps. Aortic stenosis can occur in a bicuspid aortic valve as well as a tricuspid aortic valve. The calcification develops as nodules within the sinus of Valsalva (Figure 7.34A). If fusion at the commissure has occurred, chronic rheumatic aortic valvulitis should be considered (Figure 7.34B).

ASSOCIATION WITH SUDDEN DEATH

Aortic stenosis leads to cardiac hypertrophy, which is associated with a risk for sudden death.

BICUSPID AORTIC VALVE

AUTOPSY FINDINGS

In most cases, the bicuspid aortic valve is formed by incomplete separation at a commissure, usually the commissure between the left and right sinuses of Valsalva, resulting in a midline raphe (Figure 7.35A). In this situation the two aortic valve cusps are dissimilar in

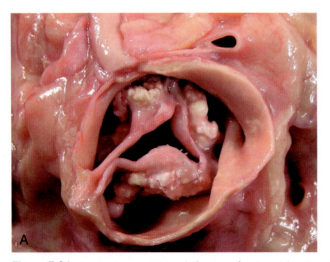
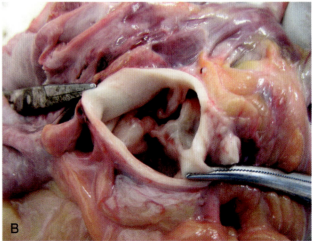

Figure 7.34. Aortic stenosis. (A) is calcification of a tricuspid aortic valve, with deposition of calcium on the sinus side of the cusps. (B) was chronic rheumatic aortic valvulitis, with fusion present at all three commissures.

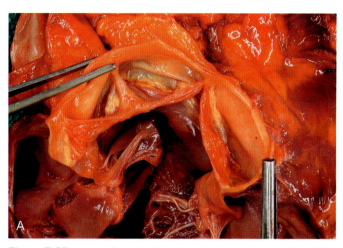
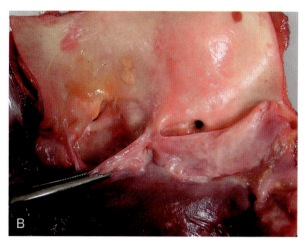

Figure 7.35. Bicuspid aortic valve. (**A**) is the more common form of bicuspid aortic valve, with a midline raphe from incomplete separation at a commissure. (**B**) is a true bicuspid aortic valve, with two cusps of equal size.

size, with one larger than the other. Rarely, just two separate cusps will form, each being the same size as the other (ie, a true bicuspid aortic valve) (Figure 7.35B).

> **FAQ:** Is a bicuspid aortic valve associated with sudden death?
>
> **Answer:** While aortic stenosis due to a bicuspid aortic valve can cause cardiac hypertrophy, which is a risk factor for sudden death, the valvular abnormality itself is not well associated with an increased risk for sudden death.

MYXOMATOUS MITRAL VALVE

AUTOPSY FINDINGS

The mitral valve leaflets will be redundant or ballooned toward the atrium (Figure 7.36A and B). The adjacent endocardium may be fibrotic, and it is possible for chordae tendineae to be ruptured. Microscopic examination will reveal a thinned fibrosa

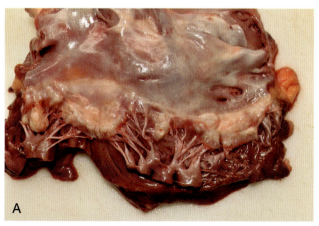
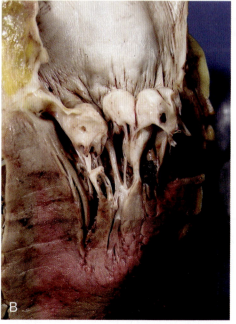

Figure 7.36. Myxomatous mitral valve. The redundancy or ballooning of the leaflets can vary from mild (**A**) to prominent (**B**). As redundancy of the mitral valve leaflets is also an age-related change, separating the true disease state from the age-related state can be a challenge, although in age-related myxoid change, the edges of the leaflets appear to be the most involved, while the disease state appears to more diffusely involve the entire leaflet.

layer and an expanded spongiosa layer.[27] A myxomatous mitral valve is the pathologic condition responsible for the clinical diagnosis of mitral valve prolapse.

ASSOCIATION WITH SUDDEN DEATH

Individuals with a myxomatous mitral valve are at risk for a sudden cardiac death.[99,100]

POTENTIAL MIMICS

With age, some redundancy of the mitral valve leaflets can occur, which does not indicate a disease process. Documenting whether the redundancy involves the entire leaflet or just the free edge may help distinguish between age-related change and a disease process.

CHRONIC RHEUMATIC MITRAL VALVULITIS

AUTOPSY FINDINGS

There is thickening of the mitral valve leaflets and fusion and shortening of the chordae tendineae (Figure 7.37). Microscopic examination will reveal fibrosis, but not Aschoff nodules, which are only associated with the acute stages of rheumatic fever.

POTENTIAL MIMIC

A muscular chorda can occur, which is a single thick mitral valve chorda tendinea (Figure 7.38), which could mimic a mild case of chronic rheumatic mitral valvulitis.[83,101]

> **FAQ:** Can autopsy identify dysfunctional valves (ie, those that are regurgitant or stenotic)?
>
> **Answer:** Assessing the functionality of valves at autopsy is challenging. The identification of stenosis is easier than the identification of insufficiency/regurgitation, as the pathologic changes are more demonstrative of the dysfunction. One method to help assess for stenosis or regurgitation is to examine the function of the valves while filling the chambers with water (eg, fill the left ventricle through the aorta and compress the heart, watching the function of the aortic valve). Normal functioning valves will most often close and prevent backflow. Also, with a regurgitant valve, a retrograde jet of blood is produced that can strike the endocardium and ultimately lead to a patch of fibrosis—this subvalvular patch of focal fibrosis can help identify regurgitation (Figure 7.39).

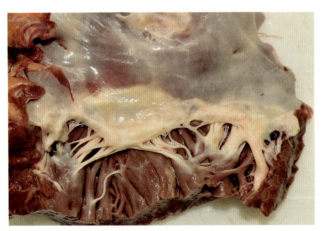

Figure 7.37. Chronic rheumatic mitral valvulitis. Classically, there is fusion, thickening, and shortening of the mitral valve chordae. The leaflets can also be thickened and the valve can be stenotic.

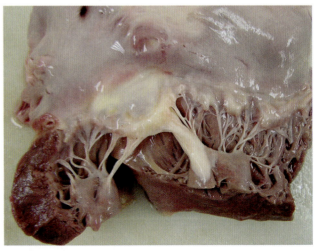

Figure 7.38. Single thickened chorda tendinea. A single chorda tendinea may represent a muscular chorda and not a mild case of chronic rheumatic mitral valvulitis. Microscopic examination of a cross section of the condition can reveal muscle.

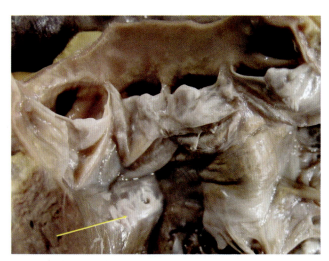

Figure 7.39. Near true quadricuspid aortic valve with regurgitation. While all four cusps appear similar in size in the image, the middle two share a fused commissure. Inferior to the valve is a patch of fibrosis on the endocardial surface (arrow). A cardiologist present at the time the heart was cut confirmed a clinical history of aortic regurgitation.

ENDOCARDITIS

AUTOPSY FINDINGS

On the valve cusps/leaflets will be vegetations (Figure 7.40A). If the endocarditis is bacterial in origin, microscopic examination will reveal the vegetations to be composed of fibrin and clusters of bacteria, with inflammatory cells in the myocardium adjacent to the valve (Figure 7.40B). If the condition is instead marantic endocarditis, the vegetations would be sterile. Fungal endocarditis can also occur. Evidence of septic emboli can be identified at autopsy, which can include Janeway lesions (Figure 7.40C); Osler nodes; splinter hemorrhages (Figure 7.40D); petechiae (Figure 7.40E); and pale white-tan lesions or hemorrhagic lesions in the lung, liver, heart (Figure 7.40F), spleen (Figure 7.40G), kidney, and other organs, which represent septic emboli. Emboli to the brain (Figure 7.40H) can cause intracerebral hemorrhage, which, if the hemorrhage occurs in a child, could be mistaken for inflicted injury.

ASSOCIATIONS OF ENDOCARDITIS

Endocarditis of the tricuspid valve is commonly associated with intravenous drug use; however, endocarditis of the tricuspid valve can occur for reasons other than drug use, and intravenous drug users can develop endocarditis of essentially any of the four cardiac valves (Figure 7.41A and B).

> **PEARLS & PITFALLS**
>
> Postmortem clots are commonly found in the heart at the time of autopsy and could potentially mimic endocarditis; however, postmortem clots can easily occur in combination with true endocarditis and if care is not used in rinsing away the postmortem clots, the vegetations can potentially be dislodged and the diagnosis of endocarditis missed at autopsy.

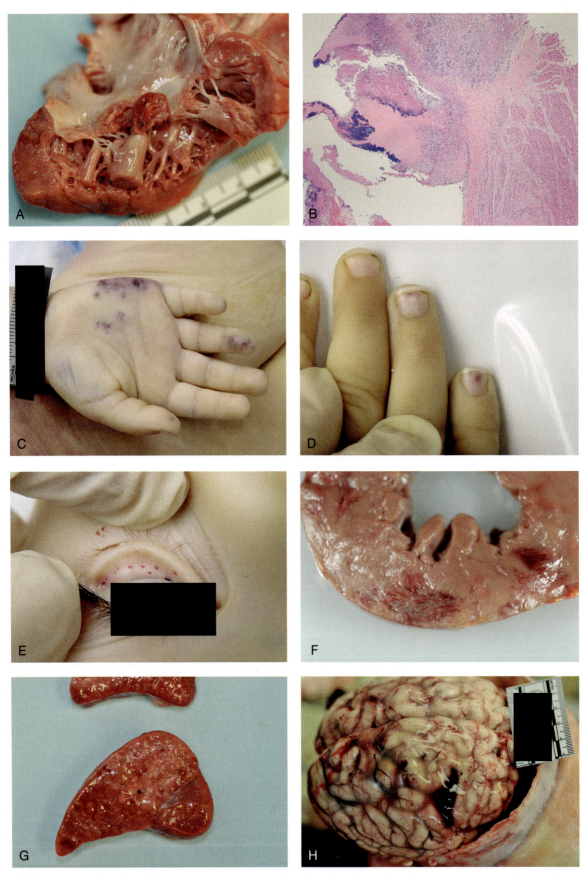

Figure 7.40. Features of endocarditis. Bacterial, marantic, and fungal endocarditis will produce vegetations on the cusps/leaflets (**A**). With an infectious endocarditis, organisms will be present, such as the bacteria in (**B**) (low power). Features of endocarditis include Janeway lesions (**C**), which, in a child, could be mistaken for abusive injuries, splinter hemorrhages (**D**), petechiae in a variety of locations (**E**), and septic emboli, often with areas of necrosis, including to the heart, spleen, and brain (**F-H**).

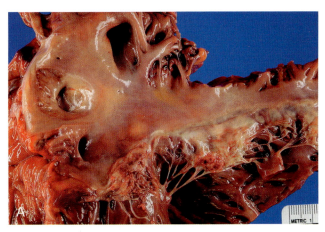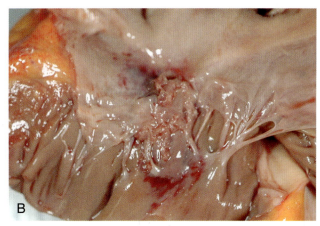

Figure 7.41. Tricuspid valve endocarditis. Both (**A** and **B**) are tricuspid valve endocarditis. (**A**) is from a decedent who used intravenous drugs, whereas (**B**) was from an individual with no known history or evidence at the death scene of intravenous drug use and negative findings upon toxicologic analysis of the blood.

PERICARDITIS

AUTOPSY FINDINGS

With pericarditis, there will be a pericardial effusion, which can be watery and yellow colored, fibrinous (Figure 7.42A), purulent (Figure 7.42B), or hemorrhagic. Depending upon the etiology of the pericarditis, microscopic examination can reveal fibrin, inflammatory cells, red blood cells, and potentially tumor, if the cause of the pericarditis is a neoplasm.

ETIOLOGIES OF PERICARDITIS

Pericarditis can occur secondary to a viral infection (and may be associated with concomitant myocarditis), myocardial infarction, renal failure, metastatic tumor, and even a delayed reaction to an aortic dissection (eg, one in which only a small amount of blood leaked into the pericardial sac). Purulent pericarditis is most commonly associated with pulmonary infection but may also be associated with infections of the soft tissue or bone.[102,103] While the infection of the lung would easily be identified with a standard autopsy, identification of a soft tissue or bone infection would require a more detailed examination. A urinary tract infection is another potential source for a purulent pericarditis.[103]

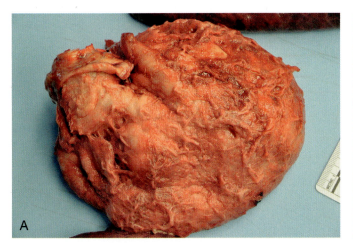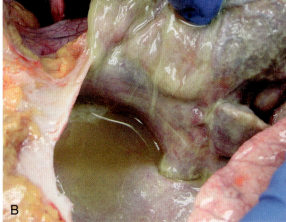

Figure 7.42. Pericarditis. Fibrinous pericarditis (**A**) can be associated with a variety of etiologies. Microscopic examination will reveal fibrin and a mild infiltrate of inflammatory cells. With purulent pericarditis (**B**), a more prominent neutrophilic component to the inflammatory infiltrate would be expected.

MYOCARDITIS

AUTOPSY FINDINGS

While inflammation of the heart (ie, a myocarditis) can cause the heart to have a pale appearance, the accurate gross diagnosis of a myocarditis is essentially not possible unless there is well-developed patchy pallor, which gives the heart a mottled appearance (ie, the pallor would be dispersed between the subendocardium and myocardium, and does not involve only the subendocardial region). Microscopic examination of the myocardium will reveal inflammatory infiltrates (Figure 7.43A), commonly lymphocytic if the causative agent is viral. Associated with the inflammatory infiltrates will be cardiac myocyte necrosis (Figure 7.43B). The Dallas criteria describe active myocarditis as inflammation associated with cardiac myocyte damage, and describe borderline myocarditis as inflammation in the absence of cardiac myocyte damage.[90] If the inflammatory infiltrate is eosinophilic and centered on the vasculature, a hypersensitivity myocarditis is most likely, which is often due to a drug reaction (Figure 7.43C). Inflammatory infiltrates in myocarditis, in addition to lymphocytic and eosinophilic, can also be neutrophilic or giant cell.[104] Use of the immunohistochemical stains, leukocyte common antigen and CD3, may also be utilized to assist with the diagnosis of myocarditis; however, Grasmeyer and Madea indicate that immunohistochemical studies should not supplant standard H&E criteria.[105,106]

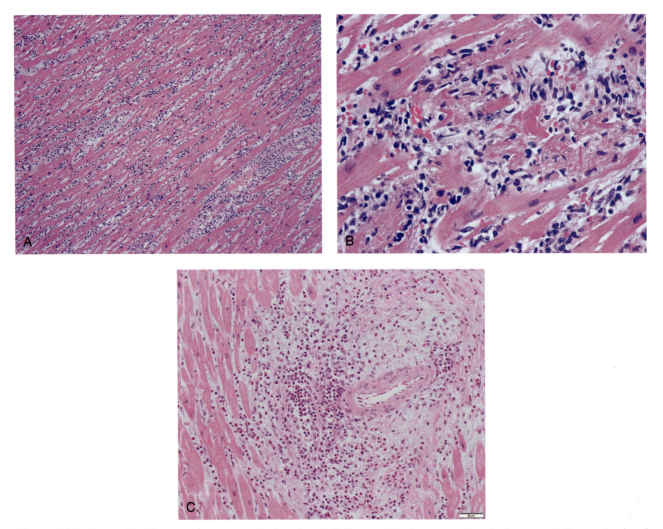

Figure 7.43. Myocarditis. There can be an extensive lymphocytic infiltrate within the myocardium (**A**, low power). Contraction band necrosis and disrupted cardiac myocytes, with fibrinlike/fibrinouslike necrosis present, indicate cardiac myocyte damage (**B**, high power). Hypersensitivity myocarditis is commonly drug-related and is identified by perivascular eosinophils (**C**, low power). Ischemic injury can occur in hypersensitivity myocarditis.

MIMICS OF MYOCARDITIS

Sarcoidosis can mimic a giant cell myocarditis; however, in a giant cell myocarditis, the inflammatory infiltrate is giant cells, and not granulomas, which should allow for the separation of the two entities (Figure 7.44).

> **FAQ:** How much of an inflammatory infiltrate is required to determine that the myocarditis was the cause of death?
>
> **Answer:** While myocarditis can be a primary cause of death, myocarditis has also been described as an incidental finding in decedents with another cause of death[107] (Figure 7.45). Kytö et al and Bonsignore et al found that myocarditis was often over-diagnosed at the time of autopsy.[108,109] In support of Kytö et al, De Salvia et al indicate that caution regarding the diagnosis of myocarditis is appropriate when the findings are not conclusive.[108,110] du Long reviewed 79 cases with inflammation of the heart and divided them into three groups: (1) those with a non-natural cause of death, (2) those with myocarditis but also another competing cause of death, and (3) those with myocarditis but no other competing cause of death.[111] Based upon their review, du Long et al determined that only a diffuse inflammatory infiltrate allowed distinctions between the groups.[111] To objectively determine the degree of myocarditis, Kitulwatte et al describe a classification scheme for marked myocarditis and mild myocarditis based upon the number of foci of inflammation.[112]
>
> On any given case in which myocarditis is identified, the forensic pathologist will have to use the totality of the scene investigation, including medical history, and autopsy findings to determine whether or not the inflammation of the heart represents the cause of death, bearing in mind that myocarditis can be an incidental finding and not necessarily the cause of death.

PEARLS & PITFALLS

If a lymphocytic myocarditis is identified at autopsy, one likely underlying cause is a viral infection. Serum from the autopsy can be tested for antibodies to confirm the presence of a virus.[113] Serologic studies in decedents with a viral encephalitis can also be used to identify the causative organism.[114]

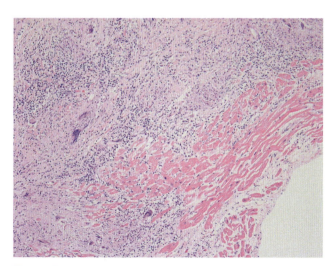

Figure 7.44. Sarcoidosis of the heart (low power). While like a giant cell myocarditis, giant cells are present in sarcoidosis, there are also granulomas and fibrosis, which would not be present with giant cell myocarditis.

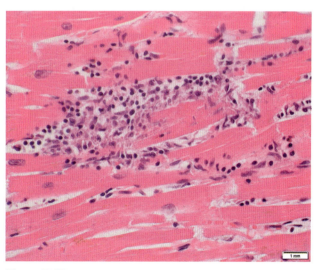

Figure 7.45. Myocarditis not as a cause of death. In Figure 7.45 is an inflammatory infiltrate associated with coagulative necrosis of a cardiac myocyte, which would fulfill the criteria for myocarditis (high power); however, this lesion was identified in an individual who died as the result of a suicidal gunshot wound.

CARDIOMYOPATHIES

AUTOPSY FINDINGS

The three classic forms of cardiomyopathy are hypertrophic, dilated, and restrictive, each of which could be identified during a forensic autopsy.[27] Hypertrophic cardiomyopathy characteristically has a thickened interventricular septum and a patch of fibrosis of the endocardium in the aortic outflow tract that corresponds to the anterior leaflet of the mitral valve. Microscopic examination will reveal myocardial disarray and fibrosis (Figure 7.46A). In a dilated cardiomyopathy, the heart has a globular (ie, rounded) overall shape and has dilation

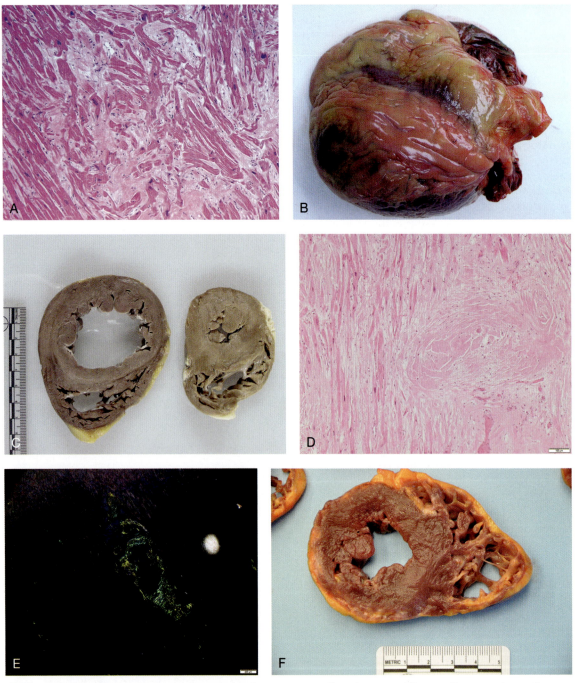

Figure 7.46. Cardiomyopathies. (**A**, low power) reveals the characteristic myofiber disarray and fibrosis of hypertrophic cardiomyopathy. In dilated cardiomyopathy, the external shape can be described as globular (ie, rounded) (**B**). When comparing a dilated heart to a non-dilated heart (**C**), the difference is apparent. Amyloid is one cause for a restrictive cardiomyopathy. Amyloid deposits can be interstitial or vascular (**D**, medium power). Congo Red staining can be used for confirmation (**E**, medium power). Arrhythmogenic right ventricular cardiomyopathy will have a dilated right ventricle with a thinned, fat infiltrated, and fibrotic wall, with microscopic examination characteristically revealing adipose tissue, fibrosis, and lymphocytes (**F**).

of the chambers (Figure 7.46B and C). The heart weight will be increased but the wall thickness will be normal (ie, eccentric hypertrophy). Microscopic examination of the heart reveals non-specific findings, such as fibrosis and cardiac hypertrophy. Restrictive cardiomyopathy can be suspected grossly based upon the myocardium being pale and/or firmer than normal; however, microscopic examination would be necessary to confirm the presence of fibrosis, hemosiderin deposits, amyloid (Figure 7.46D and E), or another underlying cause.

Another form of cardiomyopathy is arrhythmogenic right ventricular cardiomyopathy, which, upon gross examination, is identified by a dilated and thinned right ventricular wall, with fibrosis and fat deposition (Figure 7.46F). Microscopic examination will reveal adipose tissue, fibrosis, and lymphocytes. With arrhythmogenic right ventricular cardiomyopathy, plakoglobin staining may be useful as an adjunct test for the diagnosis.[115]

ASSOCIATION WITH SUDDEN DEATH

All four forms of cardiomyopathy (hypertrophic, dilated, restrictive, and arrhythmogenic right ventricular) are associated with sudden death.

MIMICS OF CARDIOMYOPATHY

A tangential section through the interventricular septum can easily mimic hypertrophic cardiomyopathy grossly. To prevent this artifact, sectioning from the inferior surface of the heart can best allow for visualization of the atrioventricular groove and facilitate sections parallel to the groove. Microscopic examination of the heart can reveal myofiber disarray in a variety of conditions other than hypertrophic cardiomyopathy, including at the junction between the right and left ventricles, and adjacent to areas of fibrosis (Figure 7.47A). Decomposition leads to dilation of the cardiac chambers, which can easily mimic a dilated cardiomyopathy. In older individuals some amount of fat deposition in the wall of the right ventricle is a common incidental finding at autopsy, especially of the anterior wall, and does not equate to a diagnosis of arrhythmogenic right ventricular cardiomyopathy (Figure 7.47B).

> **FAQ:** How can cardiac dilation be identified at autopsy?
>
> **Answer:** While the chamber diameter can be measured at the time of autopsy, decomposition will lead to ventricular dilation and impair the ability to accurately determine whether or not a chamber is dilated. If the heart is enlarged and the wall thickness is normal, the presumed diagnosis could be eccentric hypertrophy, which would indicate a dilated heart unless decomposition was present.

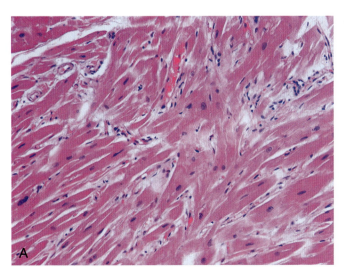 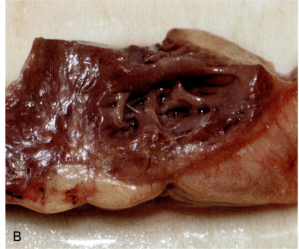

Figure 7.47. Mimics of cardiomyopathies. Histologic sampling of the junction of the right and left ventricle at the inferior surface of the heart will reveal myofiber disarray (**A**, high power). Fat infiltration of the anterior and inferior walls of the right ventricle is a common autopsy finding in older individuals. In (**B**), the anterior wall of the right ventricle is infiltrated with adipose tissue.

> **PEARLS & PITFALLS**
>
> If a cardiomyopathy is suspected, saving a purple top tube of blood from autopsy for potential genetic testing should be considered. While the expense of cardiac genetic testing has diminished over recent years, for many offices the routine use of cardiac genetic testing is still cost-prohibitive; however, in certain cases, based upon office policies and the preferences of the forensic pathologist, genetic testing, if performed, may yield useful information for surviving family members.

CORONARY ARTERY ANOMALIES ASSOCIATED WITH SUDDEN CARDIAC DEATH

AUTOPSY FINDINGS: ANOMALOUS ORIGIN OF A CORONARY ARTERY

The left anterior descending and circumflex coronary arteries can arise independently from the left sinus, the left main coronary artery can arise from the right sinus of Valsalva, the right coronary artery can arise from the left sinus of Valsalva (Figure 7.48A and B), and a coronary artery can arise from the pulmonary artery or the aorta. In addition, all three coronary arteries (right, left anterior descending, and circumflex coronary artery) can arise from one ostium, or the left main and right coronary arteries can arise from a single stem coronary artery (ie, a single coronary artery).[116,117]

ASSOCIATION WITH SUDDEN DEATH

The mortality rate for an anomalous coronary artery arising from the pulmonary artery is about 90% by 1 year of age, but survival into later adulthood is possible.[118] Anomalous origin of the coronary artery from the aorta has also been associated with sudden death.[119-121] When the left coronary artery arises anomalously from the right coronary artery sinus and has an intramural course in the aorta or passes between the aorta and the pulmonary artery, the condition has been associated with cardiac symptoms and sudden death.[121-123]

The pathologic association of anomalous origin of a coronary artery from the pulmonary artery with sudden death is clear as the coronary artery carries deoxygenated blood and is clearly linked with death at a young age; however, the association with sudden death of the other anomalies listed is not as clear, as survival into adulthood is common, and each anomaly can be an incidental finding at autopsy, in a decedent with another obvious cause of death. Thus, with each, the finding of the anomalous origin of the coronary artery at autopsy may represent simply an anatomic variant or may represent the etiology for sudden death, the difference of which will have to be determined by the forensic pathologist.[124]

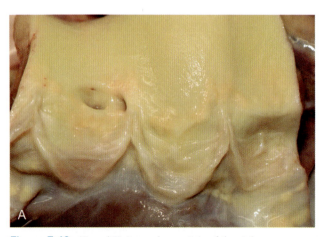
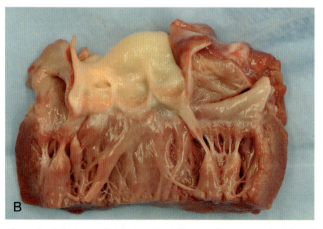

Figure 7.48. (**A** and **B**) Anomalous origin of the right coronary artery from the left sinus of Valsalva. Both figures illustrate an incidental anomalous origin of the coronary artery.

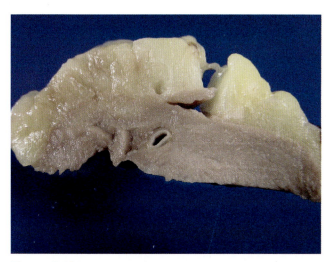

Figure 7.49. Tunneling of the coronary artery. While a common incidental finding at autopsy, tunneling has been associated with clinical symptoms and may be a cause of sudden death. Documenting the extent of the tunneling (ie, depth and length of the tunneled segment) is important.

AUTOPSY FINDINGS: TUNNELING/BRIDGING OF CORONARY ARTERY

A segment of coronary artery will run within the myocardium (Figure 7.49). In documenting the extent of tunneling, the forensic pathologist can measure the length of the segment of the coronary artery that is tunneled and the depth to which the vessel is tunneled in the myocardium.

ASSOCIATION WITH SUDDEN DEATH

While the significance of tunneling has been debated, the condition has been associated with myocardial ischemia and the risk for sudden cardiac death.[125-127]

LIPOMATOUS HYPERTROPHY OF THE INTERATRIAL SEPTUM

AUTOPSY FINDINGS

The interatrial septum is thickened and appears fatty (Figure 7.50A and B). Gay et al, in their study of 12 individuals with the pathologic change, saw an average thickness of 2.6 cm, and used 1.0 cm as a minimal low cutoff for the diagnosis of the condition.[128] The

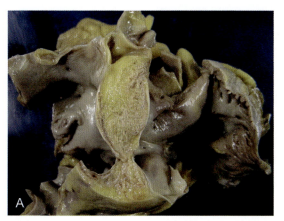
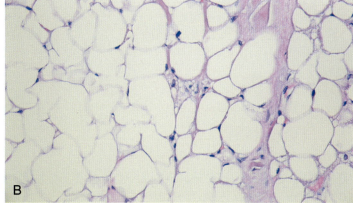

Figure 7.50. Lipomatous hypertrophy of the interatrial septum. The interatrial septum is thickened by adipose tissue (**A**), which microscopically can include fetal adipose tissue, fibrosis, inflammation, and entrapped cardiac myocytes (**B**, high power).

authors saw thicknesses as great as 7.0 cm.[128] Microscopic findings include mature adipose tissue associated with fetal adipose tissue, inflammation, fibrosis, and entrapped myocardial fibers with cytologic atypia.[128]

ASSOCIATION WITH SUDDEN DEATH

Lipomatous hypertrophy of the interatrial septum has been associated with sudden death, but it is often an incidental autopsy finding, most commonly identified in obese middle age or older individuals.[128-131]

NON-ISCHEMIC LEFT VENTRICULAR SCAR[132]

AUTOPSY FINDINGS

Gross examination will reveal a thin rim in the left ventricular free wall that is sub-endocardial or mid-myocardial (Figure 7.51A). Microscopic examination will reveal fibrosis or fibroadipose tissue and can have associated inflammation (Figure 7.51B). Right ventricular involvement is common. The condition is associated with no coronary artery lesions.

ASSOCIATED WITH SUDDEN DEATH

Non-ischemic left ventricular scar is a common cause of sudden death during sports and in younger individuals.[132]

LESIONS OF THE CARDIAC CONDUCTION SYSTEM

INTRODUCTION

While microscopic examination of the cardiac conduction system does not have to be performed in all autopsies, this specialized examination can provide useful information in the investigation of sudden death. Even in sudden deaths not of primary cardiac origin, examination of the cardiac conduction system can potentially help to better understand the mechanism of death. Tan et al examined 21 pediatric patients with either sudden death or known cardiac dysrhythmias and found abnormalities of the cardiac conduction system in 18, and concluded that examination of the cardiac conduction system revealed useful information.[133] In addition, Cohle et al had similar results, finding atrioventricular nodal dysplasia (seven cases) and mesothelioma of the atrioventricular node (four cases) in 11 of

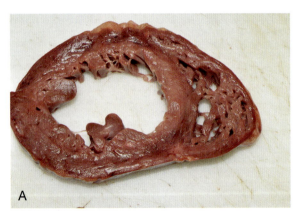
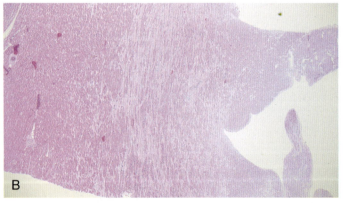

Figure 7.51. Non-ischemic left ventricular scar. While not obvious in (**A**), sectioning of the heart revealed a coarse texture and there was subendocardial pallor. Microscopic examination revealed a band of sub-endocardial fibrosis (**B**, low power), which was interstitial in location and enveloped cardiac myocytes. The decedent had no significant past medical history and there was no coronary artery atherosclerosis.

82 autopsy cases with no identifiable cause of death upon gross or microscopic examination at autopsy, which included toxicologic analysis.[134] In addition to potentially harboring an independent primary cause of death (eg, a mesothelioma), the cardiac conduction system can also exhibit abnormalities in other disease processes, and provide a possible mechanism for death in that decedent. For example, in a decedent with thrombotic thrombocytopenic purpura (TTP), microthrombi could be identified in the nodal vasculature. Nerantzis et al found changes in the atrioventricular node (fat infiltration, fibrous tissue, inflammation, and/or intimal proliferation of the vessel) in heroin addicts.[135]

ATRIOVENTRICULAR NODAL ARTERY DYSPLASIA

AUTOPSY FINDINGS

Microscopic examination of the atrioventricular node will reveal an atrioventricular nodal artery wall that is thick and disorganized with narrowing of the lumen of the vessel (Figure 7.52A and B). The change can be better examined with a Movat pentrachrome stain.[136]

ASSOCIATION WITH SUDDEN DEATH

The literature is mixed regarding the association of atrioventricular nodal artery dysplasia and sudden death. Based upon their study of 27 cases with 17 controls, Burke et al originally identified dysplasia of the atrioventricular nodal artery and associated it with sudden death.[136] However, based upon their study of 100 cases, Zack et al determined that the changes associated with atrioventricular nodal dysplasia were too common to merit the diagnosis of the condition.[137]

INCIDENTAL AND OTHER MICROSCOPIC FINDINGS IN THE HEART

CLUSTERS OF LYMPHOCYTES

Kitulwatte et al examined the hearts in 100 individuals who clearly died traumatic deaths and found scant inflammatory foci in 48 hearts, mild inflammation in 13, and moderate inflammation in three.[138]

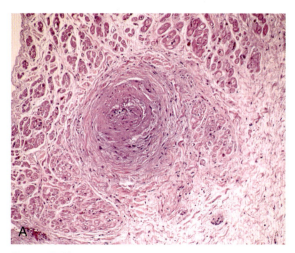
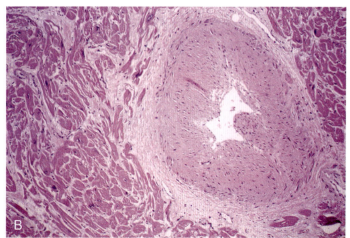

Figure 7.52. Atrioventricular nodal artery dysplasia. (**A** and **B**, high power) each illustrate a separate atrioventricular nodal artery with variable thickening and disorganization of the wall.

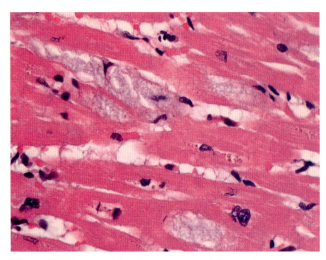

Figure 7.53. Basophilic degeneration of the cardiac myocytes. Several cardiac myocytes in the image have a pale myxoid discoloration and foamy texture of the cytoplasm (high power).

BASOPHILIC DEGENERATION

Affected cardiac myocytes will have a significant portion of the cytoplasm replaced with a blue-gray acellular substance (Figure 7.53). Basophilic degeneration is a very common finding, present in essentially all older decedents.[139]

CONTRACTION BAND NECROSIS

While contraction band necrosis (Figure 7.54A) is associated with ischemic injury, the change can also occur secondary to resuscitation efforts, and would represent an incidental finding. Artifact of sectioning and the normal anatomy of intercalated disks can potentially be misinterpreted as contraction band necrosis (Figure 7.54B).

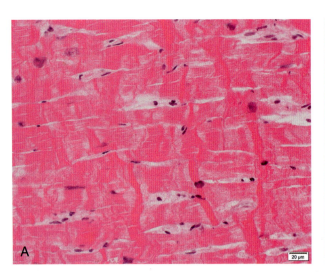
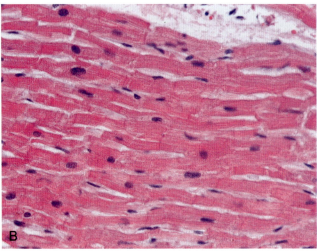

Figure 7.54. Contraction band necrosis and mimics. Contraction bands appear as discrete intermittently spaced dark eosinophilic bands that traverse the short axis of the cardiac myocyte (A, high power). Intercalated disks, which can be misinterpreted as contraction bands, are evenly spaced and each disk is regular in size and shape compared to the variability of contraction bands (B, high power).

NATURAL DISEASE OF THE RESPIRATORY SYSTEM

INTRODUCTION

At autopsy the most commonly encountered natural diseases of the respiratory system include various aspects of smoking-related disease (ie, anthracosis, smoker's lung, emphysema), other obstructive lung disease (eg, asthma), pulmonary thromboemboli and complications, pneumonia, and interstitial lung disease.

PNEUMONIA

AUTOPSY FINDINGS

A bacterial pneumonia involves one lobe (ie, lobar pneumonia) (Figure 7.55A and B) or more than one lobe in a patchy distribution (ie, bronchopneumonia) (Figure 7.55C); however, forensic pathologists can also encounter pneumonia due to viral, mycobacterial, or fungal organisms. Depending upon the cause of the pneumonia and its time course, microscopic examination could reveal a wide range of findings. Alveolar airspaces filled with neutrophils could be more frequently seen when the pneumonia has a bacterial cause or when the pneumonia is related to aspiration (Figure 7.55D); whereas interstitial inflammation with lymphocytes as the main cell type could be more frequently seen when the pneumonia has a viral cause (Figure 7.55E and F).

Associated with inflammatory infiltrates in pneumonia are a variety of findings that can be identified in the lungs depending upon the cause of the pneumonia and its time course. These findings include pulmonary edema, pulmonary hemorrhage, diffuse alveolar damage with hyaline membranes (Figure 7.55G and H), fibrinous exudates in the alveolar airspaces (Figure 7.55I), and fibrinous plugs in the alveolar airspaces. When appropriate, cultures, Gram stains, acid-fast stains, and silver stains may help the forensic pathologist identify the general type of organism responsible for the pneumonia.

POTENTIAL MIMICS OF PNEUMONIA

Lividity will cause a dark red or purple discoloration of the pulmonary parenchyma and could, based just upon visual examination and palpation, potentially mimic pneumonia (Figure 7.56). While not a mimic of pneumonia, when the center of a patch of pulmonary edema in an alveolar airspace does not survive processing, leaving a rim of pulmonary edema against the alveolar septum, this microscopic change can mimic hyaline membranes. The edema fluid has a smoother texture than the proteinaceous texture of the hyaline membranes.

> **PEARLS & PITFALLS**
>
> Often pneumonia will be present in the lung but is not visible grossly as the affected lung parenchyma looks the same as the unaffected surrounding lung. However, the lung parenchyma with the pneumonia will be more solid upon palpation due to the alveolar airspaces being filled with neutrophils, edema fluid, or protein exudates. The best way to assess for the presence of pneumonia at the time of autopsy is palpation. Palpation will allow for the detection of areas of consolidation that might otherwise go undetected via visual inspection.

> **PEARLS & PITFALLS**
>
> Examination of the lung may provide additional support for a drug overdose. When opioid drugs are the etiology of the overdose, the time course for death is often somewhat delayed, and microscopic foci of pneumonia may occur.

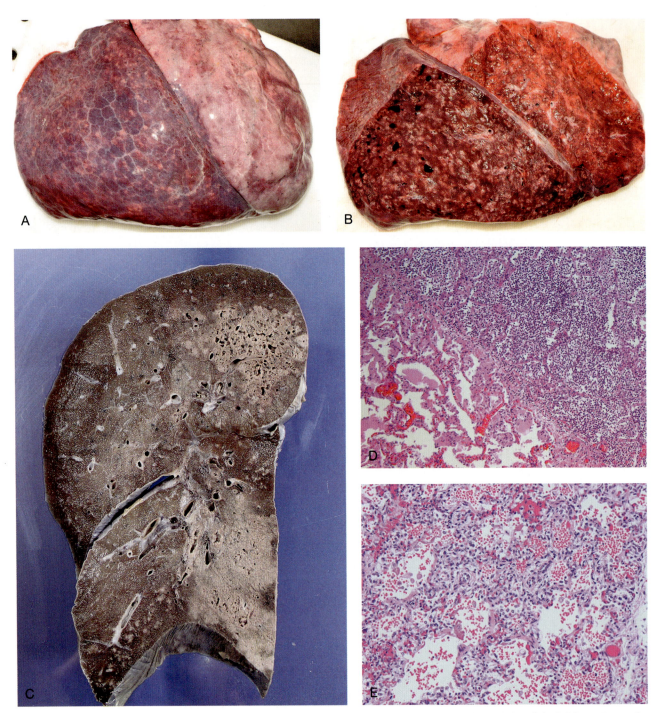

Figure 7.55. Pneumonia, types and features. (**A** and **B**) illustrate a lobar pneumonia, involving the lower lobe of the left lung. Externally, the entire lobe is discolored compared to the upper lobe; however, this appearance can be mimicked by lividity. Sectioning reveals a firm parenchyma with a discolored parenchyma with focal tan areas and exudation of a cloudy fluid. Microscopic examination can confirm the diagnosis. (**C**) illustrates a bronchopneumonia, with patchy involvement of both the upper and lower lobes. Necrosis is also present, creating widened spaces within the areas of consolidation. (**D**) (medium power) is a view of bronchopneumonia, with the upper right corner alveolar airspaces filled with neutrophils, and the lower left corner alveolar airspaces essentially empty. (**E** and **F**) are interstitial pneumonia. In (**E**, high power), the alveolar septa are expanded and have increased cellularity. There is also focal fibrin deposition in the adjacent airspace. (**F**, low power) is interstitial pneumonia centered on the larger airways. The diagnosis of an interstitial pneumonia can be challenging, but assisted by consultation with other pathologists, viral testing (culture or other method) at autopsy, and immunohistochemical studies. In infants, large aggregates of lymphocytes are common findings adjacent to larger airways and should not be misinterpreted as an interstitial pneumonia. (**G** and **H**, high power) illustrate hyaline membranes. (**I**, high power) is proteinaceous material filling the alveolar airspaces.

Figure 7.55f-i (continued)

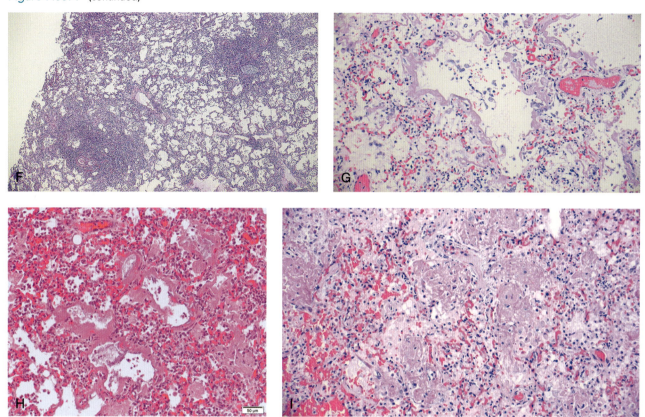

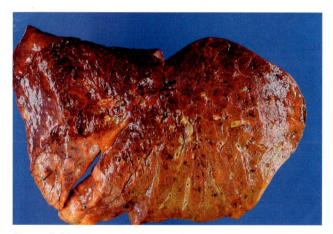

Figure 7.56. Posterior lividity mimicking pneumonia. The dark red-purple discoloration produced by lividity with its resultant increased firmness can mimic a pneumonia. If necessary, microscopic examination will easily distinguish the two conditions.

ASPIRATION PNEUMONIA

AUTOPSY FINDINGS

On gross examination, aspiration pneumonia would appear similar to other forms of pneumonia, with a palpable area of firmness in the pulmonary parenchyma. Upon microscopic examination, within the airspaces, vegetable matter and/or skeletal muscle would be present. Associated with the food material in the airway would be a neutrophilic infiltrate (Figure 7.57).

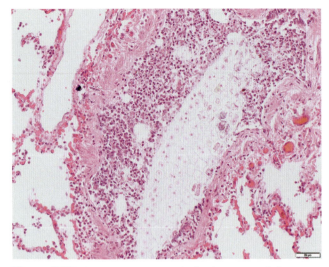

Figure 7.57. Aspiration pneumonia. In the center of the airway is a fragment of vegetable matter. Surrounding the fragment of vegetable matter are neutrophils, indicating the body is reacting to the presence of the vegetable matter (high power). Fragments of skeletal muscle can also be identified associated with aspiration pneumonia.

MIMICS

Agonal aspiration or postmortem migration of food from the gastrointestinal tract to the pulmonary parenchyma can mimic aspiration pneumonia; however, the lack of a neutrophilic infiltrate in response to the food material will help separate a significant aspiration pneumonia from agonal/postmortem movement of food material.

EMPHYSEMA

AUTOPSY FINDINGS

Grossly the lung parenchyma will appear to have enlarged airspaces and, with significant loss, can appear like a spiderweb (Figure 7.58A and B). Associated with the loss of pulmonary parenchyma can be air filled blebs of the pleural surface. These air filled blebs can also occur independently of significant gross changes within the pulmonary parenchyma. If the diagnosis of emphysema is not made grossly, the diagnosis most likely should not be made microscopically, as normal anatomy, sectioning artifact, and other factors could mimic emphysema. Microscopic features of emphysema can include fragments of alveolar septa in the airspaces (Figure 7.58C).

PEARLS & PITFALLS

If the emphysematous changes are present throughout the entire lung as opposed to being confined mostly to the upper portions, the diagnosis of α_1-antitrypsin deficiency should be considered. For this condition, microscopic examination of the liver is warranted to determine if intracellular protein inclusions are present in the periportal hepatocytes. A PAS stain, with and without diastase, will help identify the accumulations.

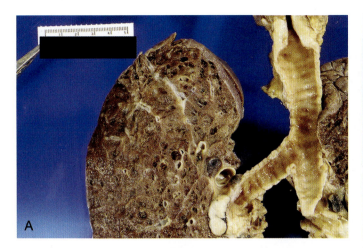
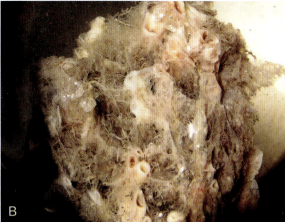
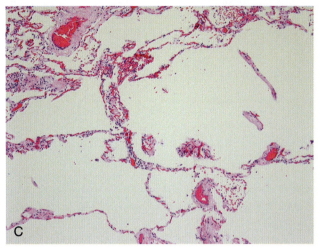

Figure 7.58. Emphysema. Grossly, emphysema will appear as enlarged airspaces, often in the upper lobes (**A**) as smoking is the most common cause of emphysema, and the smoke rises to the upper lobes after being inhaled. Putting the lung tissue in water can help better define the tissue loss as the water will fill and subsequently expand the airspaces making it easier to appreciate the amount of tissue loss (**B**). A microscopic feature of emphysema is fragments of alveolar septa in the middle of an airspace (**C**, high power).

> **PEARLS & PITFALLS**
>
> Spontaneous rupture of a pleural bleb can lead to a pneumothorax and potentially death.[140] Pleural blebs can occur unrelated to smoking and emphysematous changes in the parenchyma itself.

ASTHMA

AUTOPSY FINDINGS

When an individual dies as the result of status asthmaticus, the lungs will be hyperinflated, even to the point where lividity cannot pool within the parenchyma due to the tension and the lungs will have the normal pink-tan appearance. The hyperinflated lungs will touch across the midline and can press against and be indented by the ribs (Figure 7.59A). Sections through the lungs can reveal mucous plugging of the airways. Microscopic examination, which is best done by sampling more proximal regions of the lung, will reveal the characteristic features of asthma, including smooth muscle hypertrophy, thickening of the basement membrane region of the airway, hyperplasia of mucous glands, and an eosinophilic infiltrate (Figure 7.59B). Charcot-Leyden crystals can also be identified (Figure 7.59C). Charcot-Leyden crystals can be identified with other hypereosinophilic conditions and are not specific to asthma.

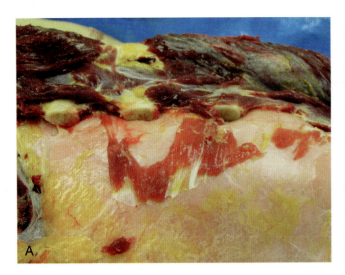
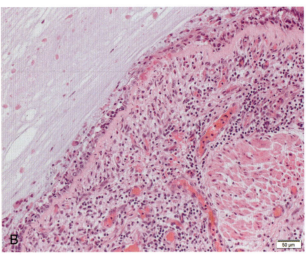
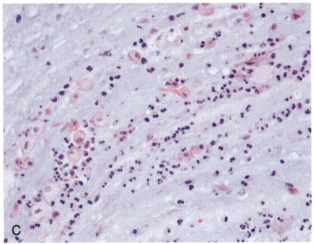

Figure 7.59. Asthma. Grossly, in a lethal case of asthma, the lung will be hyperinflated, and can be tense, similar to a balloon, indenting against the ribs and preventing blood from pooling in the lungs, giving the lung its normal pink appearance because of the absence of lividity (**A**). Microscopically, there will be mucous plugging in the airways, thickened basement membrane, an eosinophilic infiltrate, and smooth muscle hypertrophy (**B**, medium power). Mucous plugging can also be found grossly. Charcot-Leyden crystals can be identified (**C**, high power).

INCIDENTAL MICROSCOPIC FINDINGS IN THE LUNG

CORPORA AMYLACEA

Concretions similar to those found in the prostate can be found in the lung (Figure 7.60A).

LENTILS

A specific type of foreign material that is occasionally found in the lung (Figure 7.60B). The finding is derived from leguminous vegetable matter and could be mistaken for a parasitic infection.[141,142]

PULMONARY CHEMODECTOMA (MESOTHELIAL-LIKE REST)

Incidental findings, which are associated with past pulmonary thromboemboli, that are occasionally found in the lung (Figure 7.60C).[143]

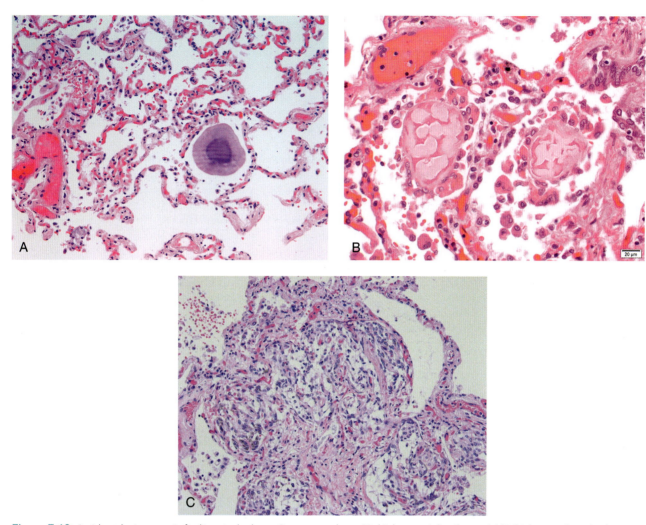

Figure 7.60. Incidental microscopic findings in the lung. Corpora amylacea (**A**, high power), lentil material (**B**, high power), and pulmonary chemodectomas (or meningothelial-like rests) (**C**, high power) can all be identified in the lung on microscopic examination. Lentil material can be also associated with aspiration pneumonia, and would, in that situation, be a significant finding.

NATURAL DISEASE OF THE HEPATOBILIARY SYSTEM

INTRODUCTION

At autopsy, the most commonly encountered natural diseases of the hepatobiliary system include cholelithiasis, cirrhosis of the liver and its various complications (including esophageal varices and ascites), and fatty liver. Incidental masses of the liver are common, with the mass most often being a cavernous hemangioma, bile duct adenoma, or von Meyenburg complex.

DIFFUSE FATTY LIVER

AUTOPSY FINDINGS

While the liver at autopsy commonly has patchy areas of steatosis (a yellow discoloration) that involve a small percentage of the overall volume, with diffuse fatty liver, the entire liver will have a yellow or pale tan-yellow appearance (Figure 7.61A and B). Often, the liver will have a greasy texture, which corresponds to the extensive fat deposition in the hepatocytes, and a segment of liver placed into formalin can float. Microscopic examination can reveal a variety of findings. The steatosis can be macrovesicular steatosis, microvesicular steatosis (Figure 7.61C), or a mixture of both, and can be associated with ballooning degeneration of the hepatocytes (Figure 7.61D and E), Mallory hyaline (Figure 7.61F-G), a neutrophilic infiltrate, including a rimming of a steatotic vacuole with neutrophils (Figure 7.61H), and bile stasis. Fatty liver is most commonly associated with alcohol use, diabetes mellitus, and obesity.

FAQ: Is diffuse fatty liver a cause of death?

Answer: Several authors have described sudden death in individuals with a diffuse fatty liver. For example, Randall described sudden death in individuals with essentially the only significant autopsy finding being that of a fatty liver.[144,145] Yuzuriha described sudden death associated with fatty liver in eleven individuals, with microvesicular steatosis being a prominent change.[146] To diagnose sudden death associated with diffuse fatty liver in chronic alcoholics, it is preferable to have a certain pattern present with several negative findings. Sudden unexplained death associated with chronic alcoholism can be diagnosed in decedents with a history of alcohol abuse, but with no obvious competing cause of death, no evidence of acute alcohol toxicity or alcoholic ketoacidosis, a morphologically normal heart, and a fatty liver.[147,148] The exact mechanism of sudden death associated with diffuse fatty liver is uncertain. Although some authors have indicated that non-alcoholic fatty liver disease (NAFLD) is well associated with atrial fibrillation, but only minimally with ventricular fibrillation, other authors have indicated that non-alcoholic fatty liver disease is a cause of elongated QTc interval and is associated with cardiac dysrhythmias and could be a risk for sudden death.[149-152]

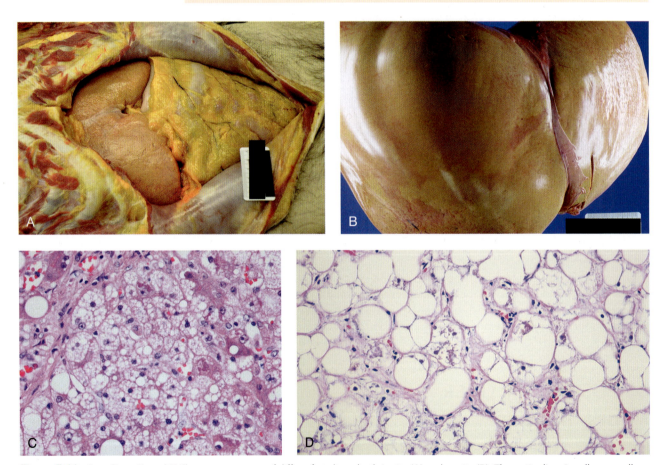

Figure 7.61. Fatty liver. (**A** and **B**) illustrate two cases of diffuse fatty liver, both in situ (**A**) and ex situ (**B**). The entire liver is yellow or yellow-tan discolored. Microvesicular steatosis can vary from hepatocytes with several small vacuoles to hepatocytes that are filled with innumerable small vacuoles and have a foamy texture (**C**, high power). With ballooning degeneration, the hepatocytes are enlarged and rounded (**D** and **E**, high power). Mallory's hyaline, or Mallory-Denk body, will be darkly eosinophilic ropy condensations within the hepatocyte (**F** and **G**, high power). With steatohepatitis, a fat vacuole will be rimmed with neutrophils (**H**, high power).

Figure 7.61 (continued)

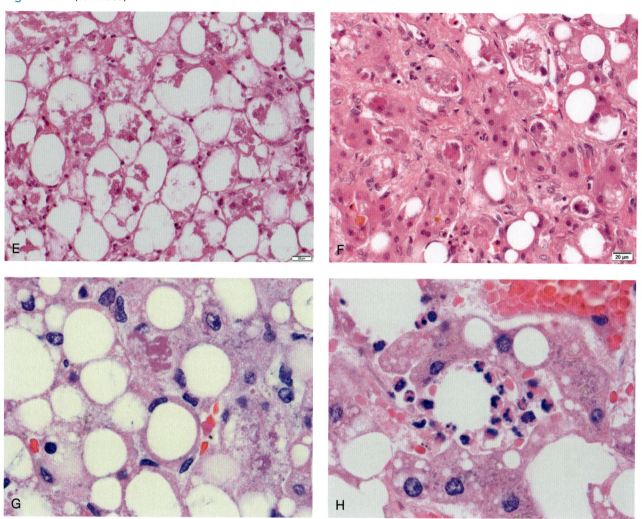

POTENTIAL MIMICS

If a body has sustained significant injury and lost a great deal of blood, the liver can have a pale tan appearance due to the relative absence of blood within the vessels and sinusoids in the liver, which can mimic a diffuse fatty liver. Microscopic examination will allow for easy separation of these two conditions if necessary (Figure 7.62).

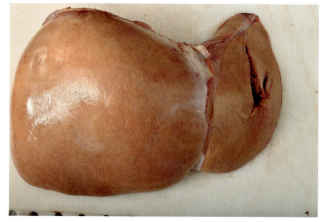

Figure 7.62. Fatty liver mimic. Although the liver in Figure 7.62 looks similar in appearance to the liver in Figure 7.61B, this individual had extensive bleeding after a wound, with resultant pallor of internal organs. Microscopic examination can easily distinguish the two conditions if necessary.

CIRRHOSIS OF THE LIVER

AUTOPSY FINDINGS

Cirrhosis is a nodular effacement of the hepatic parenchyma, which can be due to a variety of causes, including alcohol abuse, viruses (hepatitis B, C, or D), hemochromatosis, and autoimmune hepatitis. Cirrhosis can be described as micronodular or macronodular. With macronodular cirrhosis, the liver has nodules that are greater than 3 mm in diameter (Figure 7.63A-C). Microscopic examination will reveal a nodular effacement of the parenchyma, and potentially the underlying etiology (eg, iron deposition). While cirrhosis of the liver is commonly associated with alcohol abuse, routine screening of decedents with cirrhosis of the liver for hepatitis can identify undiagnosed hepatitis C infections with some frequency.

POTENTIAL MIMICS

With steatosis, in some cases, the lobular architecture of the liver is highlighted, which can mimic micronodular cirrhosis. Microscopic examination will allow for separation of the two conditions. And, the opposite is true, with gross examination of the liver sometimes not revealing cirrhosis, but with microscopic examination revealing the nodularity. Decomposition with gas formation can, if the liver is only viewed superficially, mimic cirrhosis; however, these two conditions are easily separated with closer inspection of the organ.

PEARLS & PITFALLS

If a decedent has both cirrhosis and emphysema, the diagnosis of α_1-antitrypsin deficiency should be considered. Microscopic examination of the liver may reveal the PAS positive, diastase resistant intra-hepatocyte protein globules in the periportal hepatocytes (Figure 7.64).

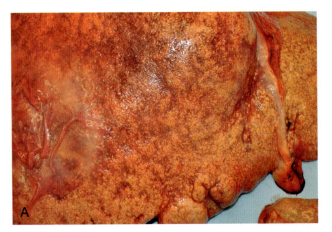
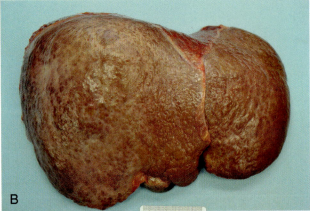
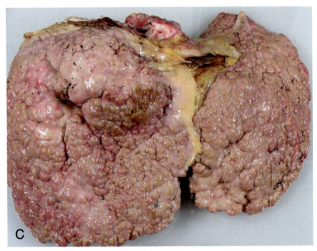

Figure 7.63. Cirrhosis. (**A-C**) represent the variation in size of the liver nodules in cirrhosis, varying from micronodular (**A**) to macronodular (**C**).

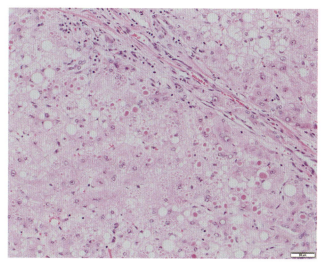

Figure 7.64. α₁-Antitrypsin deficiency. Intra-hepatocyte protein globules in the periportal hepatocytes (high power).

COMPLICATIONS OF CIRRHOSIS

Individuals with end-stage liver disease and cirrhosis can develop scleral icterus and jaundice, splenomegaly, esophageal varices (Figure 7.65A), which can lead to gastrointestinal bleeding and death, caput medusae (Figure 7.65B), which are dilated vascular channels

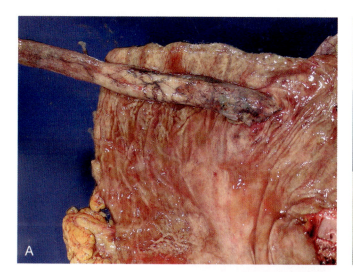
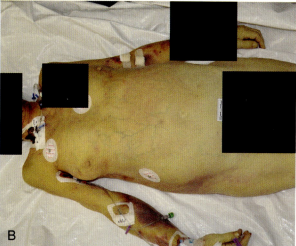
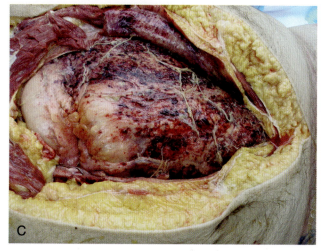

Figure 7.65. Complications of cirrhosis. Complications of cirrhosis include esophageal varices (A), caput medusae (B), and spontaneous bacterial peritonitis (C). Inversion of the esophagus can help identify esophageal varices, which can vary from subtle to quite obvious.

in the skin, and ascites. Normally ascitic fluid is watery, clear, and pale yellow; however, individuals with ascites can develop spontaneous bacterial peritonitis, which may be due to bacterial contamination of the ascitic fluid (Figure 7.65C). Cirrhosis is a risk factor for the development of hepatocellular carcinoma.

> **FAQ:** Is cirrhosis of the liver a risk factor for bleeding?
>
> **Answer:** While cirrhosis has in the past been strongly associated with a propensity for bleeding as the liver is the main source of production of important clotting factors, more recent studies indicate that cirrhosis of the liver produces pro-coagulant effects as well as anticoagulant effects, with the liver re-balancing the body's hemostatic function.[153] The result is a complex situation.[154-161] In any given case, a forensic pathologist should use caution before determining that just because cirrhosis was present that the decedent was more likely to bleed easier than normal.

> **PEARLS & PITFALLS**
>
> While varices associated with portal hypertension due to cirrhosis of the liver most commonly are associated with the esophagus, they can occur in other locations (ie, ectopic varices) such as the bladder, small and large intestine, hilum of the lung, the mesenteric, omental, or periumbilical veins, and even the gallbladder.[162-167] While ectopic varices in the stomach and intestine could lead to gastrointestinal bleeding, ectopic varices in the mesentery or omentum could lead to a hemoperitoneum.[168] Rupture of the umbilical vein, which can recanulate within the round ligament (ie, the ligamentum teres), can occur secondary to portal hypertension, leading to a hemoperitoneum[169] (Figure 7.66).

> **FAQ:** Is cirrhosis of the liver associated with sudden cardiac death?
>
> **Answer:** Cirrhotic cardiomyopathy is a condition found in individuals with no known cardiac disease who have reduced stress induced contractility and/or impaired relaxation in diastole. These cardiac alterations are associated with electrophysiological abnormalities that can lead to sudden cardiac death.[170] Ben Hammouda el al. reported the sudden death of an individual from cirrhotic cardiomyopathy while engaged in work activities.[170] Other than cirrhotic cardiomyopathy, cirrhosis is a potential risk factor for arrhythmia due to a variety of other mechanisms including induced cardiac ion channel changes, impaired drug metabolism, and electrolyte and metabolic abnormalities including those due to hepatorenal syndrome, and others.[171] In addition, impaired drug metabolism in decedent's with cirrhosis may be a consideration when interpreting toxicology results. Whether or not a forensic pathologist will utilize cirrhosis as a sole cause of death without another significant condition (eg, esophageal bleeding) would be at their discretion.

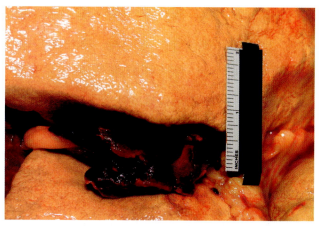

Figure 7.66. Rupture of umbilical vein in round ligament (ie, ligamentum teres). This patient with cirrhosis had a hemoperitoneum, and the round ligament was found to be suffused with hemorrhage. An umbilical vein that had reopened secondary to portal hypertension and subsequently ruptured was the source.

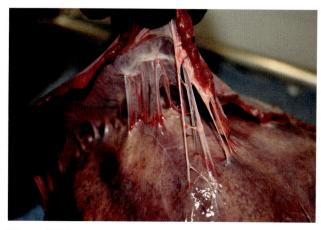

Figure 7.67. Fitz-Hugh-Curtis syndrome. Adhesions between the liver and diaphragm, which are often compared to violin strings in appearance.

FITZ-HUGH-CURTIS SYNDROME

AUTOPSY FINDINGS

Adhesions between the diaphragm and liver (Figure 7.67) form in individuals most often associated with a past *Neisseria gonorrhoeae* or *Chlamydia trachomatis* infection.

ACUTE CHOLECYSTITIS

AUTOPSY FINDINGS

The wall of the gallbladder can be thickened and hemorrhagic or otherwise discolored (Figure 7.68A). Microscopic examination would reveal infiltrates of neutrophils in the wall. Acute cholecystitis has a relatively high mortality rate of around 4% and so can be encountered at a forensic autopsy as the cause of death.[172,173] If acute cholecystitis is identified, dissection of the biliary tree may reveal an obstruction (Figure 7.68B).

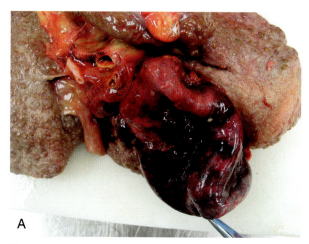
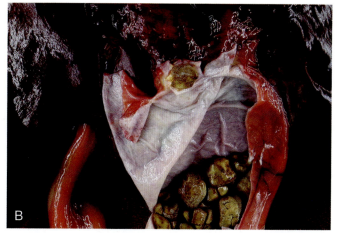

Figure 7.68. Acute cholecystitis. In (**A**), the wall of the gallbladder is thickened and hemorrhagic, with a neutrophilic infiltrate identified microscopically. In (**B**), which is a different gallbladder, there is a stone impacted in the outlet of the gallbladder.

ACUTE PANCREATITIS

AUTOPSY FINDINGS

The pancreas can be hemorrhagic, or have areas of discoloration secondary to necrosis (such as small yellow areas), or both (Figure 7.69A-C). The omentum and mesentery can have punctate foci of fat necrosis (Figure 7.69D). Microscopic examination of the pancreas will reveal necrosis and a neutrophilic infiltrate (Figure 7.69E). While Cullen sign and Grey Turner sign are associated with pancreatitis (Figure 7.69F and G), Birnaruberl et al found skin changes in only 3 of 20 cases of fatal pancreatitis.[174] Cullen sign and/or Grey Turner sign have also been associated with acute appendicitis, acute pyelonephritis, ruptured abdominal aortic aneurysm, splenic rupture, ectopic pregnancy, and other conditions.[175-179] Complications of acute pancreatitis include diffuse alveolar damage and pulmonary edema, peritonitis, disseminated intravascular coagulation, and sepsis.[180] Given the serious nature of the condition, acute pancreatitis can be a cause of sudden death.[181]

RISK FACTORS FOR ACUTE PANCREATITIS

From 405 autopsied cases of acute pancreatitis, Renner et al determined that the main causes of acute pancreatitis were chronic alcoholism, gallstones in the common bile duct, and post abdominal surgery.[182] Less common causes were viral hepatitis, drugs, and the postpartum state. In addition, the authors identified that diabetes mellitus was a risk factor for acute pancreatitis. Increased intracranial pressure, acute fatty liver of pregnancy, and systemic lupus erythematosus have also been associated with the development of acute pancreatitis.[183-185]

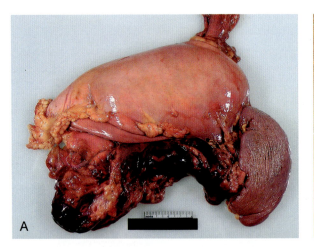
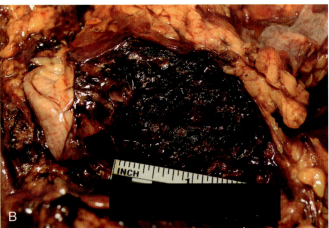
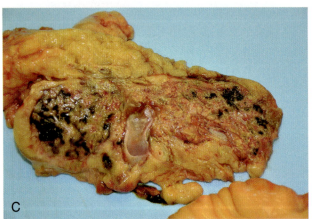
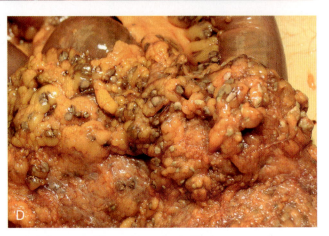

Figure 7.69. Acute pancreatitis. (**A** and **B**) are acute hemorrhagic pancreatitis, from two different autopsies. In (**B**), the pancreas was essentially completely suffused with blood and expanded to approximately twice its normal size. (**C**) is acute pancreatitis, with more prominent necrosis and less hemorrhage. (**D**) is fat necrosis in the omentum, which can accompany pancreatitis. (**E**) is a high power image of acute pancreatitis, with a neutrophilic infiltrate. (**F**) is Cullen sign, which is a periumbilical hemorrhagic discoloration associated with acute pancreatitis. (**G**) is Grey Turner sign, which is hemorrhagic discoloration of the flanks and also associated with acute pancreatitis.

Figure 7.69 (continued)

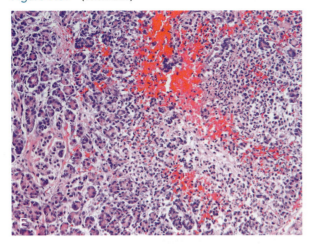
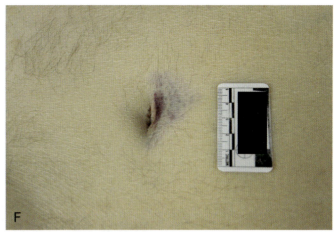
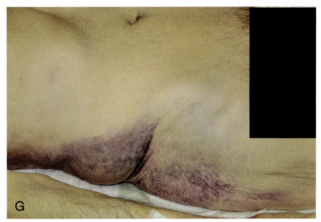

> **PEARLS & PITFALLS**
>
> A common postmortem change in the pancreas is hemorrhage, which can potentially be confused with acute hemorrhagic pancreatitis (Figure 7.70A). Occasionally postmortem foci of autolysis will be easily identified grossly, producing punctate yellow spots, which can also mimic pancreatitis (Figure 7.70B). Microscopic analysis can identify whether or not inflammation is present and confirm the diagnosis of acute pancreatitis.

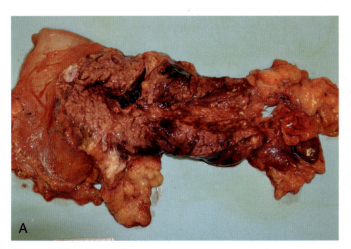
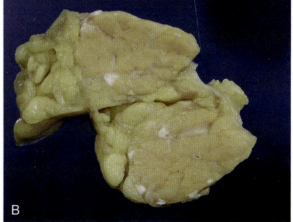

Figure 7.70. Mimics of acute pancreatitis. Decomposition commonly produces hemorrhage within the pancreas, which can be relatively extensive and mimic acute hemorrhagic pancreatitis (A). Focal prominent areas of autolysis can produce chalkylike areas in the parenchyma and mimic acute pancreatitis (B). Microscopic examination in both cases revealed no neutrophilic infiltrate.

CAVERNOUS HEMANGIOMA

AUTOPSY FINDINGS

The gross appearance of the tumor is a well-circumscribed dark red spongy mass in the parenchyma; however, there can be areas of fibrosis. The size can vary from a few millimeters to >10 cm or more (Figure 7.71A and B). The microscopic appearance of the tumor is most frequently large spaces separated by fibrous septa and filled with red blood cells (eg, a cavernous hemangioma). Cavernous hemangiomas are common findings at autopsy.

ASSOCIATION WITH SUDDEN DEATH

It is possible for the rupture of a cavernous hemangioma to occur and result in a hemoperitoneum.[186]

OTHER INCIDENTAL LIVER MASSES

Both bile duct adenomas and bile hamartomas (von Meyenburg complex) are common incidental findings in the liver.[187] Focal nodular hyperplasia (FNH) is also relatively common.

AUTOPSY FINDINGS

Both bile duct adenomas and von Meyenburg complexes will be identified in the liver as a small (most often <1 cm) tan-white sub-capsular mass (Figure 7.72A). Microscopic examination will reveal small back-to-back glands in a bile duct adenoma (Figure 7.72B) and dilated spaces interspersed with fibrous tissue in a bile hamartoma (von Meyenburg complex) (Figure 7.72C). There is no bile production in a bile duct adenoma; however, a bile duct hamartoma often produces bile. Both lesions are well-circumscribed and both are benign. FNH is a well-circumscribed mass with a central scar (Figure 7.72D). Microscopic examination reveals changes that appear just like cirrhosis (ie, "focal cirrhosis").

NATURAL DISEASE OF THE GENITOURINARY SYSTEM

INTRODUCTION

At autopsy, the most commonly encountered natural diseases of the genitourinary system include arterial and arteriolar nephrosclerosis, acute and chronic pyelonephritis, uterine leiomyomas, and renal masses (including adrenal gland rests, renal adenomas, and renal cell carcinomas).

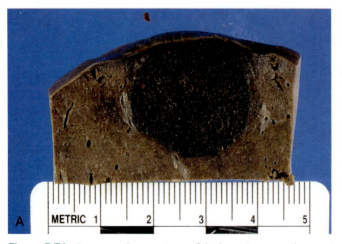
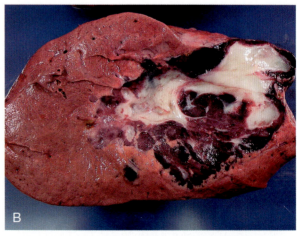

Figure 7.71. Cavernous hemangioma of the liver. Cavernous hemangiomas of the liver are easily identified grossly, being a well-circumscribed dark red spongy mass (**A**). Cavernous hemangiomas of the liver can become quite large and can have areas of fibrosis (**B**).

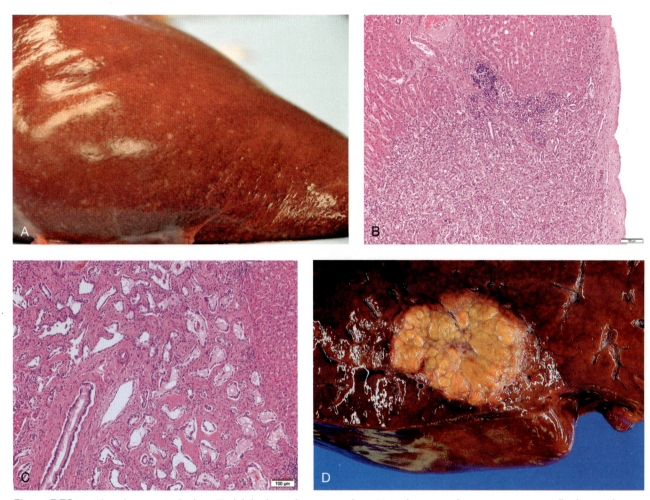

Figure 7.72. Incidental masses in the liver. Both bile duct adenomas and von Meyenburg complexes present as a small sub-capsular tan-white mass, which can be numerous and mimic a metastatic neoplasm (**A**). Bile duct adenomas are small glands back-to-back with no bile formation (**B**, low power) and von Meyenburg complexes (**C**, medium power) are dilated spaces with a fibrous background and with bile production (although essentially none is present in the image). Focal nodular hyperplasia is a tan-white or tan-yellow mass with a central scar (**D**).

NEPHROSCLEROSIS

AUTOPSY FINDINGS

Arterial nephrosclerosis presents as focal remote cortical infarcts, producing patchy loss of cortex, whereas arteriolar nephrosclerosis presents as a diffuse granular cortical surface (Figure 7.73A), with microscopic examination revealing tubular atrophy and globally sclerotic glomeruli, often with admixed clusters of lymphocytes. Vessels have a homogeneous eosinophilic acellular thickening (ie, hyaline arteriolosclerosis) (Figure 7.73B), which is the same appearance as affected vessels in decedents with diabetes mellitus.

> **FAQ:** How do you distinguish between chronic pyelonephritis and remote cortical infarcts?
>
> **Answer:** Chronic pyelonephritis is associated with a dilated calyceal system, cortical defects at the renal poles, and the microscopic finding of thyroidization of the tubules; however, in any given case without clinical history, definitively distinguishing between the two conditions may be problematic.

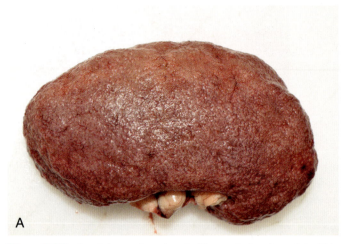
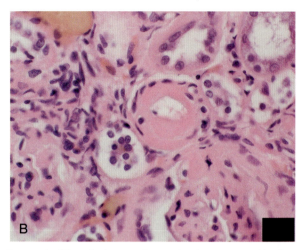

Figure 7.73. Arteriolar nephrosclerosis. The cortical surface of the kidney is granular (**A**) and microscopic examination can reveal hyaline arteriolosclerosis (**B**, high power).

ACUTE PYELONEPHRITIS

AUTOPSY FINDINGS

The gross appearance can vary from scattered few millimeter yellow spots in the cortex to a completely friable cortex. When the acute pyelonephritis manifests as yellow spots in the cortex, they can be discrete circular abscesses or more ill-defined yellow areas (Figure 7.74A-C). Microscopic examination will reveal infiltrates of neutrophils in the cortex, with tubules containing neutrophils.

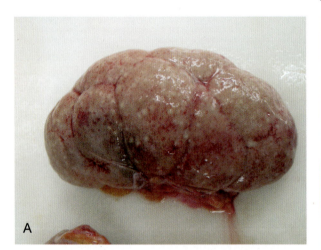
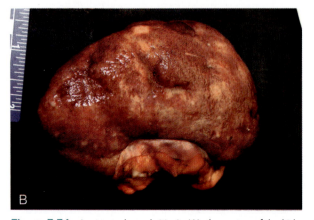
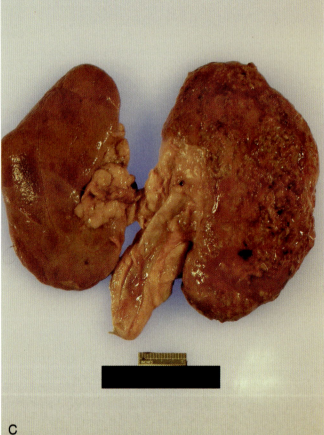

Figure 7.74. Acute pyelonephritis. In (**A**), the cortex of the kidney has numerous few millimeter discrete yellow spots, which are abscesses. In (**B**), although some lesions similar to those in (**A**) are present, many are larger and have more indistinct boundaries and inconsistent shapes. In (**C**), the kidney on the right side of the image has a friable completely involved cortex, whereas the kidney on the left side is unaffected, illustrating the role of vesicoureteral reflux in the development of acute pyelonephritis.

ASSOCIATION WITH SUDDEN DEATH

While individuals with acute pyelonephritis would most likely be symptomatic and seek medical care, if untreated, the disease process has a relatively high mortality rate, with about 15% of those patients developing sepsis or septic shock and dying.[188]

FOURNIER GANGRENE

AUTOPSY FINDINGS

Fournier gangrene is a necrotizing soft tissue infection involving the genital, perianal, and perineal region, which has a mortality rate of around 8%, and can affect both adults and children.[189,190] Gross examination would reveal discoloration and breakdown of skin (Figure 7.75). Microscopic examination would reveal necrosis and a neutrophilic infiltrate.

INCIDENTAL RENAL MASSES

ADENOMA

Often small neoplasms are identified, and these usually have a papillary architecture.

RENAL CELL CARCINOMA

Of the variants, clear cell carcinoma is the most commonly encountered, and will have a yellow and red gross appearance, and a microscopic appearance of clear cells on a delicate fibrovascular architecture.

ADRENAL GLAND REST

Occasionally small (<0.5-1.0 cm) yellow sub-capsular masses will be identified, which, upon microscopic examination are found to be normal adrenal cortical tissue.

RENOMEDULLARY INTERSTITIAL CELL TUMOR

Commonly found in the medulla, these tumors are small (<1 cm) well-circumscribed white nodules, which on microscopic examination are a paucicellular fibrous mass (Figure 7.76A and B).

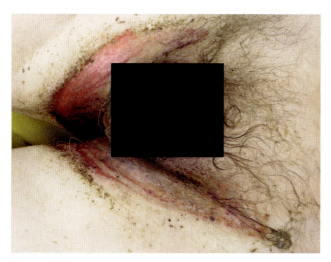

Figure 7.75. Fournier gangrene. In the femoral region, there is red discoloration and breakdown of the skin.

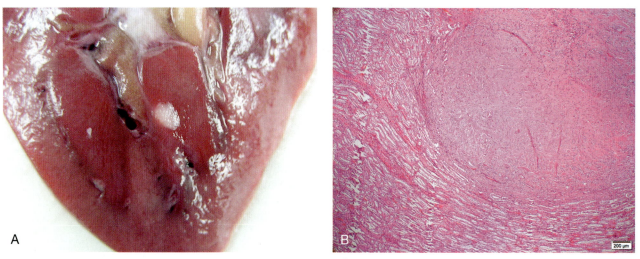

Figure 7.76. Renomedullary interstitial cell tumor. Small well-circumscribed white mass in the renal medulla (**A**), which is a paucicellular fibrous proliferation (**B**, low power).

NATURAL DISEASE OF THE ENDOCRINE SYSTEM

INTRODUCTION

At autopsy the most commonly encountered natural diseases of the endocrine system include complications of diabetes mellitus, pituitary gland infarction (most commonly associated with cerebral edema), Hashimoto thyroiditis, papillary carcinoma of the thyroid gland, and adrenal gland hypertrophy.

FEATURES OF DIABETES MELLITUS

AUTOPSY FINDINGS

While diabetes mellitus is an endocrine disease of the pancreas, its effects are found in multiple organ systems. Upon external examination, acanthosis nigricans (Figure 7.77A) and peripheral ulcers of the extremities are findings associated with diabetes mellitus. Upon internal examination, coronary artery atherosclerosis, black esophagus, hepatic steatosis, and Wischnewski spots (in diabetic ketoacidosis) are associated with diabetes mellitus (Figure 7.77B). Microscopic features associated with diabetes mellitus are nodular glomerulosclerosis (ie, Kimmelstiel-Wilson lesion), vacuolation of the basilar portion of the proximal convoluted tubules in the kidney (in diabetic ketoacidosis), and islet cell amyloidosis (in type II diabetes mellitus) (Figure 7.77C-F).

INFARCTION OF THE PITUITARY GLAND

AUTOPSY FINDINGS

Grossly the gland may appear pale. Microscopic examination will reveal coagulative necrosis of the gland. At the rim may be histologically viable cells (Figure 7.78).

ASSOCIATION

While pituitary gland infarction is commonly associated with Sheehan syndrome, which occurs in pregnant females, cerebral edema that has been present for at least a short period of time (eg, a decedent who dies after a short hospitalization and brain death) is a fairly common cause of infarction of the pituitary gland.

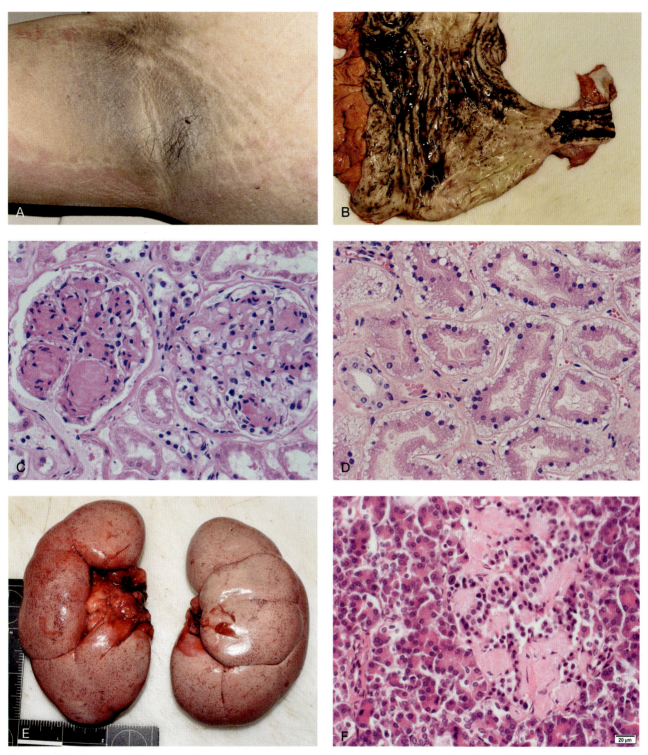

Figure 7.77. Features of diabetes mellitus. Acanthosis nigricans is black discoloration of the skin of the axillae, which can also be present with gastrointestinal malignancies (**A**). In (**B**), the decedent had both a black esophagus and Wischnewski spots, both associated with diabetic ketoacidosis. Nodular glomerulosclerosis (ie, Kimmelstiel-Wilson lesion) is characteristic for diabetes mellitus. If necessary a Congo Red stain could rule out amyloidosis (**C**, high power). Sub-nuclear vacuolation of the proximal convoluted tubules of the kidney, a feature of diabetic ketoacidosis (**D**, high power), can be suspected grossly when the kidney is pale or yellow discolored, and in the absence of exsanguination (**E**). In type II diabetes mellitus, amyloidosis of the islets can occur (**F**, high power).

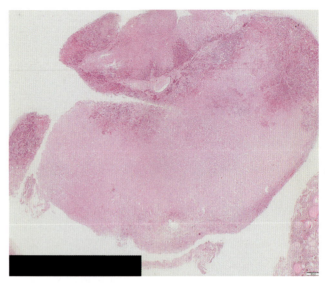

Figure 7.78. Pituitary gland infarct. Most of the gland is pale and eosinophilic, representing coagulative necrosis, with a rim of histologically viable cells preserved at the rim (low power).

HASHIMOTO THYROIDITIS

AUTOPSY FINDINGS

The gross examination will reveal a diffusely tan or focally tan thyroid gland, which also can be more firm than normal and can have a nodular texture. Microscopic examination will reveal clusters of lymphocytes, often with germinal centers, and large eosinophilic follicular cells (Hurthle cell or oncocytic change). In addition, the parenchyma can be fibrotic and nodular.

> **FAQ:** Is Hashimoto thyroiditis associated with sudden death?
>
> **Answer:** Myxedema coma, in which individuals will have systemic non-pitting edema, is life threatening and thus could present at forensic autopsy.[191] A prolonged QTc has been associated with both overt and subclinical hypothyroidism, which could potentially predispose to sudden death.[192,193] A case report does describe sudden death associated with Hashimoto thyroiditis, but the individual also had thymus hyperplasia.[194]

PHEOCHROMOCYTOMA

AUTOPSY FINDINGS

A pheochromocytoma appears as a dusky red nodule centered on the adrenal medulla. Microscopic examination will reveal a zellballen pattern (ie, cell nests), with most cells having a neuronlike appearance, with prominent nucleoli, and some cells will have more rounded and speckled appearance.[187]

> **FAQ:** What is the significance of adrenal gland hypertrophy?
>
> **Answer:** A mild hypertrophy of the adrenal gland, with a thickened and vaguely nodular cortex, is not an uncommon finding at autopsy (Figure 7.79). Adrenal gland hypertrophy is due to increased adrenocorticotropic hormone, which may result from stress or be secondary to failure of the feedback mechanism.[195,196] While adrenal gland hypertrophy can be a secondary process as just described, bilateral adrenal gland hyperplasia as well as an adenoma can be a source of primary aldosteronism, leading to hypertension and the subsequent effects of hypertension.[197]

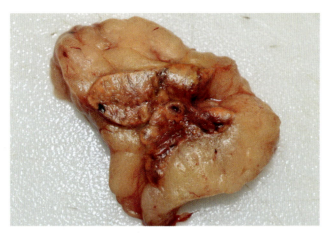

Figure 7.79. Hypertrophy of the adrenal gland. The cortex is thickened and the normal discrete linear yellow cortex is not present. The thickened adrenal gland cortex can include well-defined nodules, or just be a generalized process.

INCIDENTAL FINDINGS

MYELOLIPOMA

A myelolipoma is an incidental tumor infrequently found in the adrenal gland that is composed of adipose tissue and hematopoietic cells (Figure 7.80A and B). The tumor is benign but could be misinterpreted grossly as a pheochromocytoma. Histologic examination will easily separate the two conditions.

BLACK THYROID

A black thyroid gland is associated with minocycline therapy[198] (Figure 7.81A). Microscopic examination can reveal aggregates of brown-black pigment in the colloid and similar colored pigment in the epithelial cell[199] (Figure 7.81B). Black thyroid can potentially lead to hypothyroidism.[199]

NATURAL DISEASE OF THE GASTROINTESTINAL SYSTEM

INTRODUCTION

At autopsy commonly encountered natural diseases of the gastrointestinal system are Barrett esophagus, black esophagus, salmon patches, peptic ulcers of the duodenum and stomach, ischemic colitis, and colonic diverticula.

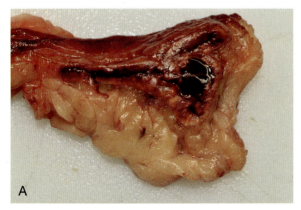
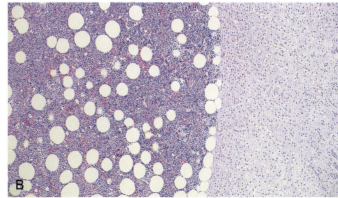

Figure 7.80. Myelolipoma. While the red mass centered on the medulla could potentially mimic a pheochromocytoma (**A**), microscopic examination reveals the mass to be composed of hematopoietic cells admixed with adipose tissue (**B**, low power).

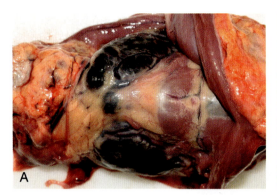 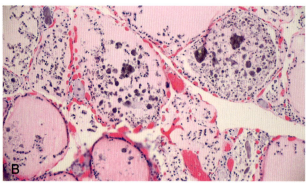

Figure 7.81. Black thyroid gland. Gross examination reveals a darkly discolored thyroid gland (**A**), with microscopic examination revealing aggregates of brown-black pigment (**B**, medium power).

> **PEARLS & PITFALLS**
>
> A gastrointestinal hemorrhage is often suspected based upon the scene investigation, with copious red blood (undigested) or black tarry stools (digested blood) present at the scene, often on the bed, on the floor, in the decedent's underwear, or in the toilet. Upon opening the abdominal cavity, the finding of distended and blue-purple or dark red discolored loops of bowel can suggest a gastrointestinal hemorrhage, with the discoloration caused by blood in the lumen of the intestine (Figure 7.82A and B). To find the cause of the gastrointestinal hemorrhage, the length of the gastrointestinal tract should be opened, until a source is identified. It should be considered that what appears as a gastrointestinal hemorrhage could also have originated from the oropharyngeal or nasopharyngeal region. Common causes of gastrointestinal hemorrhage at autopsy include esophagitis (which can be bacterial, viral, or fungal), black esophagus, Mallory-Weiss laceration (Figure 7.83), and peptic ulcer.

> **PEARLS & PITFALLS**
>
> If upon opening the peritoneal cavity, either pus or hemorrhage is found, it is best if the contents of the peritoneal cavity are inspected in-situ to identify the source of the hemorrhage or exudate. If a purulent exudate is present, possible sources would include diverticulitis, a perforation of the intestines (which could be due to inflammatory bowel disease or another condition), appendicitis, and perforated peptic ulcer among other conditions. If hemorrhage is present, possible sources would be a perforated peptic ulcer, hemorrhagic pancreatitis, splenic rupture, a bleeding tumor (eg, cavernous hemangioma of the liver, hepatocellular carcinoma of the liver), and ruptured ectopic pregnancy, among other conditions. If the source of the hemorrhage or purulence is not identified prior to removal of the organs, the source may be obscured and not identified during dissection of the organs, especially if the source of the pus or hemorrhage is a region not typically closely dissected (eg, a splenic artery aneurysm).

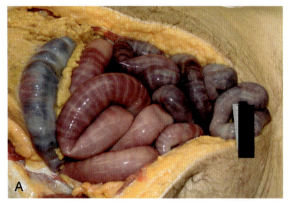 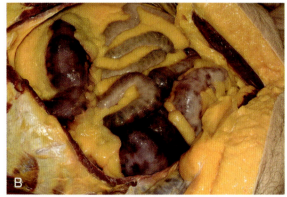

Figure 7.82. Gastrointestinal hemorrhage. In situ, loops of the small intestine have a dark red discoloration at the serosal surface in (**A** and **B**). This appearance was from blood in the lumen of the small intestine. The source must be identified. Also, postmortem decomposition and ischemic injury can also produce discoloration at the serosal surface.

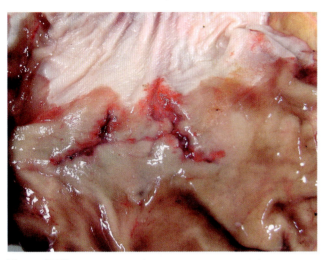

Figure 7.83. Mallory-Weiss laceration. A laceration that occurs at the gastroesophageal junction, most often associated with vomiting.

ESOPHAGEAL INLET PATCH (SALMON PATCH)

AUTOPSY FINDINGS

In the upper esophagus, one or more patches of the mucosa with a tan-pink discoloration can be identified.[200] Microscopic examination will reveal ectopic gastric mucosa[200] (Figure 7.84A-C).

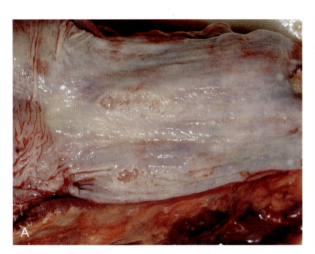
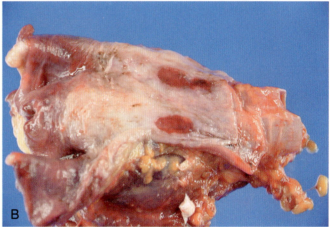
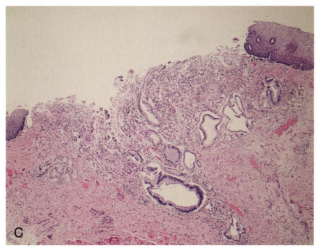

Figure 7.84. Esophageal inlet patch (ie, salmon patch). In the proximal esophagus are small red-pink discolorations of the mucosa (**A** and **B**). Microscopic examination reveals gastric mucosa (**C**, low power).

POTENTIAL MIMICS

The lesions in the upper esophagus can look somewhat like a tear and could mimic an esophageal intubation that caused damage to the esophageal mucosa.

BARRETT ESOPHAGUS

AUTOPSY FINDINGS

The gross appearance will be tails of mucuslike epithelium extending upward into the esophageal squamous epithelium. Residual islands of squamous epithelium may be present within the tongues of gastriclike mucosa. Microscopic examination will reveal intestinal-type epithelium (ie, metaplasia) with goblet cells.

> **PEARL & PITFALL**
>
> It is very common at autopsy to see tongues of gastric-appearing mucosa extend superior to the gastroesophageal junction (Figure 7.85A-C). Microscopic examination can reveal a variety of changes, and quite often intestinal-type epithelium is not present, indicating that a diagnosis of Barrett esophagus at autopsy should not be dependent upon the gross examination only. Given that Barrett esophagus is a single layer of delicate mucosa, the finding may also be very sensitive to postmortem changes and not easily identified at forensic autopsy.

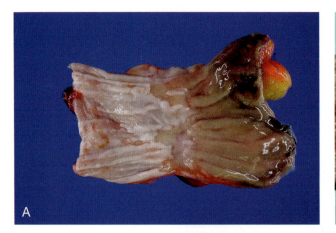
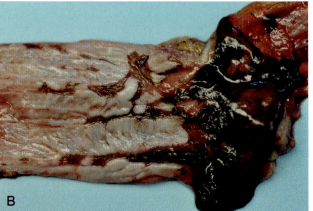
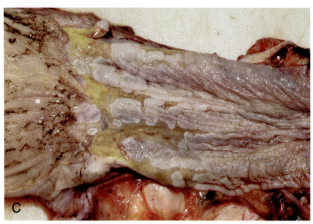

Figure 7.85. Gross features of Barrett esophagus. In (**A-C**), tongues of gastric-type epithelium extend proximal to the gastroesophageal junction, with islands of residual squamous epithelium present. In (**C**), microscopic examination revealed fibrosis and no intestinal-type epithelium.

BLACK ESOPHAGUS (ACUTE ESOPHAGEAL NECROSIS)

AUTOPSY FINDINGS

The condition can vary from longitudinal black discolorations of the esophageal mucosa to black discoloration of the entire esophageal mucosa (Figure 7.86A and B). Microscopic examination of the esophagus will reveal a necrosis/loss of the squamous mucosa, and aggregates of finely stippled yellow-black pigment (ie, digested blood) on the mucosa surface along with a neutrophilic infiltrate in the wall (Figure 7.86C).

ASSOCIATIONS

Black esophagus is associated with diabetes mellitus and hypothermia, and can have a relatively high mortality rate.[201] Black esophagus has also been reported in chronic alcoholism, alcoholic ketoacidosis, and recent COVID-19 infection.[202-204]

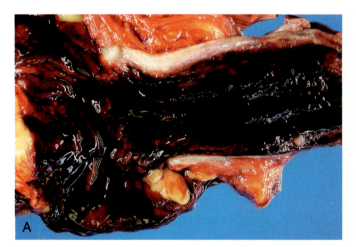
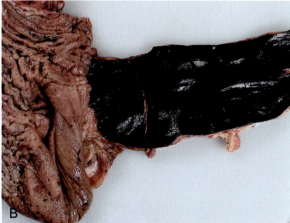
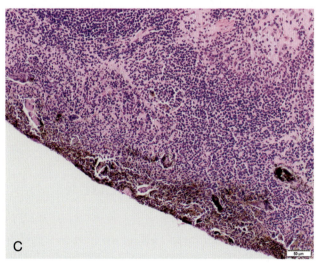

Figure 7.86. Black esophagus. In (**A** and **B**), the mucosa is either nearly completely (**A**) or completely (**B**) black discolored. In (**B**), just proximal to the gastroesophageal junction is a pink-red line, this is an artifact of dissection as the stomach with some attached esophagus and the proximal esophagus were removed in two segments, leading to transection of the esophagus at this point. In (**C**), the mucosa is absent and replaced with a layer of inflammatory cells, including mostly neutrophils, and with aggregates of finely stippled yellow-black pigment, which is hemolyzed blood (low power).

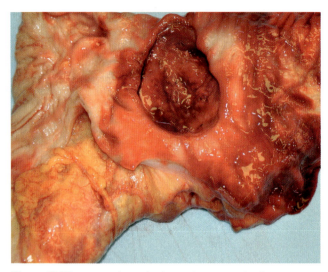

Figure 7.87. Peptic ulcer. The lesion has a punched-out appearance. Associated with a peptic ulcer can be hemorrhage in the gastrointestinal tract, or peritonitis.

PEPTIC ULCER

AUTOPSY FINDINGS

In the gastric or duodenal wall will be a cavitary punched-out defect (Figure 7.87). With a peptic ulcer, the wall of the cavity will be fibrotic. If the rim of the cavity is heaped up, a neoplasm might be present. If the peptic ulcer is bleeding, microscopic examination of the ulcer may reveal the underlying damaged vessel.

ISCHEMIC COLITIS

AUTOPSY FINDINGS

A hemorrhagic or other discoloration of the colon, which is often at the ileocecal junction and associated with hypotension (Figure 7.88A and B). Microscopic examination will reveal extravasated red blood cells in the colonic mucosa (Figure 7.88C).

POTENTIAL MIMIC

Phlegmonous colitis, which is associated with cirrhosis of the liver, has extensive neutrophilic inflammation of the wall, which can produce a red discoloration and potentially mimic ischemic colitis[205] (Figure 7.89).

INTESTINAL DIVERTICULA

AUTOPSY FINDINGS

Out-pouchings occur in the wall of the intestine, most frequently the distal colon, but potentially anywhere along the length of the colon. Diverticula can also occur in the small intestine. A Meckel diverticulum, which occurs in the distal small intestine and can harbor ectopic gastric or pancreatic tissue, can be an uncommon location for an ulcer and subsequent bowel perforation.

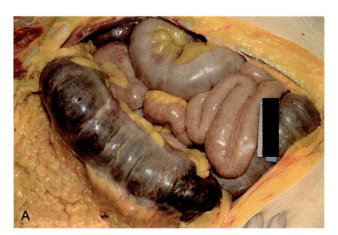
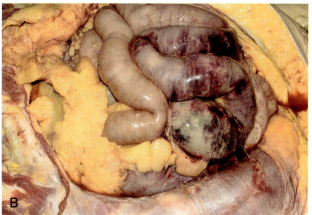
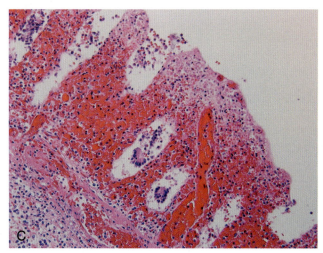

Figure 7.88. Ischemic colitis. Centered at the cecum is discoloration of the large intestine (**A** and **B**). Caution must be taken to not call decompositional changes as ischemic injury, as decomposition will also produce a discoloration of the colon most often centered on the cecum. A microscopic examination can separate the two conditions, as ischemic injury is associated with extravasated red blood cells in the mucosa (**C**, high power).

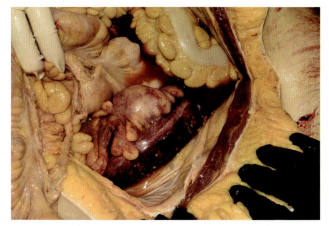

Figure 7.89. Phlegmonous colitis. Phlegmonous colitis can produce a red discoloration of the large intestine and mimic ischemic colitis; however, the wall of the colon is markedly thickened from the neutrophilic infiltrate.

GREEN COLON

AUTOPSY FINDINGS

It is not uncommon to find bright green or green-turquoise discoloration of the serosal surface of the bowel centered in the region of the cecum. This discoloration most likely results from dyes within the food recently eaten by the decedent or from dyes in medication or other ingested substance (Figure 7.90).[206]

POTENTIAL MIMIC

Decomposition will cause green discoloration of the colon centered on the cecum also, but the green discoloration is a dark green hue.

FAQ: With a forensic autopsy, should the small and large intestine be opened?

Answer: With the absence of hemorrhage or inflammation in the peritoneal cavity, with no evidence of a gastrointestinal hemorrhage at the scene or during the autopsy, and with the serosal surface of the intestinal tract appearing normal, the likelihood of finding anything of significance (eg, related to the cause of death) by opening the gastrointestinal tract would be highly unlikely; however, some forensic pathologists, depending upon their personal preference or office policies, may open the entire gastrointestinal tract in all forensic autopsies. In deaths occurring in-custody, opening the intestinal tract to search for swallowed drug packages may be useful.

PEARLS & PITFALL

With increasing postmortem interval, the normal rugal folds of the gastric mucosa will flatten out, presumably due to the effects of the now uncontrolled gastric acids and other secretions in the stomach. This flattening of the gastric mucosa can mimic atrophic gastritis. The change can also result in perforation of the stomach (Figure 7.91).

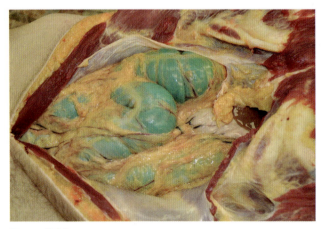

Figure 7.90. Green colon. The discoloration is most likely from dye within a substance ingested by the decedent.

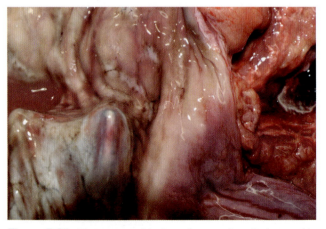

Figure 7.91. Postmortem thinning of stomach wall. A very thin area near the gastroesophageal junction was identified in this decomposed individual. While perforation did not occur, the region was translucent, and forceps placed against the serosal surface are easily identifiable from the mucosal surface.

NATURAL DISEASE OF THE HEMATOLYMPHOID SYSTEM

INTRODUCTION

Hematologic disorders can be difficult to assess at the time of autopsy; however, some gross and microscopic manifestations can occur. For example, if the disease forms a mass, such as a lymphoma, the diagnosis can often be made at the time of autopsy. Unfortunately, evaluation of the peripheral blood is more difficult at the time of autopsy; however, histologic examination of the bone marrow, which can reveal cellular infiltrates, can assist.

DISSEMINATED INTRAVASCULAR COAGULATION

AUTOPSY FINDINGS

While disseminated intravascular coagulation (DIC) is most commonly encountered in the hospital in patients who have multi-organ failure, when pathologic conditions have a quick time course (eg, acute promyelocytic leukemia), DIC may present at forensic autopsy. Grossly, DIC can cause petechiae. Microscopically, microthrombi will be identified. The glomeruli of the kidney (Figure 7.92), the alveolar septal capillaries of the lungs, and the sinusoids of the liver are good locations to check for the presence of microthrombi.

THROMBOTIC THROMBOCYTOPENIC PURPURA/ HEMOLYTIC UREMIC SYNDROME

AUTOPSY FINDINGS

The autopsy findings for TTP and hemolytic uremic syndrome (HUS) would be essentially the same as those for DIC (ie, microthrombi). The main distinguishing feature between the two disease processes, that is, the presence or absence of coagulation abnormalities, cannot be reliably determined in the postmortem period; however, while TTP is a primary disorder that arises on its own, DIC is a secondary disorder related to another condition (eg, sepsis). If no evidence of an underlying disorder can be identified through autopsy or available history, TTP or HUS are the potential etiology for the microscopic findings. TTP would be more likely to present with central nervous system findings, whereas HUS is more likely to present with renal findings.

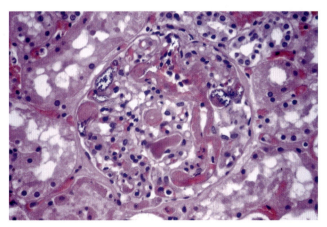

Figure 7.92. Microthrombi in kidney. This individual had disseminated intravascular coagulation (DIC). Microthrombi are present in glomerular capillary loops (high power). Also present are bacterial cocci, with sepsis being the underlying cause of the DIC.

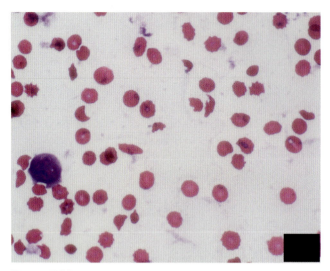

Figure 7.93. Schistocytes. This postmortem smear from a decedent with TTP revealed schistocytes (high power).

> **PEARL & PITFALL**
>
> If a hematolymphoid disease process is suspected, blood and bone marrow smears can be performed at the time of autopsy and later stained with a Wright-Giemsa or other appropriate stain to assess the hematopoietic cells (Figure 7.93). In addition, flow cytometry can be performed on postmortem blood to best help delineate a hematologic malignancy if that determination is necessary to the forensic autopsy.

> **PEARL & PITFALL**
>
> While often not examined microscopically, retaining a segment of bone, either from a rib or the vertebral column, both of which can be easily acquired at the time of autopsy, especially in cases where no cause of death is identified at the time of autopsy, can be a useful tissue to save for future examination.

FIBROSIS OF THE SPLENIC CAPSULE (SUGAR SPLEEN)

AUTOPSY FINDINGS

Gamna-Gandy bodies, which are composed of fibrosis, hemosiderin, and calcium, can underlie the dense fibrosis of the splenic capsule (Figure 7.94A and B). Gamna-Gandy

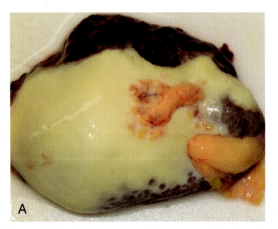
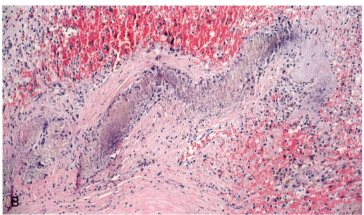

Figure 7.94. Sugar spleen and Gamna-Gandy bodies. The surface of the spleen has a thick white fibrotic coating (**A**). Underlying the fibrotic coating were Gamna-Gandy bodies (**B**, medium power).

bodies are associated with portal hypertension.[207] Fibrosis of the splenic capsule has been associated with cor pulmonale.[208]

> **PEARL & PITFALL**
>
> At autopsy, it can be easy to forget to examine the body cavities after the organs are removed. In some cases, pathologic conditions of the psoas muscle may be the cause of death. Türk et al and Tavone et al reported fatal iliopsoas hemorrhage in individuals, which was often associated with anti-coagulant therapy.[209,210] Psoas muscle abscess can also be associated with death.[211]

> **FAQ:** Is the manner of death associated with a hip fracture natural or accident?
>
> **Answer:** Hip fractures are a common terminal event for elderly individuals, and, often, will be certified as a natural death by the clinical physician. However, if an individual falls, fractures their hip, and subsequently dies, if the hip fracture is believed to have contributed to their death, the manner of death is best certified as accident. If it is believed that the individual was walking, fractured their hip because of a natural disease processes (eg, osteoporosis or metastatic disease) and then fell, the manner of death could be considered natural. Of course, distinguishing between the two situations could be difficult.

NATURAL DISEASE OF THE MUSCULOSKELETAL SYSTEM

INTRODUCTION

At the time of forensic autopsy, most of the musculoskeletal system remains unexamined, as it would involve dissection of the extremities, which is mostly avoided unless necessary (eg, documenting the pathway of a projectile or injuries caused by a stab wound), and thus, unless the disease process is present in the neck musculature, the intercostal musculature, the iliopsoas muscle, or the visible portion of the axial skeleton, the disease process is unlikely to be diagnosed at autopsy.

PREGNANCY-RELATED DEATHS

INTRODUCTION

Common causes of death in pregnancy include pulmonary thromboembolism, amniotic fluid embolism, primary postpartum hemorrhage, infections, complications of hypertension including pre-eclampsia and eclampsia, acute myocardial infarction, endocarditis, peripartum cardiomyopathy, long QT syndrome, and aortic and coronary artery dissection.[212,213] In addition, pregnant females can sustain all types of causes of death that non-pregnant individuals sustain, including traumatic causes (eg, blunt force injuries, gunshot wounds) and natural causes.

CHECKLIST of Conditions to Consider at Maternal Autopsy[214]
- ☐ Air embolus
- ☐ Amniotic fluid embolism
- ☐ Aortic and coronary artery dissections
- ☐ Ectopic pregnancy
- ☐ Peripartum cardiomyopathy
- ☐ Pulmonary thromboembolus

- Venous sinus thrombosis
- Placenta accreta
- Acute endometritis
- Pre-eclampsia and eclampsia
- Disseminated intravascular coagulation associated with pre-eclampsia, amniotic fluid embolism, gram-negative septicemia, and incompatible transfusion reactions
- Acute fatty liver of pregnancy
- Rupture of the uterus, either traumatic or associated with previous Cesarean section

AMNIOTIC FLUID EMBOLISM

AUTOPSY FINDINGS

While the gross examination of the organs would not reveal any significant findings, the microscopic examination of the lungs would reveal fetal squamous cells in the maternal vasculature.

ACUTE FATTY LIVER OF PREGNANCY

AUTOPSY FINDINGS

Examination of the liver will reveal steatosis, which, by microscopic examination, is mostly microvesicular steatosis.

ACUTE ENDOMETRITIS-MYOMETRITIS

AUTOPSY FINDINGS

The inner lining of the uterus can appear hemorrhagic. Depending upon the extent of the endometritis-myometritis, the wall of the uterus may also be discolored. Intra-uterine swabs may help identify the causative organism, which can include *Streptococcus pyogenes*, with resultant toxic shock syndrome toxin production.[215] Microscopic examination can reveal transmural inflammation, bacterial overgrowth, and necrosis.

PLACENTA ACCRETA, PLACENTA INCRETA, PLACENTA PERCRETA

AUTOPSY FINDINGS

Placenta accreta, placenta increta, and placenta percreta represent abnormal attachment of the placenta directly to the myometrium, with ingrowth into and potentially through the uterine wall. With rupture of the uterine wall, hemorrhage and/or peritonitis could occur and cause death.

PERIPARTUM CARDIOMYOPATHY

AUTOPSY FINDINGS

Gross examination of the heart would reveal features of a dilated cardiomyopathy.[216] The history will be that the decedent developed symptoms of heart failure during the last month of pregnancy or within 5 months post partum, but there is no evidence or history of a pre-existing heart disease and the cause of the cardiomyopathy is indeterminant.[217] Peripartum cardiomyopathy and dilated cardiomyopathy share some genetic defects.[217]

PRE-ECLAMPSIA/ECLAMPSIA

AUTOPSY FINDINGS

Microscopic examination reveals vascular lesions including perivascular edema, hemorrhage, small vessel thrombosis, and necrosis in the brain, periportal/portal necrosis associated with hepatic arterial medial necrosis in the liver, and glomerular endotheliosis in the kidney.[218]

HELLP SYNDROME

AUTOPSY FINDINGS

In HELLP syndrome (Hemolysis, Elevated Liver enzymes, and Low Platelets) the features of the disease would require antemortem testing or antemortem blood for testing to make an accurate diagnosis; however, HELLP syndrome is associated with hepatic rupture (Figure 7.95) and with certain histologic findings including periportal coagulation necrosis and hemorrhages, which are demarcated from the adjacent uninvolved liver by fibrin, combined with a lack of inflammatory cell infiltrate or steatosis in the liver, bloodless glomeruli in the kidney, and cigar-shaped capillary loops, all of which may allow for the diagnosis to be made postmortem.[219-221]

ECTOPIC PREGNANCY

AUTOPSY FINDINGS

A ruptured ectopic pregnancy will be identified with a hemoperitoneum, and the source being a hemorrhagic nodule or other mass most often in the pelvis (Figure 7.96A). Microscopic examination of the mass will reveal placental villi and/or fetal parts (Figure 7.96B).

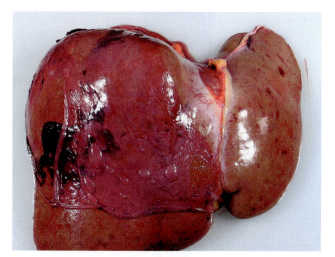

Figure 7.95. Subcapsular hemorrhage in pregnant female with HELLP syndrome. While the hemorrhage was apparent in-situ, no in-situ photo was taken and the hemorrhage was disrupted with removal of the liver from the body. However, the capsule overlying the right lobe of the liver can be seen to be disrupted with residual sub-capsular hemorrhage.

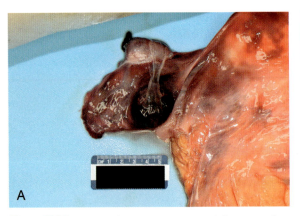
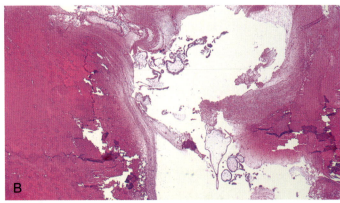

Figure 7.96. Ruptured ectopic pregnancy. Adherent to the ovary and fallopian tube is a small red soft mass (**A**). Microscopic examination revealed chorionic villi (**B**, low power). The gross and microscopic photographs are courtesy of Sunil Prashar, MD.

NEAR MISSES

Near Miss #1: While the classic Duret hemorrhage is a midline linear hemorrhage in the brainstem and while the classic hypertensive-type hemorrhage is a globular hemorrhage in the brainstem there is overlap in the appearance of the two forms of brainstem hemorrhage (Figure 7.97A and B). Assessing for cerebral edema and evidence of herniations may help determine the form of hemorrhage that is present; although, a small hypertensive-type brainstem hemorrhage could lead to cerebral edema, leading to the development of a Duret hemorrhage, and thus an overlap of the two conditions.

Near Miss #2: Small cerebral hemorrhages can have a significant impact. This individual was found outside in the winter, but immediately adjacent to his trailer and shelter, which raised the question of why he was unable to get out of the cold. Autopsy revealed a tiny cerebellar hemorrhage, which could have made him unable to coordinate his movement, and led to his inability to seek shelter from the elements (Figure 7.98A and B).

Near Miss #3: Ruptured caput medusae can present as a stab wound of the abdomen.[222,223] In a similar situation, a skin tumor, such as squamous cell carcinoma, can ulcerate and subsequently hemorrhage profusely and mimic a traumatic injury.

Near Miss #4: When estimating degree of stenosis in the cross section of a coronary artery (Figure 7.99, low power), it must be remembered to not include the thickness of

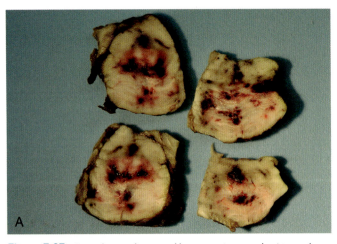
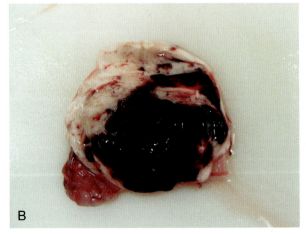

Figure 7.97. Duret hemorrhage and hypertensive-type brainstem hemorrhage. (**A**) is a Duret hemorrhage but not the characteristic midline hemorrhage. (**B**) is a classic globular hypertensive-type brainstem hemorrhage.

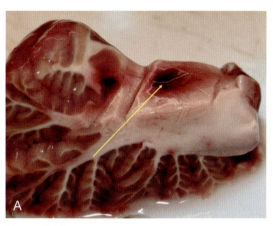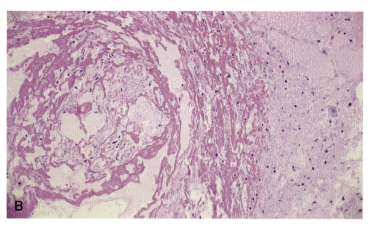

Figure 7.98. Small cerebellar hemorrhage. In the white matter of the peduncle is a small hemorrhage (arrow, **A**). Given the somewhat decomposed nature of the body after being frozen and thawed, a microscopic section confirmed the presence of fibrin (**B**, medium power), and the hemorrhage was considered antemortem and not a postmortem artifact.

the media in that determination. In the vessel in the image, the atherosclerosis produces a measured 40% stenosis of the artery if the media is excluded from the estimated area, but a measured 68% stenosis if the media is included in the estimated area.

Near Miss #5: While a myocardial rupture secondary to an acute myocardial infarct is usually a catastrophic event, with a rapid death due to the quick accumulation of fluid blood in the pericardial sac, with a tiny perforation, the process can be delayed. This individual had a hemorrhagic fibrinous pericarditis secondary to a near pinpoint perforation of the inferior wall of the left ventricle secondary to an acute myocardial infarct (Figure 7.100A-D).

Near Miss #6: Swiss cheese brain, a postmortem artifact, can mimic lacunar infarcts. Swiss cheese brain is an artifact of decomposition gas formation, which can be seen in an unfixed brain but usually requires fixation to preserve the shape (Figure 7.101A and B). However, lacunar infarcts are usually single or a few in number (Figure 7.101C), whereas Swiss cheese artifact normally produces numerous cavitary defects in the cerebral parenchyma.

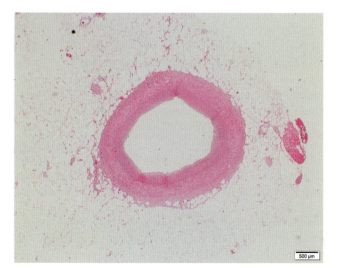

Figure 7.99. Cross section of coronary artery with atherosclerotic plaque. Incorrectly considering the medial thickness in the estimate of the degree of stenosis would result in an over-estimation of the percentage stenosis of the vessel, in this case by nearly 30%.

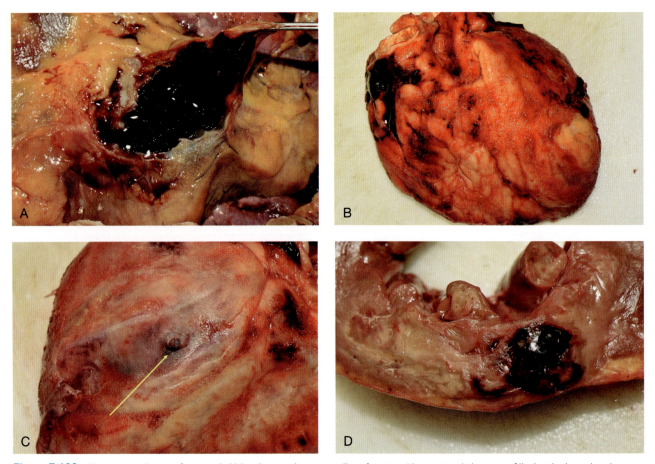

Figure 7.100. Slow accumulation of pericardial blood secondary to small perforation. The pericardial sac was filled with clotted and apparently organizing blood (**A**). The epicardial surface of the heart had a fibrinous, slightly hemorrhagic exudate (**B**). The inferior surface of the left ventricle had a relatively pinpoint perforation of the myocardium (arrow, **C**). A cross section of this region revealed hemorrhage within the wall and evidence of the recent myocardial infarct (**D**).

Near Miss #7: In some situations, the distinction between a fatty liver and cirrhosis can be difficult based only upon gross examination, and what appears nodular on gross examination may not be nodular on microscopic examination (Figure 7.102). Microscopic examination can easily determine whether or not cirrhosis is present.

Near Miss #8: At autopsy, a layer of fibrinous brown-red discolored tissue in the right pleural cavity was identified at autopsy (Figure 7.103A). The first impression was an exuberant healing reaction to rib fractures; however, the pleural was completely stripped from the ribs, revealing no fractures. Microscopic examination identified a mesothelioma (Figure 7.103B).

Near Miss #9: Within the brainstem, small clusters of pinpoint hemorrhage are sometimes identified. While the lesion could be mistaken for trauma, microscopic examination will often reveal dilated small vessels (Figure 7.104A and B).

Near Miss #10: Dried red-black fluid on the face around the mouth is highly suggestive of a gastrointestinal hemorrhage (Figure 7.105), with vomiting or purging of digested blood from the stomach; however, this individual had no identifiable source of a gastrointestinal bleed. The dried fluid on the face was due to hemorrhagic pulmonary edema.

CHAPTER 7 NATURAL DISEASE AT AUTOPSY   161

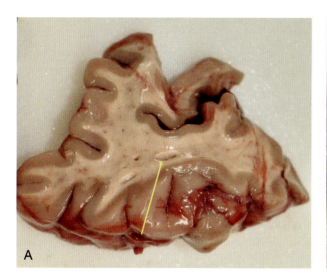
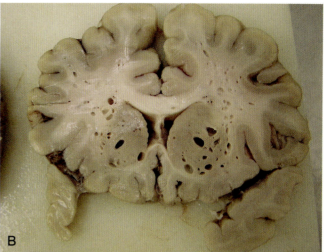
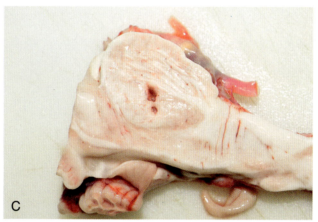

Figure 7.101. Lacunar infarct vs Swiss cheese brain. Although less common to see without fixation, Swiss cheese artifact can be identified (arrow) in a decomposed unfixed brain (**A**); however, fixation tends to preserve the artifact much better (**B**). With Swiss cheese artifact, the lesions tend to be multiple and not concentrated in certain locations, whereas lacunar infarcts tend to be single or few in number and are most often found in or near the basal ganglia or the brainstem (**C**).

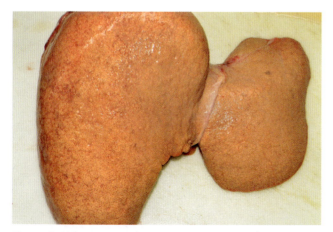

Figure 7.102. Cirrhosis or not. Although the liver appears to have micronodular cirrhosis, sometimes fat accumulation will accentuate the normal lobular architecture of the liver, and appear cirrhotic. Microscopic examination will confirm.

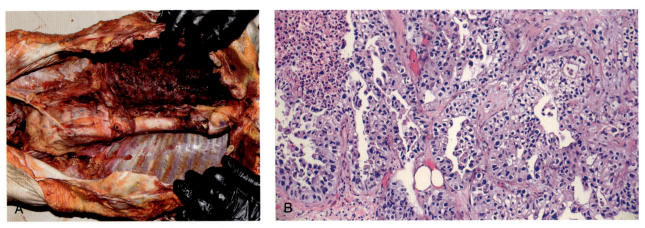

Figure 7.103. Mesothelioma of the right pleural cavity. Gross examination revealed a shaggy red-brown fibrinous exudate–like substance lining the right pleural cavity (**A**). Microscopic examination identified a mesothelioma (**B**, high power).

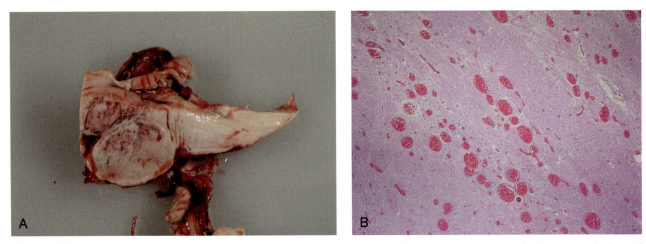

Figure 7.104. Vascular anomaly in brainstem. Gross examination revealed a cluster of pinpoint hemorrhages in the brainstem, which could be misinterpreted as trauma (**A**). Microscopic examination reveals dilated blood vessels (**B**, low power).

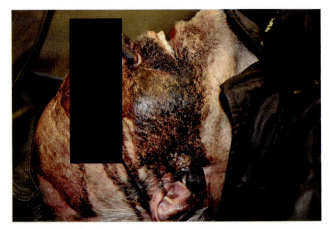

Figure 7.105. Hemorrhagic pulmonary edema mimicking GI bleeding. The dried dark red-black fluidlike substance on the face could easily mimic a GI bleed; however, no source of a GI bleed was identifiable upon dissection and the lungs were congested and hemorrhagic.

References

1. NAME Standards Committee. *Forensic Autopsy Performance Standards*. National Association of Medical Examiners; 2020.
2. Nashelsky MB, Lawrence CH. Accuracy of cause of death determination without forensic autopsy examination. *Am J Forensic Med Pathol*. 2003;24(4):313-319.
3. Gill JR, Scordi-Bello IA. Natural, unexpected deaths: reliability of a presumptive diagnosis. *J Forensic Sci*. 2010;55(1):77-81.
4. Roberts WC, Khan OS. Massive cardiomegaly (>1000 g heart) and obesity. *Am J Cardiol*. 2020;125(2):277-281.
5. Saab J, Salvatore SP. Evaluating the cause of death in obese individuals: a ten-year medical autopsy study. *J Obes*. 2015;2015:695374.
6. Byard RW. The complex spectrum of forensic issues arising from obesity. *Forensic Sci Med Pathol*. 2012;8(4):402-413.
7. Haque AK, Gadre S, Taylor J, Haque SA, Freeman D, Duarte A. Pulmonary and cardiovascular complications of obesity: an autopsy study of 76 obese subjects. *Arch Pathol Lab Med*. 2008;132(9):1397-1404.
8. Pi-Sunyer FX. The obesity epidemic: pathophysiology and consequences of obesity. *Obes Res*. 2002;10:97S-104S.
9. Kumar V, Abbas AK, Aster JC. *Robbins Basic Pathology*. 10th ed. Elsevier; 2018.
10. Byard RW, Tan L. Buried penis and morbid obesity. *Forensic Sci Med Pathol*. 2022;18(2):205-208.
11. Šteiner I, Krbal L. Is obesity a risk factor for coronary atherosclerosis? *Cesk Patol*. 2022;58(2):112-114.
12. Rodríguez-Flores M, Rodríguez-Saldaña J, Cantú-Brito C, Aguirre-García J, Alejandro GG. Prevalence and severity of atherosclerosis in different arterial territories and its relation with obesity. *Cardiovasc Pathol*. 2013;22(5):332-338.
13. Huber C, Hunsaker DM, Hunsaker JC III. The relationship between elevated body mass index and lethal ischemic heart disease: an eleven-year retrospective review of medical examiners' adult autopsies in Kentucky. *J Ky Med Assoc*. 2005;103(3):93-101.
14. Poirier P, Després JP. Obésité et maladies cardiovasculaires [obesity and cardiovascular disease]. *Med Sci*. 2003;19(10):943-949.
15. McGill HC Jr, McMahan CA, Herderick EE, et al. Obesity accelerates the progression of coronary atherosclerosis in young men. *Circulation*. 2002;105(23):2712-2718.
16. Hookana E, Junttila MJ, Puurunen VP, et al. Causes of nonischemic sudden cardiac death in the current era. *Heart Rhythm*. 2011;8(10):1570-1575.
17. Paratz ED, Ashokkumar S, van Heusden A, et al. Obesity in young sudden cardiac death: rates, clinical features, and insights into people with body mass index >50 kg/m^2. *Am J Prev Cardiol*. 2022;11:100369.
18. Vega RS, Adams VI. Suffocation in motor vehicle crashes. *Am J Forensic Med Pathol*. 2004;25(2):101-107.
19. Zhou C, Byard RW. Factors and processes causing accelerated decomposition in human cadavers - an overview. *J Forensic Leg Med*. 2011;18(1):6-9.
20. Jung E, Ryu HH, Ro YS, Cha KC, Shin SD, Hwang SO. Interactions between sleep apnea and coronary artery disease on the incidence of sudden cardiac arrest: a multi-center case-control study. *Yonsei Med J*. 2023;64(1):48-53.
21. Patel M, Yarlagadda H, Upadhyay S, et al. Disturbed sleep is not good for the heart: a narrative review. *Curr Cardiol Rev*. 2023;19(3):1-7. doi:10.2174/1573403X19666221130100141
22. Yeghiazarians Y, Jneid H, Tietjens JR, et al. Obstructive sleep apnea and cardiovascular disease: a scientific statement from the American Heart Association. *Circulation*. 2021;144(3):e56-e67.
23. Heilbrunn E, Ssentongo P, Chinchilli VM, Ssentongo AE. Sudden death in individuals with obstructive sleep apnoea: protocol for a systematic review and meta-analysis. *BMJ Open*. 2020;10(8):e039774.
24. Zhang M, Li L, Fowler D, et al. Causes of sudden death in patients with obstructive sleep apnea. *J Forensic Sci*. 2013;58(5):1171-1174.
25. Mirra SS, Heyman A, McKeel D, et al. The consortium to establish a registry for Alzheimer's disease (CERAD). Part II. Standardization of the neuropathologic assessment of Alzheimer's disease. *Neurology*. 1991;41(4):479-486.

26. Lunardi P. Lobar hemorrhages. *Front Neurol Neurosci.* 2012;30:145-148.
27. Kumar V, Abbas AK, Aster JC. *Robbins and Kumar Basic Pathology.* 11th ed. Elsevier; 2023.
28. Macdonald RL, Schweizer TA. Spontaneous subarachnoid haemorrhage. *Lancet.* 2017;389(10069):655-666.
29. Gonsoulin M, Barnard JJ, Prahlow JA. Death resulting from ruptured cerebral artery aneurysm: 219 cases. *Am J Forensic Med Pathol.* 2002;23(1):5-14.
30. Hillbom M, Kaste M. Alcohol intoxication: a risk factor for primary subarachnoid hemorrhage. *Neurology.* 1982;32(7):706-711.
31. Hillbom M, Kaste M. Does alcohol intoxication precipitate aneurysmal subarachnoid haemorrhage? *J Neurol Neurosurg Psychiatry.* 1981;44(6):523-526.
32. Portunato, Landolfa MC, Botto M, Bonsignore A, De Stefano F, Ventura F. Fatal subarachnoid hemorrhage during sexual activity: a case report. *Am J Forensic Med Pathol.* 2012;33(1):90-92.
33. Teunissen LL, Rinkel GJ, Algra A, van Gijn J. Risk factors for subarachnoid hemorrhage: a systematic review. *Stroke.* 1996;27(3):544-549.
34. Yamada M, Itoh Y, Otomo E, Hayakawa M, Miyatake T. Subarachnoid haemorrhage in the elderly: a necropsy study of the association with cerebral amyloid angiopathy. *J Neurol Neurosurg Psychiatry.* 1993;56(5):543-547.
35. Rinkel GJ, van Gijn J, Wijdicks EF. Subarachnoid hemorrhage without detectable aneurysm. A review of the causes. *Stroke.* 1993;24(9):1403-1409.
36. Zubkov AY, Sanghvi AN, Cloft HJ, Wijdicks EFM, Rabinstein AA. Subarachnoid hemorrhage as a presentation of basilar artery dissection. *Neurocrit Care.* 2007;7(2):165-168.
37. Nicastro N, Schnider A, Leemann B. Anaplastic medullary ependymoma presenting as subarachnoid hemorrhage. *Case Rep Neurol Med.* 2013;2013:701820.
38. Shah AK. Non-aneurysmal primary subarachnoid hemorrhage in pregnancy-induced hypertension and eclampsia. *Neurology.* 2003;61(1):117-120.
39. Kinoshita H, Ayaki T, Maki T, Goda N, Yoshizawa A, Takahashi R. Non-aneurysmal subarachnoid hemorrhaging: a rare cause of death in a patient with multiple system atrophy. *Intern Med.* 2019;58(11):1643-1644.
40. Given CAII, Burdette JH, Elster AD, Williams DWII. Pseudo-subarachnoid hemorrhage: a potential imaging pitfall associated with diffuse cerebral edema. *AJNR Am J Neuroradiol.* 2003;24(2):254-256.
41. Platt A, Collins J, Ramos E, Goldenberg FD. Pseudosubarachnoid hemorrhage: a systematic review of causes, diagnostic modalities, and outcomes in patients who present with pseudosubarachnoid hemorrhage. *Surg Neurol Int.* 2021;12:29.
42. Mularski A, Żaba C. Fatal meningococcal meningitis in a 2-year-old child: a case report. *World J Clin Cases.* 2019;7(5):636-641.
43. Horita T, Kosaka N, Takaoka S, et al. Three autopsy cases of non-meningococcal Waterhouse-Friderichsen syndrome with hypoplastic spleen or post-splenectomy status. *Tohoku J Exp Med.* 2022;258(4):287-301.
44. de Souza A, Desai PK. More often striatal myelinolysis than pontine? A consecutive series of patients with osmotic demyelination syndrome. *Neurol Res.* 2012;34(3):262-271.
45. Unuma K, Harada K, Nakajima M, et al. Autopsy report on central pontine myelinolysis triggered by vomiting associated with digoxin intoxication. *Forensic Sci Int.* 2010;194(1-3):e5-e8.
46. Winkelman MD, Galloway PG. Central nervous system complications of thermal burns. A postmortem study of 139 patients. *Medicine (Baltimore).* 1992;71(5):271-283.
47. Skullerud K, Andersen SN, Lundevall J. Cerebral lesions and causes of death in male alcoholics. A forensic autopsy study. *Int J Legal Med.* 1991;104(4):209-213.
48. Yarid NA, Harruff RC. Globus pallidus necrosis unrelated to carbon monoxide poisoning: retrospective analysis of 27 cases of basal ganglia necrosis. *J Forensic Sci.* 2015;60(6):1484-1487.
49. Alquist CR, McGoey R, Bastian F, Newman WIII. Bilateral globus pallidus lesions. *J La State Med Soc.* 2012;164(3):145-146.
50. Ku CH, Huang WH, Hsu CW, et al. Incidence rate and predictors of globus pallidus necrosis after charcoal burning suicide. *Int J Environ Res Public Health.* 2019;16(22):4426.
51. Al-Afasy HH, Al-Obaidan MA, Al-Ansari YA, et al. Risk factors for multiple sclerosis in Kuwait: a population-based case-control study. *Neuroepidemiology.* 2013;40(1):30-35.

52. Butler MLMD, Dixon E, Stein TD, et al. Tau pathology in chronic traumatic encephalopathy is primarily neuronal. *J Neuropathol Exp Neurol*. 2022;81(10):773-780.

53. Iverson GL, Gardner AJ, Shultz SR, et al. Chronic traumatic encephalopathy neuropathology might not be inexorably progressive or unique to repetitive neurotrauma. *Brain*. 2019;142(12):3672-3693.

54. Rushing EJ, Barnard JJ, Bigio EH, Eagan KP, White CLIII. Frequency of unilateral and bilateral mesial temporal sclerosis in primary and secondary epilepsy: a forensic autopsy study. *Am J Forensic Med Pathol*. 1997;18(4):335-341.

55. Liu Z, Mikati M, Holmes GL. Mesial temporal sclerosis: pathogenesis and significance. *Pediatr Neurol*. 1995;12(1):5-16.

56. Bote RP, Blázquez-Llorca L, Fernández-Gil MA, Alonso-Nanclares L, Muñoz A, De Felipe J. Hippocampal sclerosis: histopathology substrate and magnetic resonance imaging. *Semin Ultrasound CT MR*. 2008;29(1):2-14.

57. Whitney R, Donner EJ. Risk factors for sudden unexpected death in epilepsy (SUDEP) and their mitigation. *Curr Treat Options Neurol*. 2019;21(2):7.

58. Zhuo L, Zhang Y, Zielke HR, et al. Sudden unexpected death in epilepsy: evaluation of forensic autopsy cases. *Forensic Sci Int*. 2012;223(1-3):171-175.

59. Sköldenberg B. Herpes simplex encephalitis. *Scand J Infect Dis Suppl*. 1996;100:8-13.

60. Rogde S, Kerty E, Skullerud K. Significance of inflammatory changes in the brainstem in forensic autopsy cases. *Forensic Sci Int*. 1999;104(2-3):105-115.

61. Turillazzi E, Bello S, Neri M, Riezzo I, Fineschi V. Colloid cyst of the third ventricle, hypothalamus, and heart: a dangerous link for sudden death. *Diagn Pathol*. 2012;7:144.

62. Byard RW, Moore L. Sudden and unexpected death in childhood due to a colloid cyst of the third ventricle. *J Forensic Sci*. 1993;38(1):210-213.

63. Lagman C, Rai K, Chung LK, et al. Fatal colloid cysts: a systematic review. *World Neurosurg*. 2017;107:409-415.

64. Ackerman MJ, Giudicessi JR. Post-Mortem cardiovascular implantable electronic device interrogation: clinical indications and potential benefits. *J Am Coll Cardiol*. 2016;68(12):1265-1267.

65. Riesinger L, Fichtner S, Schuhmann CG, et al. Postmortem interrogation of cardiac implantable electrical devices may clarify time and cause of death. *Int J Legal Med*. 2019;133(3):883-888.

66. Prahlow JA, Guileyardo JM, Barnard JJ. The implantable cardioverter-defibrillator. A potential hazard for autopsy pathologists. *Arch Pathol Lab Med*. 1997;121(10):1076-1080.

67. Räder SB, Zeijlemaker V, Pehrson S, Svendsen JH. Making post-mortem implantable cardioverter defibrillator explantation safe. *Europace*. 2009;11(10):1317-1322.

68. Westaby JD, Miles C, Chis Ster I, et al. Characterisation of hypertensive heart disease: pathological insights from a sudden cardiac death cohort to inform clinical practice. *J Hum Hypertens*. 2022;36(3):246-253.

69. Kokubo Y, Matsumoto C. Hypertension is a risk factor for several types of heart disease: review of prospective studies. *Adv Exp Med Biol*. 2017;956:419-426.

70. Verdecchia P, Angeli F, Cavallini C, et al. Sudden cardiac death in hypertensive patients. *Hypertension*. 2019;73(5):1071-1078.

71. Xue JJ, Wang TQ, Jia YQ, et al. Statistical analysis of the heart and lung mass in forensic anatomical cases and its forensic significance. *Fa Yi Xue Za Zhi*. 2019;35(6):651-656.

72. Schenk KE, Heinze G. Age-dependent changes of heart valves and heart size. *Recent Adv Stud Cardiac Struct Metab*. 1975;10:617-624.

73. Hiyoshi Y, Omae T, Hirota Y, Takeshita M, Ueda K, Katsuki S. Clinicopathological study of the heart and coronary arteries of autopsied cases from the community of Hisayama during a 10 yr period—III. Heart weight. *J Chronic Dis*. 1978;31(5):329-336.

74. Howell TH. Heart weights among octogenarians. *J Am Geriatr Soc*. 1981;29(12):572-575.

75. Romppanen T, Seppä A, Roilas H. Ischemic heart disease and heart weight. *Cardiology*. 1983;70(4):206-212.

76. Molina DK, DiMaio VJ. Normal organ weights in men: part I—the heart. *Am J Forensic Med Pathol*. 2012;33(4):362-367.

77. Molina DK, DiMaio VJ. Normal organ weights in women: part I—the heart. *Am J Forensic Med Pathol*. 2015;36(3):176-181.

78. Schoppen ZJ, Balmert LC, White S, et al. Prevalence of abnormal heart weight after sudden death in people younger than 40 years of age. *J Am Heart Assoc*. 2020;9(18):e015699.
79. Basso C, Michaud K, d'Amati G, et al. Cardiac hypertrophy at autopsy. *Virchows Arch*. 2021;479(1):79-94.
80. Kakimoto Y, Asakura K, Osawa M. Cutoff value for hypertrophic heart weight in the Japanese population. *Leg Med*. 2021;48:101831.
81. Tracy RE. Association of cardiomegaly with coronary artery histopathology and its relationship to atheroma. *J Atheroscler Thromb*. 2011;18(1):32-41.
82. Jiangping S, Zhe Z, Wei W, et al. Assessment of coronary artery stenosis by coronary angiography: a head-to-head comparison with pathological coronary artery anatomy. *Circ Cardiovasc Interv*. 2013;6(3):262-268.
83. Sheppard M, Davies MJ. *Practical Cardiovascular Pathology*. Arnold; 1998.
84. Markwerth P, Bajanowski T, Tzimas I, Dettmeyer R. Sudden cardiac death-update. *Int J Legal Med*. 2021;135(2):483-495.
85. Basso C, Aguilera B, Banner J, et al. Guidelines for autopsy investigation of sudden cardiac death: 2017 update from the Association for European Cardiovascular Pathology. *Virchows Arch*. 2017;471(6):691-705.
86. Holmström L, Juntunen S, Vähätalo J, et al. Plaque histology and myocardial disease in sudden coronary death: the Fingesture study. *Eur Heart J*. 2022;43(47):4923-4930.
87. Farthing WH Jr, Shirani J. Coronary artery intimal hyperplasia, occlusive platelet thrombus, and fatal myocardial infarction in an intravenous cocaine user. *Cardiovasc Pathol*. 1995;4(3):215-219.
88. Bhavsar T, Hayes T, Wurzel J. Epicardial coronary artery intimal smooth muscle hyperplasia in a cocaine user. *World J Cardiol*. 2011;3(10):337-338.
89. Cohle SD. Fatal coronary artery intimal hyperplasia due to amphetamine use. *Cardiovasc Pathol*. 2013;22(3):e1-e4.
90. Buja LM, Butany J. *Cardiovascular Pathology*. 4th ed. Elsevier; 2016.
91. Padera RF. Pathologic evaluation of cardiovascular medical devices. *Surg Pathol Clin*. 2012;5(2):497-521.
92. Bradshaw SH, Kennedy L, Dexter DF, Veinot JP. A practical method to rapidly dissolve metallic stents. *Cardiovasc Pathol*. 2009;18(3):127-133.
93. Haque K, Bhargava P. Abdominal aortic aneurysm. *Am Fam Physician*. 2022;106(2):165-172.
94. Koyama Y, Miura M, Kobayashi T, et al. A registry study of Kawasaki disease patients with coronary artery aneurysms (KIDCAR): a report on a multicenter prospective registry study three years after commencement. *Eur J Pediatr*. 2023;182(2):633-640.
95. Chakraborty A, Johnson JN, Spagnoli J, et al. Long-term cardiovascular outcomes of multisystem inflammatory syndrome in children associated with COVID-19 using an institution based algorithm. *Pediatr Cardiol*. 2023;44(2):367-380.
96. Kang N, Choi KH, Kim SM, Kim DK, Sung K, Choi DC. Giant coronary artery aneurysm with thrombosis complicated in a patient with idiopathic hypereosinophilic syndrome. *Yonsei Med J*. 2023;64(2):148-151.
97. Schafigh M, Bakhtiary F, Kolck UW, Zimmer S, Greschus S, Silaschi M. Coronary artery aneurysm rupture in a patient with polyarteritis nodosa. *JACC Case Rep*. 2022;4(22):1522-1528.
98. Erdogan M, Ozgur DS, Akkuzu G, Bes C. A giant coronary artery aneurysm in a patient with Behçet's syndrome. *Rheumatology*. 2022;61(11):e354-e355.
99. Han HC, Parsons SA, Teh AW, et al. Characteristic histopathological findings and cardiac arrest rhythm in isolated mitral valve prolapse and sudden cardiac death. *J Am Heart Assoc*. 2020;9(7):e015587.
100. Vriz O, Landi I, Eltayeb A, et al. Mitral valve prolapse and sudden cardiac death in athletes at high risk. *Curr Cardiol Rev*. 2023;19(3):86-100. doi:10.2174/1573403X19666221220163431
101. Krawczyk-Ożóg A, Hołda MK, Bolechała F, et al. Anatomy of the mitral subvalvular apparatus. *J Thorac Cardiovasc Surg*. 2018;155(5):2002-2010.
102. Abdel-Haq N, Moussa Z, Farhat MH, Chandrasekar L, Asmar BI. Infectious and noninfectious acute pericarditis in children: an 11-year experience. *Int J Pediatr*. 2018;2018:5450697.
103. Nehme F, Gitau J, Liu J. Purulent pericarditis as a complication of bacteraemic *Enterococcus faecalis* urinary tract infection. *BMJ Case Rep*. 2017;2017:bcr2017219498.

104. Li L, Zhang Y, Burke A, et al. Demographic, clinical and pathological features of sudden deaths due to myocarditis: results from a state-wide population-based autopsy study. *Forensic Sci Int.* 2017;272:81-86.
105. Dettmeyer R, Schlamann M, Madea B. Immunohistochemical techniques improve the diagnosis of myocarditis in cases of suspected sudden infant death syndrome (SIDS). *Forensic Sci Int.* 1999;105(2):83-94.
106. Grasmeyer S, Madea B. Immunohistochemical diagnosis of myocarditis on (infantile) autopsy material: does it improve the diagnosis? *Forensic Sci Med Pathol.* 2015;11(2):168-176.
107. Sakai J, Moriya T, Takahashi S, Hashiyada M, Funayama M. An infantile case of asphyxia with coincidental myocarditis. *Leg Med.* 2009;11(6):291-293.
108. Kytö V, Saukko P, Lignitz E, et al. Diagnosis and presentation of fatal myocarditis. *Hum Pathol.* 2005;36(9):1003-1007.
109. Bonsignore A, Palmiere C, Buffelli F, et al. When is myocarditis indeed the cause of death? *Forensic Sci Int.* 2018;285:72-76.
110. De Salvia A, De Leo D, Carturan E, Basso C. Sudden cardiac death, borderline myocarditis and molecular diagnosis: evidence or assumption? *Med Sci Law.* 2011;51(suppl 1):S27-S29.
111. du Long R, Fronczek J, Niessen HWM, van der Wal AC, de Boer HH. The histopathological spectrum of myocardial inflammation in relation to circumstance of death: a retrospective cohort study in clinical and forensic autopsies. *Forensic Sci Res.* 2022;7(2):238-246.
112. Kitulwatte ID, Kim PJ, Pollanen MS. Sudden death related myocarditis: a study of 56 cases. *Forensic Sci Med Pathol.* 2010;6(1):13-19.
113. Griffiths PD, Hannington G, Booth JC. Coxsackie B virus infections and myocardial infarction. Results from a prospective, epidemiologically controlled study. *Lancet.* 1980;1(8183):1387-1389.
114. Berklite L, Mitchell S, Wheeler SE. Large viral meningoencephalitis CSF serologic panel lacks utility in clinical decisions and outcomes. *Clin Biochem.* 2022;109-110:17-22.
115. Munkholm J, Andersen CB, Ottesen GL. Plakoglobin: a diagnostic marker of arrhythmogenic right ventricular cardiomyopathy in forensic pathology? *Forensic Sci Med Pathol.* 2015;11(1):47-52.
116. Dimitrova IN, Gaydarski L, Landzhov B, et al. Variant origin of three main coronary ostia from the right sinus of Valsalva: report of a rare case. *Folia Morphol (Warsz).* 2022. doi: 10.5603/FM.a2022.0092
117. Gowda RM, Khan IA, Undavia M, Vasavada BC, Sacchi TJ. Origin of all major coronary arteries from left sinus of Valsalva as a common coronary trunk: single coronary artery—a case report. *Angiology.* 2004;55(1):103-105.
118. Niu M, Zhang J, Ge Y, Hu X, Liu Z, Wu J. Acute myocardial infarction in the elderly with anomalous origin of the left coronary artery from the pulmonary artery (ALCAPA): a case report and literature review. *Medicine (Baltim).* 2022;101(48):e32219.
119. Molossi S, Agrawal H. Clinical evaluation of anomalous aortic origin of a coronary artery (AAOCA). *Congenit Heart Dis.* 2017;12(5):607-609.
120. Benson PA. Anomalous aortic origin of coronary artery with sudden death: case report and review. *Am Heart J.* February 1970;79(2):254-257.
121. Montaña-Jimenez LP, Molossi S, Masand P, et al. Intramural course of an anomalous left coronary artery is not always associated with a slit-like ostium. *Cardiol Young.* 2023;17:1-3.
122. Amioka N, Nakamura K, Matsuo N, et al. Repeated syncope during exercise as a result of anomalous origin of left coronary artery with intramural aortic course in a teenage boy. *Tex Heart Inst J.* 2022;49(6):e217677.
123. Karikalan S, Sharma M, Chandna MK, Chandna H, Surani S. A rare case of anomalous origin of left anterior descending artery from right coronary ostium. *Cureus.* 2021;13(10):e18966.
124. D'Ascenzi F, Valentini F, Pistoresi S, et al. Causes of sudden cardiac death in young athletes and non-athletes: systematic review and meta-analysis. Sudden cardiac death in the young. *Trends Cardiovasc Med.* 2022;32(5):299-308.
125. Murtaza G, Mukherjee D, Gharacholou SM, et al. An updated review on myocardial Bridging. *Cardiovasc Revasc Med.* 2020;21(9):1169-1179.
126. Lee MS, Chen CH. Myocardial bridging: an up-to-date review. *J Invasive Cardiol.* 2015;27(11):521-528.
127. Santucci A, Jacoangeli F, Cavallini S, d'Ammando M, de Angelis F, Cavallini C. The myocardial bridge: incidence, diagnosis, and prognosis of a pathology of uncertain clinical significance. *Eur Heart J Suppl.* 2022;24(suppl I):I61-I67.

128. Gay JD, Guileyardo JM, Townsend-Parchman JK, Ross K. Clinical and morphologic features of lipomatous hypertrophy ("massive fatty deposits") of the interatrial septum. *Am J Forensic Med Pathol*. 1996;17(1):43-48.

129. Hejna P, Janík M. Lipomatous hypertrophy of the interatrial septum: a possibly neglected cause of sudden cardiac death. *Forensic Sci Med Pathol*. 2014;10(1):119-121.

130. Arbarello P, Maiese A, Bolino G. Case study of sudden cardiac death caused by lypomatous hypertrophy of the interatrial septum. *Med Leg J*. 2012;80(Pt 3):102-104.

131. O'Connor S, Recavarren R, Nichols LC, Parwani AV. Lipomatous hypertrophy of the interatrial septum: an overview. *Arch Pathol Lab Med*. 2006;130(3):397-399.

132. di Gioia CR, Giordano C, Cerbelli B, et al. Nonischemic left ventricular scar and cardiac sudden death in the young. *Hum Pathol*. 2016;58:78-89.

133. Tan SY, Fritsch MK, White S, Arva NC. Dissecting the cardiac conduction system: is it worthwhile? *Pediatr Dev Pathol*. 2020;23(6):413-423.

134. Cohle SD, Suarez-Mier MP, Aguilera B. Sudden death resulting from lesions of the cardiac conduction system. *Am J Forensic Med Pathol*. 2002;23(1):83-89.

135. Nerantzis CE, Couvaris CM, Pastromas SC, Marianou SK, Boghiokas ID, Koutsaftis PN. Histological findings of the atrioventricular conductive system in street heroin addicts, victims of sudden unexpected death. *J Forensic Sci*. 2013;58:S99-S104.

136. Burke AP, Subramanian R, Smialek J, Virmani R. Nonatherosclerotic narrowing of the atrioventricular node artery and sudden death. *J Am Coll Cardiol*. 1993;21(1):117-122.

137. Zack F, Kutter G, Blaas V, Rodewald AK, Büttner A. Fibromuscular dysplasia of cardiac conduction system arteries in traumatic and nonnatural sudden death victims aged 0 to 40 years: a histological analysis of 100 cases. *Cardiovasc Pathol*. 2014;23(1):12-16.

138. Kitulwatte IDG, Edirisinghe PAS. Study on existence of inflammation in the myocardium in unequivocal acute traumatic deaths. *J Forensic Leg Med*. 2020;75:102055.

139. Tamura S, Takahashi M, Kawamura S, Ishihara T. Basophilic degeneration of the myocardium: histological, immunohistochemical and immuno-electronmicroscopic studies. *Histopathology*. 1995;26(6):501-508.

140. Liu Z, Liu Y, Wu M, Zhu X, Xu X. Sudden unexpected death due to spontaneous pneumothorax caused by ruptured bilateral pulmonary bullae. *J Forensic Sci*. 2021;66(6):2499-2503.

141. Marom EM, McAdams HP, Sporn TA, Goodman PC. Lentil aspiration pneumonia: radiographic and CT findings. *J Comput Assist Tomogr*. 1998;22(4):598-600.

142. Oertel L, Gressel A, Tortel MC, et al. Be careful with lentils! About a forensic observation. *Int J Legal Med*. 2021;135(1):323-327.

143. Kuroki M, Nakata H, Masuda T, et al. Minute pulmonary meningothelial-like nodules: high-resolution computed tomography and pathologic correlations. *J Thorac Imaging*. 2002;17(3):227-229.

144. Randall B. Fatty liver and sudden death. A review. *Hum Pathol*. 1980;11(2):147-153.

145. Randall B. Sudden death and hepatic fatty metamorphosis. A North Carolina survey. *J Am Med Assoc*. 1980;243(17):1723-1725.

146. Yuzuriha T, Okudaira M, Tominaga I, et al. Alcohol-related sudden death with hepatic fatty metamorphosis: a comprehensive clinicopathological inquiry into its pathogenesis. *Alcohol Alcohol*. 1997;32(6):745-752.

147. Sorkin T, Sheppard MN. Sudden unexplained death in alcohol misuse (SUDAM) patients have different characteristics to those who died from sudden arrhythmic death syndrome (SADS). *Forensic Sci Med Pathol*. 2017;13(3):278-283.

148. Templeton AH, Carter KL, Sheron N, Gallagher PJ, Verrill C. Sudden unexpected death in alcohol misuse—an unrecognized public health issue? *Int J Environ Res Public Health*. 2009;6(12):3070-3081.

149. Ballestri S, Lonardo A, Bonapace S, Byrne CD, Loria P, Targher G. Risk of cardiovascular, cardiac and arrhythmic complications in patients with non-alcoholic fatty liver disease. *World J Gastroenterol*. 2014;20(7):1724-1745.

150. Chen Z, Liu J, Zhou F, et al. Nonalcoholic fatty liver disease: an emerging driver of cardiac arrhythmia. *Circ Res*. 2021;128(11):1747-1765.

151. Chung TH, Shim JY, Lee YJ. Nonalcoholic fatty liver disease as a risk factor for prolonged corrected QT interval in apparently healthy Korean women. *J Gastrointestin Liver Dis*. 2020;29(1):59-64.

152. Ameri M, Mehrpisheh S, Memarian A, Balvayeh P. Sudden death due to association between NAFLD and cardiovascular changes in a 37-year-old man: a case report. *Acta Med Iran*. 2016;54(4):283-285.

153. Kujovich JL. Coagulopathy in liver disease: a balancing act. *Hematology Am Soc Hematol Educ Program*. 2015;2015:243-249.

154. Park SB, Jeon JW, Shin HP. The risk of endoscopy-related bleeding in patients with liver cirrhosis: a retrospective study. *Medicina*. 2023;59(1):170.

155. Harrison MF. The misunderstood coagulopathy of liver disease: a review for the acute setting. *West J Emerg Med*. 2018;19(5):863-871.

156. Saner FH, Abeysundara L, Hartmann M, Mallett SV. Rational approach to transfusion in liver transplantation. *Minerva Anestesiol*. 2018;84(3):378-388.

157. Li J, Han B, Li H, et al. Association of coagulopathy with the risk of bleeding after invasive procedures in liver cirrhosis. *Saudi J Gastroenterol*. 2018;24(4):220-227.

158. Janko N, Majeed A, Commins I, Kemp W, Roberts SK. Procedural bleeding risk, rather than conventional coagulation tests, predicts procedure related bleeding in cirrhosis. *Eur J Gastroenterol Hepatol*. 2022;34(2):192-199.

159. Ruberto MF, Piras MS, Sorbello O, et al. Chronic intravascular coagulation in liver cirrhosis predicts a high hemorrhagic risk. *Eur Rev Med Pharmacol Sci*. 2021;25(17):5518-5524.

160. Ballantine A, Martin D, Thakrar SV. The coagulopathy of liver disease: a shift in thinking. *Br J Hosp Med*. 2021;82(6):1-9.

161. Zermatten MG, Fraga M, Moradpour D, et al. Hemostatic alterations in patients with cirrhosis: from primary hemostasis to fibrinolysis. *Hepatology*. 2020;71(6):2135-2148.

162. Angelo C, Tan A, Halegoua-De Marzio D, Fenkel JM. Hematuria leads to a new diagnosis of cirrhosis. *Case Rep Gastroenterol*. 2022;16(2):446-451.

163. Broussard KA, Rockey DC. Bleeding ectopic varices: clinical presentation, natural history, and outcomes. *J Investig Med*. 2022;70(5):1280-1284.

164. Flynn K, Chung K, Brooke T, Keung J. Ectopic variceal bleeding from chronic superior mesenteric vein thrombosis after hemorrhagic pancreatitis. *Clin Case Rep*. 2022;10(4):e05731.

165. Zhu K, Zhang W, Shao W, Ding J, Ma C. Report of a case of cirrhotic portal hypertension with ectopic varices in the bilateral pulmonary hilar. *DEN Open*. 2022;2(1):e99.

166. Wongjarupong N, Said HS, Huynh RK, Golzarian J, Lim N. Hemoperitoneum from bleeding intra-abdominal varices: a rare, life-threatening cause of abdominal pain in a patient with cirrhosis. *Cureus*. 2021;13(10):e18955.

167. San Juan López C, Lázaro Sáez M, Hernández Martínez Á, López González J, Vega Sáenz JL. Bleeding from gallbladder varices in a patient with an unknown liver cirrhosis. An exceptional entity. *Rev Esp Enferm Dig*. 2019;111(9):723-724.

168. Edula RG, Qureshi K, Khallafi H. Hemorrhagic ascites from spontaneous ectopic mesenteric varices rupture in NASH induced cirrhosis and successful outcome: a case report. *World J Gastroenterol*. 2014;20(25):8292-8297.

169. Goldstein AM, Gorlick N, Gibbs D, Fernández-del Castillo C. Hemoperitoneum due to spontaneous rupture of the umbilical vein. *Am J Gastroenterol*. 1995;90(2):315-317.

170. Ben Hammouda S, Grayaa M, Njima M, et al. Sudden death due to cirrhotic cardiomyopathy: an autopsy case report. *J Forensic Leg Med*. 2022;89:102369.

171. Mozos I. Arrhythmia risk in liver cirrhosis. *World J Hepatol*. 2015;7(4):662-672.

172. González-Castillo AM, Sancho-Insenser J, Miguel-Palacio M, et al. Risk factors for complications in acute calculous cholecystitis. Deconstruction of the Tokyo guidelines. *Cir Esp*. 2023;101(3):170-179.

173. Dean DE, Jamison JM, Lane JL. Spontaneous rupture of the gall bladder: an unusual forensic diagnosis. *J Forensic Sci*. 2014;59(4):1142-1145.

174. Birnaruberl CG, RiBe M, Kettner M, Schnabel A, Ramsthaler F, Verhoff MA. So-called skin signs in acute pancreatitis. *Arch Kriminol*. 2016;238(1-2):42-56.

175. Kashiwagi R, Shimamura Y, Imamura K. Uncommon etiology of Cullen's sign and Grey Turner sign. *J Gen Fam Med*. 2022;23(4):282-283.

176. Singh G, Mittal A, Panwar VK, Ghorai R, Upadhyay A. Acute pyelonephritis with Cullen's sign masquerading as pancreatitis. *Cureus*. 2022;14(3):e23222.

177. Armour RH, Clifton MA, Marsh CH. Balloon catheter contol of a ruptured abdominal aortic aneurysm in a patient with Cullen's sign. *Br J Surg*. 1978;65(5):350.

178. Chung MA, Oung C, Szilagyi A. Cullen's sign: it doesn't always mean hemorrhagic pancreatitis. *Am J Gastroenterol*. 1992;87(8):1026-1028.

179. Wright WF. Cullen sign and Grey Turner sign revisited. *J Am Osteopath Assoc*. 2016;116(6):398-401.

180. Tsokos M, Braun C. Acute pancreatitis presenting as sudden, unexpected death: an autopsy-based study of 27 cases. *Am J Forensic Med Pathol*. 2007;28(3):267-270.

181. Tümer AR, Dener C. Diagnostic dilemma of sudden deaths due to acute hemorrhagic pancreatitis. *J Forensic Sci*. 2007;52(1):180-182.

182. Renner IG, Savage WTIII, Pantoja JL, Renner VJ. Death due to acute pancreatitis. A retrospective analysis of 405 autopsy cases. *Dig Dis Sci*. 1985;30(10):1005-1018.

183. Eichelberger MR, Chatten J, Bruce DA, Garcia VF, Goldman M, Koop CE. Acute pancreatitis and increased intracranial pressure. *J Pediatr Surg*. 1981;16(4 suppl 1):562-570.

184. Moldenhauer JS, O'brien JM, Barton JR, Sibai B. Acute fatty liver of pregnancy associated with pancreatitis: a life-threatening complication. *Am J Obstet Gynecol*. 2004;190(2):502-505.

185. Bruijn JA, van Albada-Kuipers GA, Smit VT, Eulderink F. Acute pancreatitis in systemic lupus erythematosus. *Scand J Rheumatol*. 1986;15(4):363-367.

186. Bel Hadj M, Marzougui M, Ben Abdeljelil N, Dhouieb R, Zakhama A, Chadly A. Spontaneous rupture of a hepatic cavernous hemangioma: a rare case of sudden unexpected death. *Am J Forensic Med Pathol*. 2020;41(2):138-140.

187. Molavi DW. *The Practice of Surgical Pathology: A Beginner's Guide to the Diagnostic Process*. Springer; 2008.

188. Ruiz-Mesa JD, Marquez-Gomez I, Sena G, et al. Factors associated with severe sepsis or septic shock in complicated pyelonephritis. *Medicine (Baltimore)*. 2017;96(43):e8371.

189. He R, Li X, Xie K, Wen B, Qi X. Characteristics of Fournier gangrene and evaluation of the effects of negative-pressure wound therapy. *Front Surg*. 2022;9:1075968.

190. Bayileyegn NS, Tareke AA. Fournier's gangrene in an eight-day-old male neonate, a case report. *Int J Surg Case Rep*. 2022;94:106982. doi:10.1016/j.ijscr.2022.106982

191. Yoshinaka A, Akatsuka M, Yamamoto S, Yamakage M. Sudden cardiac arrest associated with myxedema coma due to undiagnosed hypothyroidism: a case report. *BMC Endocr Disord*. 2021;21(1):229.

192. Bakiner O, Ertorer ME, Haydardedeoglu FE, Bozkirli E, Tutuncu NB, Demirag NG. Subclinical hypothyroidism is characterized by increased QT interval dispersion among women. *Med Princ Pract*. 2008;17(5):390-394.

193. Galetta F, Franzoni F, Fallahi P, et al. Changes in heart rate variability and QT dispersion in patients with overt hypothyroidism. *Eur J Endocrinol*. 2008;158(1):85-90.

194. Radojevic N, Medenica S, Vujosevic S, Savic S. Sudden unexpected death associated with Hashimoto's thyroiditis and thymic hyperplasia. *Med Leg J*. 2017;85(2):111-112.

195. Harvey PW, Sutcliffe C. Adrenocortical hypertrophy: establishing cause and toxicological significance. *J Appl Toxicol*. 2010;30(7):617-626.

196. Aarella VG, Mudenha ET, Okpe A, Fernando DJ. Acute transient stress induced adrenal hypertrophy and adrenal medullary hyperactivity. *Eur J Case Rep Intern Med*. 2016;3(1):000257.

197. Monticone S, D'Ascenzo F, Moretti C, et al. Cardiovascular events and target organ damage in primary aldosteronism compared with essential hypertension: a systematic review and meta-analysis. *Lancet Diabetes Endocrinol*. 2018;6(1):41-50.

198. Bann DV, Goyal N, Crist H, Goldenberg D. Black thyroid. *Ear Nose Throat J*. 2014;93(10-11):E54-E55.

199. Tsokos M, Schröder S. Black thyroid: report of an autopsy case. *Int J Legal Med*. 2006;120(3):157-159.

200. Behrens C, Yen PP. Esophageal inlet patch. *Radiol Res Pract*. 2011;2011:460890. doi:10.1155/2011/460890

201. Živković V, Nikolić S. The unusual appearance of black esophagus in a case of fatal hypothermia: a possible underlying mechanism. *Forensic Sci Med Pathol*. 2013;9(4):613-614.

202. Unuma K, Harada K, Funakoshi T, Uemura K. Sudden death of an alcoholic elderly man with acute esophageal necrosis (black esophagus). *Forensic Sci Int*. 2011;212(1-3):e15-e17.

203. Kanamori K, Koyanagi K, Nakamura K, et al. Thoracoscopic esophagectomy for stenosis of thoracic esophagus due to acute esophageal necrosis associated with alcoholic ketoacidosis. *Asian J Endosc Surg*. 2023;16(3):518-522. doi:10.1111/ases.13158

204. Jeican II, Inişca P, Gheban BA, et al. Asymptomatic esophageal necrosis in a patient with recent COVID-19: the first case diagnosed through autopsy. *Medicina (Kaunas)*. 2023;59(1):154.
205. Gilbert JD, Byard RW. Lethal phlegmonous colitis. *Med Sci Law*. 2018;58(3):186-188.
206. Boutilier RG, Murray SK, Walley VM. Green colon: an unusual appearance at autopsy. *Arch Pathol Lab Med*. 2000;124(9):1397-1398.
207. Sagoh T, Itoh K, Togashi K, et al. Gamna-Gandy bodies of the spleen: evaluation with MR imaging. *Radiology*. 1989;172(3):685-687.
208. Zipfel E, Zschoch H, Poley F. Die Bedeutung der Milzkapselfibrose und der Periossplenitis cartilaginea für die postmortale Diagnostik von Hypertonie und Cor pulmonale [The consequences of fibrosis of spleen capsule and perisplenitis cartilaginea for the postmortem diagnosis of hypertension and cor pulmonale (author's transl)]. *Zentralbl Allg Pathol*. 1978;122(1-2):23-24.
209. Türk EE, Verhoff MA, Tsokos M. Anticoagulant-related iliopsoas muscle bleeding leading to fatal exsanguination: report of two autopsy cases. *Am J Forensic Med Pathol*. 2002;23(4):342-344.
210. Tavone AM, Giuga G, Attanasio A, et al. A rapid fatal outcome of iliopsoas hematoma: clinical and autopsy findings. *J Investig Med High Impact Case Rep*. 2022;10:23247096221111760. doi:10.1177/23247096221111760
211. Grayaa M, Ben Jomaa S, Saadi S, et al. A missed psoas abscess diagnosis: a forensic case report. *Forensic Sci Med Pathol*. 2022;18(3):240-243.
212. Christiansen LR, Collins KA. Pregnancy-associated deaths: a 15-year retrospective study and overall review of maternal pathophysiology. *Am J Forensic Med Pathol*. 2006;27(1):11-19.
213. Herbst J, Winskog C, Byard RW. Cardiovascular conditions and the evaluation of the heart in pregnancy-associated autopsies. *J Forensic Sci*. 2010;55(6):1528-1533.
214. Rushton DI, Dawson IM. The maternal autopsy. *J Clin Pathol*. 1982;35(9):909-921.
215. Riad M, Thottacherry E, Crawley C, Phillip-Abraham N, Ibrahim F. Invasive Group A streptococcal postpartum endometritis associated with multi-organ infarctions: an uncommon case presentation and literature review. *Postgrad Med*. 2020;132(6):526-531.
216. Aroney C, Khafagi F, Boyle C, Bett N. Peripartum cardiomyopathy: echocardiographic features in five cases. *Am J Obstet Gynecol*. 1986;155(1):103-106.
217. Bhattacharyya A, Basra SS, Sen P, Kar B. Peripartum cardiomyopathy: a review. *Tex Heart Inst J*. 2012;39(1):8-16.
218. Hecht JL, Ordi J, Carrilho C, et al. The pathology of eclampsia: an autopsy series. *Hypertens Pregnancy*. 2017;36(3):259-268.
219. Dubey S, Rani J. Hepatic rupture in preeclampsia and HELLP syndrome: a catastrophic presentation. *Taiwan J Obstet Gynecol*. 2020;59(5):643-651.
220. Sujirachato K, Srisont S, Peonim V. HELLP syndrome in pregnancy as a cause of sudden unexpected death and spontaneous hepatic rupture: a medico-legal autopsy case report. *J Med Assoc Thai*. 2012;95(4):614-617.
221. Tsokos M, Longauer F, Kardosová V, Gavel A, Anders S, Schulz F. Maternal death in pregnancy from HELLP syndrome. A report of three medico-legal autopsy cases with special reference to distinctive histopathological alterations. *Int J Legal Med*. 2002;116(1):50-53.
222. Frigiolini F, Lo Pinto S, Caputo F, et al. Fatal hemorrhage from a periumbilical wound: Stabbing or hemorrhage from a caput medusae? *J Forensic Sci*. 2021;66(1):393-397.
223. Bahner DRJr, Holland RWIII. Exsanguinating hemorrhage from a caput medusae: cutaneous variceal bleeding. *J Emerg Med*. 1992;10(1):19-23.

ASPHYXIA 8

CHAPTER OUTLINE

Introduction   174

Specific Forms of Asphyxia Causing Failure of Oxygen to Reach the Lung   178
- Introduction   178
- Smothering   178
  - Description   178
  - Pattern at Autopsy   180
- Choking   180
  - Description   180
  - Pattern at Autopsy   180
- Mechanical Asphyxia/Traumatic Asphyxia/Positional Asphyxia   181
  - Description   181
  - Pattern at Autopsy   183
- Vitiated Atmosphere/Suffocating Gases   183
  - Description   183
  - Pattern at Autopsy   183
- Entrapment   183
  - Description   183
  - Pattern at Autopsy   183
- Traumatic Asphyxia Combined With Smothering   183
  - Description   183
  - Pattern at Autopsy   183

Specific Forms of Asphyxia Causing External Compression of the Neck   184
- Hanging   184
  - Description   184
  - Pattern at Autopsy   184
- Strangulation   190
  - Description   190
  - Pattern at Autopsy   191

Other Specific Forms Of Asphyxia   193
- Carbon Monoxide Poisoning   193
  - Description   193
  - Pattern at Autopsy   193
- Drowning   195
  - Description   195
  - Pattern at Autopsy   195
  - Freshwater Versus Salt Water Drowning   197

Near Misses   197

INTRODUCTION

Asphyxia results from the impaired ventilatory exchange of oxygen and carbon dioxide and can be due to a variety of general mechanisms.[1] One way to categorize the general mechanisms that lead to asphyxia is as follows: external compression of the chest; external obstruction of the mouth and nose; internal obstruction within the mouth, pharynx, larynx, or tracheobronchial tree; external compression of the neck; and interference with gas exchange.[2] Interference of gas exchange is a fairly broad mechanism and could potentially include situations in which not enough oxygen is present in the environment (eg, a plastic bag over the head filled with helium gas) or where the exchange of oxygen at a cellular level is obstructed (eg, carbon monoxide poisoning). Another more general way to categorize the causes of asphyxia by mechanism would be simply those forms that lead to failure of oxygen to reach the lungs and those forms that are due to external compression of the neck. The term "suffocation," which is a general term used in association with asphyxial-type deaths, has been used both to describe conditions that cause obstruction at the level of the nose and mouth and conditions that cause the failure of oxygen to reach the blood.[2-5]

While asphyxia itself leaves no characteristic findings that can be identified at autopsy, certain features found during a postmortem examination have been associated with asphyxia in the past including cyanosis, petechiae, postmortem fluidity of the blood, congestion and edema of the lungs, and dilation of the right-sided chambers of the heart, but these findings are non-specific and occur in a range of conditions other than asphyxial deaths.[2,6-8]

Each of the specific types of asphyxia, to be discussed below (eg, hanging, strangulation), is associated with a variable pattern of scene and autopsy findings, the pattern of which can help a forensic pathologist identify the cause of death; however, there is also much overlap and, in many situations, no characteristic findings other than those found during the scene investigation are available to the pathologist to determine the cause and manner of death (ie, the autopsy findings alone would not allow the pathologist to identify the cause of death without considering the scene investigation findings).

KEY FEATURES: General Mechanisms of Asphyxia

- External compression of the chest
- External obstruction of the mouth and nose
- Internal obstruction of the mouth, pharynx, larynx, or tracheobronchial tree
- External compression of the neck
- Interference with gas exchange, which can include displacement of oxygen from the environment, depletion of oxygen from the environment, or impairment of cellular exchange of oxygen

CHECKLIST for Evaluation of an Asphyxial Death (in addition to those for a general forensic autopsy)

- ☐ Conduct or advocate for a careful scene investigation, including the investigator determining whether or not breathing would have been difficult in the position in which the body was found
- ☐ Examine the conjunctivae, peri-orbital skin, and oral mucosa for petechiae
- ☐ Examine the skin of the neck for abrasions and contusions
- ☐ Conduct an in situ layer-by-layer dissection of the anterior neck musculature
- ☐ Ex situ dissection of the muscles following an in situ layer-by-layer dissection can allow for better visualization of some areas of the neck
- ☐ Examine the soft tissue adjacent to the hyoid bone and thyroid cartilage for hemorrhage, using radiography (if necessary), inspection, and palpation; examine the hyoid bone and thyroid and cricoid cartilages
- ☐ Reflect the musculature from the posterior surface of the superior horns of the thyroid cartilage to allow for better visualization of the cartilage
- ☐ Remove and dissect the tongue
- ☐ Depending upon the circumstances, consider a posterior neck dissection
- ☐ In the case of strangulation or suspected strangulation, swab the neck for DNA and obtain a sexual activity kit as evidence

FAQ: Is there an autopsy finding that is specific for asphyxia?

Answer: No, there is no autopsy finding that is specific for asphyxia.[9] In addition, resuscitation introduces artifacts that essentially cannot be distinguished from changes associated with asphyxial-type deaths (eg, hemorrhage in the neck musculature associated with intubation attempts).[8] In the past, fluid blood and congestion have been used as markers for asphyxia; however, these findings are not specific as they are found with other conditions as well. In addition, their identification can be subjective. Other features that have been associated with asphyxia include hemorrhages under the epicardium and the visceral pleura, hemorrhages in the sternocleidomastoid muscles at their attachment to the sternum, ruptures of the intima of the common carotid artery (Amussat sign), and ruptures of the ligaments and the disk between vertebrae with hemorrhage (Simon sign).[10] Other than just gross autopsy findings, research studying the specificity of various molecular markers for asphyxia has been performed. For example, Bartschat et al identified decreased concentration of calbindin-D28k in the cerebellum in acute hypoxia.[11] Nogami et al identified immunoreactivity of nuclei in the medulla for c-fos as a potential marker for asphyxia.[12] Cecchi et al identified that hypoxic deaths are associated with an increased expression of HIF1-alpha.[13] Palmiere and Tani et al determined that elevated concentrations of thyroid hormones (T3 and T4) may indicate hypoxia/ischemia.[14,15] Quan et al found that intranuclear ubiquitin immunoreactivity of the substantia nigra neurons was induced by asphyxiation and drowning.[16] However, none of these methods is routinely employed in the diagnosis of asphyxial-type deaths. In addition to these studies of various molecular markers, research regarding features identified on standard hematoxylin and eosin staining has been conducted to determine the feasibility of using these findings to assist in the diagnosis of asphyxia. In this regard, the presence of congestion, septal hemorrhage, ductal over-insufflation, alveolar hemorrhage, and other features may assist with the diagnosis of asphyxia.[17] While frequently associated with asphyxial-type deaths (eg, strangulation), petechiae are a purely mechanical phenomenon and not the result of hypoxia.[18] Therefore, the presence of petechiae should not be used to confirm asphyxia as a cause of death, and the absence of petechiae does not rule out an asphyxial death.

Because of the lack of specific autopsy findings to indicate a death due to asphyxia, asphyxial deaths are only identified when scene investigation in combination with autopsy findings identifies the mechanism for the asphyxia (eg, identification of a plastic bag over the head at the scene in the case of a smothering or identification of injuries to the neck organs in the case of a strangulation).

PEARLS & PITFALLS

The presence of petechial hemorrhages (Figure 8.1A-E) in the conjunctivae (or on the oral mucosa or peri-orbital skin) is frequently associated with asphyxial-type deaths (eg, strangulation); however, petechial hemorrhages are not a sign of asphyxia, but are instead a mechanical phenomenon.[18] In the case of strangulation, petechiae are produced by intermittent pressure on the arteries and veins, with occlusion of the veins but not the arteries at the same time, leading to overfilling of capillaries and subsequent rupture, which produces the petechiae. In hanging, most frequently, both arteries and veins in the neck supplying the face are occluded, which results in no petechiae being formed as there is no blood flow to or from the face through the anterior neck vasculature. Petechiae can also develop in non-asphyxial-type events (Figure 8.2) as a result of sudden natural death (eg, cardiac death) and as a result of a face-down position (Figure 8.3A-C), with lividity overfilling capillaries and leading to rupture with subsequent development of petechial hemorrhages, sometimes termed Tardieu spots.[19,20] Resuscitation is not considered a cause of petechiae by some authors.[21]

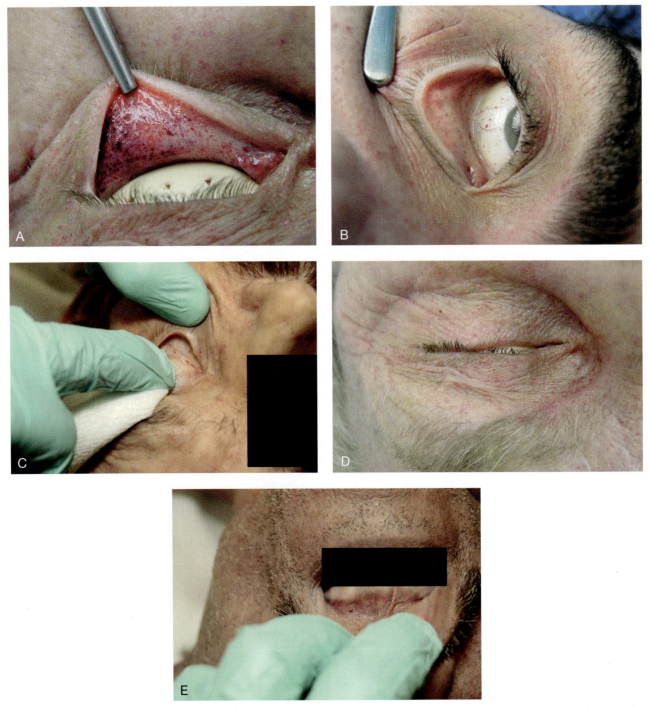

Figure 8.1. Petechial hemorrhages. While petechial hemorrhages can be quite obvious upon examination, in some cases, they must be searched for more diligently. (**A**) illustrates florid petechial hemorrhages of the conjunctivae. While both the palpebral and bulbar conjunctivae can exhibit petechiae, petechial hemorrhages are most commonly found on the inferior bulbar conjunctivae. (**B**) illustrates less florid petechial hemorrhages, but both the bulbar and the palpebral conjunctivae exhibit the hemorrhages. (**C**) illustrates conjunctival petechial hemorrhages, but in a less florid distribution than in (**A**). (**D**) illustrates peri-orbital petechiae, which can be quite subtle. (**E**) illustrates a patch of oral mucosal hemorrhages.

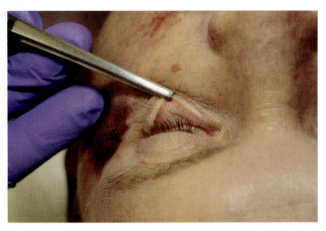

Figure 8.2. Petechiae associated with seizure-related death. The decedent died as the result of a witnessed seizure and, at autopsy, had some petechiae of the inferior palpebral conjunctivae.

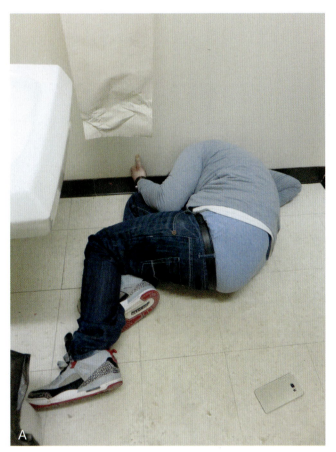
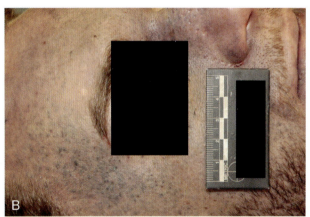
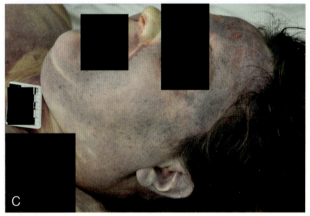

Figure 8.3. Petechiae due to a face-down position. The decedent was found face-down in a bathroom (**A**). Examination of the peri-orbital regions revealed florid petechiae (**B**). In (**C**), the decedent was also face-down for a significant period of time resulting in the formation of petechial hemorrhages.

> **PEARLS & PITFALLS**
>
> The vasculature of the conjunctivae can become congested, which can mimic petechiae to an untrained observer. Congested vessels will have a branching pattern, whereas petechiae are pinpoint hemorrhages (Figure 8.4A-C).

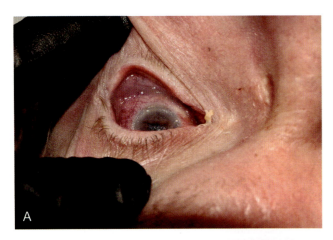
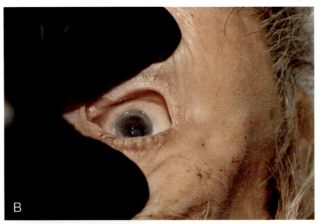
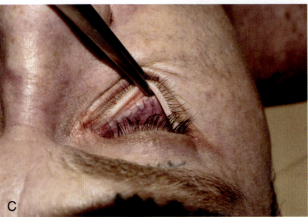

Figure 8.4. Congested conjunctivae. (**A** and **B**) are both from the same decedent. Due to body position, the left eye was congested, whereas the right eye was not, offering a chance for comparison and contrast in the same body. (**C**) is another example of congestion of the conjunctivae. While clearly in a branching vascular pattern, this congestion can be mistaken for petechial hemorrhages.

> **PEARLS & PITFALLS**
>
> In any sudden unexpected death where choking is a possibility, the airway from the tongue to the lungs should be examined. An abscess at the base of the tongue can cause airway obstruction, but can be subtle at the time of autopsy (Figure 8.5A-D).

SPECIFIC FORMS OF ASPHYXIA CAUSING FAILURE OF OXYGEN TO REACH THE LUNG

INTRODUCTION

While there are variable classification schemes for categorizing asphyxial deaths, with terminology not used consistently, the below categories are derived mainly from Sauvageau and Boghossian.[8,22]

SMOTHERING

Description

In smothering, an object prevents air from entering the nose or mouth (eg, a plastic bag over the head) (Figure 8.6).

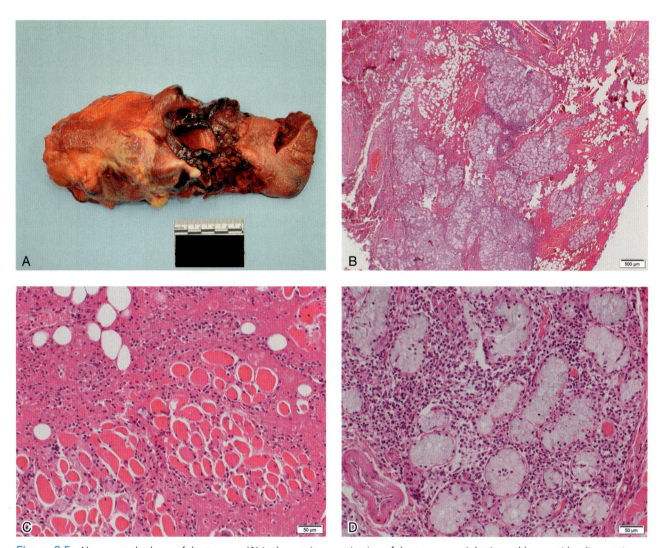

Figure 8.5. Abscess at the base of the tongue. (A) is the ex situ examination of the tongue, epiglottis, and larynx with adjacent tissue. Removal of the neck organs was difficult and the region around the epiglottis is swollen and black discolored, but serial sections of the base of the tongue did not clearly reveal an abnormality. (B-D) are microscopic sections of the tongue. (B), a low power view of the tongue (H&E stain), reveals an infiltrative cellular process and hemorrhage. (C and D), higher power views of the tongue (H&E stain), reveal infiltrates of neutrophils in the muscle (C) and the salivary glands (D).

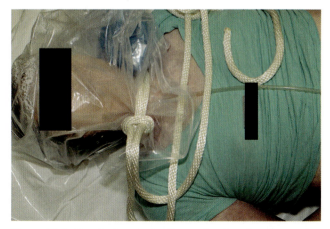

Figure 8.6. Smothering. In the figure, the decedent has a plastic bag placed over the head, which is secured with a rope, which would illustrate a smothering. However, the decedent also introduced gas underneath the plastic bag, which would have produced a vitiated atmosphere.

Pattern at Autopsy

In the case of a smothering, unless the causative object is in place, no specific pattern of findings is usually identified at autopsy.[23] If the smothering was caused by another person (eg, someone held a pillow over the decedent's nose and mouth until they died), autopsy may identify injuries of the peri-oral skin, lips, or oral mucosa (from pressure against this region of the body), or fibers from the object placed over the nose and mouth may be found in the nose or mouth.

CHOKING

Description

In choking, an object or anatomic defect blocks or otherwise obstructs the airway and prevents air from entering the lungs (Figure 8.7A-D). While choking most commonly occurs in infants/children and elderly individuals, adult decedents with a history of psychiatric illness, esophageal disease, mental retardation, and neuromuscular disorders are also at risk.[24] Choking can be non-natural or natural in origin. For example, both a piece of meat that is aspirated by an intoxicated individual and then lodges in the larynx (ie, an accidental death) and swelling associated with epiglottitis (ie, a natural death) could cause choking. Rarely, a large amount of a small substance (eg, sand or grain) is aspirated, filling the airways and causing death.[25] Aspiration of oral and nasopharyngeal secretions in those who have neuromuscular impairment can also obstruct the airway.[26]

Pattern at Autopsy

In the case of choking, examination of the airway will reveal the foreign object trapped within and occluding the airway. However, emergency medical services may have removed object in the airway, often a bolus of food, prior to autopsy, in which case confirmation of the presence

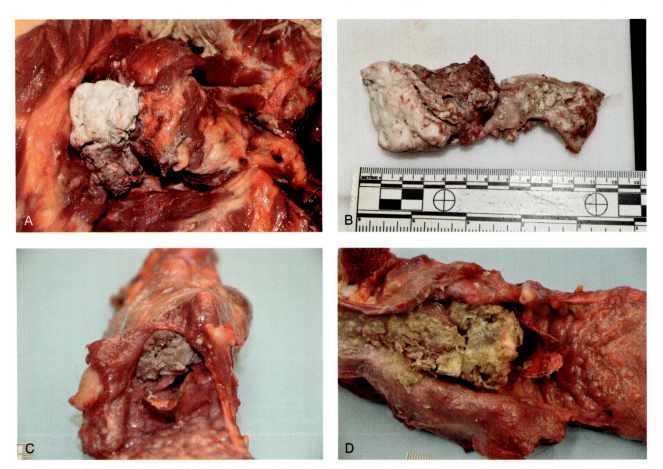

Figure 8.7. Choking. In (**A** and **B**), the decedent choked on a large fragment of steak. (**A**) is an in situ view. During removal of the neck organs from the body, the fragment of steak was identified. The reflected skin of the neck is to the left of the image and the thoracic inlet is to the right of the image. (**B**) is the fragment of steak removed from the body. In (**C** and **D**), the decedent choked on meat in a sandwich. (**C**) shows the bolus of meat impacted at the upper end of the esophagus, but impinging upon the airway, thus causing choking. (**D**) shows the esophagus opened with the bolus of meat at the upper end.

of the foreign object must be obtained from medical records. In the case of occlusion of the airway due to edema or other natural disease process, the epiglottis, larynx, and trachea must be closely examined to identify the pathologic process responsible for the choking. If airway inflammation is identified as the underlying etiology for the asphyxia, an allergic reaction is a distinct possibility. The diagnosis of an allergic reaction is most often done by testing for serum tryptase as well as the specific IgE against the suspected antigen (eg, wasp venom).[27]

> **PEARLS & PITFALLS**
>
> It is common for individuals to aspirate food material during the agonal phase (Figure 8.8). Such aspiration does not necessarily represent the cause of death unless it could be shown that the bolus of aspirated food material caused a significant obstruction, and even then, the reason for the aspiration should be considered as the underlying cause of death.

MECHANICAL ASPHYXIA/TRAUMATIC ASPHYXIA/POSITIONAL ASPHYXIA

Description

While the terms "mechanical asphyxia"/"traumatic asphyxia"/"positional asphyxia" are used interchangeably by some authors, some list traumatic asphyxia and positional asphyxia as a type of mechanical asphyxia, whereas others consider mechanical and traumatic asphyxia as interchangeable, but distinct from positional asphyxia.[3,4,28] In mechanical/traumatic asphyxia, compression of the chest impairs ventilation by obstructing expansion of the lungs, or compression of the head against the chest obstructs the airway, which also leads to impaired ventilation. Both mechanisms can lead to asphyxia. Scene investigation is important to correctly identify traumatic asphyxia. In mechanical/traumatic asphyxia, the decedent is trapped and not able to extricate themselves from their location (Figure 8.9A-C). In positional asphyxia, like traumatic asphyxia, there is also compression of the head against the chest, which obstructs the airway, or compression of the chest, both of which lead to asphyxia (Figure 8.9D and E). However, in positional asphyxia, in contrast to mechanical/traumatic asphyxia, the decedent is not trapped in their position and could easily extricate themselves from the asphyxial environment, but, because they are alcohol or drug impaired, they do not voluntarily move. Once again, scene investigation is a vital component of the correct identification of the cause of death in these situations.

The mechanism of asphyxiation in positional asphyxia could also be a head-down position, with the abdominal contents pressing against the diaphragm.[29] The classic scene pattern for a traumatic asphyxia is an individual in a vehicular accident who is compressed in the cab between the steering wheel/dashboard and the car seat because of compaction of the driving compartment (see Figure 8.9A). The classic scene pattern for a positional asphyxia is an intoxicated individual who falls off a bed and wedges between the bed and the wall, unable to breathe.

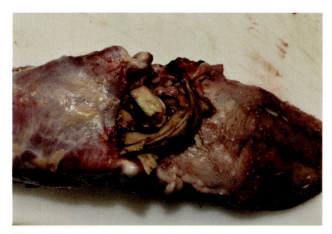

Figure 8.8. Agonal aspiration of food. The decedent died as the result of a gunshot wound. The finding of a large bolus in the nasopharynx illustrates how individuals can aspirate a large bolus of food during the agonal phase, with the aspiration unrelated to their cause of death.

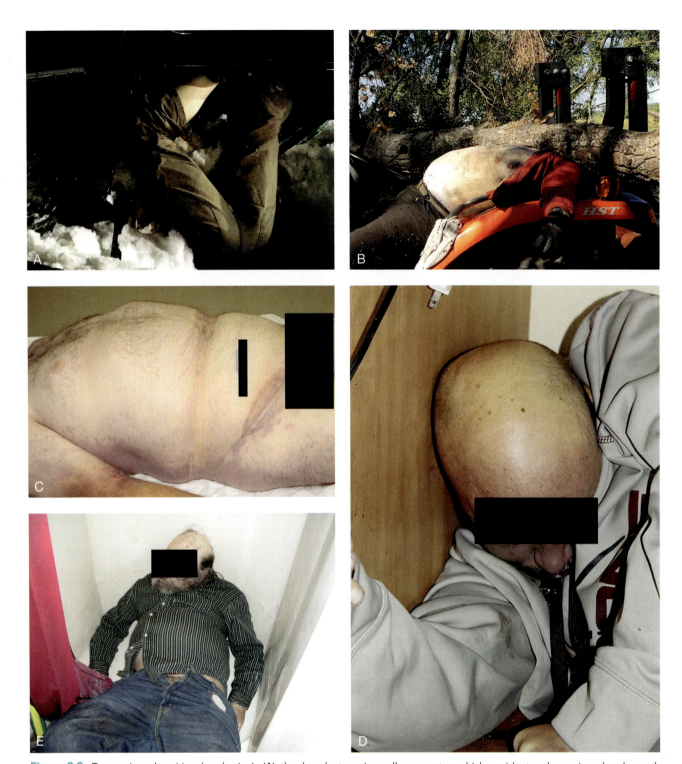

Figure 8.9. Traumatic and positional asphyxia. In (**A**), the decedent was in a roll-over motor vehicle accident and was pinned underneath the roof of the vehicle, which would cause a traumatic asphyxia. In this case, autopsy did not identify any lethal blunt force injuries. In (**B**), the decedent was working on their ranch on a tractor and fell a tree on top of themselves, which lead to a traumatic asphyxia. The log is across the chest of the individual, pinning them in the seat of the tractor. In (**C**), the individual was pinned in a motor vehicle accident, with the point of compression being the abdomen, with a narrow compressed band of skin visible in a horizontal band. In (**D**), the decedent was alcohol impaired and collapsed against a dresser. The individual was only unable to extricate themselves from the position because of the alcohol impairment, thus illustrating positional asphyxia. In (**E**), the decedent entered the bathroom to urinate after drinking and fell backward into the shower. The decedent's head is pinned against the chest, leading to obstruction of the airway and asphyxiation. If not intoxicated, the decedent could have moved from the position and not asphyxiated.

Pattern at Autopsy

Mechanical/traumatic asphyxia can produce a characteristic pattern of autopsy findings. With compression of the chest at a certain level, blood flow to the heart is impaired, leading to engorgement and rupture of vessels, producing florid petechiae of the face, neck, and upper trunk above the level of compression of the chest (Figure 8.10A-C); however, not all cases of traumatic asphyxia have such a characteristic finding.[30] In positional asphyxia, other than the scene investigation, autopsy findings are not characteristic.

VITIATED ATMOSPHERE/SUFFOCATING GASES

Description

Vitiated atmosphere (meaning spoiled atmosphere)/suffocating gases is an environment where the air is filled with some substance that renders breathing in of oxygen not possible (eg, propane gas in a basement). The mechanism of this form of asphyxia can also be considered as due to a reduced amount of oxygen in the environment secondary to displacement of the oxygen by another gas.[31]

Pattern at Autopsy

In the case of a vitiated atmosphere, no specific pattern of autopsy findings is identified, and the diagnosis would rest upon scene investigation (combined with a negative autopsy that identified no other competing cause of death) and toxicologic analysis of the decedent's blood, with some causative substances, such as propane, detectable through toxicologic analysis.

ENTRAPMENT

Description

Similar to a vitiated atmosphere in that the underlying mechanism is reduced oxygen available to breathe, entrapment occurs when an individual enters into an environment in which oxygen becomes depleted by their presence and cannot be replaced. Older versions of refrigerators used to become locked and if a child climbed inside and closed the door, they could asphyxiate. The mechanism of this form of asphyxia can also be considered as due to a reduced amount of oxygen in the environment secondary to consumption of the oxygen.[31]

Pattern at Autopsy

In the case of an entrapment, no specific pattern of autopsy findings is identified, and the diagnosis would rest upon scene investigation (combined with an autopsy that identified no other competing cause of death).

TRAUMATIC ASPHYXIA COMBINED WITH SMOTHERING

Description

DiMaio and Molina describe a specific type of asphyxial death in which traumatic asphyxia is combined with smothering.[3] One specific example is overlay, in which an infant sleeping with adults, other children, or pets is rolled over onto, leading to asphyxia, which would be a combination of traumatic asphyxia (a body on top of the infant) and smothering (covering of the infant's nose and oral orifice). A second specific example is burking, in which an individual would sit on the chest of another individual, who was usually intoxicated, and then place something over that intoxicated individual's mouth and nose, leading to asphyxiation.

Pattern at Autopsy

Other than the potential injuries of the peri-oral skin, lips, or oral mucosa (from pressure against this region of the body) and the potential for fibers from the object placed over the face being found in the nose or mouth, there are no specific patterns to be identified at autopsy, which would indicate traumatic asphyxia combined with smothering. As traumatic asphyxia is a component of the death, petechial hemorrhages can be present; however, given the non-specific nature of petechiae, without further findings or investigative information, the diagnosis cannot reliably be made solely from the autopsy findings.

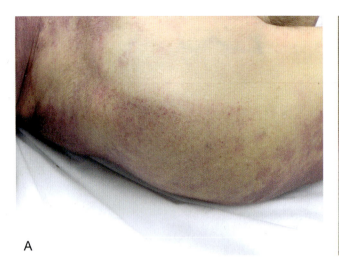
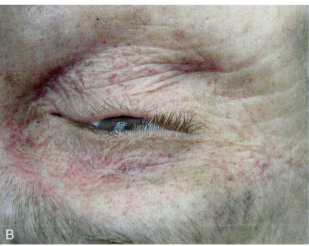
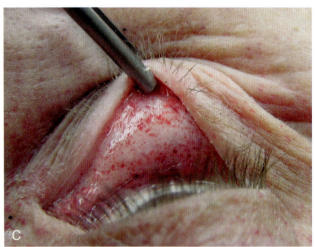

Figure 8.10. Traumatic asphyxia underneath car. The decedent in the figure was pinned underneath a car and had features at autopsy from the compression. (**A**) illustrates petechiae on the shoulder, with a horizontal line of demarcation. With mechanical/traumatic asphyxia, the characteristic autopsy finding is congestion and petechiae of the face, neck, and upper trunk (assuming the point of compression is the chest). (**B** and **C**) illustrate the florid peri-orbital (**B**) and conjunctival (**C**) petechiae present at autopsy.

SPECIFIC FORMS OF ASPHYXIA CAUSING EXTERNAL COMPRESSION OF THE NECK

HANGING

Description

The decedent's body weight or head weight provides the force that leads to asphyxia. In hanging, most often, the weight of the body against a rope or other object around the neck leads to occlusion of the vessels in the neck, most often both arteries and veins, leading to asphyxia. In a judicial hanging, the mechanism of death is different, with death occurring due to fracture of the neck and resultant damage to the spinal cord at the level of the atlas and axis.[3]

Pattern at Autopsy

In a hanging, the most classic autopsy findings are a lack of conjunctival petechiae, lack of external or internal injuries of the neck, and a ligature furrow on the skin of the neck, which normally cants upward toward the point of suspension (Figure 8.11A-I). However, external and internal injuries can occur. If the ligature were to slip during its placement or afterward, the skin can be abraded (Figure 8.12). When the ligature slips, arterial blood can escape through, and with resultant venous but not arterial compression, petechiae can occur (Figure 8.13A and B). Internal injuries, including fractures of the hyoid bone or thyroid cartilage, can also occur (Figure 8.14A and B). In their review of 102 cases of suicidal hanging, Kurtulus et al found fractures of neck structures in 69 cases.[32] Sharma et al found fractures of the hyoid bone in 21% of hanging deaths and fractures of the thyroid cartilage in 17% of hanging deaths.[33] Simon sign (hemorrhage into the anterior aspect of the intervertebral disks of the lumbar region) can also be seen with hanging.[34,35]

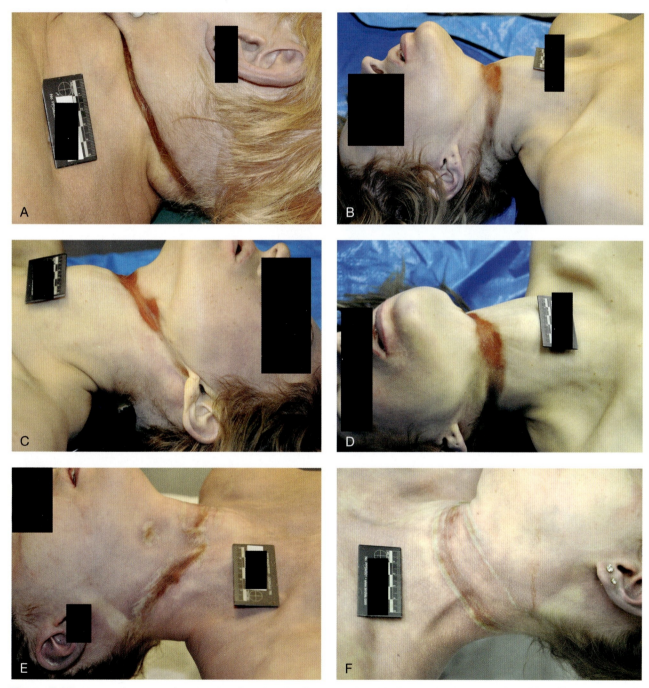

Figure 8.11. Ligature furrow in a hanging. In a hanging, the furrow produced by the ligature's compression of the skin is often a well-defined linear depression in the skin with dried orange-yellow surfaces and no injuries on the adjacent skin (**A**). In a hanging death, often the furrow is lower on one side of the neck than the other (**B** and **C**) and most frequently crosses the anterior surface of the neck above the laryngeal prominence (**D**). As a variety of objects can be used for the ligature, including electric cords, ropes, belts, and even chains, the ligature furrow will not always be a well-defined linear compression, and can instead have irregular edges (**E**). While often the ligature furrow encompasses the circumference of the neck only once, sometimes it will be wrapped more than once, creating two or more furrows (**F**). Lividity can enhance the appearance of the furrow as the lividity will not fill into areas that are compressed (**G**). In this regard, if the decedent were to collapse onto a rope or cord, with the cord compressing the neck, a pseudo-furrow could be created and mimic a hanging when no hanging occurred. Depending upon the nature of the ligature (eg, thin electrical cord vs broad blanket) and the time from the hanging to discovery of the body, the prominence of the furrow varies, and can, oftentimes, be indistinct (**H**). Often, the ligature furrow will not be circumferential and the posterior surface of the neck will be minimal involved (**I**).

Figure 8.11a-i (continued)

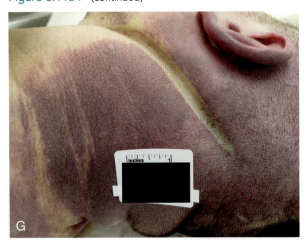
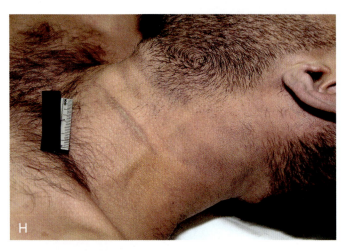
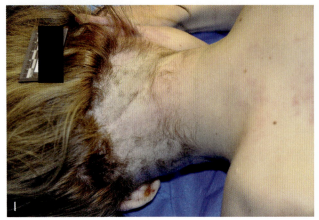

> **FAQ:** Is the furrow produced by the noose an abrasion of the skin?
>
> **Answer:** Histologic examination of the furrow in the skin produced by the noose indicates that the furrow is compressed squamous epithelium (Figure 8.15A and B).

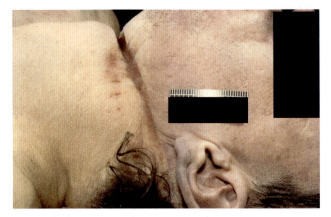

Figure 8.12. Abrasion of the skin adjacent to ligature furrow. On the skin inferior to the furrow on the neck are some parallel thin linear abrasions. If the cord or other object used to facilitate the hanging slips during placement or shortly thereafter, the result can be abrasions on the neck, which would be misinterpreted as a simulated suicide.

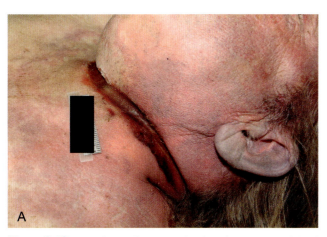 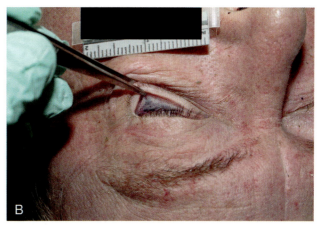

Figure 8.13. Petechiae in hanging. The decedent's cause of death was a hanging. The ligature furrow is prominent on the neck (**A**); however, examination of the conjunctivae revealed petechiae (**B**).

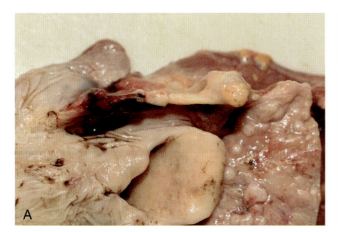 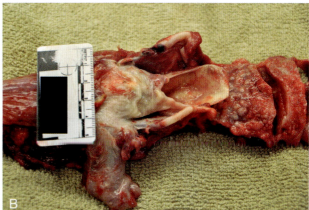

Figure 8.14. Fractures of the thyroid cartilage in hanging. (**A**) reveals a fracture of the left superior horn of the thyroid cartilage. (**B**) reveals bilateral fractures of the superior thyroid horns. In both cases, the fractures occurred during a hanging.

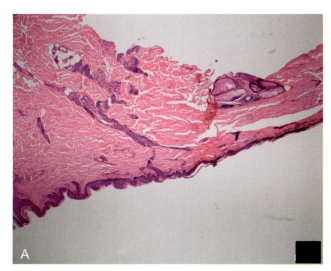 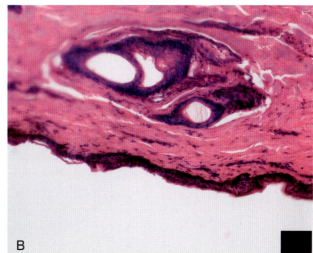

Figure 8.15. Microscopic appearance of furrow in hanging death. (**A**) reveals the transition between the involved and uninvolved skin, with the involved skin (ie, the furrow) on the right side of the image appearing thinner (low power, H&E). (**B**), a higher power view of the involved skin, reveals the epidermis to be intact but, along with the dermis, compressed (high power, H&E).

PEARLS & PITFALLS

The lividity pattern present on the body may provide information as to the position of the body (Figure 8.16A-C), with individuals who are suspended, standing, or kneeling having prominent lividity of the lower extremities and pallor of the upper portions of the body.

PEARLS & PITFALLS

While rare, homicidal hangings can occur. Sauvageau identified four homicidal hangings in 251 cases of hanging and considered this number artificially high.[36] Russo et al identified one homicidal hanging in 260 cases of hanging.[37] For a homicidal hanging to occur, the decedent could potentially be rendered unconscious and then hanged to simulate a suicide, or the decedent could be strangled to death, or killed in another fashion, and then hanged to simulate a suicide.[38] In the first scenario, separating a homicide from a suicide at autopsy would be challenging as the first event (ie, the rendering of the decedent unconscious) would not necessarily leave distinguishing marks; however, in the second scenario (ie, a preceding strangulation or other lethal event), a thorough autopsy examination may allow for features of the strangulation or other lethal event to be identified. However, that being said, distinguishing a homicidal hanging made to simulate a suicide can be very challenging and definitely requires a careful correlation of autopsy findings with scene investigation.[39-41] In distinguishing a true hanging suicide from a simulated suicide, comparison of the texture of the noose with the texture of the furrow on the neck could be of use (Figure 8.17A and B). For example, the texture created in the furrow in the skin from a smooth electrical cord

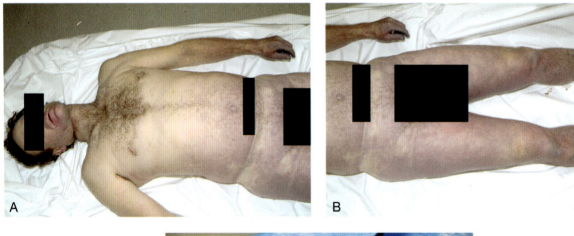

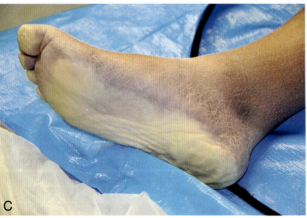

Figure 8.16. Lividity pattern in hanging. In (**A** and **B**), the prominent lividity in the lower abdomen and lower extremities, and the relative pallor of the upper trunk and head and the absence of lividity on the knees, indicates the decedent was likely standing or was suspended. In (**C**), the absence of lividity on the bottom of the feet indicates that the feet were pressed against something. The decedent in (**C**) (different than the decedent in **A** and **B**) was standing when they hanged themselves.

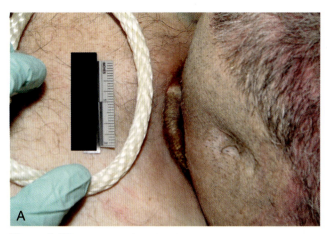 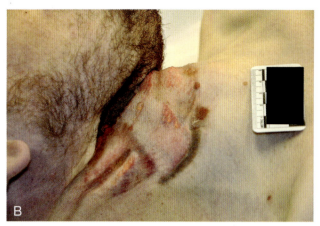

Figure 8.17. Impression from ligature. Both (**A** and **B**) reveal a distinct pattern in the furrow. In (**A**), the decedent hanged themselves with a rope and, in (**B**), the decedent used a belt with holes. The skin was pressed into the holes in the belt, creating the regularly interspersed discolored elevations on the skin surface.

used as a noose would be different than the texture created in the furrow in the skin from a rope, with the first furrow being smooth and the second being more undulating. If a ligature strangulation occurs using one type of object and then the body is staged to appear as a hanging using a second and different object, the texture of the furrow in some locations may reveal a discrepancy. In addition, while the furrow from the noose in a suicidal hanging most often cants upward to the point of suspension, in a ligature strangulation, it is often horizontal on the neck.

PEARLS & PITFALLS

Some individuals are or may be trained to incapacitate people rapidly with various forms of chokeholds (eg, police officers or bouncers at bars may have such training). Such an individual could rapidly incapacitate another person, leaving no or only very subtle signs of a struggle and then subsequently hang them to make the death appear as a suicide. During the investigation, especially if other circumstances are suspicious, determining whether or not anyone who knew the decedent has such an ability may be useful in helping to determine the cause and manner of death.

SAMPLE NOTES: DESCRIPTION OF NOOSE FURROW ON THE NECK

"Circumferentially on the neck is a furrow, which reaches a high point on the left side of the neck, just posterior to the ear, at 6 inches below the top of the head. The furrow varies from ¼ inch in width anterior and on the right side of the neck, to ½ inch in width behind the left ear. The furrow crosses the anterior surface of the neck above the laryngeal prominence of the thyroid cartilage."

Another method is to measure from the top of the head to the furrow at four points on the neck: front of neck, posterior surface of neck, below the inferior attachment of the left ear, and below the inferior attachment of the right ear.

PEARLS & PITFALLS

When removing the noose from around the neck, the integrity of the knot should be retained (ie, the noose should not be removed by untying the knot). And, in some cases, there is no actual knot in the noose (eg, if a belt is used, and the belt buckle and fastener are used as the knot). The knot can be retained by cutting the noose opposite the side of the knot. The site where the noose is cut can be marked with zip ties (Figure 8.18A and B). A zip tie can also be used to secure the knot region itself, if it is of a design that will loosen when the noose is removed from the neck (eg, a belt secured with the buckle) (Figure 8.18C).

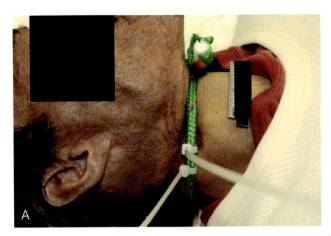
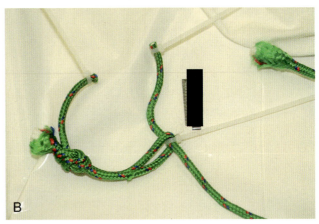
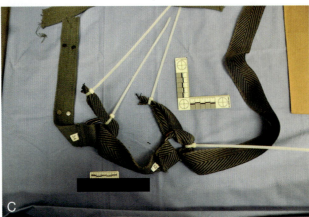

Figure 8.18. Removal of a ligature to preserve the knot for evidence purposes. In (**A** and **B**), the decedent hanged themselves with a climbing-type rope. Zip ties were used to identify a point on the opposite side of the neck from the knot region (**A**). The rope was then cut between the zip ties (**B**). In addition, a third zip tie was used to secure the knot region of the ligature. Often, the knot region is not fixed and would be lost if the area was not fastened in such a manner. In (**C**), the decedent used a corded belt, with passage through metal loops forming the suspension point on the neck. The belt at the loops was secured with zip ties and the location where the belt was cut from the neck was identified with two zip ties.

STRANGULATION

Description

A force other than the decedent's body weight or head weight applied to the body leads to asphyxia. Two forms of strangulation are ligature and manual. In manual strangulation, an attacker used their hands, elbow, or even knee to asphyxiate the decedent, whereas in ligature strangulation, an object, such as a belt or rope, is used to apply pressure to the decedent's neck.

PEARLS & PITFALLS

While ligature strangulation more commonly indicates a homicide as the manner of death, ligature strangulation can also occur in suicides. Jackson and Paul reported a suicidal ligature strangulation where cable ties were used.[42] Lin et al reported a suicidal ligature strangulation where rubber bands were used.[43] Even though an individual can commit suicide via ligature strangulation (Figure 8.19A and B), they technically should not be able to do so via manual strangulation, as upon becoming unconscious, the pressure to the neck would be released and blood flow restored.

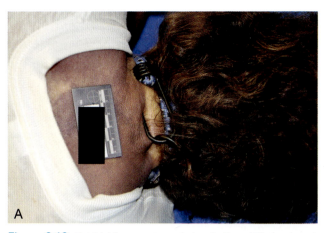 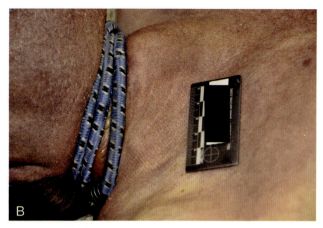

Figure 8.19. Suicidal ligature strangulation. In (**A** and **B**), the decedent used a bungee cord to commit suicide. He was found in a room with a note on the door indicating his intent. The bungee cord was wrapped a few times around the neck and secured posterior with the two metal hooks.

Pattern at Autopsy

In a strangulation, the most classic autopsy findings are conjunctival petechiae, external injuries of the neck (including abrasions and contusions), and internal injuries of the neck (including hemorrhage into the musculature of the neck, potentially both anterior and posterior, hemorrhage in the tongue, hemorrhage in the prevertebral musculature and fascia, and fractures of the hyoid bone and/or thyroid and cricoid cartilages) (Figure 8.20A-H). Although commonly associated with strangulation, not all victims of strangulation will have petechial hemorrhages.[44] While fractures of the hyoid bone and thyroid cartilage can occur in both a hanging and a strangulation, fractures of the cricoid cartilage are much more specific for strangulation. Godin et al found fractures of neck structures in 23.4% of 231 hanging cases, but no fractures of the cricoid cartilage, whereas fractures of the cricoid cartilage were found in 20.6% of homicidal strangulations (of 52 cases).[45] Fractures of the neck structures can also occur in agonal falls.[46] A rare finding associated with strangulation is otorrhagia, which is identifiable hemorrhage within the external auditory canal; however, otorrhagia has also been identified in positional asphyxia.[47-49]

PEARLS & PITFALLS

Of importance to remember is that postmortem lividity can mimic the features of a strangulation.[50,51] Also, injuries of the oral mucosa, the posterior pharynx, the epiglottis, the piriform recess, the larynx and trachea, the strap muscles, and the skin of the neck can be caused by resuscitation measures and could mimic strangulation.[52]

PEARLS & PITFALLS

Histologic examination of the thyroid cartilage may potentially reveal findings that were not identified grossly, including hemorrhage and features of a delayed mechanism of death (eg, fibrin and neutrophilic infiltrates).[53] Pollanen also discusses the utility of the identification of subepithelial laryngeal hemorrhage, intralaryngeal hemorrhage, and intracartilaginous laryngeal hemorrhage in the diagnosis of strangulation.[9]

PEARLS & PITFALLS

The findings in a homicidal strangulation can be highly variable, from a neck with numerous abrasions and contusions, and possibly even linear scratches consistent with fingernail marks, combined with extensive hemorrhage in the underlying musculature and fractures of the hyoid bone and thyroid cartilage to no external findings and only a few hemorrhages in the anterior neck musculature. As such, strangulation-type deaths can easily be missed and forensic pathologists must have a higher index of suspicion for such a death and carefully weigh the investigative findings with the autopsy findings to determine whether or not a strangulation has occurred.

> **PEARLS & PITFALLS**
> Triticeous cartilage, which is a small segment of cartilage found in the thyrohyoid ligament, can, upon palpation, mimic a fracture; however, no hemorrhage is present as would be an expected finding with a recent fracture (Figure 8.21).

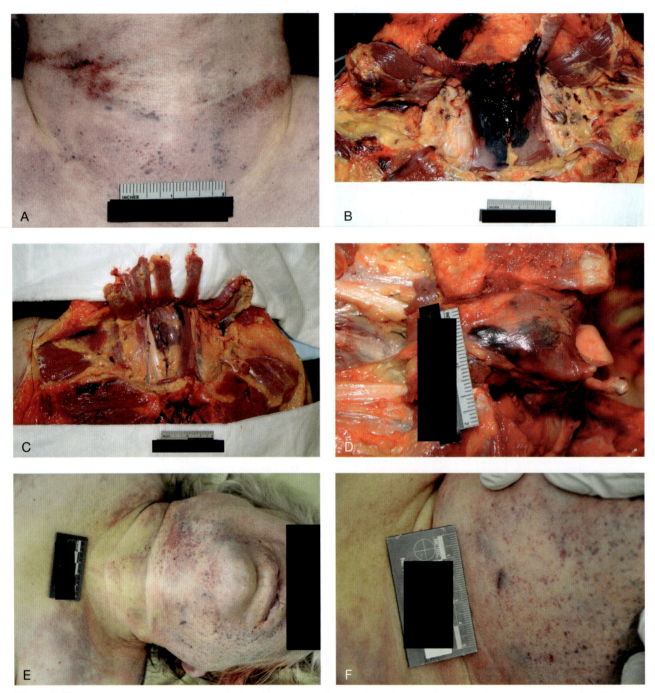

Figure 8.20. Features of strangulation. (**A** and **B**) are from a young female who was manually strangled by her significant other. (**A**) shows patchy abrasions and contusions of the skin of the neck. (**B**) shows extensive hemorrhage in the anterior neck musculature. When individuals struggle against the attack, it is more likely that more damage will occur, leading to more injuries of the neck. (**C** and **D**) are also from a female who was strangled by her significant other. In contrast to the previous two images, there is less extensive hemorrhage in the neck musculature. Compression of the neck organs against the cervical vertebral column can lead to hemorrhage in the prevertebral fascia and adjacent musculature. (**E-H**) are from an elderly woman who was strangled by her husband. (**E**) illustrates some contusions of the neck and extensive petechial hemorrhages of the face. (**F**) is a close-up view of the neck and on the left side of the jawline is a linear abrasion, which could represent a fingernail mark. (**G**) shows the relatively minimal hemorrhage in the anterior neck musculature. (**H**) shows the tongue with numerous scattered hemorrhages. Cross section of the tongue revealed numerous hemorrhages in the musculature.

Figure 8.20 (continued)

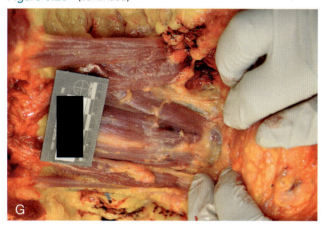
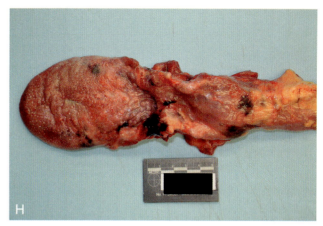

> **PEARLS & PITFALLS**
>
> In the case of homicidal asphyxia, more than one mechanism can be used. Lupascu et al describe a homicide using smothering, strangulation, and traumatic asphyxia with compression of the chest.[54]

OTHER SPECIFIC FORMS OF ASPHYXIA

CARBON MONOXIDE POISONING

Description

The most common form of asphyxia in the United States due to the presence of a potentially lethal gas is likely carbon monoxide poisoning. Although carbon monoxide exposure is frequently the cause of death in house fires, exposure to exhaust fumes from a motor vehicle or a grill in a confined space will also lead to carbon monoxide poisoning.

Pattern at Autopsy

With carbon monoxide poisoning, the lividity will have a characteristic cherry red coloration (Figure 8.22A and B). Blood internally will be lighter red in coloration than in a typical forensic autopsy, and tissue from a carbon monoxide poisoning that is placed into formaldehyde will retain the lighter coloration and can stain the formaldehyde. A cherry red discoloration can also be caused by refrigeration and cyanide poisoning.

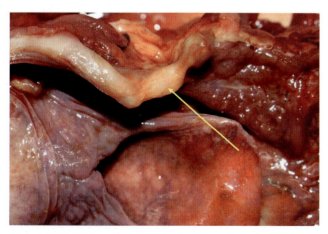

Figure 8.21. Triticeous cartilage. Triticeous cartilages are small fragments of cartilage in the thyrohyoid ligament (arrow), which are commonly found at autopsy and can be unilateral or bilateral. As triticeous cartilage can be misinterpreted as a break in the thyroid cartilage, it can potentially be misinterpreted as a fracture; however, unlike a fracture, no hemorrhage is found in the surrounding soft tissue.

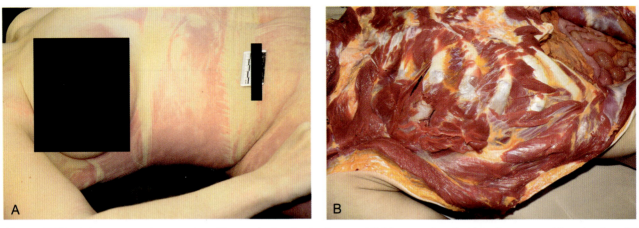

Figure 8.22. Carbon monoxide poisoning. (**A**) reveals the classic cherry red lividity associated with carbon monoxide poisoning. (**B**) reveals the relative pallor of the skeletal muscle. Although the muscle is not pink, it is much more light red than the typical appearance of postmortem skeletal tissue.

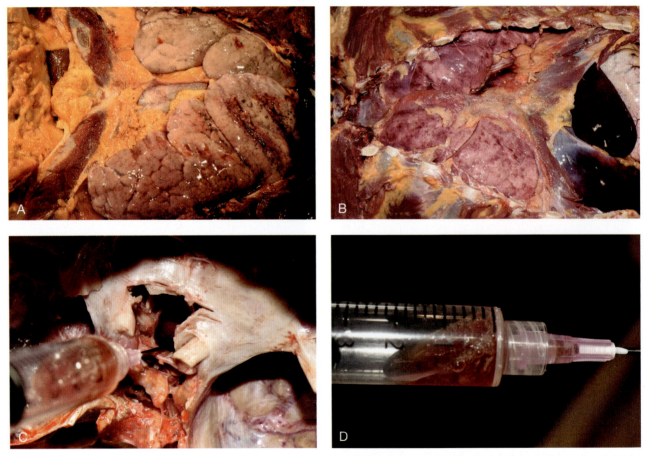

Figure 8.23. Features of drowning. (**A** and **B**) illustrate the hyperinflation of the lungs often found in individuals who have drowned. The lungs completely fill the pleural cavities and oftentimes touch in the midline. (**C** and **D**) illustrate water in the sphenoid sinus. The sphenoid sinus can easily be accessed at autopsy by chipping away the bone anterior to the sella turcica. (**E**) shows an oral foam cone. Oral foam cones are most commonly associated with drowning and drug overdoses, but can occur in a range of other conditions. (**F**) shows wrinkling of the skin of the palms. Wrinkling of the skin of the palms and soles is commonly found in bodies recovered from the water. This change is associated with immersion and does not indicate a drowning. If an individual dies in a shower, with the water running, even though they did not drown, the hands and feet may show the same change.

Figure 8.23 (continued)

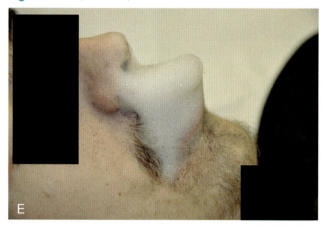
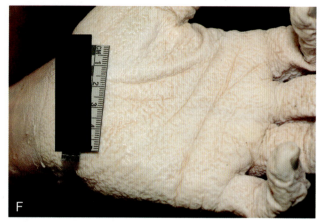

> **PEARLS & PITFALLS**
>
> Other gases, such as methane, helium, chloroform, and propane, are associated with chemical asphyxia; however, the mechanism is often due to displacement of the oxygen in the environment unlike carbon monoxide poisoning, which is due to irreversible binding of the carbon monoxide to hemoglobin, thus impairing oxygenation of tissues.[55-57]

DROWNING

Description

An individual is submerged in water, leading to asphyxia.

Pattern at Autopsy

While the autopsy findings are not diagnostic, several findings are characteristically associated with drowning. The finding of foam in the airways and hyperinflated lungs is probably the best combination for the diagnosis of drowning, but is not specific.[58,59] Foam in the airways is a feature of drowning, but can also be seen in opioid overdose and heart failure and can be diminished or obliterated by resuscitation and prolonged immersion.[58] The foam can also form in internal airways postmortem, but external foam does not arise postmortem.[60] Hyperinflated lungs (ie, lungs that are well-inflated and fill their respective pleural cavity and often touch in the midline) are often present in individuals who have drowned, being present in around 99% of drowning cases; however, the finding can be diminished or obliterated by resuscitation and decomposition and can be found in other conditions.[58] Hemorrhage in the petrous ridge of the temporal bones and water in the stomach are associated with drowning but are non-specific (Figure 8.23A-F). Grass, leaves, and/or mud can be identified in the airways. Paltauf spots are subpleural hemorrhages associated with drowning, which appear as petechial hemorrhages, but are larger and not as well defined as Tardieu spots.[61]

In their study, Okuda et al used five criteria to diagnose drowning: history of recovery from water, foam in the airway, watery fluid (>0.5 mL) in the sphenoid sinus, hyperinflated lungs, and watery fluid in the stomach contents, with not all cases of drowning having all five features.[62] Based upon the above information, the veracity of the quote "Death by drowning remains one of the most difficult diagnosis in forensic medicine." is easily proven.[59]

> **PEARLS & PITFALLS**
>
> Hemorrhage in the neck musculature can be encountered in drowning victims. The origin of this hemorrhage is controversial; however, Carter et al identified neck hemorrhage in about 10% of cases, with no explanation, with the etiology described as most likely hypostasis, but also possibly violent neck movements occurring during the drowning process.[63]

PEARLS & PITFALLS

Peri-orbital and conjunctival petechial hemorrhages have been described as a feature of pediatric drownings; however, the peri-orbital petechiae occur in less than 15% of drownings and become less prevalent when the time period from death to examination is >24 hours.[64]

KEY FEATURES Associated With Water Immersion and/or Drowning[58,65]
- Wrinkling of the skin of the hands and feet
- Nasal/oral foam cone and foam in the airway internally
- Hyperinflated lungs (ie, emphysema aqueosum)
- Fluid in the sinuses (Svechnikov sign)
- Hemorrhage in the petrous ridge
- Pleural effusions
- Subpleural hemorrhage (Paltauf spots)
- Splenomegaly
- Water in the stomach (Wydler sign)

FAQ: What is meant when it is said that drowning is a diagnosis of exclusion?

Answer: When a body is found in water, while drowning is a distinct possibility as the cause of death, other causes of death must be excluded. Following a homicide, bodies can be thrown into a body of water in the hopes of disposing of the body and preventing its discovery. While certain autopsy findings are associated with drowning (eg, hyperinflated lungs, hemorrhage in the petrous ridges, water in the stomach), they are not specific enough to identify drowning as a cause of death, unless other competing causes of death are ruled out; thus, drowning is a diagnosis of exclusion.

FAQ: If an individual has a natural event and dies prior to entering the water, can this be determined at autopsy?

Answer: Whether the decedent simply had a cardiac event and collapsed into the water or whether they had a cardiac event while swimming must be considered. Unfortunately, as the findings of a drowning are non-specific, to absolutely exclude drowning in the case of a body found in the water with only natural disease, unless that natural disease is definitive and would have caused death quickly (eg, an aortic dissection with rupture into the pericardial sac or a ruptured berry aneurysm), it is most likely best to defer to drowning as the cause of death, causing the manner of death to be accident. When drowning occurs likely related to a cardiac event, it is also important to consider the possibility of long QT syndrome.

PEARLS & PITFALLS

When individuals drown in a body of moving water, such as a creek or river, the tumbling of the body can cause injuries of the body, including contusions and abrasions, and the water can forcibly remove some or all of the clothing from the body. A nude or semi-nude and apparently beaten individual found in a river or creek is not necessarily a victim of a homicide (Figure 8.24A and B).

PEARLS & PITFALLS

Aspiration of water from the sphenoid sinus can help determine whether or not a body was submerged. Whereas this finding would not be of much use if the body was known to have been in the water, it could be of great importance in the investigation if the body was not known to have been submerged in the water, but drowning is a possibility. For example, if a husband reports he found his wife unresponsive on the floor of the bathroom, and investigation reveals a bathtub full of water, the identification of water in the sphenoid sinus at autopsy could be of significance to the investigation. Fluid within the sphenoid sinus can also be cerebrospinal fluid.[66]

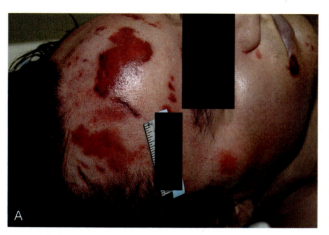 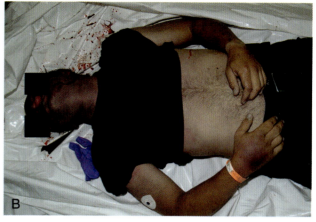

Figure 8.24. Blunt force injuries associated with drowning. The decedent was found in the water with numerous blunt force injuries including abrasions and lacerations of the head (**A**). The autopsy did not identify any lethal internal injuries and the decedent had an oral foam cone (**B**). The injuries of the face were caused during the process of drowning or shortly thereafter.

PEARLS & PITFALLS

Bathtub drownings present a challenging scenario for forensic pathologists. As the drive to breathe is significant, bathtub drownings are most often accidental and proceeded by unconsciousness, with risk factors such as cardiovascular disease, drug or alcohol use, or seizure disorders being common contributory conditions and with the heat of the water contributing to a cardiac dysrhythmia or hypotension.[2,62] If none of these factors is present, any bathtub drowning should be thoroughly investigated to rule out the possibility of a homicide. Bathtub drowning suicides do occur, however. In the five cases they reviewed, Murayama identified factors for suicidal intent in bathtub suicides as follows: suicidal intent identified and reported to investigators by a witness to such intent, a suicide note, if clothing was worn by the decedent, or the presence of a mechanism to ensure the suicide.[67] The author has seen a bathtub drowning suicide where the individual broke out the tiles above the faucet handles in the bathtub, and inserted his feet into the resulting hole, which would impair his ability to lift his head out of the water. A toxic concentration of his anti-depressant medication was also identified.

Freshwater Versus Salt Water Drowning

Based upon the differences in the water and the resultant effects on the body (eg, water movement in the body due to hypertonic salt water or hypotonic freshwater), autopsy findings may help distinguish the two types of drowning. Analysis of sodium, chloride, and magnesium concentrations in the sphenoid sinus can potentially be used to distinguish a freshwater drowning from a saltwater drowning.[68] While the weight of the brain and lungs in individuals who have drowned in salt water are higher than in those who have drowned in freshwater, because, in lungs, the salt water causes fluid to be drawn from the vasculature into the alveoli due to osmotic effects, Girela-Lopez et al indicate that the body mass index and degree of decomposition affect the weights to a greater degree.[69]

NEAR MISSES

Near Miss #1: While fractures of the hyoid bone and thyroid and cricoid cartilage are associated with strangulation, they can occur in other situations as well. In Figure 8.25, the individual sustained bilateral fracture of the superior horns of the thyroid cartilage, which can occur due to blunt force injuries.

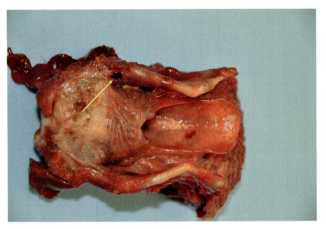

Figure 8.25. Bilateral fractures of the superior horns of the thyroid cartilage. The fracture of the left side is most distinct in the photograph (arrow).

Near Miss #2: The features of strangulation can be difficult to interpret in a non-decomposed body, let alone a decomposed body; however, close examination of the body in combination with information from the scene investigation can still allow for the diagnosis to be made (Figure 8.26A-H). This case also shows how without good investigation that a strangulation with relatively subtle features could easily be missed at autopsy.

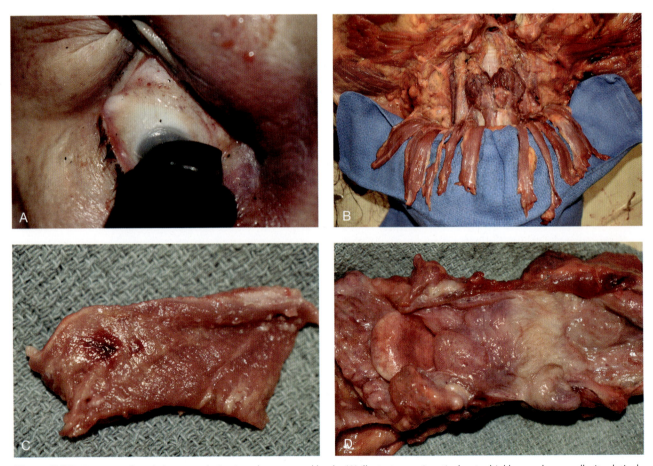

Figure 8.26. Features of a subtle strangulation in a decomposed body. (**A**) illustrates conjunctival petechial hemorrhages, albeit relatively sparse in distribution. (**B**) was the layered neck dissection performed during the autopsy. No hemorrhage was identified. (**C**) shows a contusion in the tongue. (**D**) is the resected tongue and neck organs. At the junction of the greater horns of the hyoid bone and the tips of the superior horns of the thyroid cartilage is hemorrhage. (**E**) reveals a fracture of the right superior horn of the thyroid cartilage. Although the hemorrhage in the soft tissue surrounding the fracture is most often apparent, removal of the soft tissue from the posterior surface of the superior horns during dissection can aid in identification of a fracture. (**F-H**) are photos of the external surface of the neck, which reveal faint contusions and abrasions. The effects of decomposition, including discoloration and skin slippage, can obscure significant findings.

Figure 8.26 (continued)

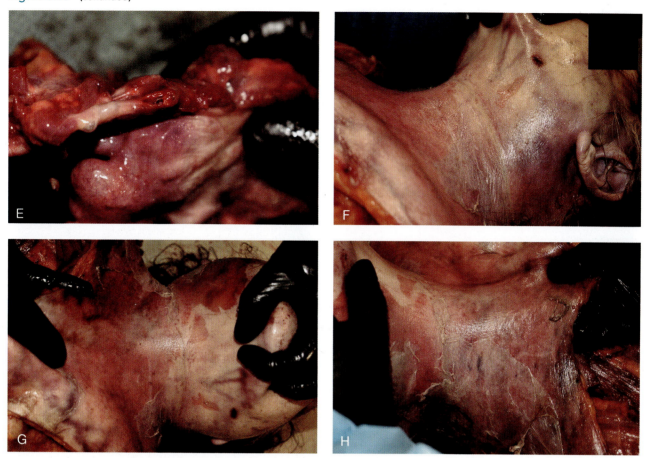

Near Miss #3: Lividity and congestion combined with other factors can mimic hanging and strangulation. The presence of a medical device (eg, an oral endotracheal tube) or a linear object (eg, an electrical cord) pressing on the neck can inhibit the formation of lividity and could potentially be confused with a furrow or ligature mark (Figure 8.27A). This is especially important to consider if the pathologist has not seen scene photographs and is unaware of how the body was found or what objects were found in association with the body (eg, if the decedent was found collapsed on the floor, but with their neck entangled with a computer cord). The formation of the lividity itself, when associated with creasing of the neck, can create artifacts that could be misidentified as a furrow or ligature mark (Figure 8.27B).

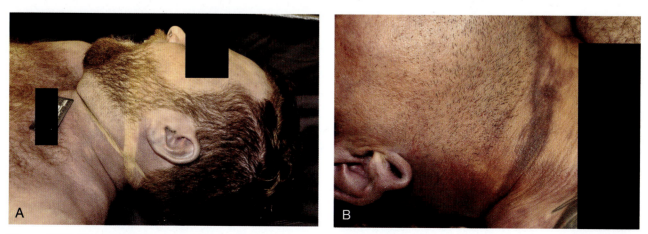

Figure 8.27. Change of lividity potentially mimicking a furrow or ligature mark. In (**A**), the lividity developed after placement of an endotracheal tube, which left strips of pallor on the neck. (**B**) illustrates a linear mark on the neck, which was due to lividity, with no indication from the scene investigation or autopsy that a hanging or other compression of the neck occurred. (**C** and **D**) both are from bodies found face-down and have marked development of Tardieu spots on the skin of the neck, which could be misinterpreted as trauma.

Figure 8.27 (continued)

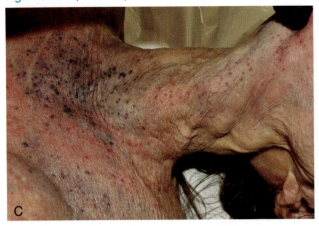
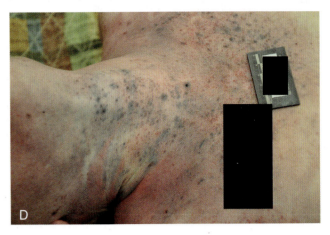

Tardieu spots, which can occur in areas of lividity, could potentially be misinterpreted as trauma (Figure 8.27C and D). While the term "Tardieu spots" is used in literature to describe this phenomenon (ie, punctate hemorrhages in areas of lividity),[3] Necas et al indicate that the term should only be applied to the subpleural and subepicardial and thymic hemorrhages.[3,61]

Near Miss #4: If an individual hangs themselves with a broad soft object, such as a blanket, or if they are found quickly enough after the hanging has occurred, or some combination of those two factors, it is possible for no ligature furrow to be present on the neck at the time of autopsy (Figure 8.28A-D). Correction identification of the cause and manner of death in such a situation would require good correlation with the scene investigation and the known circumstances of the death.

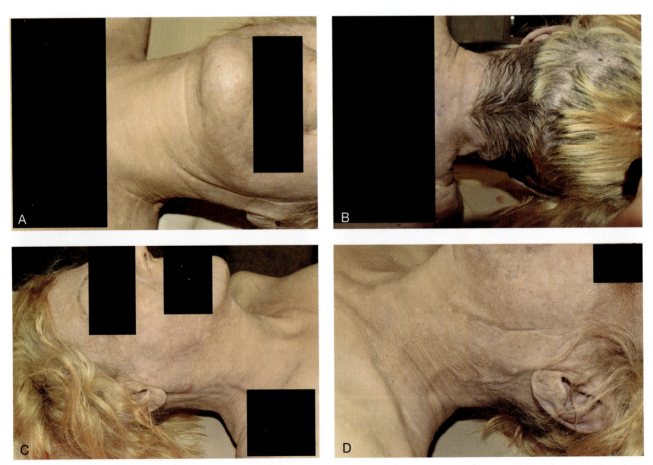

Figure 8.28. Hanging with no ligature furrow. This individual hanged themselves in their jail cell with a section of a blanket, and was relatively immediately found after the hanging occurred. At autopsy, no ligature furrow was identified on the skin of the neck (**A-D**).

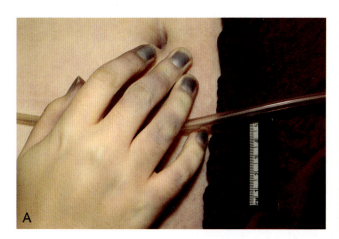
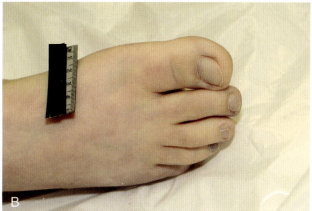
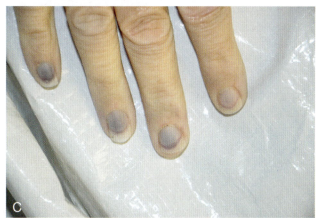

Figure 8.29. Blue discoloration of the nail beds at autopsy. (**A** and **B**) exhibit blue discoloration of the fingernail beds, but pale tan coloration of the toenail beds. (**C**) shows blue discoloration of some fingernail beds, but pale tan color of other fingernail beds.

Near Miss #5: Cyanosis has been listed as one of the autopsy findings in asphyxial deaths, and in a living individual, blue discoloration of the fingernail beds would be associated with cyanosis (Figure 8.29A); however, blue discoloration of the fingernail beds at autopsy is not a reliable sign of asphyxia. In this body, while the fingernail beds are blue, the toenail beds are pale tan (Figure 8.29A and B). In a different body, some of the fingernail beds were blue and some were tan (Figure 8.29C).

References

1. Hensyl WR, Felscher H, eds. *Stedman's Medical Dictionary*. 25th ed. Williams and Wilkins; 1990.
2. Fisher RS, Petty CS. *Forensic Pathology: A Handbook for Pathologists*. National Institute of Law Enforcement and Criminal Justice, Law Enforcement Assistance Administration, US Department of Justice (Grant to College of American Pathologists, NI 71-118G); 1977.
3. DiMaio VJM, Molina DK. *DiMaio's Forensic Pathology*. 3rd ed. CRC Press; 2022.
4. Dolinak D, Matshes E, Lew E. *Forensic Pathology: Principles and Practice*. Elsevier Academic Press; 2005.
5. Saukko P, Knight B. *Knight's Forensic Pathology*. CRC Press; 2016.
6. Gordon I. The medicolegal aspects of rapid deaths initiated by hypoxia and anoxia. *Leg Med Annu*. 1975;1975:29-47.
7. Byard R. Issues in the classification and pathological diagnosis of asphyxia. *Aust J Forensic Sci*. 2011;43(1):27-38.
8. Puschel K, Turk E, Lach H. Asphyxia-related deaths. *Forensic Sci Int*. 2004;144(2-3):211-214.
9. Pollanen MS. Subtle fatal manual neck compression. *Med Sci Law*. 2001;41(2):135-140.
10. Doichinov ID, Doichinova YA, Spasov SS, Marinov ND. Suicide by unusual manner of hanging. A case report. *Folia Med (Plovdiv)*. 2008;50(1):60-62.

11. Bartschat S, Fieguth A, Könemann J, Schmidt A, Bode-Jänisch S. Indicators for acute hypoxia—an immunohistochemical investigation in cerebellar Purkinje-cells. *Forensic Sci Int*. 2012;223(1-3):165-170.
12. Nogami M, Takatsu A, Endo N, Ishiyama I. Immunohistochemical localization of c-fos in the nuclei of the medulla oblongata in relation to asphyxia. *Int J Legal Med*. 1999;112(6):351-354.
13. Cecchi R, Sestili C, Prosperini G, et al. Markers of mechanical asphyxia: immunohistochemical study on autoptic lung tissues. *Int J Legal Med*. 2014;128(1):117-125.
14. Palmiere C, Tettamanti C, Scarpelli MP, Rousseau G, Egger C, Bongiovanni M. Postmortem biochemical investigation results in situations of fatal mechanical compression of the neck region. *Leg Med*. 2018;30:59-63.
15. Tani N, Ishikawa M, Watanabe M, Ikeda T, Ishikawa T. Thyroid-related hormones as potential markers of hypoxia/ischemia. *Hum Cell*. 2020;33(3):545-558.
16. Quan L, Zhu BL, Ishida K, et al. Intranuclear ubiquitin immunoreactivity of the pigmented neurons of the substantia nigra in fatal acute mechanical asphyxiation and drowning. *Int J Legal Med*. 2001;115(1):6-11.
17. Delmonte C, Capelozzi VL. Morphologic determinants of asphyxia in lungs: a semiquantitative study in forensic autopsies. *Am J Forensic Med Pathol*. 2001;22(2):139-149.
18. Ely SF, Hirsch CS. Asphyxial deaths and petechiae: a review. *J Forensic Sci*. 2000;45(6):1274-1277.
19. Schroder AS, Muller F, Gehl A, Sehner S, Anders S. Post-mortem development of conjunctival petechiae following temporary prone position. *Forensic Sci Int*. 2012;223(1-3):e53-e55.
20. Lasczkowski G, Risse M, Gamerdinger U, Weiler G. Pathogenesis of conjunctival petechiae. *Forensic Sci Int*. 2005;147(1):25-29.
21. Maxeiner H, Jekat R. Resuscitation and conjunctival petechial hemorrhages. *J Forensic Leg Med*. 2010;17(2):87-91.
22. Sauvageau A, Boghossian E. Classification of asphyxia: the need for standardization. *J Forensic Sci*. 2010;55(5):1259-1267. doi:10.111/j.1556-4029.2010.01459.x.
23. Haddix TL, Harruff RC, Reay DT, Haglund WD. Asphyxial suicides using plastic bags. *Am J Forensic Med Pathol*. 1996;17(4):308-311.
24. Aissaoui A, Salem NH, Chadly A. Unusual foreign body aspiration as a cause of asphyxia in adults: an autopsy case report. *Am J Forensic Med Pathol*. 2012;33(3):284-285.
25. Benomran FA, Hassan AI. Accidental fatal asphyxiation by sand inhalation. *J Forensic Leg Med*. 2008;15(6):402-408.
26. Prahlow JA, Prahlow TJ, Rakow RJ, Prahlow ND. Case study: asphyxia caused by inspissated oral and nasopharyngeal secretions. *Am J Nurs*. 2009;109(6):38-43; quiz 51.
27. Tse R, Wong CX, Kesha K, et al. Postmortem tryptase cut-off level for anaphylactic death. *Forensic Sci Int*. 2018;284:5-8.
28. Spitz WU, Diaz FJ. *Spitz and Fisher's Medicolegal Investigation of Death*. 5th ed. Charles C. Thomas; 2020.
29. Chmieliauskas S, Mundinas E, Fomin D, et al. Sudden deaths from positional asphyxia: a case report. *Medicine (Baltimore)*. 2018;97(24):e11041.
30. Byard RW, Wick R, Simpson E, Gilbert JD. The pathological features and circumstances of death of lethal crush/traumatic asphyxia in adults—a 25-year study. *Forensic Sci Int*. 2006;159(2-3):200-205.
31. Byard RW, Jensen LL. Fatal asphyxial episodes in the very young: classification and diagnostic issues. *Forensic Sci Med Pathol*. 2007;3:177-181.
32. Kurtulus A, Yonguc GN, Boz B, Acar K. Anatomopathological findings in hangings: a retrospective autopsy study. *Med Sci Law*. 2013;53(2):80-84.
33. Sharma BR, Harish D, Sharma A, Sharma S, Singh H. Injuries to neck structures in deaths due to constriction of neck, with a special reference to hanging. *J Forensic Leg Med*. 2008;15(5):298-305.
34. Tawil M, Serinelli S, Gitto L. Simon's sign: case report and review of the literature. *Med Leg J*. 2022;90(1):52-56.
35. Nikolić S, Zivković V, Juković F, Babić D, Stanojkovski G. Simon's bleedings: a possible mechanism of appearance and forensic importance-a prospective autopsy study. *Int J Legal Med*. 2009;123(4):293-297.
36. Sauvageau A. True and simulated homicidal hangings: a six-year retrospective study. *Med Sci Law*. 2009;49(4):283-290.

37. Russo MC, Verzeletti A, Piras M, De Ferrari F. Hanging deaths: a retrospective study regarding 260 cases. *Am J Forensic Med Pathol*. 2016;37(3):141-145.
38. Sharma L, Khanagwal VP, Paliwal PK. Homicidal hanging. *Leg Med*. 2011;13(5):259-261.
39. Pollak S, Thierauf-Emberger A. Homicidal assault to the neck with subsequent simulation of self-hanging. *Forensic Sci Int*. 2015;253:e28-e32.
40. Monticelli FC, Brandtner H, Kunz SN, Keller T, Neuhuber F. Homicide by hanging: a case report and its forensic-medical aspects. *J Forensic Leg Med*. 2015;33:71-75.
41. Geisenberger D, Pollak S, Thierauf-Emberger A. Homicidal strangulation and subsequent hanging of the victim to simulate suicide: delayed elucidation based on reassessment of the autopsy findings. *Forensic Sci Int*. 2019;298:419-423.
42. Jackson NR, Paul ID. An unusual method of suicide: cable ties. *Am J Forensic Med Pathol*. 2020;41(3):223-226.
43. Lin Z, Kondo T, Sato Y, Ohtsuji M, Takayasu T, Ohshima T. An autopsy case of suicidal strangulation with four looped rubber bands. *Nihon Hoigaku Zasshi*. 1997;51(3):231-234.
44. Thomsen AH, Leth PM, Hougen HP, Villesen P. Asphyxia homicides in Denmark 1992-2016. *Int J Leg Med*. 2022;136(6):1773-1780. doi:10.1007/s00414-022-02787-0
45. Godin A, Kremer C, Sauvageau A. Fracture of the cricoid as a potential pointer to homicide. A 6-year retrospective study of neck structures fractures in hanging victims. *Am J Forensic Med Pathol*. 2012;33(1):4-7.
46. Bux R, Padosch SA, Ramsthaler F, Schmidt PH. Laryngohyoid fractures after agonal falls: not always a certain sign of strangulation. *Forensic Sci Int*. 2006;156(2-3):219-222.
47. Barranco R, Tettamanti C, Bonsignore A, Ventura F. Otorrhagia in strangulations: an important but often underestimated finding in forensic pathology. *J Forensic Sci*. 2022;67(4):1739-1742.
48. Loughney E, Kemp WL. Homicide-suicide: a homicidal asphyxiation misinterpreted as a gunshot wound at the scene. *Am J Forensic Med Pathol*. 2020;41(4):321-323.
49. Bugelli V, Campobasso CP, Angelino A, Gualco B, Pinchi V, Focardi M. Postmortem otorrhagia in positional asphyxia. *Am J Forensic Med Pathol*. 2020;41(3):217-219.
50. Amadasi A, Tsokos M, Bushmann CT. Differential diagnosis on discolorations of the skin in a case of suspected positional asphyxia. *Forensic Sci Med Pathol*. 2019;15(4):671-674.
51. Pollanen MS. Forensic pathology and the miscarriage of justice. *Forensic Sci Med Pathol*. 2012;8(3):285-289.
52. Raven KP, Reay DT, Harruff RC. Artifactual injuries of the larynx produced by resuscitative intubation. *Am J Forensic Med Pathol*. 1999;20(1):31-36.
53. Rajs J, Thiblin I. Histologic appearance of fractured thyroid cartilage and surrounding tissues. *Forensic Sci Int*. 2000;114(3):155-166.
54. Lupascu C, Lupascu C, Beldiman D. Mechanical asphyxia by three different mechanisms. *Leg Med*. 2003;5(2):110-111.
55. Byard RW, Wilson GW. Death scene gas analysis in suspected methane asphyxia. *Am J Forensic Med Pathol*. 1992;13(1):69-71.
56. Grassberger M, Krauskopf A. Suicidal asphyxiation with helium: report of three cases. *Wien Klin Wochenschr*. 2007;119(9-10):323-325.
57. Allan AR, Blackmore RC, Toseland PA. A chloroform inhalation fatality—an unusual asphyxiation. *Med Sci Law*. 1988;28(2):120-122.
58. Schneppe S, Dokter M, Bockholdt B. Macromorphological findings in cases of death in water: a critical view on "drowning signs." *Int J Leg Med*. 2021;135(1):281-291.
59. Piette MHA, DeLetter EA. Drowning: still a difficult autopsy diagnosis. *Forensic Sci Int*. 2006;163(1-2):1-9.
60. Reijnen G, Vos P, Buster M, Reijnders U. Can pulmonary foam arise after postmortem submersion in water? An animal experimental pilot study. *J Forensic Leg Med*. 2019;61:40-44.
61. Necas P, Hejna P. Eponyms in forensic pathology. *Forensic Sci Med Pathol*. 2012;8(4):395-401. doi:10.1007/s12024-012-9328-z
62. Okuda T, Wang Z, Lapan S, Fowler DR. Bathtub drowning: an 11-year retrospective study in the state of Maryland. *Forensic Sci Int*. 2015;253:64-70.
63. Carter N, Ali F, Green MA. Problems in the interpretation of hemorrhage into neck musculature in cases of drowning. *Am J Forensic Med Pathol*. 1998;19(3):223-225.

64. Somers GR, Chiasson DA, Taylor GP. Presence of periorbital and conjunctival petechial hemorrhages in accidental pediatric drowning. *Forensic Sci Int*. 2008;175(2-3):198-201.
65. Stephenson L, Van den Heuvel C, Byard RW. The persistent problem of drowning—a difficult diagnosis with inconclusive tests. *J Forensic Leg Med*. 2019;66:79-85.
66. Tamakawa Y, Hanafee WN. Cerebrospinal fluid rhinorrhea: the significance of an air-fluid level in the sphenoid sinus. *Radiology*. 1980;135(1):101-103.
67. Murayama M, Takahashi Y, Sano R, et al. Characterization of five cases of suspected bathtub suicide. *Leg Med*. 2015;17(6):576-578.
68. Hayakawa A, Terazawa K, Matoba K, Horioka K, Fukunaga T. Diagnosis of drowning: electrolytes and total protein in sphenoid sinus liquid. *Forensic Sci Int*. 2017;273:102-105.
69. Girela-Lopez E, Beltran-Aroca CM, Dye A, Gill JR. Epidemiology and autopsy findings of 500 drowning deaths. *Forensic Sci Int*. 2022;330:111137.

BLUNT FORCE INJURIES 9

CHAPTER OUTLINE

Introduction 206
Types of Blunt Force Injuries 206
- Abrasions 206
- Contusions 209
- Lacerations 211
- Fractures 214

Pattern Interpretation of Blunt Force Injuries 214

Blunt Force Injuries of the Head 219

Subgaleal Hemorrhage 219

Cranial Fractures 223

Types of Cranial Fractures 223
- Linear Fracture 223
- Stellate (or Complex) Fracture 224
- Depressed Fracture 224
- Ring Fracture 225
- Basilar Fracture 225
- Comminuted Fracture 227
- Diastatic Fracture 227

Extra-Cerebral Hemorrhage 228
- Epidural Hemorrhage 228
- Subdural Hemorrhage 230
- Subarachnoid Hemorrhage 235

Traumatic Injuries of the Brain 239

Type of Contusions 240
- Coup Contusions 240
- Contre-Coup Contusions 240
- Fracture Contusions 242
- Herniation Contusions 242
- Intermediary Contusions 246
- Gliding Contusions 246

Blunt Force Injuries of the Neck 250
Blunt Force Injuries of the Trunk 252
Blunt Force Injuries of the Extremities 255
Fractures 255
Specific Fracture Types 257
Extent: Incomplete vs Complete Fracture 258
- Incomplete Fractures 258
  - Bow 258
- Torus/Buckle Fracture 259
- Greenstick Fracture 259

Complete Fracture: Fracture Type Based Upon Direction 259
- Transverse Fracture 259
- Oblique Fracture 260
- Longitudinal Fracture 261
- Spiral Fracture 261

Other Fracture Types 261
- Comminuted Fracture 261
- Butterfly Fracture 261
- Segmental Fracture 262
- Avulsion Fracture 263

Timing of Bone Trauma 264
- Antemortem Fractures 265
- Postmortem Fractures 265
- Perimortem Injuries 265

Near Misses 268

INTRODUCTION

The distinction between blunt and sharp force injuries can be seen as a categorical description and not as an acknowledgment of two types of force, with blunt force injuries including abrasions, contusions, lacerations, and fractures. These four types of blunt force injuries are not mutually exclusive and often occur together (Figure 9.1). For example, the margins of a laceration are often abraded, and abrasions and contusions are commonly admixed at the same site (eg, a contused abrasion). When a portion of the body is partially or completely separated from the body by blunt force, the term avulsion or partial avulsion can be used (Figure 9.2A1-B). An avulsion of the upper extremity from the body would be a combination of laceration and fracture, and abrasions and contusions may also be present. Blunt force injuries are caused by impacts of a broad or fairly broad object against the body, or impacts of the body against a broad or fairly broad object or surface (eg, a floor, a foot, a baseball bat), whereas sharp force injuries are caused by impacts to the body with (or against) a much narrower object (eg, a knife, a machete).

TYPES OF BLUNT FORCE INJURIES

ABRASIONS

Description: While by definition, an abrasion is removal of superficial layers of the skin or a mucosal surface,[1,2] some authors indicate that involvement through the epidermis and dermis and into the muscle and bone is also possible.[3,4]

Mechanism: Abrasions occur when contact with an object essentially rubs off a portion of the skin, which could involve only the superficial epidermis or extend to the deeper epidermis, full thickness through the epidermis and into the dermis, and even through the dermis and possibly into the underlying fascia and adipose tissue. Although with the complete loss of a significant patch of skin in its entirety, avulsion is more fitting of a term. As blood vessels are present only in the dermis and not the epidermis, injury that only involves the epidermis should not produce significant hemorrhage. If the application of force is tangential to the surface of the skin, a brush burn type abrasion will develop (Figure 9.3A and B).[2] If the application of force is perpendicular to the skin, a patterned injury can develop (ie, the shape of the object creates an imprint on the skin in the form of an abrasion) (Figure 9.4A-D).[2]

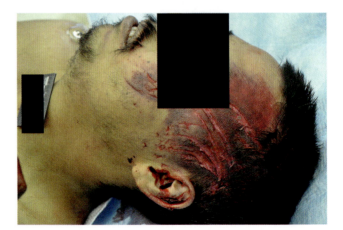

Figure 9.1. Abrasion, contusion, and lacerations of the face. Centered at the left temple and lateral to the left eye is a contiguous patch of parallel superficial lacerations associated with abrasion, which is best seen on the left side of the forehead, and contusion, which is the dark purple discoloration of the skin at the inferior aspect of the wound complex.

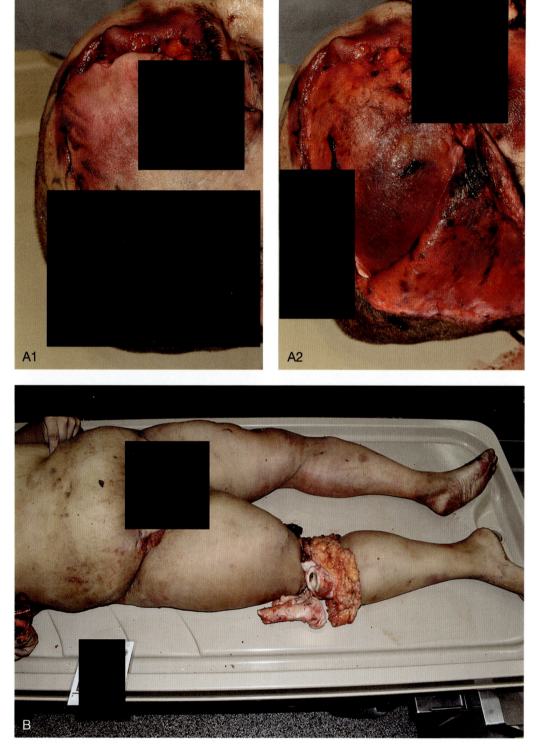

Figure 9.2. Partial avulsion of scalp. (**A1**) is with the affected segment of scalp in its relatively normal location. (**A2**) is with the partially avulsed segment of scalp reflected, revealing the underlying cranium. This is an example of a partial avulsion, as the scalp is partially torn from its attachments but overall still remains attached to the cranium. (**B**) shows a complete avulsion of the right leg from the body, with the separation occurring at the region of the right knee.

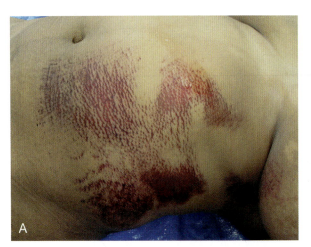 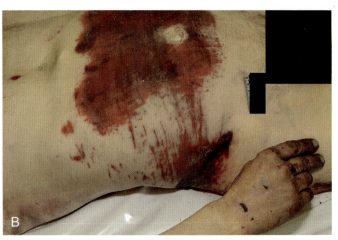

Figure 9.3. Brush-burn type abrasion. In (**A**), on the left side of the trunk is an abrasion. The large patches of absent epidermis are consistent with a brush-burn type abrasion, which is due to tangential contact of the body against a broad surface (eg, the ground). In (**B**), on the right side of the trunk is a large brush-burn type abrasion.

PEARLS & PITFALLS

To potentially allow for the determination of the direction of the application of force to the skin that produced an abrasion, examine the edges of the lesion. Piled epidermis may occur at the edge opposite the direction of force (ie, similar to a snowplow, the epidermis will pile up at the end of the application of force).[3,4] While this concept in a mechanistic approach is useful because this finding could assist in the understanding of the nature of abrasions on the body, its application is often limited[2] (comment: in the author's experience, the ability to distinguish piled epidermis on one edge of an abrasion vs another edge usually is not possible, or is, at least, very subjective in interpretation).

PEARLS & PITFALLS

If a patterned abrasion or patterned contusion is present, photographs of the injury using an ABFO (American Board of Forensic Odontology) ruler as the size marker should be used. Using this L-shaped ruler will allow a latent prints/impression evidence examiner to compare the weapon suspected of causing the injury to the injury itself to possibly provide for a match. The use of a straight ruler in the photograph would not allow for an accurate comparison. Even if the pattern is faint, ill-defined, or inconsistent, erroring on the side that the injury is patterned and taking a photograph with the ABFO ruler will ensure that if a future match can potentially be made, that the opportunity is available (Figure 9.5).

PEARLS & PITFALLS

Postmortem insect activity can produce damage to the skin that can mimic traumatic abrasions (Figure 9.6A-C). Ants can produce a serpiginous lesion, presumably from the column that ants often travel in, but can also produce abraded parchmentlike lesions at the edge of clothing or at the edge of skin that is otherwise obstructed (ie, the exposed area of skin at the edge of something the body is pressed against).[5] Other insects, such as cockroaches, can also cause postmortem injuries to the skin.

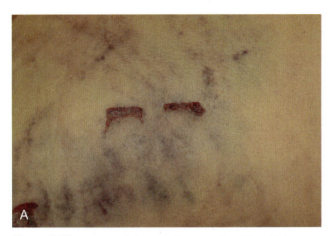

Figure 9.4A. Patterned abrasion from crowbar. The skin has two similar sized rectangular abrasions with a preserved region of skin between the two defects. This pattern was consistent with the reported use of a crowbar to inflict the blunt force injuries.

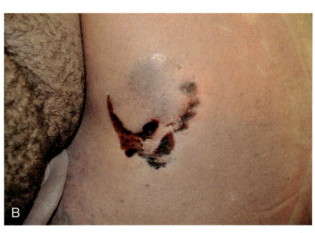

Figure 9.4B. Patterned abrasion from bite. On the shoulder of this individual is a patterned abrasion consisting of a semi-circular group of contiguous and similar sized square and rectangular abrasions. This individual was reported to have been bitten by another person.

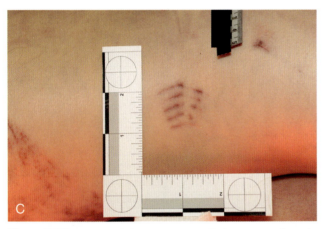

Figure 9.4C. Patterned abrasion, potentially from a tire. This individual was in an all-terrain vehicle with other persons when he fell out of the vehicle and subsequently died of blunt force injuries. Identified on the body was this patterned abrasion interpreted as representing contact with a tire; however, confirmation of the origin of the patterned injury was not done by the investigating agency.

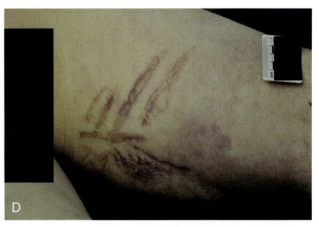

Figure 9.4D. Patterned abrasion of unknown origin. This individual died as the result of drug use, under suspicious circumstances with their significant other. Identified on the left thigh was this patterned abrasion, which was felt to possibly represent contact with an iron; however, the source of the patterned injury was never identified via investigation. Identification of patterned injuries, and documentation of their size with the ABFO ruler, will allow subsequent comparisons to suspected objects. However, in many cases, such analysis is either not needed in the investigation or not performed as no suspected weapon is identified. ABFO, American Board of Forensic Odontology.

CONTUSIONS

Description: A contusion is a local extravasation of red blood cells into the dermis or subcutaneous tissue or into the parenchyma of an internal organ, with the overlying skin or membrane remaining intact (Figure 9.7).

Mechanism: Contusions are due to damage to blood vessels, which allows blood to escape the vessel and leak into the surrounding tissue. The hemorrhage, if contained, can form a mass lesion (ie, a hematoma). If the hemorrhage is not contained by a membrane or the surrounding soft tissue, hemorrhage into a body cavity can occur, leading to extra-cerebral hemorrhage, hemothorax, hemopericardium, or hemoperitoneum, depending upon the location of initial injury. It is possible for a once-contained hemorrhage to later rupture, which can lead to a delayed death following a traumatic injury.

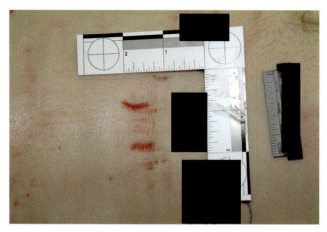

Figure 9.5. Patterned abrasion with ABFO ruler. Although the patterned abrasion in the image is faint and inconsistent, documentation with the ABFO ruler instead of a standard straight ruler will allow for potential future pattern matching, if the opportunity is available, whereas, if the photograph was taken without the ruler, such opportunity is lessened. ABFO, American Board of Forensic Odontology.

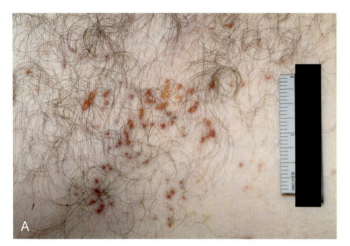
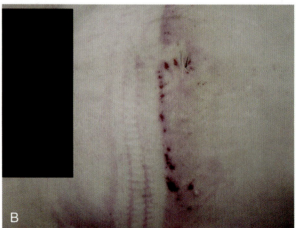
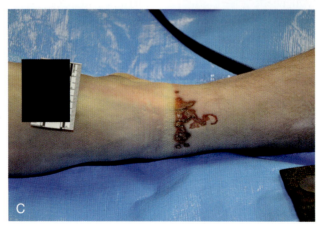

Figure 9.6. Ant bites of the skin. In (**A**), there are numerous punctate orange-yellow lesions of the skin. The discoloration is commonly associated with postmortem change, as no or minimal hemorrhage can occur at the site. These changes were due to postmortem ant bites. In (**B**), there are numerous red discolorations of the skin, which are postmortem abrasions due to ant activity. The injuries end at the waistband compression in the skin, and as such, only occurred on exposed skin, which was available for insect activity. In (**C**), there is a large patch of dried orange-red skin at the sock line. This change also is from ant activity, which was obstructed by the presence of clothing, in that the changes are only present on the exposed skin. These postmortem injuries, not taken in the context of the scene investigation and autopsy findings, could be misinterpreted as antemortem injury.

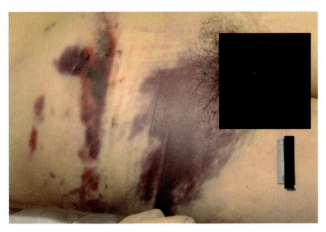

Figure 9.7. Contusion. The lower abdomen has a large purple discoloration centered just above the right femoral region. This is a large contusion that occurred in a snowmobile accident.

> **FAQ:** Can contusions occur postmortem?
>
> **Answer:** As contusions are due to the release of blood from damaged vessels and as blood is contained within vessels following death, postmortem damage to the blood vessels can allow blood to leak into the surrounding tissue; however, since no blood is circulating, the amount of blood released should be minimal. For example, after cardiopulmonary resuscitation has been performed, it is common at the time of autopsy to find rib fractures; however, often these rib fractures will have minimal or no hemorrhage in the surrounding soft tissue. In certain circumstances, though, such as postmortem damage in an area of lividity, extravasation of the blood from damaged vessels could mimic antemortem injury.[2]

> **PEARLS & PITFALLS**
>
> It is possible for postmortem lividity to mimic a contusion (and vice versa). Most frequently, however, an experienced forensic pathologist can easily distinguish postmortem lividity from a contusion. With lividity, there is no hemorrhage into the underlying adipose tissue (Figure 9.8A and B), and with a contusion, there is hemorrhage into the underlying adipose tissue (Figure 9.8C and D). If necessary, an incision into the location can allow for a conclusive determination (Figure 9.8E). Individuals who are inexperienced with postmortem changes are much more likely to mistake postmortem lividity for a contusion (Figure 9.8F).

LACERATIONS

Description: A laceration is a torn or jagged wound in the skin or internal organ.[1] Often, the linear defect is jagged and the surrounding skin has abrasion, contusion, or both (Figure 9.9).

Mechanism: A tangential blow to the skin stretches and tears the skin, or a perpendicular impact can stretch the skin or crush the skin against underlying bone leading to tearing of the skin. With a tangential blow to the skin, undermining as well as partial avulsion or complete avulsion of the skin can occur.

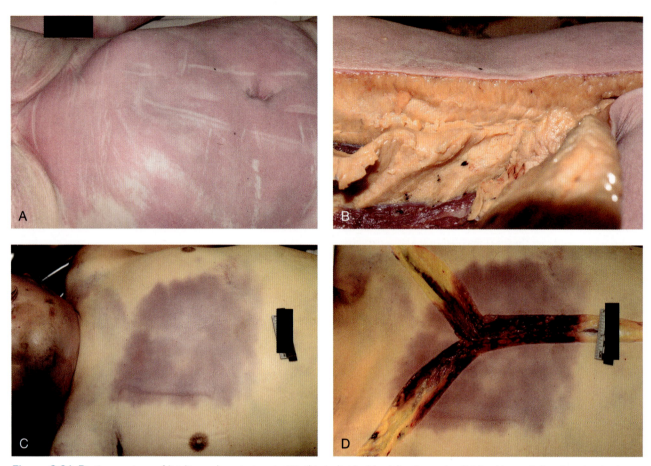

Figure 9.8A-D. Comparison of lividity and contusion. In (**A**), this individual had fixed anterior lividity (the red discoloration is due to prolonged refrigeration prior to autopsy, and is not related to carbon monoxide exposure). In (**B**), an incision into the skin and subcutaneous tissue of the anterior surface of the trunk reveals normal yellow adipose tissue, with no evidence of hemorrhage. In (**C**), this individual sustained a forceful blow to the chest, leading to a contusion. In (**D**), incision into the skin of the chest reveals hemorrhage into the adipose tissue underlying the discoloration of the skin.

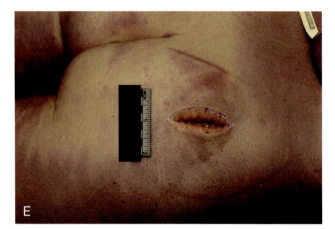

Figure 9.8E. Incision into skin to check lividity. On the buttock is some patchy purple discoloration. The incision into the skin revealed normal yellow underlying adipose tissue, which confirms the coloration in the skin is lividity and not a contusion.

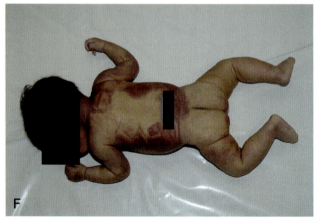

Figure 9.8F. Posterior lividity. The posterior lividity was interpreted as extensive bruising by a non-forensic pathologist physician witness.

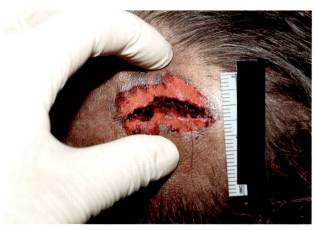

Figure 9.9. Laceration. There is a jagged tear in the skin. The surrounding skin is extensively abraded and there is a thin rim of contusion at the edge of the abrasion. The laceration has some tissue bridging.

PEARLS & PITFALLS

While in most cases, the distinction between a laceration of the skin and an incised or stab wound of the skin is straightforward, some lacerations can appear very much like a stab wound or incision (Figure 9.10), having sharp ends and non-abraded and non-contused margins. In this situation, assessing for the presence of tissue bridging can determine the nature of the wound. In a laceration, spreading open the wound will reveal strands of tissue that cross the gap (Figure 9.11). These strands of tissue are arteries, veins, nerves, and other tissue, and are referred to as tissue bridging; in an incised wound or stab wound, the weapon will sever these structures. The more superficial the injury, the more difficult it becomes to identify tissue bridging, and for very superficial wounds, the absolute determination of a linear abrasion vs a superficial laceration vs a superficial incised wound may not be possible. When there is a very superficial injury and the nature of the wound is unknown (eg, abrasion vs laceration vs incised wound), a potentially less specific term, scratch, could be used.

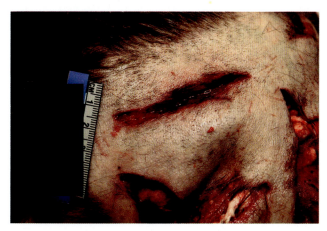

Figure 9.10. Lacerations mimicking incised wounds. The laceration has relatively sharp edges and the margins of the wound are not abraded. This wound can mimic a stab wound or incised wound.

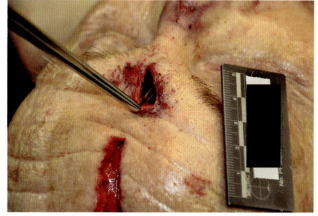

Figure 9.11. Laceration with good tissue bridging. While the first impression appearance of a laceration may mimic a stab wound or incised wound, closer examination, including opening the wound up, will reveal tissue bridging, which is strands of tissue crossing the gap in the skin created by the wound. Tissue bridging would not occur in an incised wound, as the sharp edge of the weapon would sever these strands of tissue.

FRACTURES

Description: A fracture is a break in the bone.[1]

Mechanism: Fractures can be incomplete or complete, based upon whether the fracture line completely divides the bone, and can occur due to direct or indirect force applied to the bone and will be described in detail below.

PATTERN INTERPRETATION OF BLUNT FORCE INJURIES

Interpretation of the pattern produced by blunt force injuries in the skin or internal organs is important for both being able to identify the injuries themselves and for not confusing the injury with another condition as well as for determining the circumstances under which those injuries occurred. Although not possible for every blunt force injury, evaluation of features of the wound may allow a pathologist to determine (a) the relative magnitude of force that caused the injury, (b) the object that caused the wound, and (c) the timing of the injury in relation to the time of death (ie, if the wound is antemortem, perimortem, or postmortem). For example, the appearance of the wound can be patterned and representative of the object used to inflict the injury. Correct documentation of that pattern is important to help with a future match of the injury with the object that caused the injury. The location on the body in combination with the features of the injuries can also help with the interpretation of the injury pattern. For example, the presence of a broad oblique band of abraded contusion between the lower right side of the trunk and the left shoulder is consistent with a seatbelt abrasion, which can indicate the driver of a motor vehicle involved in an accident (Figure 9.12).

> **PEARLS & PITFALLS**
>
> When a rod-shaped object strikes the skin, it will characteristically produce a central area of pallor, with a line of contusion to both sides (Figure 9.13).

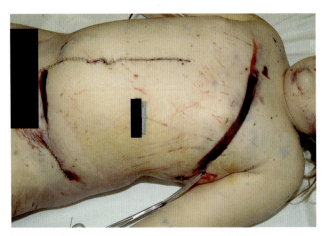

Figure 9.12. Seat belt abrasion. This young child was in a motor vehicle accident and underwent efforts to sustain her life, including placement of a chest tube and laparotomy. Extending between the right shoulder and the left side of the trunk and across the lower abdomen is a band of dried red discoloration, which was consistent with a seat belt abrasion. In addition, in the left femoral region, are stretch-type abrasions/superficial lacerations of the skin, which are consistent with a rear-impact, with the upper body thrown backward.

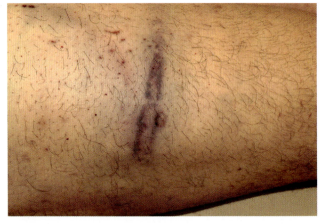

Figure 9.13. Blow from rod-type object. This individual was struck with a short pole, producing the characteristic skin findings in such an injury.

FAQ: Can the amount of force that caused an injury be accurately determined?

Answer: While generalizations regarding magnitude of force needed to cause an injury can be made (eg, avulsion of an upper extremity is much more consistent with a train accident or severe motor vehicle accident than a fall down the stairs), in any given situation, care must be used in determining how much force was required to cause an injury. One important consideration is that not only the magnitude of force, but also the area over which it is distributed is important. A less forceful blow affecting a small area can do more damage than a more forceful blow affecting a large area. The issue of whether a certain amount of force can cause a certain injury frequently arises in the investigation of infant deaths. In those situations, the scenario offered by caregivers must be compared to the injury identified to determine if the scenario offered by the caregivers is consistent with being a cause of the injuries identified at autopsy. For fractures, some research to determine the amount of force required has been performed. Porta determined that the force required to cause a fracture varies from 2,000 N to 14,100 N.[6] For reference, a 4.75 cm diameter steel pipe moving at 17.5 mph and striking a leg can generate 7,800 N of force.[6] In the case of blows with a hammer, wooden handle, or simulated fall to the floor, Sharkey et al, using porcine heads, determined that a force of greater than 4,000 N was required for fracture development.[7] In addition to the amount of force, the direction of the force is also important. For example, femoral bone has a 135 MPa ultimate tensile strength in the longitudinal direction, but only 53 MPa in the transverse direction. The ultimate compressive strength of femoral bone is 205 MPa and the ultimate shear strength is 67 MPa.[8] It is very important to remember that pathologic conditions affecting the skeletal system or the skin and subcutaneous tissue can produce a predisposition to injury development because of the inherent weakness of the tissue produced by the disease process. Conditions predisposing to fracture development include osteoporosis, rickets, tumors and other masses, and inflammation.[9] Senile ecchymoses in elderly individuals are another example of a condition acquired with age that predisposes to easier injury (Figure 9.14). With age, sun-damaged skin becomes very prone to minor trauma causing significant contusions, which can mimic inflicted trauma.

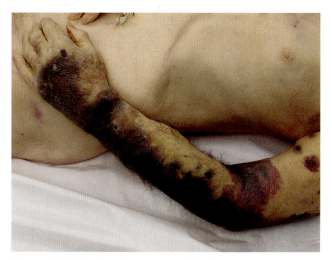

Figure 9.14. Senile ecchymoses. In elderly patients, it is common to see hemorrhagic discoloration of the skin of the upper extremities, which can be in small patches, or diffusely from the hands to the shoulder. Often, sections of associated skin are torn.

FAQ: Can contusions and abrasions be accurately dated?

Answer: For a contusion, the gross appearance of a yellow or yellow-brown coloration, which coincides with the deposition of hemosiderin within the soft tissue from the breakdown of red blood cells, indicates that an injury is antemortem. The reported timing of hemosiderin deposition varies between >18 hours and 2 to 3 or more days prior to death[2,10] (Figure 9.15A-C). Other colorations (eg, red vs purple vs blue) are not useful in dating a contusion. For an abrasion, DiMaio cites a paper from 1972 which indicates an infiltrate of neutrophils occurs at 4 to 6 hours, after which a scab forms.[2] The scab is fibrin layered on neutrophils layered on damaged collagen. For up to 18 hours after the time of injury an increasing number of neutrophils are seen. At 1 to 3 days epithelial regeneration is present and at 5 to 8 days subepithelial granulation tissue is present. Final regression occurs at 12+ days and is associated with atrophy. According to Robbins Basic Pathology, the relative steps of acute inflammation and wound repair, which would occur following an injury, are (1) an inflammatory infiltrate, with neutrophils the initial responders followed by macrophages during the next 6 to 48 hours; (2) cellular proliferation, which takes place for up to 10 days and includes epithelial cells, endothelial cells, and fibroblasts; (3) deposition of collagen and new blood vessel formation; and, finally, (4) reorganization of the collagen to produce a stable scar, which can take months to years to complete.[11] This procession can be used for a general time frame. Also, Robbins Basic Pathology describes that several factors affect tissue repair: infection, diabetes mellitus, nutritional status, use of steroids, mechanical factors (which could lead to wound dehiscence), poor perfusion, foreign bodies, type and extent of tissue injury, and location of the injury.[11] Therefore, understanding that each individual could heal following an injury in a different time frame than others, caution should be used when dating an injury, including providing a wide interval. Dolinak et al, Curran et al, and Gonzales et al recommend not providing precise dates of the time of abrasions and contusions.[12-14]

FAQ: In general, how do you distinguish an antemortem injury from a postmortem injury?

Answer: When an injury occurs prior to death while the heart is still beating, extravasated blood will accumulate at the site of injury, which will give the wound a red or red-purple coloration. When an injury occurs after death, blood extravasation will not occur, or will occur in only a minimal amount, and thus, the wound will have a different appearance, a dried yellow-orange, or yellow-brown appearance (Figures 9.16A-9.16C), which has been described as parchmentlike.[12] However, with time, an antemortem injury can dry out and resemble a postmortem injury. Also, injury to the body must occur to a depth necessary to damage blood vessels (ie, through the epidermis and into the dermis) for there to be hemorrhage associated with the injury if it is antemortem.

SAMPLE NOTES: DOCUMENTATION OF BLUNT FORCE INJURIES

While blunt force injuries can be documented in the autopsy report in a variety of ways, most, if not all reports, will have a separate injuries section. Within this separate section, once again, the injuries can be documented in a variety of ways; however, having an organized approach to the documentation of blunt force injuries allows for easy review of the report and quick identification of findings and helps prevent findings from being omitted from the report.

One general way to organize the injuries section for blunt force injuries is as follows:
  I. Blunt force injuries of the head and neck:
     A. Injuries of the skin
     B. Injuries of the subgaleal region
     C. Injuries of the cranium
     D. Extra-cerebral hemorrhages
     E. Injuries of the brain
     F. Injuries of the neck
 II. Blunt force injuries of the trunk:
     A. Injuries of the skin
     B. Injuries of the ribs, clavicles, sternum, vertebral column, and pelvis
     C. Hemorrhage in the body cavities
     D. Injuries of the internal organs
III. Blunt force injuries of the extremities:
     A. Injuries of the skin
     B. Fractures/dislocations of the skeletal system

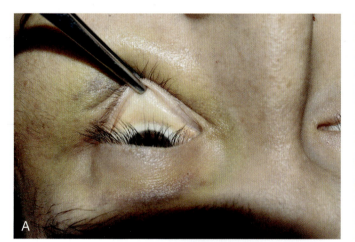
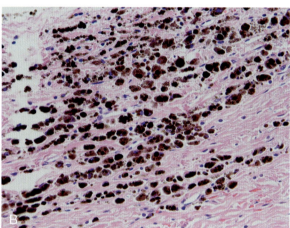
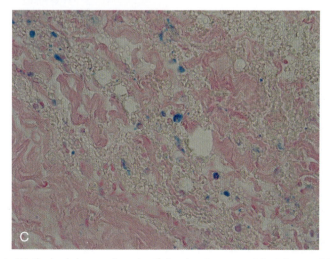

Figure 9.15. Healing contusion. In (**A**), the body has a yellow rim of discoloration around the left eye, which is the result of a healing contusion due to an assault that occurred days prior to the individual's death. Microscopic examination of the soft tissue would reveal hemosiderin (**B**), which appears as a chunky yellow-brown pigment on H&E (hematoxylin and eosin, medium power). If a more definitive identification of iron deposition is required, an iron stain should be performed. With an iron stain, the hemosiderin-laden macrophages will appear blue (**C**) (Prussian blue, lower power). An iron stain would be much more definitive for identification of iron than H&E, and, when dating an injury, the presence of any iron could at least indicate that the injury did not occur right around the time of death (within hours) and that there was some delay (within days), which may help with an investigation.

SAMPLE NOTES

When certifying the death certificate for an individual who died from blunt force injuries, some people advocate a general approach (eg, "Blunt force injuries" as the cause of death in a person with multiple blunt force injuries), whereas others advocate a more specific approach, attempting to prioritize the condition(s) that led to the individual's death (eg, "Flail chest due to multiple rib fractures," with part II, listing, "Lacerations of the extremities; dislocation of the pubic symphysis"). Which approach to use is dependent upon office policies and the training and experience of the pathologist. In a situation where there is a direct chain of events from one major pathology to another, in the background of only minor other injuries, a specific approach is most likely the better approach. For example, "Hemothorax due to aortic transection due to blunt force injuries of the chest" is better than "Blunt force injuries" to describe the same individual.

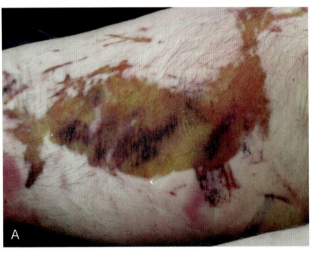

Figure 9.16A. Postmortem abrasion. On the trunk is a large patch of multiple areas of dried yellow-orange with focal red and black discoloration. This appearance is consistent with a postmortem abrasion as the lack of circulating blood does not allow hemorrhage to occur at the site, and the injury to the skin will take on a dried, parchmentlike appearance.

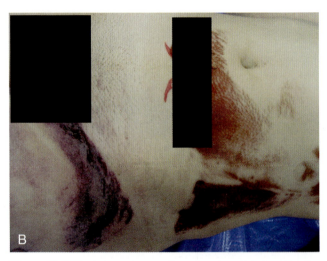

Figure 9.16B. Antemortem and postmortem injuries. On the left thigh is a red-purple discolored contused abrasion, which by appearance is consistent with having occurred antemortem. Below the umbilicus is a dried yellow-brown parchmentlike area, which is consistent with a postmortem injury.

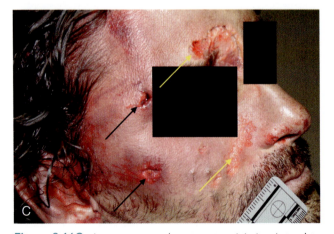

Figure 9.16C. Antemortem and postmortem injuries. Lateral to the right eyebrow and on the right cheek are antemortem lacerations (black arrows), which are associated with contusion in the surrounding skin. The bridge of the nose and to the right side of the nose have postmortem animal activity (yellow arrows). Note the pale, non-hemorrhagic edges of these lesions, which are consistent with their postmortem nature.

BLUNT FORCE INJURIES OF THE HEAD

Blunt force injuries of the head include abrasions, contusions, and lacerations of the scalp, subgaleal hemorrhage, fractures of the cranium, extra-cerebral hemorrhages, and contusions and lacerations of the brain.

PEARLS & PITFALLS

When an individual sustains a sudden cardiac death and collapses to the ground, often they will strike areas of the head where skin directly overlies bone, such as the eyebrows, the cheek, and the chin. In this case, abrasions or a laceration can occur (Figure 9.17). Scene investigation will often allow for the determination of whether such an injury was antemortem or postmortem, for when the laceration occurs after an uncontrolled fall, there is usually no or minimal blood loss apparent at the scene whereas if a scalp laceration occurs prior to death, copious bleeding often occurs. One exception to no or minimal blood being found at the scene if an injury is sustained in a terminal fall could be if the individual falls and ends up in a head-down situation. In this case, postmortem lividity would be most intense in the head and blood could easily leak from the postmortem laceration and mimic an antemortem injury.

PEARLS & PITFALLS

Individuals who have an abrasion, contusion, or laceration of the chin or neck and are found to have a basilar subarachnoid hemorrhage likely sustained an atlanto-occipital or atlanto-axial fracture or dislocation, ponto-medullary laceration (which can also be due to an atlanto-occipital or atlanto-axial fracture or dislocation), or a vertebral artery laceration (Figure 9.18A-E). If a ponto-medullary laceration is a possible finding at autopsy, care must be used in removing the brain so as to not cause artifactual tearing of the brainstem, although this most frequently seems to occur at the midbrain. Examination of the vertebral arteries can be done via radiography through contrast injection of the vertebral arteries, via dissection and direct examination, or via both methods. When a basilar subarachnoid hemorrhage is identified, it is important to determine the source of the subarachnoid hemorrhage. In the scenario described above, it is possible that the decedent had a ruptured berry aneurysm, which was the cause of death, and that the injury of the chin was just an incidental finding and not related to the cause of death. In this case, the manner of death would be natural.

PEARLS & PITFALLS

Minor blunt force injuries of the head combined with ethanol intoxication can be associated with death. At autopsy, no significant injuries of the brain are identified and the alcohol concentration, while elevated, is not within a lethal range, with the usual concentration being around 0.17 to 0.30 g/dL.[15] The mechanism is believed to be a combination of cerebral concussion induced by the head trauma, leading to apnea, and augmented by the alcohol intoxication, with neither factor, by itself, lethal but only lethal in combination.[15-17]

SUBGALEAL HEMORRHAGE

Description: Hemorrhage occurring beneath the galea-aponeurotica and superior to the periosteum (Figure 9.19), with the five layers of the scalp being the skin, the subcutaneous tissue, the galea-aponeurotica, the loose space (in which the hemorrhage is most frequently located), and the periosteum. This hemorrhage can be either identified on the cranium or the undersurface of the reflected scalp.

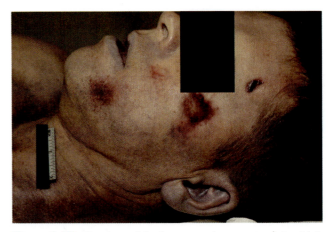

Figure 9.17. Abrasions of the face secondary to unrestrained fall. On the left side of the forehead, the left cheek, and the left side of the jaw are abrasions. These abrasions are overlying bony regions. This patient had a seizure, precipitating an unrestrained fall, which resulted in the injuries in the photo. Injuries such as this are sometimes referred to as marks of innocence, because they occurred under non-suspicious circumstances, even though injuries of the face may normally be associated with inflicted trauma, such as a punch.

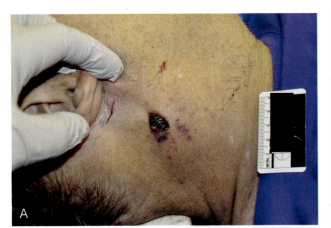

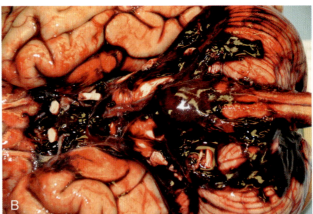

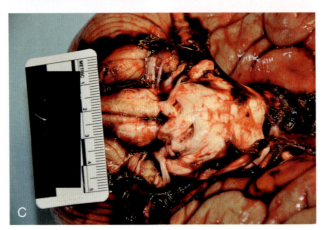

Figure 9.18A-C. Ponto-medullary laceration secondary to assault. This individual was assaulted by another person. External examination revealed minimal findings, other than a small abraded laceration on the right side of the neck (**A**). Upon opening the cranium, a prominent basilar subarachnoid hemorrhage was identified (**B**). Removal of the blood at the base of the brain revealed no aneurysm or dissection, but did identify a laceration of the ponto-medullary junction (**C**).

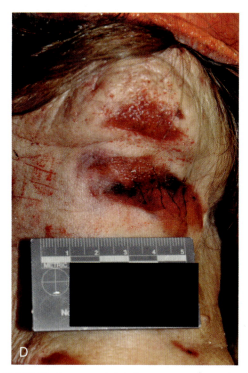 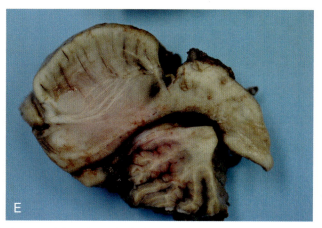

Figure 9.18D-E. Ponto-medullary laceration associated with abrasion of chin. This individual had sustained an injury of the chin by external examination (**D**), and upon internal examination was found to have a basilar subarachnoid hemorrhage with a tear at the ponto-medullary junction (**E**).

PEARLS & PITFALLS

While the external surface of the scalp itself may not show any sign of an injury, the underlying subgaleal region often will, and the location of a subgaleal hemorrhage can identify an impact site. Depending upon the nature of the death (eg, how suspicious the death is for a homicide, and how exact the pathologist needs to be as to the cause of an injury), if a subgaleal hemorrhage is identified upon reflection of the scalp, re-examination of the overlying skin surface, with shaving of hair to best examine this surface, may be useful. Photographs and careful documentation of the location of subgaleal hemorrhage may be useful in comparing the circumstances described by witnesses to the injury itself, in that the location of the subgaleal hemorrhage can mark where on the head the decedent fell or was struck.

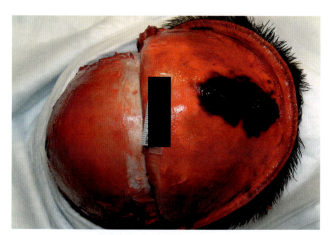

Figure 9.19. Subgaleal hemorrhage. In the midline near the parietal region of the scalp is a patch of subgaleal hemorrhage. Focal subgaleal hemorrhage like this can help identify the impact site for trauma of the head.

> **PEARLS & PITFALLS**
>
> In neonates, subgaleal hemorrhage can occur as a result of birth, and, in rare circumstances, most often when paired with a skull fracture and/or intra-cranial hemorrhage or injuries of the brain, can be a lethal condition (Figure 9.20).[18]

> **PEARLS & PITFALLS**
>
> Postmortem lividity, especially in a body that has laid on its back for a period of time with early decomposition just beginning, can have prominent subgaleal hemorrhage due to congestion, which must be distinguished from a traumatic subgaleal hemorrhage. Although the overlying hair can be shaved to examine the skin, incision into the subcutaneous tissue in this location can also assist. Since traumatic subgaleal is due to an impact, the overlying cutaneous tissue will usually have a contusion, whereas, if the collection of blood is a postmortem artifact, the overlying adipose tissue will be its normal yellow coloration.

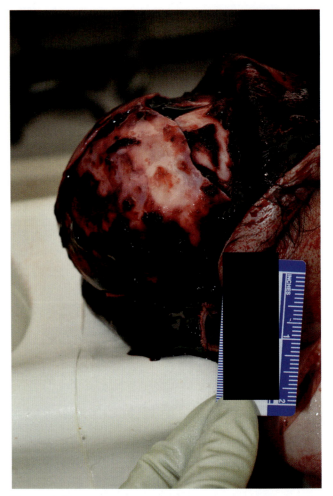

Figure 9.20. Extensive subgaleal hemorrhage in a neonate. This infant died during delivery. Underneath the scalp is extensive subgaleal hemorrhage, which at autopsy measured >100 g. There were no underlying fractures of the cranium or intra-cranial hemorrhage. In the image, what appear to be skull fractures is just overlapping of the cranial sutures.

CRANIAL FRACTURES

While both the cranium and long bones of the body can be fractured, the terminology used for fractures of the cranium is often different than that used for the long bones (ie, types of fractures of the cranium do not necessarily have an equivalent in the long bones, and vice versa). However, some similar terminology is used for fractures in both locations, such as a comminuted fracture, which can affect both the cranium and the long bones. Also, the to-be-described types of cranial fractures are not mutually exclusive. For example, the decedent can easily have a depressed fracture that is also comminuted.

TYPES OF CRANIAL FRACTURES

LINEAR FRACTURE

Description: A single fracture line with two end points (Figure 9.21).

Mechanism: Most commonly due to impact with an object of >5 cm^2 in size.[19] Possible causes of a linear fracture could include a fall, with the head striking the floor.

> **PEARLS & PITFALLS**
>
> A linear skull fracture by itself is not usually a potentially lethal condition unless paired with an underlying intra-cranial hemorrhage, such as a subdural hemorrhage or epidural hemorrhage, or injuries of the brain, such as traumatic axonal injury (TAI), lacerations, or contusions, which could develop into a lobar hemorrhage, One caveat, already described above, would be if the fracture occurred in the context of acute intoxication, then death could result.

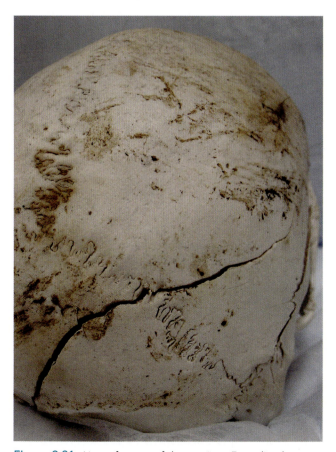

Figure 9.21. Linear fracture of the cranium. Extending between the occipital bone and the right parietal bone near the squamosal suture is a linear fracture.

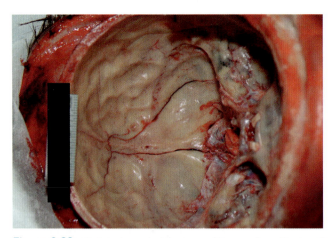

Figure 9.22. Stellate (complex) fracture of the cranium. Centered superior and posterior to the cruciform eminence is a stellate fracture of the occipital bones, with fracture lines radiating into the floors of the left and right posterior cranial fossae, as well as to the left petrous ridge and the foramen magnum.

> **PEARLS & PITFALLS**
>
> If a cranium sustains two or more injuries causing fractures, which would include blunt force injuries but also gunshot wounds and even sharp force injuries if the damage is severe enough, the injuries can potentially be sequenced. When a fracture line meets an already formed fracture line, it will stop. Therefore, the nature of the intersection of the fracture lines can be used to determine the order of the injuries.[20]

STELLATE (OR COMPLEX) FRACTURE

Description: A stellate fracture occurs when fracture lines radiate outward from a central point. Stellate fractures have three or more endpoints[1] (Figure 9.22).

DEPRESSED FRACTURE

Description: The involved segment of the bone is depressed compared to the surrounding bone (Figure 9.23A and B).

Mechanism: Most commonly due to impact with an object of <5 cm^2 in size.[19] Possible causes of depressed fractures could include a strike against the head with a hammer (Figure 9.24).

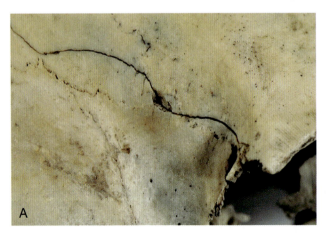
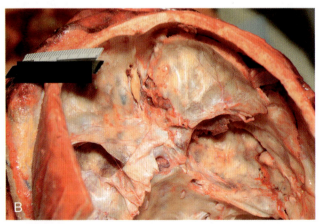

Figure 9.23. Depressed fractures of the cranium. In (**A**), the cranium has a linear fracture just posterior to the region of a zygomatic process. Contained within this linear fracture is a small area of depression, which most likely marks the impact site for the injury that caused the linear fracture. In (**B**), the cranium has an extensive and comminuted depressed fracture centered on the anterior and right side of the head, with depression of a segment of the right frontal bone, including the orbital plate, into the cranial cavity.

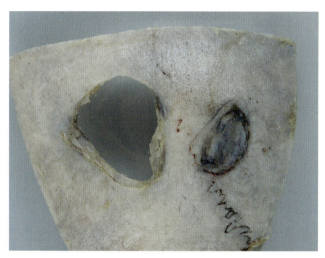

Figure 9.24. Individual assaulted with hammer. This individual was beaten with a hammer. The section of bone illustrates two impact sites. The partial thickness defect to the right side of the image is a depressed fracture, with the outer table compressed inward but the inner table still attached.

RING FRACTURE

Description: A fracture that surrounds the foramen magnum, hence the name (Figure 9.25).

Mechanism: A blow to the top of the head, which drives the cranium against the vertebral column, or a fall onto the buttocks or feet, which drives the vertebral column against the cranium.[19]

BASILAR FRACTURE

Description: A fracture of the base of the cranium, which involves the floor of anterior, middle, and/or posterior cranial fossae (Figure 9.26). Although the base of the cranium includes the floors of all fossae, most frequently, a basilar skull fracture implies a fracture of one or both of the middle cranial fossae to include the region of the sella turcica. The term hinge fracture is used to refer to cranial fractures that involve the left and right petrous ridge and sella turcica (Figure 9.27A and B).

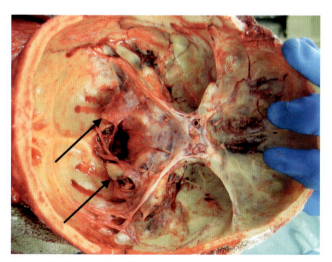

Figure 9.25. Partial ring fracture. This individual sustained severe blunt force injuries of the head. Both the left and right petrous ridges are fractured, and to the left and right sides of the foramen magnum is a displaced fracture (arrows). However, the fractures do not completely encircle the foramen magnum.

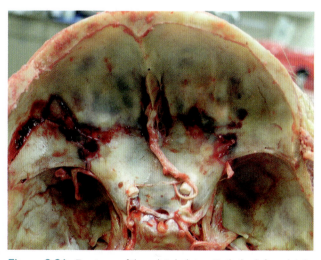

Figure 9.26. Fractures of the orbital plates. Both the left and right orbital plates (ie, the floor of the anterior cranial fossae) are fractured. Such fractures occur in a variety of circumstances including a fall on the back of the head, a gunshot wound of the head, and as a general component of cranial fractures in motor vehicle accidents and other such circumstances. Blood will often enter the upper eyelids leading to this finding at external examination.

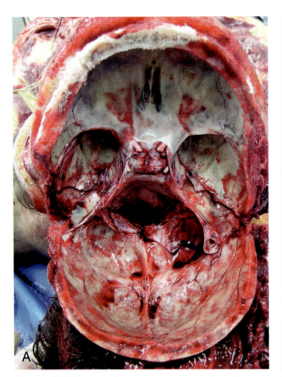
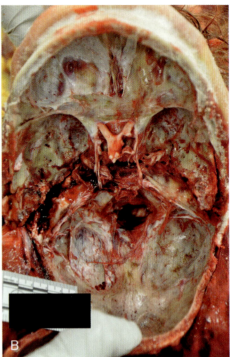

Figure 9.27. Hinge fractures. Both (**A** and **B**) illustrate a hinge fracture. The fracture line involves the floor of both middle cranial fossae and is often just anterior to the petrous ridge. The fracture line often extends through the sella turcica.

Mechanism: Fractures of the floor of the anterior cranial fossae and possibly the middle cranial fossae that are associated with contre-coup contusions of the frontal and temporal lobes result from a fall onto the back of the head and could also be considered contre-coup injuries. Hinge fractures most commonly result from injuries of high force, such as a motor vehicle accident. While hinge fractures are frequently lethal likely due to the fracture line being adjacent to the brainstem, fractures of the anterior cranial fossae are not, by themselves, usually lethal injuries.

PEARLS & PITFALLS

Fractures of the base of the cranium can often be diagnosed by external examination. Fluid blood that drains freely from the external ear canal is indicative of a fracture of the corresponding petrous ridge, as the fracture of the petrous ridge allows blood from torn vessels to enter the ear canal and drain externally. Before diagnosing a basilar skull fracture by finding fluid blood in the ear, the external ear should be cleaned and then the head turned to allow blood to drain from the external ear canal (Figure 9.28A and B). The mere presence of blood in the external ear canal could just be the product of an injury of the ear or drainage to the ear from an injury of the scalp. While hemorrhage into the upper eyelids most commonly is associated with fractures of the orbital plates (ie, the floors of the anterior cranial fossae), lacerations of the forehead can also be a cause.

PEARLS & PITFALLS

Rarely it is possible for opening of the cranium at autopsy to cause a basilar skull fracture. In this context, the injury must be correlated with the scenario and the other autopsy findings to exclude antemortem trauma.

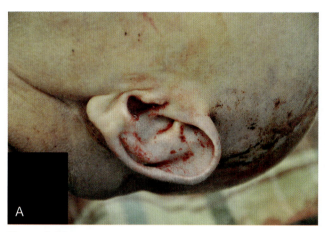 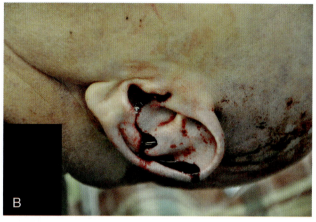

Figure 9.28. Demonstration of basilar skull fracture by external examination. To demonstrate a basilar skull fracture by external examination, first remove as much excess blood from the ear as possible (**A**), then, rotate the head to the side, and, if a basilar skull fracture is present, often fluid blood will drain from the external ear canal (**B**).

COMMINUTED FRACTURE

Description: The bone is broken into multiple fragments (Figure 9.29).

Mechanism: As opposed to a linear fracture, a comminuted fracture indicates a relatively higher magnitude of force but can also be associated with a more focal application of force.

DIASTATIC FRACTURE

Description: Separation of cranial bones at a suture (Figure 9.30A and B)

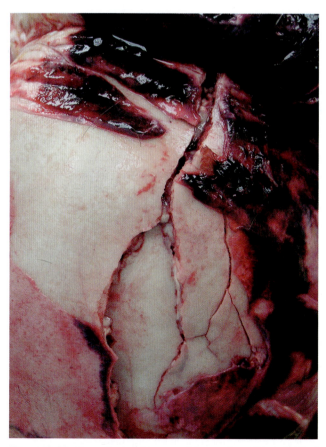

Figure 9.29. Comminuted fracture of the cranium. This individual was struck on the head with a baseball bat. In the right frontal-parietal region is a comminuted and depressed skull fracture, with brain exuded at the edges of the fracture lines.

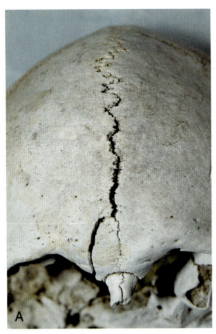 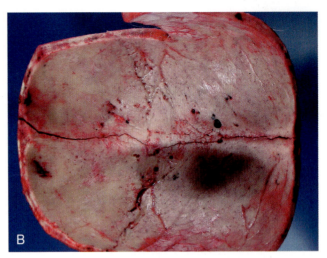

Figure 9.30. Diastatic fracture. In (**A**), there is a linear fracture of the right side of frontal region, which extends to a metopic suture, and caused a diastatic fracture of the metopic suture. In (**B**), there is a linear fracture of the midline of the frontal bone, which extends to bregma (ie, the intersection of the coronal and sagittal sutures), and causes a diastatic fracture of the sagittal suture.

Mechanism: Commonly, diastatic fractures are due to cerebral edema, with expansion of the brain within the cranial cavity pushing outward on the bone, causing the sutures to open. Other mechanisms of diastatic fracture include a traumatic fracture that extends to the suture line and forces open the suture. Diastatic fractures are commonly found in children because of the non-fused nature of the sutures; however, they can also be identified in adults.

EXTRA-CEREBRAL HEMORRHAGE

Three patterns of extra-cerebral hemorrhage occur with trauma: epidural, subdural, and subarachnoid hemorrhage. Epidural and subdural hemorrhages are easily distinguished based upon their relationship to the dura. Subdural and subarachnoid hemorrhages are also easily distinguished based upon their relationship to the arachnoid. An acute subdural hemorrhage will, once the cranium has been opened, slide from the brain, whereas the subarachnoid hemorrhage will stay tightly applied to the brain.

EPIDURAL HEMORRHAGE

Description: Circumscribed hemorrhage occurring between the dura and the cranium (as compared to a subdural hemorrhage, which is non-circumscribed). As the dura is between the hemorrhage and the brain, the hemorrhage is non-uniform in its effects on the underlying brain, exerting pressure on the gyral crests (as compared to an acute subdural hemorrhage, which is uniform in distribution, exerting pressure on the surface of the gyri equally, including within the sulci).

Mechanism: An epidural hemorrhage occurs secondary to a fracture, most commonly of the temporal bone, which tears the middle meningeal artery, leading to an arterial flow of blood, which will form a mass between the cranium and the dura (Figure 9.31A-F). The middle meningeal artery runs beneath the pterion where it is vulnerable to injury because of the relative thinness of the skull at this location. If available, the history would indicate a fall with subsequent conscious behavior (ie, a lucid interval) followed by death. In the forensic context, unfortunately, such history is often not available as the falls are usually unwitnessed or not described to another person by the person who fell prior to their death.

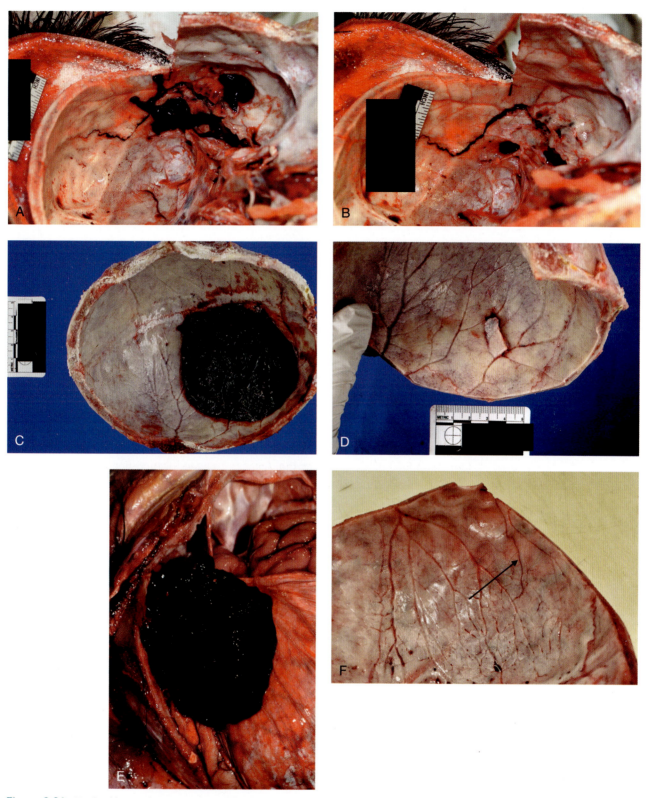

Figure 9.31. Epidural hemorrhage. In (**A** and **B**), the individual sustained lethal head injuries which included a small, not-by-itself lethal, epidural hemorrhage, however, the finding illustrates the pathologic process. In (**A**), there is hemorrhage present on the endocranial surface lateral to the petrous ridge. In (**B**), the hemorrhage has been removed, clearly revealing the fracture line through the groove for the middle meningeal artery. In (**C** and **D**), the individual died as a result of the epidural hemorrhage. (**C**) reveals the epidural hemorrhage forming a mass on the endocranial surface. (**D**) reveals the fracture of the cranium, with involvement of the groove for the middle meningeal artery, with the hemorrhage having been removed to identify the fracture. In (**E** and **F**), the individual was found unresponsive outside, with no clear historical evidence as to a reason for his collapse. At autopsy, an epidural hemorrhage was identified. (**E**) reveals the hemorrhage in the left temporal-parietal region, with the hemorrhage being in situ prior to removal of the brain. (**F**) reveals a subtle linear fracture, which crosses to the groove for the middle meningeal artery (arrow).

> **PEARLS & PITFALLS**
>
> In a fire damaged body, it is not uncommon to see cooked blood underlying the cranium. This epidural hemorrhage is artifactual and occurs secondary to the thermal effects (Figure 9.32). The overlying calvarium is also often fractured, which is artifactual secondary to thermal injury.

SUBDURAL HEMORRHAGE

Description: Hemorrhage occurring between the dura and the arachnoid, which can occur as an acute subdural hemorrhage or a chronic (organizing) subdural hemorrhage. As the hemorrhage is not constrained between two solid objects (eg, the dura and the cranium in an epidural hemorrhage), the hemorrhage can spread out more, following the gyri and sulci and is, hence, non-circumscribed.

Mechanism: A subdural hemorrhage commonly occurs secondary to tearing of a bridging vein due to a fall with the head striking the ground (Figure 9.33), and forms a mass on the undersurface of the dura (Figure 9.34). A bridging vein is a vein extending between the cortical surface and the dura. While a subdural hemorrhage is most commonly traumatic in origin, a subdural hemorrhage can also result from a natural cause. If an intracerebral hemorrhage associated with hypertension ruptures through the cortical surface of the brain, a subdural hemorrhage can arise. A ruptured arteriovenous malformation, disease-related damage to a blood vessel, or hemorrhage from a neoplasm could also potentially cause a subdural hemorrhage. While ruptured berry aneurysms are most frequently associated with subarachnoid hemorrhage, they can rarely cause subdural hemorrhage.[21]

> **PEARLS & PITFALLS**
>
> Increased age associated with cortical atrophy is a risk factor for the development of a subdural hemorrhage as the distance between the cortical surface and the dura is lengthened, which contributes to risk for rupture of a bridging vein.

> **PEARLS & PITFALLS**
>
> Based upon their relationship to the dura and underlying brain, epidural and subdural hemorrhages produce different changes and while an epidural hemorrhage, in the forensic context, is essentially always an acute finding, a subdural hemorrhage encountered at autopsy can be acute or chronic (organizing), each with different features (Table 9.1).

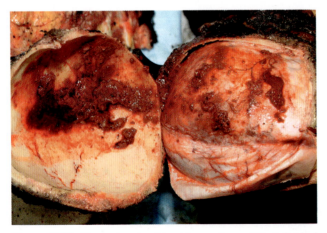

Figure 9.32. Heat-related epidural hemorrhage. This individual died in a house fire. The head was charred. Reflection of the cranium revealed an epidural hemorrhage. Unlike the clotted blood appearance of a traumatic epidural hemorrhage, the blood has a more cooked appearance and is thought to possibly be due to bubbling of the bone marrow secondary to the heat.

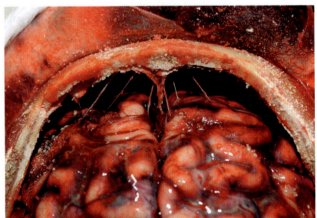

Figure 9.33. Bridging veins. With the brain retracted, the bridging veins can be seen as small thin branches between the surface of the cerebral hemisphere and the dura. The decedent had blunt force injuries of the head, including subgaleal hemorrhage and subarachnoid hemorrhage, which are visible in the image. This image is used to illustrate bridging veins and not a subdural hemorrhage.

FAQ: How do you date a subdural hemorrhage?

Answer: Various features of a subdural hemorrhage include extravasated red blood cells (Figure 9.35), fibroblast ingrowth into the red blood cells (Figure 9.36A and B), formation of a neomembrane at both the dura and arachnoid surfaces of the clot (Figure 9.37), proliferation of capillaries and medium sized thin wall vessels (Figure 9.38), hemosiderin deposition (Figure 9.39), and formation of a hyalinized neomembrane (Figure 9.40A and B). As these histologic features change over time, the microscopic examination of a subdural hemorrhage may allow for dating the time course of the hemorrhage. When obtaining a sample for histologic analysis, it is best to take a section from the edge of the hemorrhage.[12] It is also important to remember that an individual may have more than one subdural hemorrhage present (eg, an acute subdural hemorrhage occurring on a more chronic and resolving subdural hemorrhage). Van den Bos reviewed numerous forensic publications,[22-25] which all apparently derive time frames for the aging of a subdural hemorrhage from one source[26]; however, the time intervals for the various histologic changes seen in a subdural hemorrhage as it ages are different between the sources, and the changes are presumably derived from the author's own experiences.[27] Van den Bos et al provide a list of 28 histologic features and each of their time courses.[27] Table 9.2 summarizes many of these features. Identification of lymphocytes and macrophages can be done with hematoxylin and eosin (H&E) staining but is easier with immunohistochemical stains.[27] Hemosiderin-containing cells can be identified by H&E stain; however, an iron stain would be much more sensitive. While a membrane forms at both the dural and arachnoidal side of the hemorrhage, van den Bos et al indicated that tissue processing may affect the ability to examine the arachnoidal side of the membrane and, thus, its presence was left out of their assessment.[27] Hematoidin, which is a late feature of subdural organization, was found at 9 days but only identified in two cases reviewed by van den Bos et al.[27] Van den Bos et al indicate that fibroblast proliferation and the neomembrane (which is a layer at least 3 cells thick over the length of the subdural) begin at the dural side.[27] Based upon the discrepancies in the literature regarding the absolute dating of organizing subdural hemorrhages, some caution regarding determining an exact timing for their development is probably best. Van den Bos et al recommend reporting the timing as follows: liquid subdural from onset of trauma, fibrin layer at dural and arachnoidal side from hours to a half day, macrophages from 1/2 to 1 day, hemosiderin containing macrophages (as identified with iron stain) at less than 1 week, proliferation of capillaries at about 1 week, medium sized thin walled vessels at 1 to 2 weeks, neomembrane of the whole dural thickness from 2 weeks, and a hyalinized neomembrane at 1 month or more.[27] However, even these general time frames are not without fail (Figure 9.41).

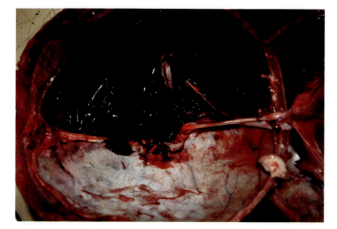

Figure 9.34. Subdural hemorrhage. The calotte has been reflected backward after sawing of the cranium, with the subdural hemorrhage forming a mass underneath the dura, which is visible on the left side. When an individual dies from an acute subdural hemorrhage, the hemorrhage is not adherent to the dura and upon reflection of the cranium, the hemorrhage will often slide from the arachnoid surface. Capturing the finding with photography prior to complete removal of the top of the cranium can allow for recording of the hemorrhage in situ.

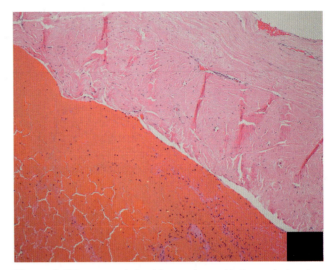

Figure 9.35. Acute subdural hemorrhage. Underneath the dura is a layer of extravasated red blood cells. There is no layer of fibrin underneath the dura (hematoxylin and eosin, medium power).

TABLE 9.1: Comparison and Contrast of Epidural Hemorrhage and Acute and Chronic (Organizing) Subdural Hemorrhages

	Epidural Hemorrhage	Acute Subdural Hemorrhage	Chronic (Organizing) Subdural Hemorrhage
Circumscribed	Yes	No	Yes
Flattening of gyri underlying hemorrhage	Yes	No	Yes
Midline shift	Yes	Yes	No

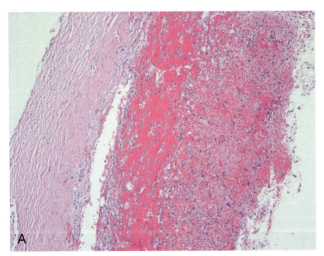
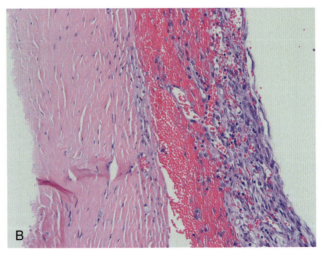

Figure 9.36. Organizing subdural hemorrhage. Both (**A** and **B**) exhibit fibroblast ingrowth into the subdural hemorrhage. While the fibroblast ingrowth begins at the dural surface of the clot, it will eventually involve the full thickness of the clot (hematoxylin and eosin, medium power).

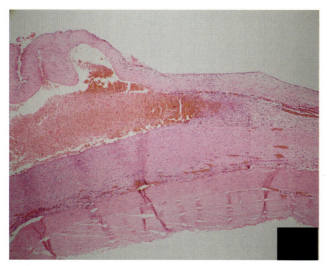

Figure 9.37. Organizing subdural hemorrhage. The image illustrates the neomembrane at the dural surface and at the arachnoidal surface meeting at the edge of the hemorrhage. Between the two neomembranes are red blood cells (hematoxylin and eosin, low power).

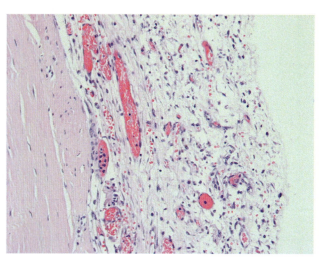

Figure 9.38. Organizing subdural hemorrhage. At the dural surface is a neomembrane of essentially the same thickness as the dura. The neomembrane is composed of granulation tissue (loose fibrosis and capillaries) (hematoxylin and eosin, high power).

PEARLS & PITFALLS

While epidural and subarachnoid hemorrhages, when encountered at autopsy, are almost always acute, with the exception of residual subarachnoid hemorrhage or hemosiderin staining of the arachnoid associated with remote contusions, subdural hemorrhage in various stages of resolution can be encountered at autopsy. In an acute subdural hemorrhage, the blood will be unattached to the dura, whereas in a chronic subdural hemorrhage, the blood will be attached to the dura. In an acute subdural hemorrhage, the cortical surface at the site of the hemorrhage will retain its convoluted texture, whereas in a chronic subdural hemorrhage, the cortical surface at the site of the hemorrhage can be flattened (Figures 9.42A-B, 9.43A, and 9.43B). With a chronic subdural hemorrhage, the membrane formed by organization of the hemorrhage can often be peeled from the inner surface of the dura (Figure 9.44).

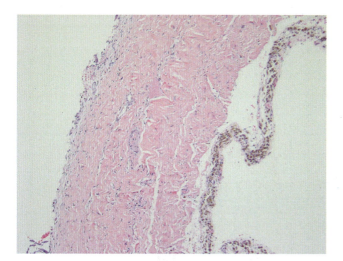

Figure 9.39. Organizing subdural hemorrhage. At the dural surface is a thin layer of loose fibrosis and an abundance of hemosiderin-laden macrophages. The first appearance of hemosiderin-laden or hemosiderin-containing macrophages occurs much earlier in the time course of organization and using an iron specific stain would be more sensitive to its presence than just H&E (hematoxylin and eosin, medium power).

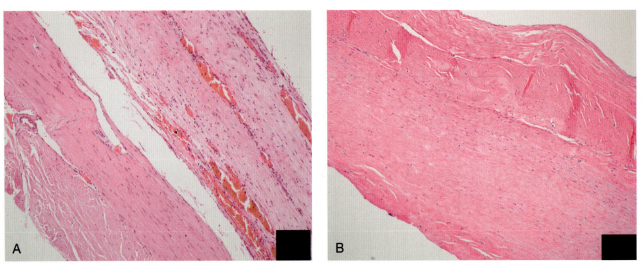

Figure 9.40. (A and B) Organized subdural hemorrhage. Ultimately a subdural hemorrhage will organize into a fibrous neomembrane (hematoxylin and eosin, medium power).

> **PEARLS & PITFALLS**
>
> When subdural blood is present, it is good to collect the blood for toxicologic analysis. Since the subdural blood was outside the normal blood flow, the concentration of drugs in the subdural blood may more accurately represent the toxicologic status of the decedent at the time the injury occurred, as, when a subdural hemorrhage alone is the cause of death, the individual will have a delayed period between the time of the injury and the time of their death, and the concentration of drugs in the blood may have decreased (or increased, if there was use/consumption following the injury). However, the author has seen a case where an individual was hospitalized with a subdural hemorrhage; an alcohol concentration obtained at the time of hospital admission was 0.395 g/dL. The individual died several days later. The subdural blood was retained for toxicologic analysis, which revealed an ethanol concentration of 0.05 g/100 mL and medications given during the hospitalization were present in the subdural blood, including ketamine.

TABLE 9.2: Features for Dating a Subdural Hemorrhage[27]

Feature	Timing
Liquid subdural	0-24 h
Fibrin layer at dural and arachnoidal side	3 h-14 d
Neutrophils	2 h-45 d (usually <10 d)
Macrophages	12 h-9 d (usually >1 d)
Fibroblasts enter clot	15 h-12 d
Hemosiderin-containing macrophages in dural half	16 h-30 d (usually >4 d)
Fragmented nuclei	15 h (usually >2 d)
Liquefaction of red blood cells	3-7 d
Free iron	4 d
Proliferation of capillaries	5 d
Neomembrane <1/2 dural thickness	7 d
Hemosiderin-laden macrophages in entire membrane	10 d
Fibrous neomembrane	10 d
Hyalinized neomembrane	27 d

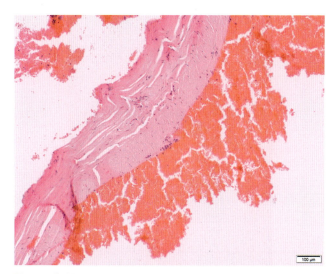

Figure 9.41. Acute subdural hemorrhage. The microscopic section of the subdural hemorrhage exhibits extravasated red blood cells underneath the dura. The known time frame for this subdural hemorrhage was 6 days; however, no fibrin layer is visible between the dura and the hemorrhage, a finding which is supposed to represent a time course of hours to a half day. The image may not be representative of the actual aging of the subdural hemorrhage, or it may represent an area of re-bleeding, and thus looks younger than the known age of the subdural hemorrhage. However, it illustrates that aging of a subdural hemorrhage is most likely best done with several sections to best identify the features of the hemorrhage, and conservatively, accepting that each individual and each subdural can organize at a different rate than the published norm (hematoxylin and eosin, medium power).

SUBARACHNOID HEMORRHAGE

Description: Hemorrhage underneath the arachnoid (Figure 9.45A-C).

Mechanism: Subarachnoid hemorrhage can occur both due to traumatic injuries, presumably due to tearing of vessels underneath the arachnoid, or natural disease processes, such as rupture of a berry aneurysm, rupture of an arteriovenous malformation, or dissection of the vertebral artery.

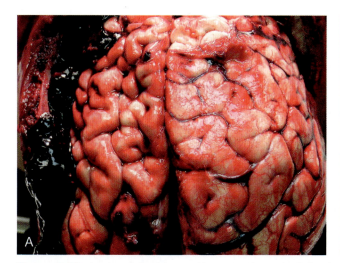
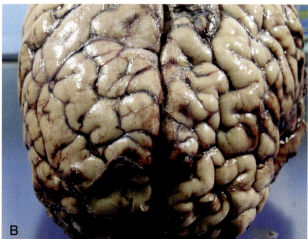

Figure 9.42. Acute subdural hemorrhage. In (**A**), on the left side of the cranial cavity is a space-occupying subdural hemorrhage. Underneath the subdural hemorrhage, the cerebral hemisphere retains its gyral pattern, but on the opposite side of the brain, the cerebral hemisphere is pushed against the dura, which flattens the gyri and effaces the sulci, giving the surface of the brain a smooth texture. (**B**) is the same brain as (**A**) but formalin-fixed.

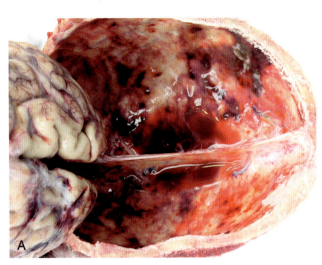

Figure 9.43A. Organizing subdural hemorrhage. Attached to the undersurface of the dura is an organizing subdural hemorrhage.

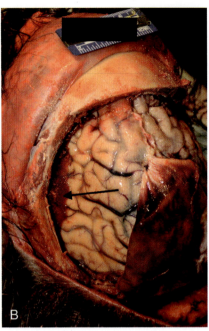

Figure 9.43B. Organizing subdural hemorrhage. At the left cerebral hemisphere is an organizing subdural hemorrhage. The organizing subdural hemorrhage is visible at the reflected dura on the right side of the image and at the edge of the cut cranium on the left side of the image (arrow). The underlying gyri are flattened and the sulci are effaced. Unlike an acute subdural hemorrhage that equally applies pressure to the cerebral hemisphere on the side of the hemorrhage, hence retaining the gyral pattern, a chronic subdural hemorrhage, which forms an underlying membrane between the hemorrhage and the gyri, pushes against this membrane leading to flattening of the gyri.

> **PEARLS & PITFALLS**
>
> With postmortem imaging becoming more and more common and with hospital imaging often routinely available to forensic pathologists, it is important to understand that several conditions can be misinterpreted as subarachnoid hemorrhage on imaging studies (ie, a pseudosubarachnoid hemorrhage). Most commonly, cerebral edema is the condition that is misinterpreted as subarachnoid hemorrhage, but hypoxic ischemic encephalopathy, venous congestion, a cerebral hemorrhage, meningitis, and cerebral infarct can also be misinterpreted as subarachnoid hemorrhage.[28]

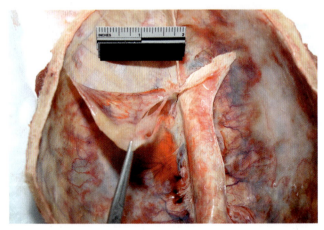

Figure 9.44. Organizing subdural hemorrhage. The organizing subdural hemorrhage can form a membrane, which can be peeled from the underlying surface of the dura.

CHAPTER 9 BLUNT FORCE INJURIES 237

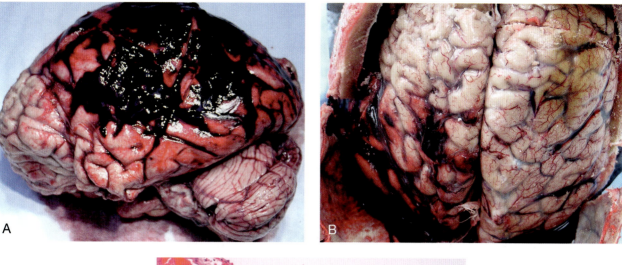

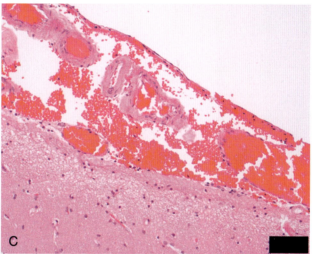

Figure 9.45. Subarachnoid hemorrhage. (**A**) has an acute subarachnoid hemorrhage at the left cerebral convexity. (**B**) illustrates an acute subarachnoid hemorrhage at the left cerebral hemisphere along the greater longitudinal fissure, which was associated with an acute subdural hemorrhage. In addition, at the right cerebral hemisphere is an organized subarachnoid hemorrhage, with the yellow discoloration due to hemosiderin deposition with resolution of the hemorrhage. (**C**) is a microscopic section of an acute subarachnoid hemorrhage, with extravasated red blood cells underneath the arachnoid membrane (hematoxylin and eosin, medium power).

PEARLS & PITFALLS

When subarachnoid hemorrhage is found at the base of the brain, two main etiologies responsible for the hemorrhage are either a ruptured berry aneurysm or vertebral artery laceration (Figure 9.46A-C). Classically, vertebral artery laceration occurs following an impact to the neck. Vertebral arteries are reportedly most prone to injury from rotational acceleration, which causes compression and tension of the vessel, instead of translational force. A punch to the face could cause rotational acceleration whereas a simple fall to the floor would be translational.[29] Identification of the source of the hemorrhage at the time of autopsy is important. Gray et al, based upon a review of 14 cases, identified that the location of the tear is most commonly intra-cranial, including the posterior apical and posterior inferior cerebellar arteries, and the authors comment that injection of the vertebral arteries with contrast can often demonstrate the location of the injury.[30] Fixation of the brain prior to examination of the circle of Willis will impair identification of an aneurysm as the blood becomes fixed, whereas removal of the subarachnoid hemorrhage with running water at the time of autopsy will facilitate discovery of a ruptured aneurysm. Examination of the vertebral artery will require either a posterior neck dissection and direct visualization of the vertebral arteries, or injection of the vertebral arteries with contrast and subsequent x-ray. In addition, computed tomography (CT) scan or magnetic resonance imaging (MRI) (if available) can help identify the vertebral artery lesion; however, all would have to be undertaken before the body was released. While a vertebral artery laceration in combination with an injury of the neck is a classic injury pattern, other circumstances can result in vertebral artery dissection including methamphetamine use. Vertebral artery laceration is commonly associated with relatively minor trauma to the head, and the victim often becomes immediately unresponsive.[31]

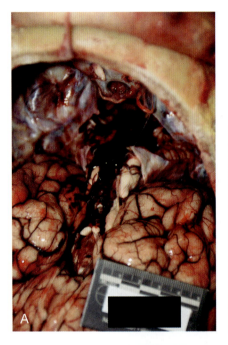
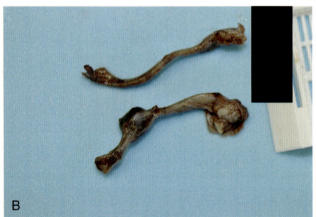
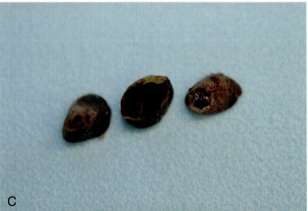

Figure 9.46. Vertebral artery dissection with pseudo aneurysm. (**A**) illustrates the hemorrhage at the base of the brain that was identified as the brain was being removed. At this time, prior to removal of the brain, the vertebral arteries can be injected with contrast to assess for the presence of a traumatic injury. (**B**) is the two segments of vertebral artery (left and right) removed via posterior neck dissection, revealing the aneurysmal dilation of the vertebral artery. (**C**) is a cross section of the aneurysmal segment of the vessel. This individual had a delayed death following a motor vehicle accident, with the vertebral artery injured at the time of the accident and completing the rupture at a later point.

FAQ: How do you physically examine the vertebral arteries in a case of suspected vertebral artery laceration?

Answer: Although the posterior neck can be dissected with removal of the surrounding bone to expose the vertebral arteries (Figure 9.47), this method, unless routinely used, can be tedious and time-consuming, with potential for artifact if the vertebral artery is damaged during the removal of the bone. Kim et al describe a method in which the dura and spinal cord are exposed, including with removal of the bone around the foramen magnum.[31] The dura surrounding the penetrating portion of the vertebral artery is cut, and the intra-cranial vertebral artery is pulled upward, with the extracranial portion of the vertebral artery cut just below the dura. The brain, spinal cord, and attached vertebral arteries are removed in one block.

TRAUMATIC INJURIES OF THE BRAIN

Traumatic injuries of the brain include contusions and lacerations. Several different types of contusions associated with different trauma scenarios include coup, contre-coup, herniation, fracture, intermediary, and gliding contusions. Lacerations are commonly associated with displaced and/or comminuted fractures of the cranium.

General pattern of contusions: Contusions occur as streaklike hemorrhages in the gray matter oriented perpendicular to the cortical surface, or as punctate hemorrhages in the gray matter or white matter. Microscopic examination will reveal clefts in the gray and white matter filled with extravasated red blood cells and often with a centrally placed vessel (Figure 9.48A and B). Identifying the distribution of the hemorrhages and their other associations best allows for the potential interpretation of their etiology as the gross and microscopic appearance of each of the types of contusions listed below is essentially the same.

PEARLS & PITFALLS

When considering the etiology of contusions it helps to consider the moving/non-moving status of the head. For coup, contre-coup, intermediary, and gliding contusions, the moving/non-moving status of the head is important. The head is non-moving in coup contusions and moving in contre-coup, intermediary contusions, and gliding contusions. For fracture and herniation contusions, the moving/non-moving status of the head is un-important, as both types of contusions can occur whether the head is moving or non-moving.

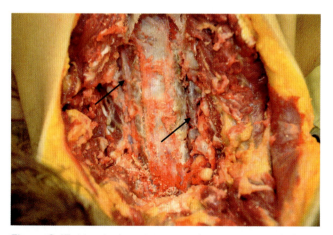

Figure 9.47. Vertebral arteries exposed via posterior neck dissection. With a careful dissection of the posterior neck, the vertebral arteries can be exposed via removal of the bone surrounding each of the vessels (arrows). Once the vessels are exposed, they can be removed and serial-sectioned to examine for injury.

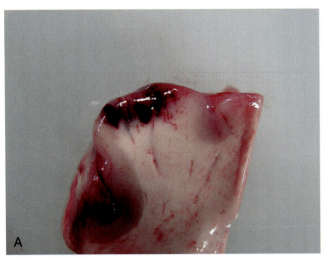
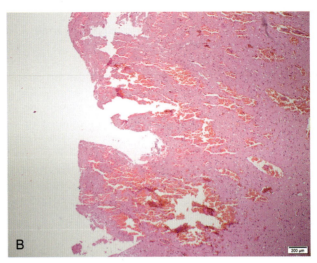

Figure 9.48. Cerebral contusion. (**A**) illustrates cerebral contusions in the gray matter, which are streaklike hemorrhages oriented perpendicular to the cortical surface. (**B**) illustrates the microscopic appearance of the cerebral contusions (hematoxylin and eosin, low power).

TYPE OF CONTUSIONS

COUP CONTUSIONS

Mechanism: Contusions that occur at the point of impact and involve a moving object striking a non-moving head.

Location: Potentially in any location where the overlying scalp and cranium could be struck.

> **PEARLS & PITFALLS**
>
> Commonly, when a head is struck by an object, a fracture will occur at or near the point of impact. This fracture can be associated with contusions, which will be described below. Therefore, if a fracture is identified overlying a brain with contusions, the fracture is usually defaulted to as the cause of the contusions. To identify true coup contusions, the contusions would have to occur at the point of impact and not be associated with a fracture of the cranium (Figure 9.49A-C).

CONTRE-COUP CONTUSIONS

Mechanism: Contusions that occur opposite the point of impact and involve a moving head striking a fixed object. With an injury occurring around the time of death, the contusions will appear as fresh hemorrhage in the cerebral parenchyma, whereas in remote contusions (ie, those occurring months to years before death), the contusion will appear as a superficial depression in the surface of the brain lined with a yellow-brown surface, which is from the deposition of hemosiderin (Figure 9.50). Microscopic examination could assist with other relative dating of the contusion (Figure 9.51A and B). The mechanism of formation of contre-coup contusions is potentially due to the fact that the brain is less dense than the cerebrospinal fluid, so, with a fall, the denser CSF will move toward the point of impact, displacing the brain toward the opposite side of the cranium where it impacts the bone, leading to contre-coup contusions.[32]

Location: Most commonly, contre-coup contusions are found on the inferior surface of the frontal lobes and the inferior surface and tips of the temporal lobes; however, occipital contusions can occur, and with a fall on the side of the head, contusions of the contralateral cerebral hemisphere can also occur. With a fall on the back of the head, contusions of the undersurface of the frontal and temporal lobes occurs (Figure 9.52). These contusions are

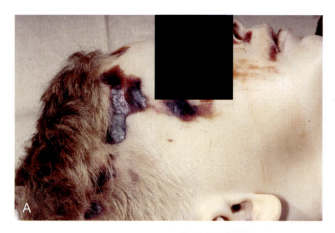
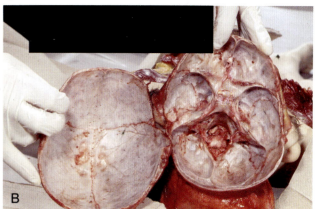
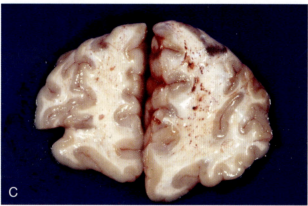

Figure 9.49. Coup contusions. This child was struck by a motor vehicle as a pedestrian. (**A**) illustrates the impact site, as exhibited by abrasions of the right side of the head. (**B**) illustrates the inner surface of the cranium, revealing no fracture. (**C**) is a cross section of the anterior portion of the brain, with contusions of the superior and anterior portion of the right frontal lobe of the brain, which would correspond to the location of the abrasions.

frequently associated with subarachnoid hemorrhage (Figure 9.53A-C). With a fall on the front of the head, contusions of the occipital lobes would occur (Figure 9.54). With a fall onto the left side of the head, contusions of the right temporal lobe and right parietal lobe would occur (Figure 9.55A and B). However, unlike with a fall on the back of the head, in which the contusions are of the temporal lobe tips and the undersurface, in a fall on the side of the head, the contusions of the opposite side temporal lobe would be on the lateral surface. The appearance of the contusion can indicate the relative time course of the contusion.

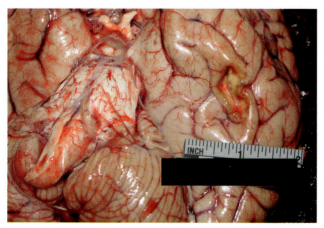

Figure 9.50. Remote contre-coup contusion. On the inferior surface of the left temporal lobe of the brain is a superficial shallow defect in the cortical surface lined by a yellow-brown discoloration.

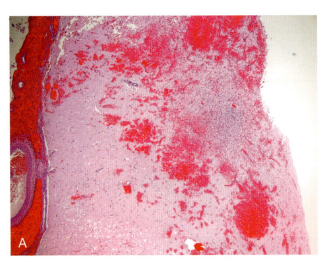
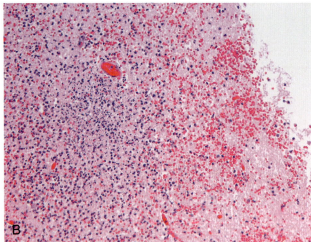

Figure 9.51. Cerebral contusion with neutrophilic infiltrate. The images (**A** is low power and **B** is high power, with both hematoxylin and eosin) are that of a cerebral contusion. The neutrophilic infiltrate would indicate that some length of time elapsed between the time of the injury and the individual's death, at least several hours, but possibly a few days.

FRACTURE CONTUSIONS

Mechanism: Occur on the cortical surface of the brain adjacent to fractures.

Location: Any location where the brain is adjacent to bone is possible.

HERNIATION CONTUSIONS

Mechanism: When herniation of the brain occurs, contusions can develop.

Locations: Commonly, herniation contusions occur on the medial surface of the temporal lobe associated with uncal herniation (Figure 9.56), on the corpus callosum associated with cingulate gyrus herniation (Figure 9.57), and on the cerebellar tonsils associated with tonsillar herniation (Figure 9.58).

> **PEARLS & PITFALLS**
>
> In the case of a gunshot wound of the head or potentially a fall or other significant traumatic injury of the head, herniations can occur quickly but are temporary. Even though the herniation can then reverse, contusions of the cortex can still occur. In the case of cerebral edema, hemorrhage of the herniated brain can occur, but a component of ischemia may be present from the pinching of the tissue obstructing blood flow.

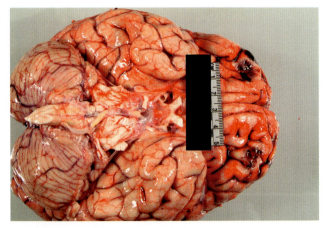

Figure 9.52. Contre-coup contusions. On the inferior surface of both the left and right frontal lobes of this brain are small patches of contusions. In this location, the most common scenario is a fall on the back of the head.

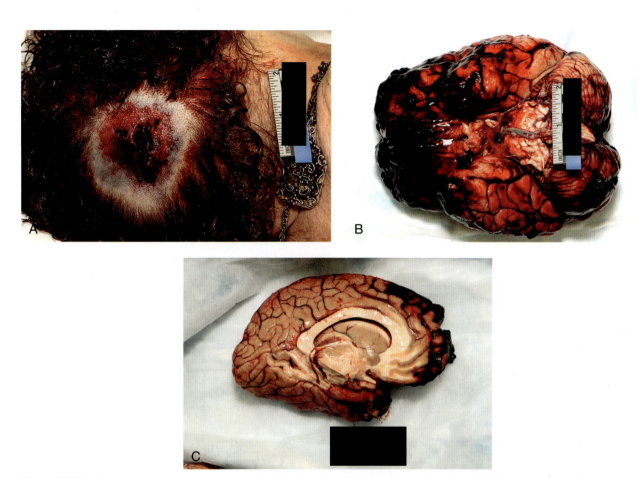

Figure 9.53. Contre-coup contusions associated with subarachnoid hemorrhage. This individual fell on the back of their head and sustained contre-coup contusions. (**A**) illustrates the impact site, with the posterior region of the scalp having an irregular laceration with a surrounding abrasion and contusion. (**B**) illustrates the inferior surface of the brain. Covering the inferior surface of the frontal and temporal lobes is prominent subarachnoid hemorrhage. The inferior surface of the temporal lobes best exhibits the contusions, which are the punctate red discolorations. (**C**) is a longitudinal section of the brain illustrating the subarachnoid hemorrhage of the frontal and temporal lobes.

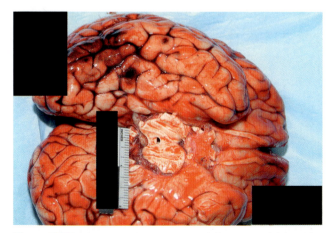

Figure 9.54. Contre-coup contusions of the occipital lobe. This individual was an unrestrained driver in a motor vehicle accident. Reflection of the scalp revealed an impact site anterior. Examination of the brain revealed a patch of subarachnoid hemorrhage and contusions on the inferior surface of the right occipital lobe, which was not otherwise explained by fractures of the cranium. These contusions would represent contre-coup contusions.

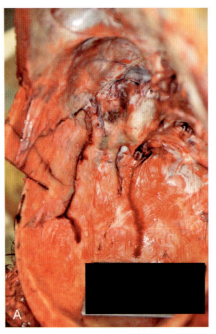
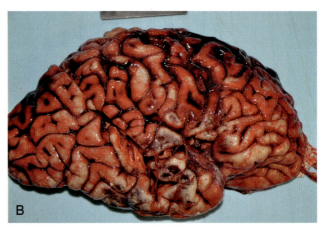

Figure 9.55. Contre-coup contusions from fall on the side of the head. This individual fell and hit the left side of their head. (**A**) illustrates the fracture on the left side of the cranium, which occurred at the impact site. (**B**) illustrates the right side of the cerebral hemisphere, with contusions of the temporal lobe present.

> **PEARLS & PITFALLS**
>
> If an individual develops contusions as a result of a traumatic incident and survives, these contusions can expand in size and produce larger hemorrhages, which can be termed lobar hemorrhages (Figure 9.59A-C). Individuals who survive the initial traumatic event and those who are anti-coagulated or who have hypertension would be at greatest risk for developing a lobar hemorrhage. The differential diagnosis for a lobar hemorrhage would include a natural disease process such as cerebral amyloid angiopathy.

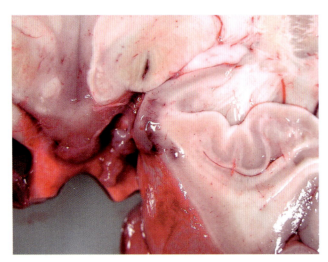

Figure 9.56. Uncal herniation contusions. At the uncus are streak-like hemorrhages in the gray matter. With significant trauma of the head, the uncus can herniate briefly, which can result in contusions. Contusions can also occur in a more slowly developing herniation; however, the fact that ischemic injury may be combined is likely.

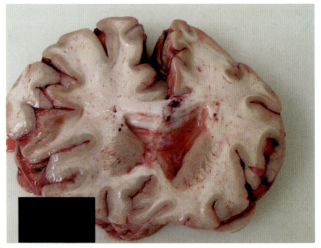

Figure 9.57. Cingulate gyrus herniation resulting in contusions of the corpus callosum. The left cingulate gyrus has herniated resulting in contusions of the corpus callosum as exhibited by the punctate red discolorations. Punctate hemorrhage in the corpus callosum can also occur in diffuse axonal injury (traumatic axonal injury). Distinguishing the two may not be possible by gross examination only; however, history may help. For example, if the cingulate herniation is secondary to a subdural hemorrhage, the source of the punctate hemorrhage in the corpus callosum is known, and diffuse axonal injury can be excluded. Also, given the fact that only the left cingulate gyrus herniated, the underlying source is most likely unilateral and not a diffuse injury.

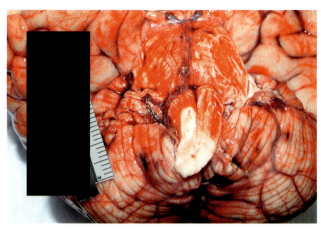

Figure 9.58. Cerebellar tonsillar herniation contusions. While this individual was shot and did not die from blunt force injuries, the image illustrates contusions of the tonsils, which are due to herniation. As with the unci described above, temporary herniation of the cerebellar tonsils can result in contusions. Examination of the surrounding brain in the image reveals a normal gyral pattern, and not flattening as would be expected if cerebral edema were the cause for the tonsillar herniation.

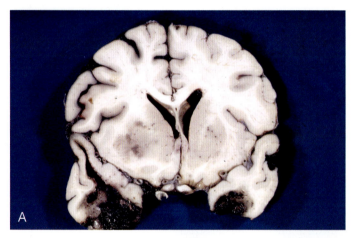

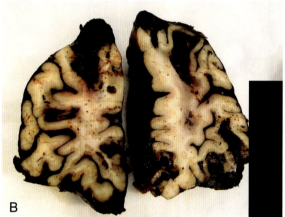

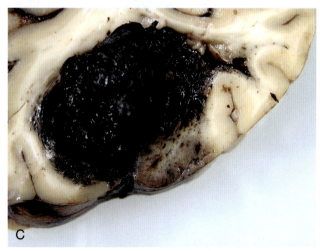

Figure 9.59. Lobar hemorrhages associated with survived blunt force injuries. (A) illustrates enlarged hemorrhages at the inferior aspect of both temporal lobes. These were contre-coup contusions that expanded with survival time into larger hemorrhages. (B) illustrates numerous expanded hemorrhages at both the superior and inferior portion of the frontal lobes as well as within the white matter. The lobar hemorrhage centered in the white matter most likely developed from a gliding contusion. (C) illustrates a close-up of the gray matter overlying a lobar hemorrhage. The lobar hemorrhage did develop in the brain of an individual who survived blunt force head injuries for a period of time. The gray matter appears to have cortical contusions overlying the lobar hemorrhage; however, duskiness secondary to ischemic injury and congestion can mimic the contusions. Gross examination can sometimes separate the two conditions as contusions affect the crests of the gyri and ischemic injury affects the gyri along the depths of the sulci. Also, contusions can tend to have a wedge shape, with the base at the apex of the gyrus. Microscopic examination may also help separate the two mechanisms.

INTERMEDIARY CONTUSIONS

Mechanism: Contusions associated with coup and contre-coup contusions[2] and/or diffuse axonal injury (DAI).[1]

Location: These contusions occur at the basal ganglia, thalamus, internal capsule, corpus callosum, and pons (Figure 9.60).

GLIDING CONTUSIONS

Mechanism: Spitz and Fisher refers to contusions on the inferior surface of the frontal lobes as gliding contusions in reference to one mechanism by which contre-coup contusions are felt to possibly develop, that is, by gliding along the orbital plates.[3] Dolinak et al and DiMaio associate gilding contusions with DAI.[2,12] Gliding contusions are due to tearing of veins to the arachnoid granulations, with the weakest point being in the white matter.[2]

Location: Occur in the white matter of the frontal lobes (Figure 9.61A-C).

Nomenclature: As DAI has two main mechanisms, the terms traumatic axonal injury and ischemic axonal injury are also used.[33] Rungruangsak describes diffuse vascular injury as a macroscopic finding, which may or may not be associated with DAI (Figure 9.62A and B).[34]

Gross appearance: Punctate hemorrhages within the corpus callosum (often splenium) and dorsolateral brainstem (Figure 9.63A-C). Grade 1 is microscopic injury only, and grades 2 and 3 are gross hemorrhages in the corpus callosum and dorsolateral brainstem, respectively.[33]

Microscopic appearance: The characteristic finding is spheroids, which can be seen on H&E (Figure 9.64); however, β-amyloid precursor protein histologic staining can identify abnormalities prior to the development of spheroids. Kalimo et al recommend sampling of anterior and posterior corpus callosum and associated parasagittal white matter from both sides of the brain, the medial portion of both temporal lobes, the bilateral thalami including the posterior limb of the internal capsule, the cerebellar hemispheres, midbrain, pons (both upper and lower), the medulla, and all the upper cervical spinal cord segments.[35]

Mechanism: TAI occurs due to accelerational forces which have a relatively long duration (eg, such as occur in a motor vehicle accident, or in a fall from a great height). A simple fall or a strike to the head very rarely causes TAI.[33]

Clinical consequence: Immediate unconsciousness (primary coma) in many cases, but usually at least a moderate disturbance of consciousness.[33]

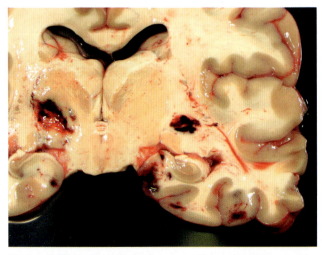

Figure 9.60. Intermediary contusions. This individual survived a motor vehicle accident for a short period of time. There are hemorrhages in the internal capsule bilaterally, and the edge of the left thalamus. In addition, there are herniation contusions of the unci. The herniation contusions of the unci are associated with cerebral edema.

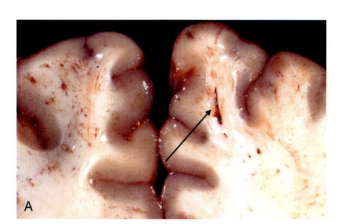
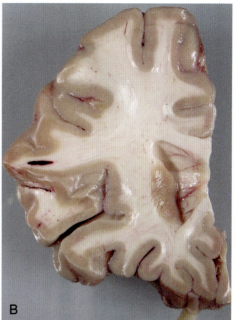
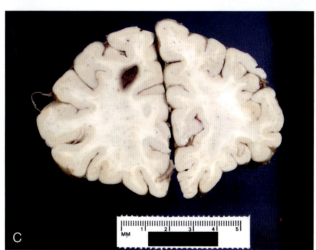

Figure 9.61. Gliding contusions in the frontal white matter. (**A**) illustrates thin streaklike gliding contusions in the frontal white matter (arrow). (**B**) illustrates a streaklike contusion in the frontal white matter, but, instead of being medial as most are, this gliding contusion is laterally placed. (**C**) is from an individual who survived for a short period of time after the head injuries. The gliding contusion has expanded, forming a small hematoma.

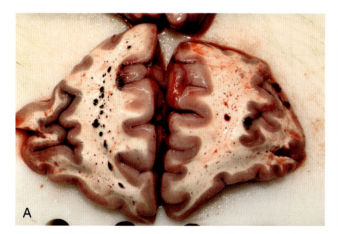
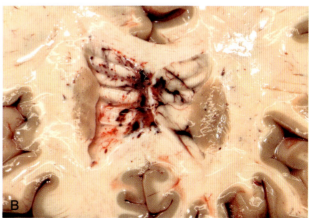

Figure 9.62. Diffuse vascular injury. In both (**A** and **B**), the decedents died as the result of a motor vehicle collision. In (**A**), there are large punctate hemorrhages in the anterior portion of the frontal lobes. In (**B**), there are large punctate hemorrhages in the genu of the corpus callosum. While hemorrhage in the corpus callosum is most commonly associated with traumatic axonal injury, the splenium is the most common location. Also, overlap between traumatic axonal injury and diffuse vascular injury exists.

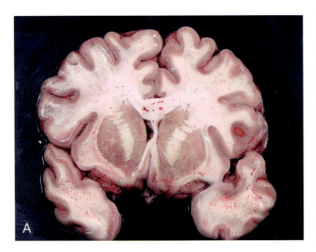
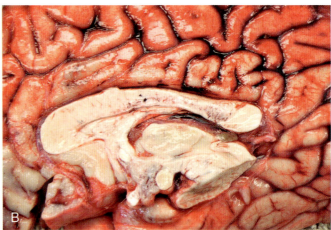
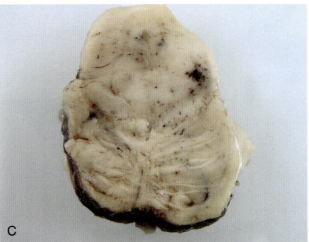

Figure 9.63. DAI/TAI. (**A**), a cross section of the brain, shows punctate hemorrhages in the corpus callosum. (**B**), a longitudinal section of the brain, shows punctate hemorrhages in the corpus callosum. (**C**), a cross section of the brainstem, shows a cluster of hemorrhages in the dorsolateral region of the pons. DAI, diffuse axonal injury; TAI, traumatic axonal injury.

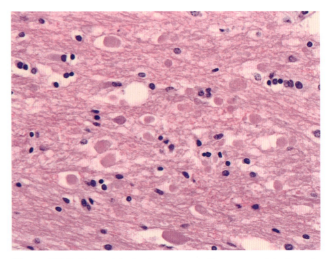

Figure 9.64. Spheroids. In the corpus callosum are globular pale eosinophilic bodies, which are called spheroids (or axonal retraction balls). These are indicative of injury to the axons, and represent accumulations of axonal proteins at the site of injury. Spheroids are associated with diffuse axonal injury of both traumatic and ischemic origin (hematoxylin and eosin, high power).

> **PEARLS & PITFALLS**
>
> Intermediary contusions can be considered the gross appearance of the effects of rotational acceleration, and DAI or TAI the microscopic effects.

> **PEARLS & PITFALLS**
>
> Both traumatic and ischemic injury can cause DAI; however, on β-amyloid precursor protein immunostaining, Davceva et al describe that trauma produces singly or small group clusters of positively stained axons (Figure 9.65), with varicosity-like swollen axons and retraction balls, whereas ischemia produces linear or geographic patterns of staining, which are often described as zigzag shaped, with no enlargement of axons (Figure 9.66).[36]

> **FAQ:** How quickly following a head injury can cerebral swelling occur?
>
> **Answer:** While cerebral edema often develops more slowly after a head injury, or other injury leading to hypoxic ischemic encephalopathy, there are reports of cerebral edema developing rapidly after the onset of trauma, with Byard presenting a case of cerebral edema that occurred almost immediately after trauma occurred, with the deceased individual having cerebral edema in the background of extensive cranial fractures and an aortic transection.[37]

SAMPLE NOTES: DOCUMENTATION OF BLUNT FORCE INJURIES OF THE HEAD

Documentation of blunt force injuries of the head can be done in a coordinated fashion by proceeding from outside to inside in layers, proceeding from external to subgaleal region to the cranium (fractures) to the extra-cerebral space (epidural, subdural, and/or subarachnoid hemorrhages) to the brain (contusions, lacerations).

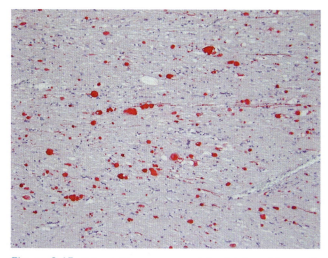

Figure 9.65. β-Amyloid precursor protein staining of traumatic axonal injury. The axons stained are individual or in small clusters and many are enlarged (β-amyloid precursor protein immunohistochemical stain, medium power).

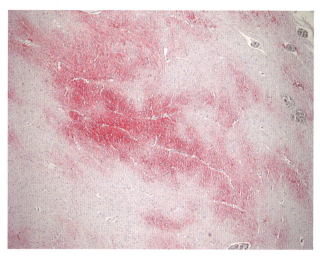

Figure 9.66. β-Amyloid precursor protein staining of ischemic axonal injury. This low power view illustrates the geographic or zigzag appearance of axonal injury due to ischemic injury. It must be remembered, however, that traumatic axonal injury and ischemic axonal injury are not mutually exclusive, and an individual with a survival period after a traumatic head injury may have both (β-amyloid precursor protein immunohistochemical stain, low power).

I. Blunt force injuries of the head
   A. There is a 2-inch laceration in the left temporal region surrounded by a 4-inch abrasion.
   B. Underlying the above-described laceration is a 10 cm patch of subgaleal hemorrhage.
   C. Extending between the left parietal bone and the left temporal bone is a 6 cm fracture that on the inner surface of the cranium crosses the path of the middle meningeal artery.
   D. Underlying the cranium on the left side of the head and external to the dura is a measured 50 mL of clotted blood.
   E. In the location of the above-described fracture are linear hemorrhages in the gray matter of the underlying parietal and temporal lobes, which are oriented perpendicular to the cortical surface.

BLUNT FORCE INJURIES OF THE NECK

Blunt force injuries of the neck include abrasions, contusions, and lacerations of the skin, hemorrhage in the underlying musculature, and fractures and dislocations. While the use of a full body imaging system (either plain film radiography, CT scan, or MRI) is most useful to examine the bony structures of the neck, this technology is either not available to most offices in the United States, or only available at high cost (eg, with contracts through a local hospital). Evaluation of the neck at autopsy can be performed in a variety of other ways. Prior to autopsy, radiographs of the neck can be obtained, and, with traction placed on the head, these radiographs can sometimes reveal a fracture or dislocation of the neck (Figure 9.67). With an atlanto-occipital or atlanto-axial dislocation, often basilar subdural and subarachnoid hemorrhage and hemorrhage within the prevertebral fascia and musculature of the upper cervical segment of the vertebral column occur, and, often, a palpable or visible dislocation is present, with the vertebral column displaced into the foramen magnum (Figure 9.68A-C). In this case, removal of the brain and removal of the neck organs,

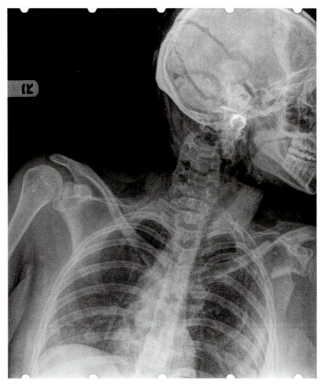

Figure 9.67. Radiograph of the neck. The vertebral column is not continuous, with a dislocation in the upper cervical region.

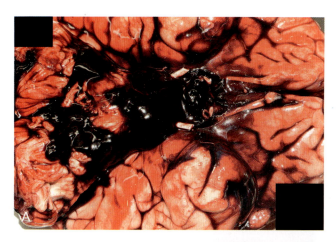
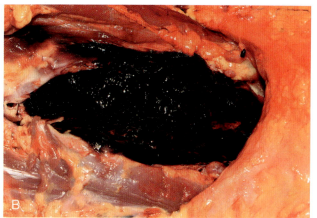
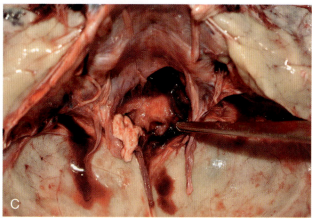

Figure 9.68. Features of atlanto-occipital dislocation. The individual in (A-C) sustained an atlanto-occipital dislocation. (A) illustrates the basilar subarachnoid hemorrhage, which can be due to tearing of the vessels of the circle of Willis or associated with laceration of the brainstem. (B) illustrates extensive hemorrhage in the prevertebral fascia and musculature of the cervical portion of the vertebral column. Hemorrhage at this location identified with removal of the neck organs can provide a clue as to the presence of a neck fracture or dislocation. (C) is of the base of the brain. The foramen magnum contains the upper portion of the cervical vertebral column, with a complete dislocation having occurred.

which are a standard part of most autopsies, is sufficient to make the diagnosis. However, in some circumstances, a more subtle neck injury is present, which requires a posterior neck dissection to identify. Dolinak and Matshes provide a good description of how to perform a posterior neck dissection.[38]

PEARLS & PITFALLS

It is not uncommon to perform an autopsy on an individual who has most likely died from a sudden cardiac event and to find a small fracture on the anterior surface of the lower cervical segment of the vertebral column associated with a small amount of hemorrhage in the prevertebral fascia (Figure 9.69A-C). Examination of the spinal cord reveals no injuries. The question is whether this injury is the result of an uncontrolled fall to the ground after a cardiac event (similar to lacerations of the face that occur in regions with underlying bone such as the orbital margins) or an antemortem neck fracture that contributed to the individual's death. Such deaths most likely need to be evaluated on a case-by-case basis to determine the significance of the injury.

PEARLS & PITFALLS

When an individual is found at the base of stairs, even if no external signs of injury are present, the best course is usually to perform an autopsy. Even if the individual has significant natural disease and would be expected to have a risk for sustaining a sudden cardiac death, the ability to completely exclude a neck injury (or head injury or bleed into a body cavity) by external examination alone is not possible.

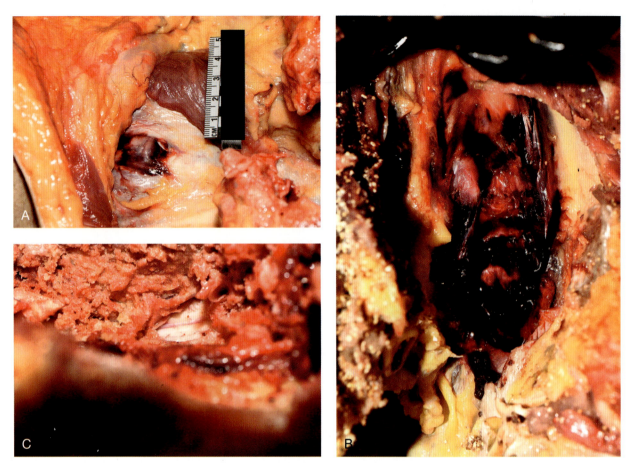

Figure 9.69. Fracture of anterior portion of cervical vertebral column near the level of the fifth cervical vertebra, with minimal hemorrhage in the surrounding soft tissue. In (**A**), whether the fracture and hemorrhage are from an agonal fall, or are the cause of death from a fall, is the primary question. The minimal hemorrhage, minimal fracture which usually only involves the anterior surface of the vertebra, and the lack of hemorrhage to the spinal cord in the background of a natural disease that could precipitate sudden death, suggest the former. In (**B**), there is more extensive hemorrhage in the prevertebral fascia and musculature and a wider dislocation at the intervertebral disk (**B**), but there was no injury of the spinal cord or hemorrhage around the spinal cord (**C**).

BLUNT FORCE INJURIES OF THE TRUNK

The organs of the trunk can sustain abrasions of the mucosal surfaces, contusions, and lacerations, and the skeletal portion of the trunk, including the clavicles, ribs, vertebral column, sternum, and pelvis, can sustain fractures and discolorations.

> **FAQ:** How much blood loss is required to cause death, and how can the amount of blood loss be determined?
>
> **Answer:** In general, a loss of 30% to 40% of the circulating blood volume is severe and a loss of >40% of the circulating blood volume will cause an individual to rapidly develop hypovolemic shock.[39] In many cases, an exact determination of the amount of blood loss is not possible due to blood loss external to the body, which is not available for quantification at the time of autopsy, and blood loss into soft tissue, such as adipose tissue, which cannot be accurately quantitated. Individuals with significant underlying natural disease, such as congestive heart failure, other forms of heart disease, or emphysema, may succumb to lesser degrees of blood loss. Multiple traumatic injuries combining to cause death must also be considered. If blood loss occurs directly into a cavity, the exact volume of blood can be measured; however, if blood loss occurs into soft

tissue (eg, the retroperitoneum or musculature of the thigh), an exact measurement of the amount of blood loss is not possible as the blood suffuses through the soft tissue. While not an exact marker of blood loss, pale conjunctivae, a reduced amount of lividity, wrinkling of the splenic capsule, and pallor of the internal organs (especially the kidneys and the liver) are consistent with blood loss (Figure 9.70A and B).[39] If individuals survive long enough to be treated in the emergency room, an antemortem measurement of hemoglobin may be available; however, in an acute blood loss situation, the concentration of hemoglobin may not accurately reflect the amount of blood loss.

PEARLS & PITFALLS

When exsanguination has occurred and attempted resuscitation has involved the administration of blood products, caution must be used in the interpretation of toxicologic findings, as the decedent's initial concentration of the drug at the time of death will be diluted by the use of fluids and blood products during resuscitation.

FAQ: How can rib fractures due to trauma and rib fractures due to cardiopulmonary resuscitation be distinguished?

Answer: Quite commonly, a body at autopsy can have fractures both due to trauma and due to cardiopulmonary resuscitation and absolute separation of the two etiologies can be problematic. Fractures associated with cardiopulmonary resuscitation tend to be located anterior and will often have little or no hemorrhage in the adjacent intercostal muscle. Rib fractures associated with trauma can be in any location (Figure 9.71A and B).

PEARLS & PITFALLS

In the examination of a body searching for a cause of death due to blunt force injuries, consider a flail chest. If three or more ribs are each fractured in two or more locations, the result can be a flail chest, which could be associated with asphyxia (Figure 9.72).

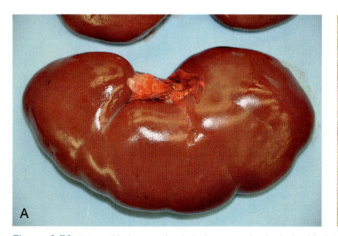
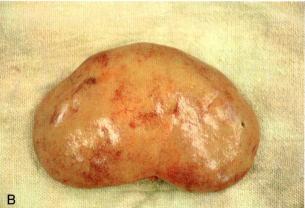

Figure 9.70. Normal kidney and pale kidney in individual who bled. (**A**) is a normal kidney, with the characteristic dark red color. (**B**) is an individual who sustained blunt force injuries and bled significantly. Compared to the kidney in image A, this kidney is much paler, as would be expected with a significant loss of blood.

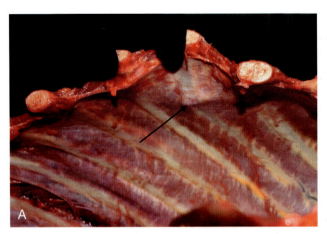
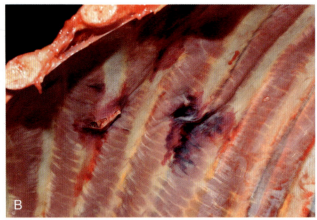

Figure 9.71. Rib fractures from CPR vs rib fractures from trauma. Both (**A** and **B**) are from the same autopsy. In (**A**), the fractures are anterior in location and associated with essentially no hemorrhage in the surrounding soft tissue (arrow). In (**B**), the fractures are lateral in location and associated with hemorrhage in the surrounding soft tissue. In this autopsy, the fractures in (**A**) were felt to be secondary to CPR and those in (**B**) were felt to be traumatic in origin, as the individual was involved in a motor vehicle accident. However, CPR could certainly be associated with displaced fractures, which are more lateral in location, and which have hemorrhage in the surrounding tissue. CPR, cardiopulmonary resuscitation.

PEARLS & PITFALLS

Blunt force injuries of the chest can lead to concussion of the heart, which is also called commotio cordis. Concussion of the heart can cause sudden death, but is not associated with any characteristic gross or microscopic change.[40] Commotio cordis is thought to be caused by ventricular fibrillation induced by a blow to the chest just before the peak of the T wave and, although rare overall, is one of the more common causes of sudden death in athletes.[41] In an individual who is struck in the chest with a blunt object, such as a baseball or hockey puck, and who subsequently sustains cardiac arrest, this condition should be considered; however, the diagnosis would require both historical information and an otherwise negative autopsy. Blunt force injuries of the chest can also lead to a cardiac contusion, which is also associated with death, and would have gross and microscopic findings (ie, focal hemorrhage in the epicardium or myocardium, dissection of the coronary artery).[42] Blunt force injuries of the chest are also associated with myocardial infarction, both with and without underlying atherosclerosis of the coronary arteries.[43]

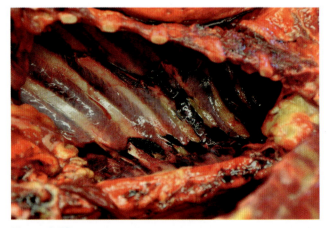

Figure 9.72. Flail chest. On the right side of the chest numerous ribs are fractured both anterior lateral and posterior lateral, with many of the rib fractures being displaced. This case represents a flail chest.

> **PEARLS & PITFALLS**
>
> Injuries of the organs of the trunk, especially the spleen and liver, are a common reason for a delayed death following a traumatic event. In such a situation, commonly what occurs is that the spleen or liver develops a subcapsular hemorrhage, which contains the hemorrhage, allowing the patient to survive; however, at some point later, the contained hemorrhage ruptures, leading to fatal blood loss.

> **PEARLS & PITFALLS**
>
> While cardiopulmonary resuscitation (CPR) is a common cause of rib fractures, such rib fractures are most commonly anterior or anterior-lateral. Posterior rib fractures are essentially always due to trauma.

SAMPLE NOTES: DOCUMENTATION OF BLUNT FORCE INJURIES OF THE TRUNK

As with the head, an organized documentation of the injuries proceeding from outside to inside can be done, describing the external surface of the trunk, followed by the skeletal system (ribs, vertebral column, and pelvis), hemorrhage into body cavities, and injuries to internal organs.

I. Blunt force injuries of the trunk:
   A. On the lateral surface of the left side of the trunk near the costal margin is a 6.5 cm purple circular contusion.
   B. Left ribs #6 to 8 are fractured lateral and associated with extensive hemorrhage into the surrounding musculature.
   C. Within the peritoneal cavity are a measured 1,000 mL of clotted and unclotted blood. Within the retroperitoneal tissue centered on the left upper quadrant of the abdomen is hemorrhage (comment: which cannot be accurately measured given its suffusion through the soft tissue).
   D. The hilum of the spleen has a 3.5 cm laceration.

BLUNT FORCE INJURIES OF THE EXTREMITIES

All four types of blunt force injuries (abrasions, contusions, lacerations, and fractures) can involve the extremities. Fractures will be discussed in detail below.

FRACTURES

To discuss fractures of the bone, it is important to understand the structure of bone and how it responds to force, as these two factors affect the development of fractures.

Composition of bone and effects on fracture development: Bone is composed of both organic materials (collagen and other proteins) and inorganic materials (hydroxyapatite crystals composed of calcium and phosphorus).[44] The organic materials give a ductile (ie, bendable) component to the bone and the inorganic materials give a brittle (ie, not bendable) component to the bone.[44] In addition, bone is a viscoelastic substance, meaning the bone responds to different types of force in a different fashion. A rapidly loaded bone has increased stiffness and greater ultimate tensile strength to failure so that failure of the bone will more represent failure of a brittle substance (ie, the bone will shatter), whereas a slowly loaded bone has decreased stiffness and lower ultimate tensile strength and failure will more represent failure of a ductile substance (ie, the bone will bend and break).[45] This viscoelastic nature (ie, different responses to different forms of loads) of the bone can affect the fracture morphology with slow loading more likely to produce linear fractures and rapid loading more likely to produce comminuted fractures.[46]

General mechanisms of fracture production: Force applied to bone is termed load. Stress is the load applied per unit of area and strain is the ratio of change in length to original length.[6,45,47] Stress can be plotted vs strain to produce a stress-strain curve. When force is initially applied, the stress (y-axis) and strain (x-axis) increase proportionally (Table 9.3). The bone deforms in proportion to the force; however, the deformation is not permanent and will reverse if the force is removed.[6,47,48] In other words, bone can bend and return to its form. This segment of the stress-strain curve is referred to as the elastic phase. At some level of stress, the bone reaches the yield point and enters the plastic phase (Table 9.3). In the plastic phase, the increase in stress is no longer proportional to the increase in strain. Instead, for a small increase in stress, there is a large increase in strain.[6,48,49] The strain produced in the bone is termed plastic deformation. Plastic deformation, unlike elastic deformation, will not reverse when the stress is removed. Therefore, plastic deformation causes a bone to permanently bend but not break. Plastic deformation of the bone will occur until the level of stress reaches the ultimate strength of the bone and fracture occurs[6,50] (Table 9.3). Also for comparison and to help explain the concepts, on the stress-strain curve, a pure brittle substance such as glass has a line that parallels the y-axis, with no change in strain produced with increasing stress, until failure is reached, whereas a pure ductile substance such as rubber has a line that parallels the x-axis, with an extensive plastic phase with minimal increase in stress prior to fracture.[6] Therefore, brittle material breaks inside or just beyond the zone of elastic deformation, while ductile material can undergo much plastic deformation before fracture occurs.[8,45,47] However, with viscoelastic material, the rate of application of the stress also affects the stress-strain curve shape, and thus, the mechanical properties of the bone.[6] With slower loading of bone, plastic deformation will occur as the bone behaves more like a ductile substance but with rapid loading of bone, which makes the bone behave more like a brittle substance, the bone will essentially shatter. This concept is important when reconstructing a skull (or other bone) that has been the object of a traumatic injury. With plastic deformation and subsequent fracture, the bone fragments often cannot be pieced back together exactly as original, whereas, in a rapidly loaded bone that essentially shatters, the bone fragments can easily be pieced back together to reform the original shape (Figure 9.73A and B).

Type of force that can fracture bone: Three primary types of force can act on bone: tensile, compression, and shear.[8] However, pure compression or pure tension acting on the shaft of a bone is rare, and bending and torsion, which are combinations of the previous three, are the most common type of force that affects bone.[6] In the bending of a shaft due to directly applied force, at the point of impact, the bone sustains compression, while on the opposite side of the shaft, the bone is subject to tension. Shearing is two forces acting on the bone, each in a different plane.[8,47,49,51] Also, force causing fractures can be either direct (applied at the site of the fracture), or indirect (applied at a point distant to the fracture).

TABLE 9.3: A Generalized Stress-Strain Curve to Illustrate Concepts

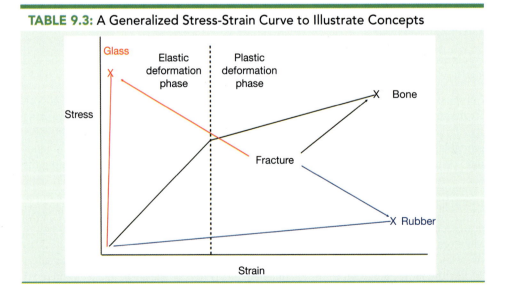

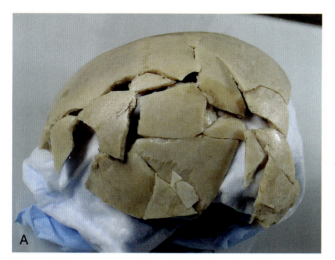

Figure 9.73A. Plastic deformation with fracture. This individual was beaten with a rock. Notice how the fragments of bone did not fit back together perfectly to re-form the cranium. With slower loading of the bone, plastic deformation (ie, permanent bending) of the bone prior to fracture can occur, which would impair re-alignment of fracture segments.

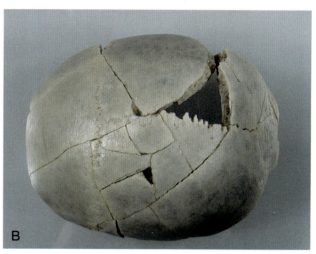

Figure 9.73B. Fracture of cranium due to rapid force loading. This individual died in a motor vehicle collision. This rapid loading of the bone essentially caused the bone to behave as a brittle substance and shatter, thus, the fracture fragments could easily be pieced back together to reform the original shape of the cranium.

Finally, the force can occur in one of two forms: dynamic or static.[47,49,51] Dynamic forces place a sudden high degree of stress on the bone, while static forces are low but constant degrees of stress.[51] Schmidt found that static and dynamic forces caused different overall fracture patterns in ribs, with static force fracturing one rib after another in different places (eg, in a circular pattern overall), and with dynamic force fracturing ribs one after the other more in a row.[52]

With regarding to mechanism by which a given force produces a certain type of fracture, adult bone is more susceptible to fracture by stretching forces (ie, tension) than by compressive forces[9,47,53-55] but is most susceptible to shearing forces.[8] Pediatric bones are more susceptible to fracture by compression than tension.[49] However, in adults, failure at the point of tension first is not universal. Love and Symes found that the ribs, especially in areas where the cortex is thin, can fail at the point of compression first, which was interpreted as buckling, or, collapse due to compressive instability.[56] Buckle fracture as used by Love and Symes is an engineering term, and does not indicate a torus fracture (as the term "buckle fracture" has also been used in the literature as an alternative for).[56] Fractures at the point of tension tend to have a billowed surface, oriented perpendicular to the long axis of the bone, while fractures at the point of compression tend to have a splintered surface, oriented parallel to the long axis of the bone.[57]

SPECIFIC FRACTURE TYPES

Fracture terminology and classification: *Stedman's Medical Dictionary* lists over 100 specific fracture names with the fracture name often derived from the specific scenario that led to the fracture (eg, boxer fracture); however, a more generalized descriptive and non-specific terminology that can be applied to bones in general can be more useful.[1] Rogers classified fractures using the six criteria of extent, integrity of skin, direction of fracture, position, number of fracture lines, and alignment of fracture ends (Table 9.4) (Figure 9.74).[47] Galloway classified fractures based upon the extent of the fracture followed by the pattern of breakage and whether direct or indirect force led to the fracture (Table 9.5).[58] The Galloway classification scheme implies knowledge of mechanism of the fracture within the terminology (eg, direct vs indirect), which often at autopsy under uncertain circumstances cannot be reliably determined.[58] Also, there is overlap within Galloway's classification scheme. Pierce et al, whose article was directed toward evaluation of fractures in children, recommended that a qualitative description of a fracture includes (1) the

TABLE 9.4: Rogers Classification of Fractures

General Criteria for Fracture Classification[47]	
Extent	Complete or incomplete
Integrity of overlying skin	Closed or open (older terms are simple and compound respectively)
Direction of fracture	Transverse, longitudinal, oblique, or spiral
Position (specific and/or general location)	eg, epiphyseal, metaphyseal, or diaphyseal, and, if diaphyseal, proximal, middle, or distal
Number of fracture lines	
Alignment of the fracture ends	Non-displaced or displaced

location of the fracture (metaphyseal, diaphyseal, and proximal, middle or distal third of shaft), (2) the line of fracture propagation (transverse, oblique, spiral, buckle/torus, corner or bucket handle), and (3) the relationship of the fracture segments (angulation, displacement, fracture separation, comminuted).[49]

EXTENT: INCOMPLETE VS COMPLETE FRACTURE

Description: An incomplete fracture does not include the entire circumference of the bone,[1] whereas a complete fracture does (Figure 9.75A and B). Incomplete fractures are more common in children than adults and the terms greenstick, torus, and bowing are used.[47] The four main types of complete fracture, which indicate the direction of the fracture, are transverse, oblique, longitudinal, and spiral.

INCOMPLETE FRACTURES

Bow

Description: A bowing fracture, which usually involves the radius or ulna, occurs when a bone is bent due to multiple micro-fractures of which none are seen on radiographs.[1] Bowing fractures are more uncommonly called bending fractures, and can occur in the radius and ulna of children after a fall. They are an example of plastic deformation of the bone.[48]

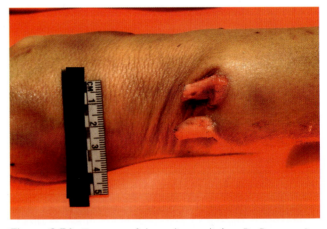

Figure 9.74. Fractures of the radius and ulna. By Rogers criteria, these fractures could be described as complete (extent), open (integrity of skin), oblique (direction of fracture), distal diaphysis (position), and displaced (alignment of fracture ends), with each fracture having one fracture line.

TABLE 9.5: Galloway Fracture Classification[58]

Extent of Fracture/Pattern of Breakage		Location of Force Causing Fracture	
Incomplete Fractures	Complete Fractures	Direct	Indirect
Bow	Transverse	Tapping	Linear
Bone bruise	Oblique	Crush	Avulsion
Torus	Spiral		Traction
Greenstick	Comminuted		Angulation
Toddlers	Butterfly		Rotational
Vertical	Segmental		Compression
Depressed			

TORUS/BUCKLE FRACTURE

Description: A torus fracture is a bulge resulting from a longitudinal compression of the bone.[1]

Mechanism: Buckle or torus fractures occur from axillary loading and are most common at the metaphysis and represent a failure due to compression at the harder cortical bone is pressed into the softer trabecular bone.[49]

GREENSTICK FRACTURE

Description: A greenstick fracture is bending of the bone with an incomplete fracture involving only the convex side of the curve.[1]

COMPLETE FRACTURE: FRACTURE TYPE BASED UPON DIRECTION

TRANSVERSE FRACTURE

Description: Johner and Wruhs define transverse as having an angle less than 30° (Figure 9.76A and B).[59]

Mechanisms: Pure tension can stretch the bone and produce a transverse fracture.[8,47,49,51,60] Bending, which includes a component of tension, curves the bone, causing compression at the concave surface and tension at the convex surface, and produces a transverse

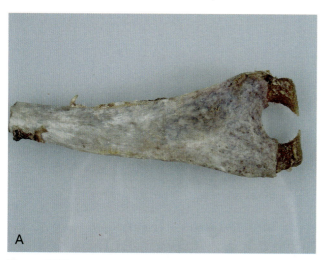
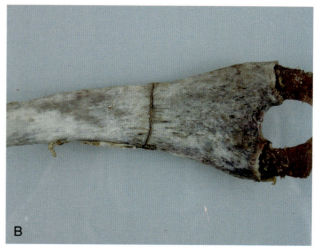

Figure 9.75. Incomplete fracture. This bifid rib has an incomplete fracture. The fracture line is visible in (**B**), but not (**A**), indicating the fracture does not completely divide the bone.

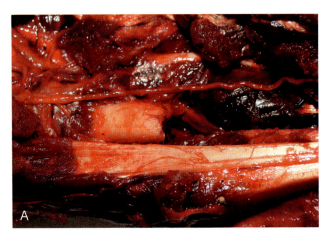
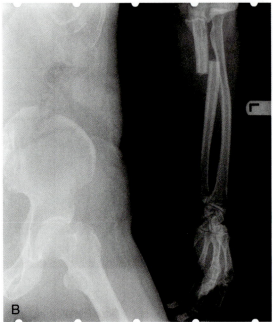

Figure 9.76. Transverse fractures. (**A** and **B**) are in situ (**A**) and radiographic images (**B**) of an ulna with a transverse fracture.

fracture.[47,49,51,53] In bending, the transverse fracture line begins opposite the point of application of force, with compression occurring at the point of application of force; however, bending resulting in transverse fractures of the shaft of long bones is rare, as there is usually a vertical load present.[47,59] Transverse fractures are a form of direct fracture.[59]

OBLIQUE FRACTURE

Description: Johner and Wruhs define oblique as having an angle greater than 30° (Figure 9.77).[59]

Mechanism: Oblique fractures are due to uneven bending or axial twisting with axial loading and, as such, oblique fractures are very common, since uneven bending or bending-compression forces on bone are common.[47,53,59] Oblique fractures are a form of direct fracture.[59]

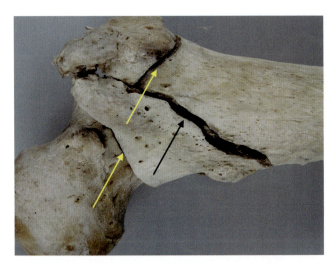

Figure 9.77. Oblique fracture of the femur. This individual with osteoporosis sustained a hip fracture. The proximal femur has an oblique fracture (black arrow). Also present at the greater trochanter and femoral neck are cuts made with the bone saw during removal of the segment of bone (yellow arrows).

LONGITUDINAL FRACTURE

Description: Longitudinal fractures extend lengthwise along the bone.

SPIRAL FRACTURE

Description: Johner and Wruhs define a spiral fracture as one that has a fracture line turning around the bone over three edges and a longitudinal line joining the proximal and distal ends of this other line.[59]

Mechanism: Torsion twists the bone and produces spiral fractures; however, pure torsion is rare, and is usually accompanied by axial compression or bending, which make a spiral fracture more oblique in appearance.[47,49,51,60] Spiral fractures are a form of an indirect fracture.[59]

OTHER FRACTURE TYPES

COMMINUTED FRACTURE

Description: A fracture resulting in multiple fragments of bone (Figure 9.78).

Mechanism: A comminuted fracture is due to either a rapid application of indirect force or direct, crushing force. The direction of forces applied may not be able to be separated out.[47]

BUTTERFLY FRACTURE

Description: A butterfly fracture is a broad triangular fracture that occurs in the diaphysis of bones[1] (Figure 9.79A-C).

Mechanism: A butterfly fracture, or Messerer fracture, is produced when the fragment on the oblique fracture is sheared off; thus, a butterfly fracture is indicative of a bending load acting on a weight-bearing extremity, although Porta reported seeing butterfly fractures in pure bending, with no axial loading (such as occurs in a weight-bearing extremity).[6,47,53,61] In a combined fracture due to bending (ie, angulation) and compression (eg, force on the femur from the weight of the trunk when an individual is standing), the bending of the bone decreases the compressive force at the convex side, but increases it at the concave side, and thus, an oblique fracture can appear at the transverse fracture.[6,47] Butterfly fractures can occur both due to torsion and bending. Butterfly fractures by torsion are the result of both indirect (torsion) and direct (bending) forces.[59] Butterfly fractures by bending, either one or several, are due to bending with compression, with one butterfly fracture occurring with low-speed impacts and two or more butterfly fractures occurring with high-speed impacts.[59]

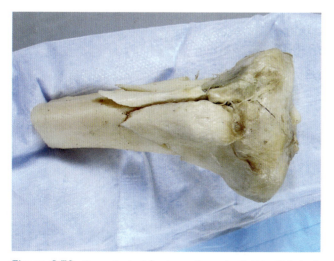

Figure 9.78. Comminuted fracture of proximal tibia. This individual was either pushed, bumped by a car, fell, or jumped off a highway overpass, and was found at the bottom. The tibia had a comminuted fracture.

> **PEARLS & PITFALLS**
> The appearance of the butterfly fracture can allow for a determination of the direction of force applied to the bone,[62] which could assist in interpretation of history provided to investigators and in correlation of the witness accounts with the autopsy findings.

SEGMENTAL FRACTURE

Description: Segmental fracture is due to four point bending and is a direct fracture. In a segmental fracture, the shaft of the bone is fracture at two locations, result in a displaced segment of bone (Figure 9.80).

Mechanism: Segmental fractures are due to high force impacts.

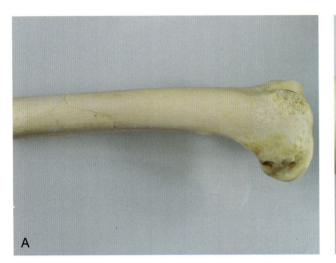
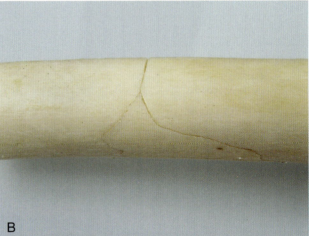
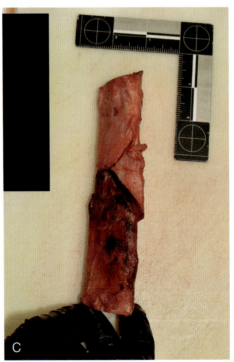

Figure 9.79. Butterfly fracture. (**A** and **B**) are an overall and a close-up of a butterfly fracture of the femur. (**C**) is a butterfly fracture of the tibia identified in an individual who was the victim of a hit and run. The butterfly fracture appears as a triangle in the bone. The broad base of the triangle is the impact site and the narrow tip is the point of tension at which the fracture begins.

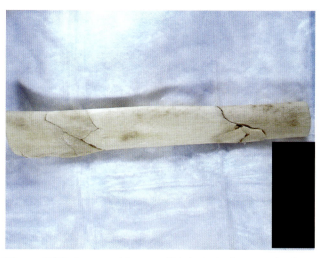

Figure 9.80. Segmental fracture. This individual was involved in a pedestrian vs motor vehicle accident, which resulted in a segmental fracture of the tibia.

AVULSION FRACTURE

Description: Rodríguez-Martín describes an avulsion fracture as a small defect that is several millimeters deep, rounded in shape, and with trabeculae at the base, which occurs at a point of muscle attachment and is due to suspension, forced positions, or electric shock.[63]

Mechanism: An avulsion fracture occurs when a tendon, ligament, or joint capsule is pulled from the bone as a result of a contracture of muscle or joint dislocation, resulting in a fragment of bone being removed from the bulk of the skeletal element.[1] The lesion does not involve a joint surface (helping to distinguish it from osteochondritis dissecans) and is most common at the humerus. Avulsion fractures (eg, the patellar tendon pulling on the tibial tuberosity) are one form of pure tension fracture that occur relatively frequently.[6]

> **PEARLS & PITFALLS**
>
> When a fractured bone is encountered at autopsy, depending upon the nature of the death, consider removal of the bone for defleshing and close examination.

> **PEARLS & PITFALLS**
>
> Fracture formation is not necessarily specific to a certain type of force. Daegling et al found that seven ribs, all with the same loading, developed fractures at basically the same location (ie, the mid-shaft), but the fracture types included complete and incomplete, and transverse, spiral, butterfly, and buckle. They used rehydrated dried bones, and could not guarantee that all seven bones had the exact same geometry or that the force was applied to each bone in the exact same manner, however.[50]

> **PEARLS & PITFALLS**
>
> The types of force-fracture pattern combinations described above are not absolute. For example, with pure bending (ie, no axial loading or torsion), Porta reports seeing oblique and butterfly fracture patterns and not just transverse fractures.[6] As might be expected, in practice, simple pure tension on a long bone in the longitudinal plane (producing a transverse fracture in the shaft) and simple pure compression of a long bone in the longitudinal plane (producing an oblique fracture) do not commonly occur.[53] The pattern of the fracture produced in the bone is determined by both extrinsic and intrinsic factors. Intrinsic factors include components and shape of the bone, bone stiffness and density, fatigue strength, and

ability of bone to absorb and dissipate energy. Extrinsic factors include direction, magnitude, rate of loading, and duration of the forces that are applied to the bone.[46,52,64] With the ribs, external factors affecting loading capacity of the thorax and thus, production of fractures, include body weight and height, the thickness of the fat layer and muscle mass, as well as the elasticity of the ribs.[52]

PEARLS & PITFALLS

Non-metric traits and anatomical variants can mimic trauma. Mann and Hunt provide an extensive list of the various skeletal findings that can mimic trauma[65] (Figure 9.81A-C).

TIMING OF BONE TRAUMA

Introduction: Fractures of the bone can be antemortem, perimortem, or postmortem. Antemortem fractures are those that definitely occurred before death. Postmortem fractures are those that definitely occurred after death. Perimortem fractures occurred around the time of death but could be up to days before death or up to weeks or months after death.[63] Sauer describes five steps to distinguish antemortem, perimortem, and postmortem fractures: (1) identification of the fracture, (2) identification of general mechanism of injury responsible for the fracture, (3) identification of any osteogenic response, (4) identification of animal activity, and (5) identification of differential staining.[66]

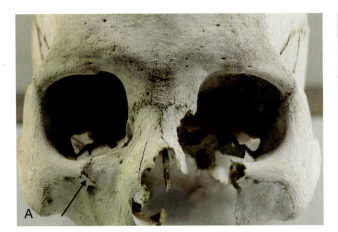
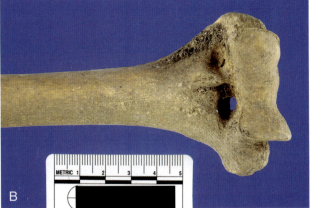
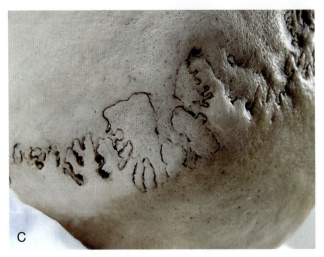

Figure 9.81. Skeletal trauma mimics. (**A**) is a right infraorbital suture extending from the zygomaticomaxillary suture to the infraorbital foramen, which could mimic a fracture (arrow). (**B**) is a septal aperture in the olecranon fossa of the humerus, which could mimic a perforating wound. (**C**) is a wormian bone. If the wormian bone falls out of the cranium, the residual space can mimic a gunshot wound.

ANTEMORTEM FRACTURES

Description: Antemortem fractures exhibit reaction to the injury (ie, attempted healing), which can include callus, fiber-bone periostitis, or an etched line parallel to the fracture line, which is indicative of periosteal uplifting.[63] Fracture healing times in the long bones are not the same as fracture healing times in the cranium, with fractures of the cranium appearing freshly fractured for a long period of time after the injury.[9]

> **FAQ:** How do you identify antemortem fractures?
>
> **Answer:** In fleshed remains, the process is much easier. Based upon the time since the injury, the bone will go through a variety of changes, including inflammatory cell infiltrate, red blood cell extravasation, and edema, which are visible for the first few days, deposition of cartilage and collagen and infilling of the fracture line in the next few weeks, and calcification of cartilage in the next few weeks.[67] In skeletonized remains, these changes, except for calcification, will be lost, but rounded fracture edges can assist. A developed callus forms relatively quickly and will be identifiable in skeletonized remains (Figure 9.82); however, the earliest stages in the healing cycle would be lost when skeletonization occurs.

POSTMORTEM FRACTURES

Description: Postmortem breakage can occur due to burial circumstances or poor recovery techniques.[63,66] In addition to fractures, postmortem warping, animal activity (Figure 9.83A and B), and bone weathering (Figure 9.84), must also be distinguished from perimortem trauma. Bone weathering is cracking, splitting, exfoliation, and fragmentation of bone exposed to the weather.

PERIMORTEM INJURIES

General features: Distinguishing perimortem from postmortem injuries is critical, as one fracture type definitely occurred after death, while the other fracture type may have occurred at the time of death and therefore can be of importance in understanding the circumstances of the death.

Perimortem fractures tend to occur in wet bone and postmortem fractures tend to occur in dry bone. Wet bone is more flexible because of its higher moisture and collagen content and should (or, may) fracture in a different manner than dry bone (Figure 9.85).[64] Wet bone is alternatively called fresh or green bone.[64] However, there are no absolute time

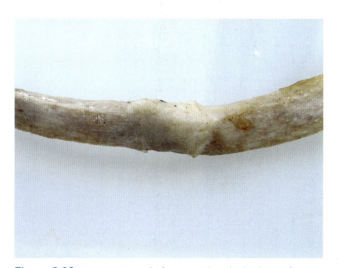

Figure 9.82. Antemortem rib fracture. The rib displays a fracture callus, which identifies the trauma as occurring prior to death.

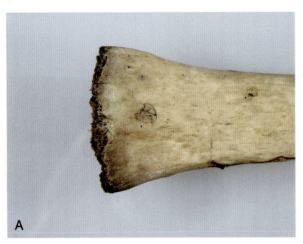 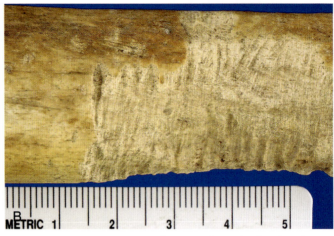

Figure 9.83. Postmortem animal activity. (**A**) is a carnivore puncture. Carnivores and omnivores will often chew the ends of the long bones, to access the marrow for nutrients. (**B**) is rodent gnawing. Rodents will often gnaw on the shaft of the long bones to access the mineral content.

frames for the transition from wet to dry bone, as the state of the bone is very dependent upon many factors including the environment in which it is placed. Bodies buried in wet environments (eg, under the water table), bodies with saponification, or bodies with retention of decompositional fluid, may retain wet bones and, with trauma, develop perimortem fractures for a long period after death.[64] After bone is dried, it is more brittle than wet bone, fracturing with less deformation due to force.[8] For example, energy delivered to a dried skull can cause crushing of the bone and complete loss of anatomic relationships, while severe trauma occurring perimortem to a wet bone can still allow for maintenance of anatomic relationships.[64] Wet bone tends to splinter, so perimortem fractures tend to have irregular edges and small fragments of bone that are attached to the fracture margin (see Figure 9.85), because the periosteum and other soft tissue was still present when the injury occurred.[63,66] In addition, wet bone can have flaking of the cortex adjacent to the fracture margin.[64] In general, the appearance of the fracture angle, the fracture edge (or, fracture surface), and the fracture outline may help distinguish perimortem and postmortem fractures. The fracture angle (the angle formed by the surface of the fracture and the surface of the cortical bone) is obtuse or acute in wet bones, whereas those in dry bones are at or nearly at, right angles.[64,68,69] The fracture edge (or, fracture surface) is the surface of the fractured end

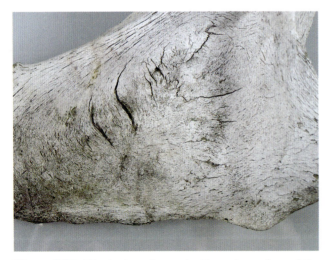 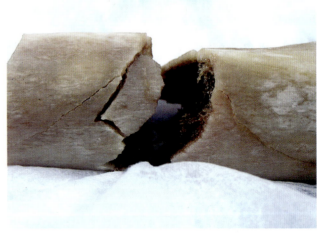

Figure 9.84. Weathering of scapula. The outer surface of the scapula is splitting, cracking, and exfoliating. Such changes in the thin body of the scapula such as long splits in the bone could mimic trauma such as a stab wound.

Figure 9.85. Example of wet bone reaction. The shaft of this bone is fractured. At the left side of the fracture is a small segment of bone that is partially bent in, but still attached to the shaft. Such a finding would be consistent with wet bone, and a perimortem fracture.

of the bone and is usually smooth, sharp, and sometimes beveled in wet bone, and irregular or jagged in dry bone.[64,69-71] However, this texture of the fracture edge may also depend upon the source of the load, with low-energy force producing a rough fracture surface as a result of spread around vascular spaces and high-energy force producing a smooth fracture surface as a result of propagation through vascular spaces.[72] Therefore, a low-energy force could produce a fracture edge that mimics a postmortem fracture, while a high-energy force could produce a fracture that is consistent with a perimortem fracture. The fracture outline is the general shape of the fractured end of the bone. Designation of fracture outline includes (1) transverse, (2) curved, and (3) intermediate.[68] Intermediate fracture outlines are those fracture outlines that are straight but oblique, or those with a stepped outline.[68]

Studies regarding timing of bone fractures: Wieberg and Wescott found that the change in fracture surface morphology (ie, fracture edge) and the change in fracture angle were significantly different with extended time since death; however, the change in fracture outline was not significantly different with time since death.[73] This finding contrasts that of Villa and Mahieu who found that differences in fracture angle and fracture outline were significant, but that differences in the fracture surface was not.[68] In other words, as the postmortem interval increased in Wieberg and Wescott, the frequency of jagged surfaces increased and the frequency of smooth surfaces decreased and the frequency of right angled fractures increased.[73] Wieberg and Wescott described that "…bones do not consistently manifest 'postmortem' characteristics until 141 days postmortem."[73] When 22 forensic anthropologists were asked to assess the timing of fractures of ten of the bones used in the study, the number of cases correctly assigned to time frame (as to antemortem, perimortem, or postmortem) ranged from 3 to 10, with those forensic anthropologists using the fracture surface morphology scoring highest.[73]

Color differences can help distinguish perimortem from postmortem fractures, with perimortem injuries showing the same patina between the margins of the fracture and the remainder of the bone[63,64,66,70,74] (Figure 9.86A and B). However, color differences are not an absolute indicator of postmortem fractures as differential staining of the cortical surface and fracture margin can be due to various factors including hemorrhage, decompositional fluids, soil, foliage (such as leaves), and dirty water, and therefore should be used cautiously.[64]

Other features of the fracture may help to distinguish perimortem from postmortem. Moraitis et al state that fracture patterning can help distinguish perimortem trauma.[70] The authors used a stellate fracture, a Le-Fort type III fracture, complex fractures with multiple lines, and butterfly fractures as examples, indicating that such fracture types would indicate a perimortem fracture. However, Ubelaker and Adams described three butterfly fractures which were postmortem in nature based upon (1) differential coloration of the fracture edge and the adjacent cortex and (2) the direction of forces producing the butterfly fractures on the left tibia and left fibula were in opposite directions, and therefore, could not have occurred in a living individual or even in articulated human remains.[74] Transverse fractures are also more common postmortem than perimortem.[60,71]

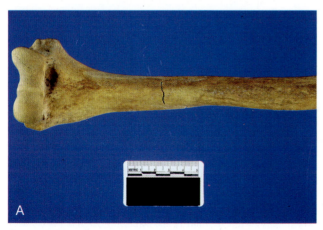 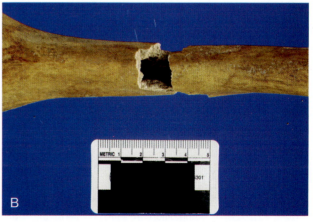

Figure 9.86. Postmortem fracture of distal humerus. The distal humerus has a fracture (**A**). However, the edges of the fracture have a different coloration than the surrounding cortical surface (**B**). If the fracture had occurred prior to death, the fracture edges would have expected to be exposed to the same conditions as the surface of the bone and should essentially be the same color.

> **PEARLS & PITFALLS**
>
> As Mann and Owsley and Ubelaker and Adams illustrate, reconstruction of the skeletal elements present into the normal orientation in a fleshed individual can help distinguish perimortem from postmortem injury.[74,75] If injuries exist that could not have possibly occurred in a fleshed individual (eg, pellet entrance wounds in the femoral head, with no corresponding exit defects in the acetabulum), the wounds must be postmortem.

NEAR MISSES

Near Miss #1: A woman who sustained blunt force injuries in a motor vehicle accident was identified to have a patch of yellow-orange with focal black discolored skin on the left breast, which was initially interpreted as a postmortem abrasion (Figure 9.87A). After sectioning into the chest wall, hemorrhage was identified in the underlying soft tissue (Figure 9.87B). A section of the skin revealed an intact epidermis, but compressed dermis (Figure 9.87C). This injury has features of both antemortem and postmortem changes and highlights the difficulty with distinguishing an antemortem injury from a postmortem injury. If the determination is an important finding in any given autopsy, microscopic examination of the skin lesion may lend additional information for rendering a decision regarding the nature of the lesion.

Near Miss #2: An investigator reported an individual had been found in the middle of the road with a stab wound of the forehead (Figure 9.88). At autopsy, examination of the wound revealed what initially appeared to be consistent with an incised wound or stab

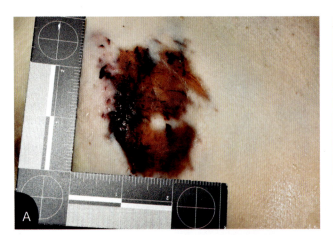
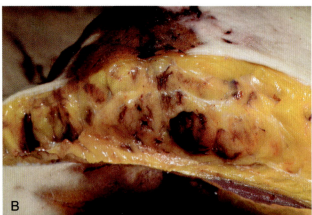
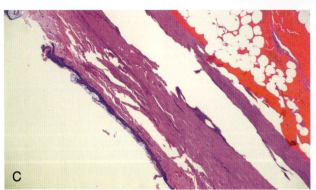

Figure 9.87. Lesion of the breast. (**A**) shows the lesion of the breast, which appears postmortem. (**B**) shows hemorrhage in the underlying soft tissue, which appears to support the injury being antemortem in origin. (**C**) is a microscopic section of the skin, which reveals a compressed dermis, but intact epidermis, which would not appear to support that the injury is an abrasion (hematoxylin and eosin, medium power).

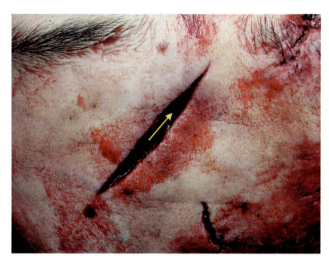

Figure 9.88. Laceration of skin. In the depths of the wound, tissue bridging is apparent (arrow).

wound, which had sharp edges and no abrasions or contusions of the surrounding skin; however, in the depths of the wound, tissue bridging was apparent, which would be inconsistent with sharp force injuries.

Near Miss #3: At autopsy some splotchy red discolorations of the skin were identified (Figure 9.89). While these findings could initially appear as small abrasions, investigators reported that the decedent had recently started a job at a body repair shop and that the red discolorations on the extremities were paint.

Near Miss #4: In skeletal remains of historical interest, the fracture in Figure 9.90 was identified. The edges of the fracture have a lighter coloration than the adjacent cortex of the bone, which would be consistent with a postmortem fracture; however, at the edge of the fracture is a small segment of still attached, but bent in bone, which would be consistent with wet bone, which would be consistent with a perimortem fracture. This finding just illustrates the potential difficulties in distinguishing perimortem and postmortem fractures. As the bone was of historical interest, the history behind the injury is unknown.

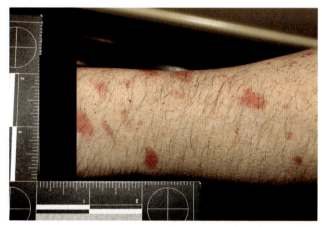

Figure 9.89. Splotches of paint on the upper extremities. A finding that could at first glance mimic abrasions.

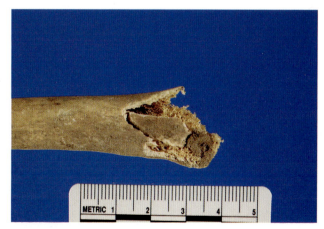

Figure 9.90. Bone with features of both perimortem and postmortem fracture. The coloration differences between the cortical surface and the fracture edge are consistent with a postmortem fracture; however, the bent in segment of bone could be interpreted as a feature of wet bone, which is consistent with a perimortem fracture.

References

1. Hensyl WR, Felscher H, eds. *Stedman's Medical Dictionary*. 25th ed. Williams and Wilkins; 1990.
2. DiMaio VJ, DiMaio D. *Forensic Pathology*. 3rd ed. CRC Press; 2022.
3. Spitz WU, Diaz FJ. *Spitz and Fisher's Medicolegal Investigation of Death: Guidelines for the Application of Pathology to Crime Investigation*, 5th ed. Charles C. Thomas; 2020.
4. Baden MM, Petty CS. Blunt trauma: specific injuries. In: Fisher RS, Petty CS, eds. *Forensic Pathology: A Handbook for Pathologists*. National Institute of Law Enforcement and Criminal Justice; 1977.
5. Byard RW, Heath KJ. Patterned postmortem ant abrasions outlining clothing and body position after death. *J Forensic Leg Med*. 2014;26:10-13.
6. Porta DJ. Biomechanics of impact injury. In: Rich J, Dean DE, Powers RH, eds. *Forensic Medicine of the Lower Extremities*. Humana Press; 2005:279-310.
7. Sharkey EJ, Cassidy M, Brady J, Gilchrist MD, NicDaeid N. Investigation of the force associated with the formation of lacerations and skull fractures. *Int J Legal Med*. 2012;126(6):835-844.
8. Turner CH, Burr DB. Basic biomechanical measurements of bone: a tutorial. *Bone*. 1993;14(4):595-608.
9. Moritz AR. *Pathology of Trauma*. Lea & Febiger; 1942.
10. Saukko P, Knight B. *Knight's Forensic Pathology*. Hodder Arnold; 2004.
11. Kumar V, Abbas AK, Aster JC. *Robbins Basic Pathology*. 10th ed. Elsevier; 2018.
12. Dolinak D, Matshes E, Lew E. *Forensic Pathology: Principles and Practice*. Elsevier Academic Press; 2005.
13. Curran WJ, McGarry AL, Petty CS. *Modern Legal Medicine, Psychiatry, and Forensic Science*: FA Davis Company; 1980.
14. Gonzales TA, Vance M, Helpern M, et al. *Legal Medicine: Pathology and Toxicology*. Appleton Century Crofts, Inc; 1954.
15. Molina DK, DiMaio VJ. Head trauma and alcohol: a lethal combination. *Am J Forensic Med Pathol*. 2015;36(4):290-292.
16. Kodikara S. A death due to concussive brain injury augmented by alcohol (case report). *Forensic Sci Med Pathol*. 2007;3(4):283-284.
17. Milovanovic AV, DiMaio VJ. Death due to concussion and alcohol. *Am J Forensic Med Pathol*. 1999;20(1):6-9.
18. Swanson AE, Veldman A, Wallace EM, Malhotra A. Subgaleal hemorrhage: risk factors and outcomes. *Acta Obstet Gynecol Scand*. 2012;91(2):260-263. doi:10.1111/j.1600-0412.2011.01300.x.
19. Pearl GS. Traumatic neuropathology. *Clin Lab Med*. 1998;18(1):39-64.
20. Viel G, Gehl A, Sperhake JP. Intersecting fractures of the skull and gunshot wounds. Case report and literature review. *Forensic Sci Med Pathol*. 2009;5(1):22-27.
21. Inokuchi G, Makino Y, Yajima D, et al. A case of acute subdural hematoma due to ruptured aneurysm detected by postmortem angiography. *Int J Legal Med*. 2016;130(2):441-446.
22. Hardman JM. Microscopy of traumatic central nervous system injuries. In: Perper JA, Wecht CH, eds.*Microscopic Diagnosis in Forensic Pathology*. Charles C Thomas; 1980:268-326.
23. Leestma JE. *Forensic Neuropathology*. Raven; 1988.
24. Oehmichen M, Auer RN, König HG. *Forensic Neuropathology and Associated Neurology*. Springer; 2006.
25. Dettmeyer RB. *Forensic Histopathology*. Springer; 2011.
26. Munro D, Merritt HH. Surgical pathology of subdural hema-toma, based on a study of one hundred and five cases. *Arch Neurol Psychiatr*. 1936;35:64-78.
27. van den Bos D, Zomer S, Kubat B. Dare to date: age estimation of subdural hematomas, literature, and case analysis. *Int J Legal Med*. 2014;128(4):631-640.
28. Shirota G, Gonoi W, Ikemura M, et al. The pseudo-SAH sign: an imaging pitfall in postmortem computed tomography. *Int J Legal Med*. 2017;131(6):1647-1653.
29. Kaiser C, Schnabel A, Berkefeld J, Bratzke H. Traumatic rupture of the intracranial vertebral artery due to rotational acceleration. *Forensic Sci Int*. 2008;182(1-3):e15-e17.
30. Gray JT, Puetz SM, Jackson SL, Green MA. Traumatic subarachnoid haemorrhage: a 10-year case study and review. *Forensic Sci Int*. 1999;105(1):13-23.

31. Kim S, Kim M, Lee BW, Kim YH, Choi YS, Seo JS. Investigation of bleeding focus in the intracranial vertebral artery with the use of posterior neck dissection method in traumatic basal subarachnoid hemorrhage. *J Forensic Leg Med*. 2015;34:151-154.

32. Drew LB, Drew WE. The Contrecoup-Coup phenomenon: a new understanding of the mechanism of closed head injury. *Neurocrit Care*. 2004;1(3):385-390.

33. Davceva N, Sivevski A, Basheska N. Traumatic axonal injury: a clinical-pathological correlation. *J Forensic Leg Med*. 2017;48:35-40.

34. Rungruangsak K, Poriswanish N. Pathology of fatal diffuse brain injury in severe non-penetrating head trauma. *J Forensic Leg Med*. 2021;82:102226.

35. Kalimo H, Saukko P, Graham D. Neuropathological examination in forensic context. *Forensic Sci Int*. 2004;146(2-3):73-81.

36. Davceva N, Janevska V, Ilievski B, Spasevska L, Popeska Z. Dilemmas concerning the diffuse axonal injury as a clinicopathological entity in forensic medical practice. *J Forensic Leg Med*. 2012;19(7):413-418.

37. Byard RW, Vink R. Speed of development of cerebral swelling following blunt cranial trauma. *J Forensic Leg Med*. 2013;20(6):598-600.

38. Dolinak D, Matshes E. *Medicolegal Neuropathology: A Color Atlas*. CRC Press; 2002.

39. Potente S, Ramsthaler F, Kettner M, Sauer P, Schmidt P. Relative blood loss in forensic medicine-do we need a change in doctrine?. *Int J Legal Med*. 2020;134(3):1123-1131.

40. Guan DW, Ohshima T, Jia JT, Kondo T, Li DX. Morphological findings of 'cardiac concussion' due to experimental blunt impact to the precordial region. *Forensic Sci Int*. 1999;100(3):211-220.

41. Lucena JS, Rico A, Salguero M, Blanco M, Vázquez R. Commotio cordis as a result of a fight: report of a case considered to be imprudent homicide. *Forensic Sci Int*. 2008;177(1):e1-e4.

42. Darok M, Beham-Schmid C, Gatternig R, Roll P. Sudden death from myocardial contusion following an isolated blunt force trauma to the chest. *Int J Legal Med*. 2001;115(2):85-89.

43. Mugadlimath A, Sane M, Yoganarasimha K, Kamath G, Koulapur V, Zine KU. Myocardial infarction and concurrent chest injuries: two case reports. *Forensic Sci Int*. 2012;217(1-3):e1-e3.

44. Burstein AH, Zika JM, Heiple KG, Klein L. Contribution of collagen and mineral to the elastic-plastic properties of bone. *J Bone Joint Surg*. 1975;57(7):956-961.

45. Reilly DT, Burstein AH. Review article. The mechanical properties of cortical bone. *J Bone Joint Surg*. 1974;56(5):1001-1022.

46. Smith OC, Peters CE. Biomechanics and the bone. In: Symes SA, ed. *Bones, Bullets, burns, Bludgeons, Blunderers, and Why. Bone Trauma Workshop Presented at 48th Annual Meeting of the American Academy of Forensic Sciences*. 1996.

47. Rogers LF. *Radiology of Skeletal Trauma*. Churchill-Livingstone; 1982.

48. Crowe JE, Swischuk LE. Acute bowing fractures of the forearm in children: a frequently missed injury. *Am J Roentgenol*. 1977;128(6):981-984.

49. Pierce MC, Bertocci GE, Vogeley E, Moreland MS. Evaluating long bone fractures in children: a biomechanical approach with illustrative cases. *Child Abuse Negl*. 2004;28(5):505-524.

50. Daegling DJ, Warren MW, Hotzman JL, Self CJ. Structural analysis of human rib fracture and implications for forensic interpretation. *J Forensic Sci*. 2008;53(6):1301-1307.

51. Ortner DJ. Trauma. In: Ortner DJ, ed. *Identification of Pathological Conditions in Human Skeletal Remains*. 2nd ed. Academic Press; 2003:119-178.

52. Schmidt G. Rib-cage injuries indicating the direction and strength of impact. *Forensic Sci Int*. 1979;13(2):103-110.

53. Alms M. Fracture mechanics. *J Bone Joint Surg*. 1961;43-B(1):162-166.

54. Reilly DT, Burstein AH. The elastic and ultimate properties of compact bone tissue. *J Biomech*. 1975;8(6):393-405.

55. Viano DC, Stalnaker RL. Mechanisms of femoral fracture. *J Biomech*. 1980;13(8):701-715.

56. Love JC, Symes SA. Understanding rib fracture patterns: incomplete and buckle fractures. *J Forensic Sci*. 2004;49(6):1153-1158.

57. Galloway A, Zephro L. Skeletal trauma analysis of the lower extremity. In: Rich J, Dean DE, Powers RH, eds. *Forensic Medicine of the Lower Extremity: Human Identification and Trauma Analysis of the Thigh, Leg, and Foot*. Humana Press; 2005:253-277.

58. Galloway A. The biomechanics of fracture production. In: Galloway A, ed. *Broken Bones: Anthropological Analysis of Blunt Force Trauma*. Charles C Thomas; 1999:35-62.

59. Johner R, Wruhs O. Classification of tibial shaft fractures and correlation with results after rigid internal fixation. *Clin Orthop Relat Res.* 1983;178:7-25.

60. Wheatley BP. Perimortem or postmortem bone fractures? An experimental study of fracture patterns in deer femora. *J Forensic Sci.* 2008;53(1):1-4.

61. Yukawa N, Kojimahara M, Green MA, Saito T, Osawa M, Takeichi S. A Messerer fracture. *Forensic Sci Int.* 1997;88(3):231-234.

62. Love JC, Wiersema JM. Skeletal trauma: an anthropological review. *Acad Forensic Pathol.* 2016;6(3):463-477.

63. Rodríguez-Martín C. Identification and differential diagnosis of traumatic lesions of the skeleton. In: Schmitt A, Cunha E, Pinheiro J, eds. *Forensic Anthropology and Medicine: Complementary Sciences from Recovery to Cause of Death.* Human Press; 2006:197-220.

64. Moraitis K, Spiliopoulou C. Identification and differential diagnosis of perimortem blunt force trauma in tubular long bones. *Forensic Sci Med Pathol.* 2006;2(4):221-229.

65. Mann RW, Hunt DR. Non-metric traits and anatomical variants that can mimic trauma in the human skeleton. *Forensic Sci Int.* 2019;301:202-224.

66. Sauer NJ. The timing of injuries and manner of death: distinguishing among antemortem, perimortem, and postmortem trauma. In: Reichs KJ, ed. *Forensic Osteology: Advances in the Identification of Human Remains.* 2nd ed. Charles C Thomas; 1998:321-332.

67. Calmar EA, Vinci RJ. The anatomy and physiology of bone fracture and healing. *Clin Ped Emerg Med.* 2002;3:85-93.

68. Villa P, Mahieu E. Breakage patterns of human long bones. *J Hum Evol.* 1991;21:27-48.

69. Wright CS. *Perimortem and Postmortem Fracture Patterns in Deer Femora.* MA thesis. University of Alabama; 2009:64.

70. Moraitis K, Ellopoulos C, Spiliopouloi C. Fracture characteristics of perimortem trauma in skeletal material. *Internet J Biol Anthropol.* 2009;3(2). doi:10.5580/20a2.

71. Shattuck RE. *Perimortem Fracture Patterns in South-central Texas: A Preliminary Investigation into the Perimortem Interval.* MA thesis. Department of Anthropology, Texas State University-San Marcos. 2010.

72. Herrmann NP, Bennett JL. The differentiation of traumatic and heat-related fractures in burned bone. *J Forensic Sci.* 1999;44(3):461-469.

73. Wieberg DAM, Wescott DJ. Estimating the timing of long bone fractures: correlation between the postmortem interval, bone moisture content, and blunt force trauma fracture characteristics. *J Forensic Sci.* 2008;53(5):1028-1034.

74. Ubelaker DH, Adams BJ. Differentiation of perimortem and postmortem trauma using taphonomic indicators. *J Forensic Sci.* 1995;40(3):509-512.

75. Mann RW, Owsley DW. Human osteology: key to the sequence of events in a postmortem shooting. *J Forensic Sci.* 1992;37(5):1386-1392.

SHARP FORCE INJURIES 10

CHAPTER OUTLINE

Introduction 274

Types of Sharp Force Injuries 274
- Stab Wound 274
  - Description 274
  - Documentation of Stab Wound 274
  - Determination of Depth of Stab Wound 278
- Incised Wound 279
  - Description 279
- Chop Wound 281
  - Description 281

Sharp Force Injuries of the Bone and Cartilage 284
- Introduction 284
- Basic Features of Bony Defects From Sharp Force Injuries 284
- Identifying Class Characteristics of Sharp Force Injuries in the Bone 286
- Other Features Used to Interpret Sharp Force Wound Characteristics 286

Near Misses 288

INTRODUCTION

The distinction between blunt and sharp force injuries can be seen as a categorical description and not as an acknowledgment of two types of force. Sharp force injuries classically include stab wounds, incised wounds, and chop wounds.

TYPES OF SHARP FORCE INJURIES

STAB WOUND

Description

A stab wound is a defect in the skin that penetrates into the body to a depth that is longer than the corresponding length of the defect in the skin (Figure 10.1). For example, while the defect at the cutaneous surface could be 2 inches in length, the depth that the knife penetrated into the body could be 6 inches. The angles are the ends or poles of the stab wound and can be sharp or blunt. The angles can also be called the extremities. The margins are the edges of the wound and are most often smooth and non-abraded. A stab wound would have an absence of tissue bridging, whereas a laceration, which can have relatively smooth and non-abraded margins and thus potentially mimic a stab wound or an incised wound, would have tissue bridging, helping to distinguish the two types of injuries. Tissue bridging is stranding of fibrous tissue, vessels, or nerves between the wound edges (ie, perpendicular to the long axis of the wound).

Documentation of Stab Wound

When documenting the stab wound, it is important to describe the angles and the margins (Figure 10.2A and B). The angles can be sharp or blunt. Sharp angles come to a point and indicate a sharp edge of a weapon, or a blunt end that tore. Blunt angles are squared off. In many cases, the shape of the angle cannot be accurately determined because of drying artifact or other changes warping the appearance, and instead of sharp or blunt can be characterized as an indeterminant or undetermined angle. The presence of a superficial incision tail at one end can help identify the sharp angle (Figure 10.3). With rare stab wounds that penetrate the cranium or another bone, the shape of the knife can be preserved and distinguishing sharp and blunt angles is easy (Figure 10.4). In addition to a description of the angles and margins, the wound can be described in relation to its plane, either horizontal or vertical or oblique.

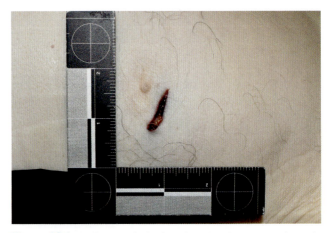

Figure 10.1. Stab wound. The length in the skin is around 1 inch, but the measured depth into the chest that the knife penetrated was several inches.

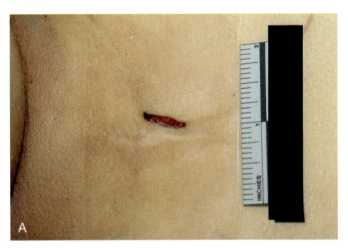 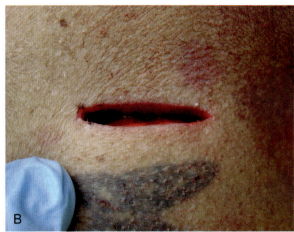

Figure 10.2. Stab wound features. In (**A**), the angle closest to the ruler is pointed, which would correspond to the sharp edge of the blade, and the angle on the opposite side is blunt, which would correspond to the edge of the knife opposite the sharp edge. In (**B**), the angle on the left side of the image is squared off (ie, blunt), and the angle on the right side of the photograph comes to a point (ie, sharp).

PEARLS & PITFALLS

As stab wounds frequently cut across lines of Langer, which produces a gaping wound, re-approximation of the wound can allow for more accurate identification of the features of the stab wound. The edges of a stab wound can easily be re-approximated with superglue or with clear plastic tape or with just fingertip pressure applied to the edges of the wound or along one edge (Figure 10.5A-G). If clear plastic tape is used, the depths of the stab wound must be as dried as much as possible, or else blood will ooze from the wound and coat the tape. Another technique is to examine the parietal pleural surface or pericardial sac, which, if involved by the stab wound, may better retain the features of the stab wound than the skin as far as blunt or sharp angles.

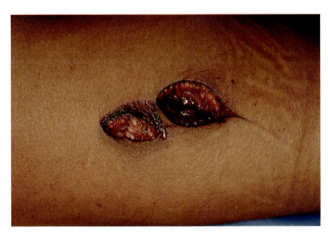 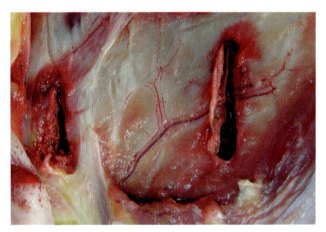

Figure 10.3. Tail to help identify the sharp angle. The decedent's extremity has two stab wounds; however, due to the gaping nature of the wounds and the drying of the edges of the wounds, distinguishing blunt from sharp at the angles is challenging. However, at the stab wound on the right side, there is a trailing tail at 3 o'clock, which would identify the sharp edge of the knife.

Figure 10.4. Stab wounds of the cranium. While the gaping of stab wounds of the skin and drying of edges can make determination of the features of the stab wound challenging to distinguish, when the stab wound involves bone, the features can be much more preserved. Figure 10.4 has two stab wounds of the cranium, with the blunt angle inferior in both, and the sharp angle superior in both, which makes identifying the orientation of the knife to the body a straightforward determination.

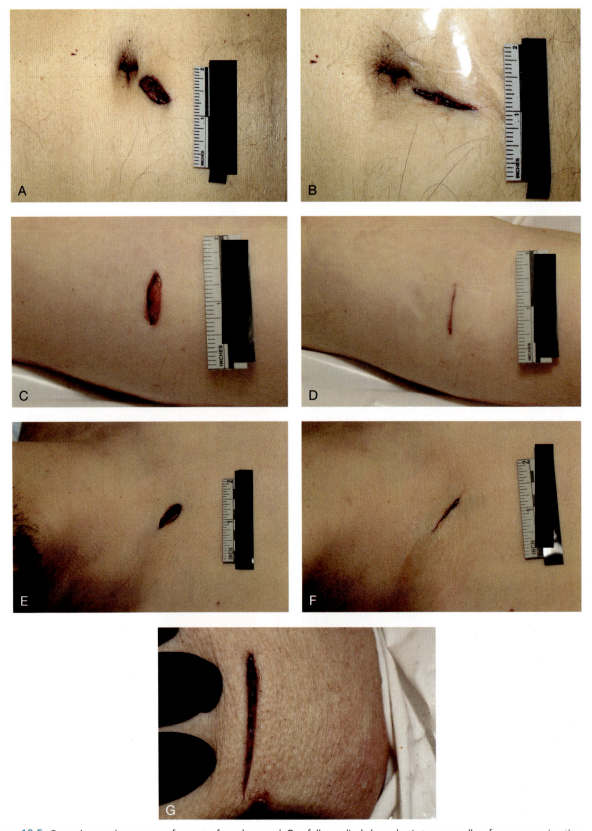

Figure 10.5. Procedures to better exam features of a stab wound. Carefully applied clear plastic tape can allow for re-approximation of the margins to better identify features of a stab wound. (**A** and **C**) are pre-application of tape and (**B** and **D**) are post-application of tape. Unfortunately, blood oozing from the wound impairs this process; however, if the wound is effectively dried, it can be performed. Superglue can also be used to re-approximate the margins of the stab wound. (**E**) is the pre-application of superglue and (**F**) is post-application of superglue. In addition, just using the fingers to re-approximate the margins of the stab wound can also work (**G**).

PEARLS & PITFALLS

Sometimes a stab wound will be "L" or "V" shaped. Whether this occurred due to overlapping separate stab wounds or a single stab wound with movement of the decedent or the knife after penetration cannot necessarily be determined (Figure 10.6A-E).

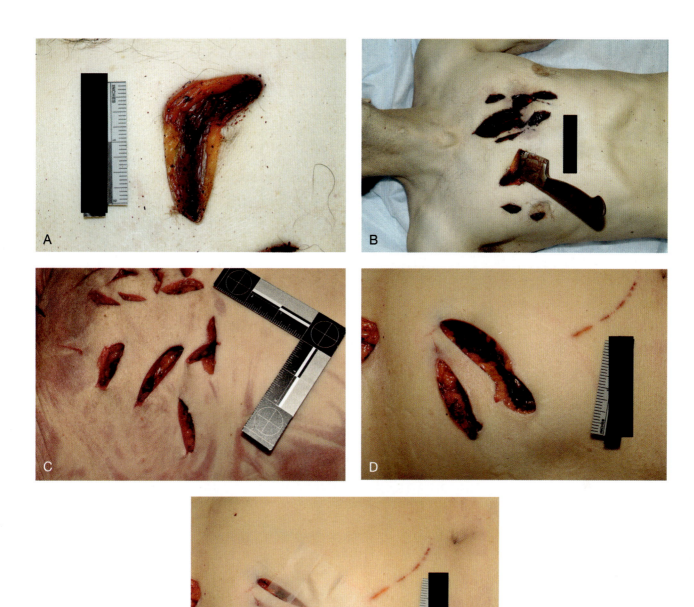

Figure 10.6. Non-linear stab wounds. When a stab wound is "L" or "V" shaped, whether the wound is overlapping separate stab wounds, or a change in orientation of the knife to the body caused by movement of the attacker or movement of the decedent, can be challenging to determine. If the weapon is known (eg, a single-edged knife) and the available angles do not match up (eg, two blunt angles on a "V" shaped wound), the injuries are overlapping. However determining the nature of the wound in all cases is difficult. The wound in (**A**) is "L"-shaped; however, in (**B**), it can be seen that the knife was in this wound when the body was discovered. (**C**) is a stab wound in an individual who was stabbed multiple times in a relatively small area of the body, and includes a likely overlapping wound. (**D** and **E**) illustrate how taping (or supergluing) a complex stab wound may help distinguish whether the wound was two overlapping stab wounds.

Determination of Depth of Stab Wound

The depth of the stab wound can potentially be determined by probing the wound, layered dissection of the wound, or computed tomography after introduction of a contrast medium.[1] While stab wounds of solid tissue, such as the extremities, have a more easily measurable depth, those stab wounds that involve the body cavities are more difficult to determine the depth of penetration, unless they end in a fixed or solid object such as the heart or vertebral column.[1]

> **FAQ:** Can the depth of a stab wound be accurately determined?
>
> **Answer:** With probing of the wound, identifying the depth of penetration can be challenging, and often the depth of penetration is a measured estimate, especially since the body has already been opened and the reflected skin must be re-approximated to measure the depth of the stab wound. If the knife produces hemorrhage in the penetrated soft tissue, and that hemorrhage abruptly ends, the depth of penetration may be more accurately measured, or, if the sharp instrument strikes bone or a solid organ, such as the liver, the depth of penetration can be more accurately determined (Figure 10.7A and B).

> **PEARLS & PITFALLS**
>
> If the pathway of the wound intersects cartilage, the segment of cartilage can be removed and preserved. Comparison of the cartilage segment to the causative weapon can potentially allow for a match.

SAMPLE NOTE: DESCRIPTION OF A STAB WOUND

On the left side of the chest is a 2 inch horizontal stab wound. The medial angle is blunt and 1/8 inch wide. The lateral angle is sharp. The wound is centered 14 inches below the top of the head, 4 inches to the left of midline, 1 inch below the level of the left nipple, and 1 inch medial to the left nipple. The stab wound perforates the chest wall at the left third interspace and penetrates into the upper lobe of the left lung. The pathway of the stab wound is front to back, and the measured depth of penetration is 5 inches.

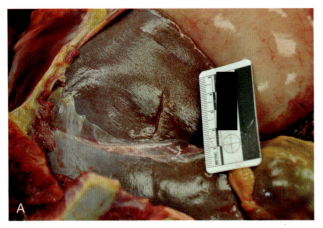
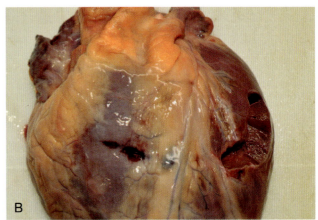

Figure 10.7. Stab wounds of the organs. When the stab wound ends in a solid organ, such as the liver or heart, determining the depth of penetration is easier as the end point of the stab wound is often more well-defined (**A** and **B**).

SAMPLE NOTE: MULTIPLE STAB WOUNDS

The documentation of multiple stab wounds (or multiple gunshot wounds) can be daunting as there could literally be hundreds of wounds. Measuring each wound and giving locating measurements (eg, distance from the top of head) for each wound would be time consuming and could end in an un-necessarily lengthy autopsy report, which can create difficulties in sorting out the vital findings. In decedents who have multiple stab wounds (Figure 10.8), the wounds can be lumped together and described as a unit. An example of such an approach, which does not correlate with the image though, is given below.

On the left side of the chest is a cluster of seventeen stab wounds, which occupy a 5 × 5 inch area. The stab wounds vary from 3/4 inch to 4 inches in size. Many have one blunt angle and one sharp angle. The blunt angles are often 1/8 inch in width. The stab wounds are predominantly oriented in a vertical plan; however, some are more oblique. The cluster of stab wounds is centered 10 inches below the top of the head, 4 inches to the left of midline, 2 inches medial to the left nipple, and 1 inch superior to the left nipple. The stab wounds perforate the left third and fourth ribs and intervening skeletal muscle, and penetrated into the upper lobe of the left lung, the lower lobe of the left lung, and the heart. The measured depth of penetration is 6 inches.

PEARLS & PITFALLS

When an individual is stabbed multiple times, there is a reasonable chance that the two individuals knew each other, to include a possible romantic/sexual relationship or an otherwise close and personal relationship (Figure 10.8). For this reason, it is often best to obtain a sexual activity kit for evidence when the cause of death is multiple stab wounds.

INCISED WOUND

Description

An incised wound penetrates into the body to a depth that is shorter than the length of the defect in the skin (Figure 10.9A and B). For example, while the defect at the cutaneous surface could be 6 inches in length, the depth that the knife penetrated into the body could be 2 inches. Incised wounds will lack tissue bridging, which can help distinguish an incised

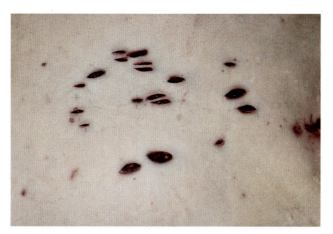

Figure 10.8. Multiple stab wounds. This individual was stabbed numerous times in a relatively small region of the chest. Describing each wound individually as far as size and location would be time-consuming and create a long complex autopsy report description. In such a situation, lumping the wounds together and describing as a group may be a reasonable approach.

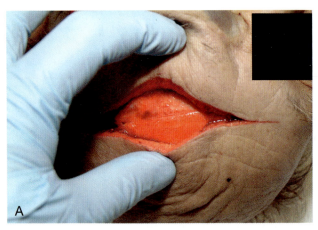
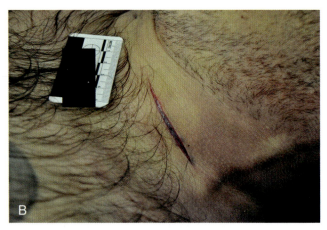

Figure 10.9. Incised wounds. (**A**) is an incised wound of the scalp, which penetrates full thickness to the cranium. The edges of the incised wound are being spread apart to show the lack of tissue bridging. (**B**) is an incised wound of the neck, which is much more superficial than the incised wound in (**A**).

wound from a laceration. The absolute distinction between a stab wound and an incised wound can, with particular injuries, be blurred, as what may initially be a stab wound can be converted to an incised wound by modifying the application of force, that is, along the body instead of into the body (Figure 10.10A and B). Also, as the exact depth of a stab wound can be difficult to determine, unlike the exact measurement of length in the skin, both measurements could be close, leading one observer to determine a stab wound and the next observer to determine an incised wound.

> **PEARLS & PITFALLS**
>
> If a decedent has an incised wound of the neck that involves a vein, the possibility of an air embolus should be considered. An air embolus can be detected through a radiograph of the chest obtained prior to autopsy. Subsequently, the heart can be opened under water.[2]

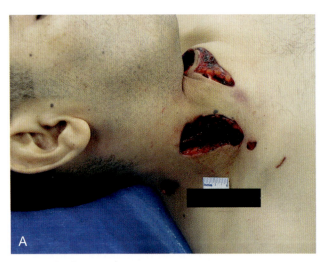
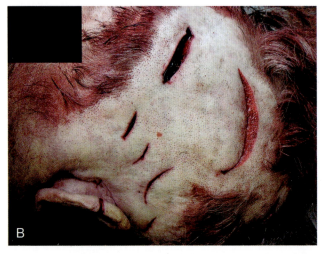

Figure 10.10. Stab wound/incised wound. In (**A**) on the right side of the neck is a wide gaping stab wound; however, given the inability to determine the exact depth into the soft tissue in many stab wounds, determining whether the wound would technically classify as a stab wound vs an incised wound may be debatable. In (**B**) on the right side of the image is a long curvilinear stab wound that has a sharp angle medial and a blunt angle lateral, however, the depth in the soft tissue may be difficult to accurately determine. These two images should just illustrate that although the definition of stab wound vs incised wound is clear, the practical application of the two terms has some overlap.

> **PEARLS & PITFALLS**
>
> It is important with stab wounds and incised wounds to, as best as possible, document the associated injuries caused by the sharp force weapon. In some cases, this is rather easy (Figure 10.11), as stab wounds across large caliber arteries leave the vessel open and often identifiable, whereas stab wounds of smaller vessels can be more difficult to identify. If possible, injection of the vasculature with contrast and subsequent radiography can help to identify injuries of the vessels. In addition to injuries of the vasculature, sharp force injuries can also cause injuries of the muscles and tendons. Identifying which muscles are so affected could potentially allow for a determination of what movements the decedent was capable of.

CHOP WOUND

Description

With a chop wound, the defect in the skin is similar to a stab wound or an incised wound, with smooth margins of the wound; however, underlying the defect in the skin are features of blunt force injuries, which may include fractures of the bone (Figure 10.12A-C). While weapons commonly associated with chop wounds include a machete or an axe, any weapon with a sharp edge can potentially produce a chop wound. For example, if a decedent is beaten with a table leg with four well-defined corners, the findings at autopsy can include chop wounds.

> **PEARLS & PITFALLS**
>
> Decedents with sharp force injuries should always have radiographs performed. If a fragment of the weapon used to cause the sharp force injuries can be identified (Figure 10.13A and B), the fragment, if recovered from the body, can subsequently be used to match a suspected weapon to the decedent (Figure 10.14). However, the identification of fragments within the body from the weapon used to cause the sharp force injuries is relatively rare. In the 58 cases that Banasr et al. reviewed, no weapon fragment was identified within the body.[3]

> **PEARLS & PITFALLS**
>
> While stab wounds that involve the bone can produce very well-defined features, such as a clearly defined sharp and blunt angle in a single-edged knife (Figure 10.15), vascular marking of the cranium can mimic an incised wound of the bone (Figure 10.16).

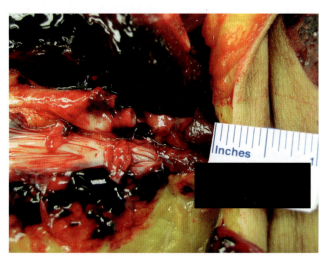

Figure 10.11. Incised wound of the carotid artery. The carotid artery has been completely transected by the weapon.

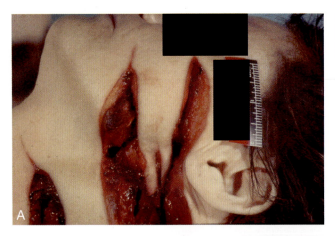
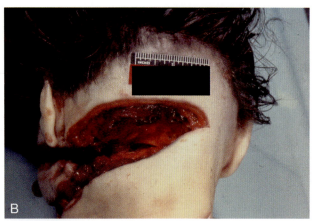
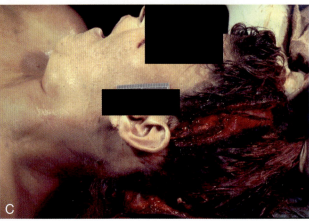

Figure 10.12. Chop wounds. (**A-C**) illustrate chop wounds. In (**C**), the wounds were caused by a boat propeller. Chop wounds often have large gaping skin wounds.

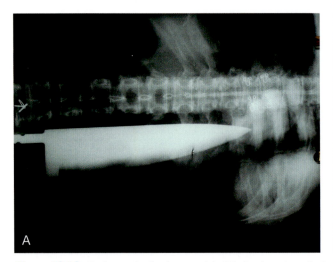
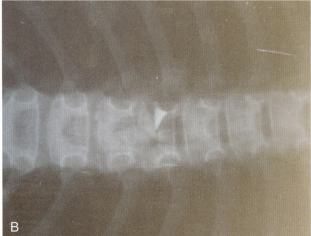

Figure 10.13. Radiograph of stab wound. In (**A**), the decedent died as the result of sharp force injuries. Although the individual was known to have been stabbed, the weapon was not known to be within the body. The radiograph is important for autopsy safety. In (**B**), the decedent was stabbed with a knife and the tip embedded and broke off in the vertebral column. Identifying the tip helps with autopsy safety, but the identification of the knife tip can also provide for crucial evidence that can help match the exact knife used in the death.

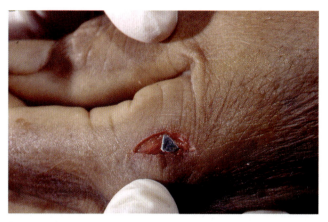

Figure 10.14. Knife tip in soft tissue. Occasionally a fragment of knife will be found in soft tissue and not within the bone.

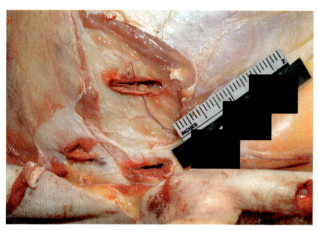

Figure 10.15. Stab wound in the bone. When a knife strikes bone, the margin and angles can be well reproduced. In two of the three defects in the cranium in Figure 10.15, the sharp angle and blunt angle are clearly seen.

> **FAQ:** Is it possible to match a specific sharp force weapon to a specific injury?
>
> **Answer:** While some features of the wound can help distinguish certain types of weapons (eg, a stab wound with one blunt and one sharp angle did not arise from a double-edged knife; and serrated knives may leave grouped parallel linear scratches from the serrations; Figure 10.17A and B), in general, many features of the stab wound will not help distinguish the weapon. For example, a 1/2 inch-wide knife could create a much larger wound in the skin depending upon how the stab wound was made, and a 5-inch long knife thrust with significant force against the abdomen could create a 10-inch-deep stab wound. Depending upon the angle of the attack, the force behind the attack, the area of the body hit by the attack, the presence or absence of movement by the attacker upon retracting the blade, or the presence or absence of movement by the victim after the knife has entered the skin can all affect the features of the wound, which makes skin changes unreliable to identify the specific weapon used. When a sharp force weapon strikes cartilage or bone, or when a sharp force weapon is used to dismember a body, marks on the cartilage and bone may assist with the identification of the weapon used. However, the best chance to match a particular knife to a wound is via recovery of a fragment of the knife within the wound, which is why all individuals who have been stabbed should have radiography performed.

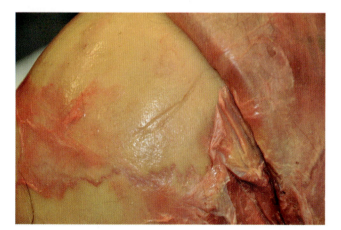

Figure 10.16. Vascular markings in the bone. Superficial grooves on the outer surface of the bone can mimic incised wounds. Vascular grooves also appear on the inner surface of the cranium; however, in this location, they should less commonly be confused with an incised wound.

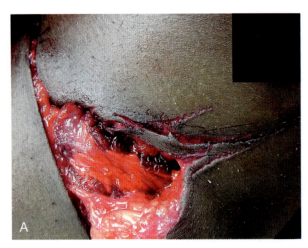
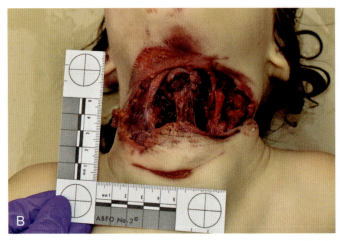

Figure 10.17. Serrated knife markings. In (**A**), on the right side of the wound is a zigzag pattern, which is consistent with a serrated knife. In (**B**), the serrated edge of the knife produced several parallel marks at the edge of the wound.

SHARP FORCE INJURIES OF THE BONE AND CARTILAGE

INTRODUCTION

When the cause of death is sharp force injuries, skeletal and cartilage injuries are relatively common. Even without the benefit of the removal of the soft tissue, Banasr et al. identified injuries to the skeletal elements and cartilage during autopsy in 53% of cases.[3]

> **PEARLS & PITFALLS**
>
> While a knife passing through cartilage can leave striations that could potentially be matched to the weapon causing the injury, Love et al. found a high error rate with this process (50%-65%) depending upon the method used.[4] Histologic examination of the bone and soft tissue may also assist in the identification of foreign particles.[5]

BASIC FEATURES OF BONY DEFECTS FROM SHARP FORCE INJURIES

General types of sharp force weapons that can leave a mark on the bone are saws, knives, and chopping weapons (eg, a machete or axe). Entry of a knife blade into the bone produces a smooth and flat cut surface. If the angle of entry is greater than 90°, the obtuse angle is smooth and the acute angle is rough and ends in fractured bone and, at the margin of the acute angle, the outer bone layer detaches in flakes. As with a gunshot wound, passage of the blade through the bone may produce large flakes.[6]

When a saw or knife strikes a bone perpendicular along the edge of the blade, the resultant defect is called a kerf.[7-9] The general features of the kerf include corners at the initial site of the cut, walls and a floor, and floor corners. Striae are the ridges produced by the saw on the wall of the kerf (Figure 10.18). While the striae can be seen with gross inspection, the use of a dissecting microscope and tangential lighting would allow for the best visualization and subsequent photographic documentation of the features. The shape of the kerf depends upon the type of weapon used. Knife blades will produce a "V"-shaped kerf floor because of their beveled edge.[9] Saw cuts will produce a squared kerf floor. Cross cut saws produce a kerf floor that in cross section resembles a "W." Saws can produce three general types of defects in the bone: superficial false start scratches (ie, a superficial defect in the bone), false start kerfs (Figure 10.19) (ie, deeper defect in the bone, but not completely through the bone), or completely sectioned bone cuts.[10]

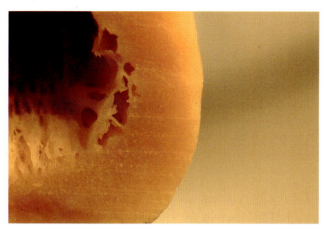

Figure 10.18. Striae on cut edge of bone. Intermittently spaced horizontal lines on the cut edge of the bone are present. These striae can provide characteristics regarding the saw that produced them in cutting the bone.

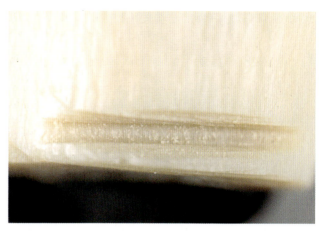

Figure 10.19. False start kerf. In Figure 10.19, the view is looking down on top of the bone. The cut edge of the bone is the inferior portion. Adjacent to the cut edge is a groove in the cortical surface, which is the false start kerf. A saw started to cut the bone at this site but was then moved to finish the cut through the bone.

Chopping (or hacking) type weapons (eg, machete, axe, or cleaver), like a knife cut wound, will, unless the wound is oriented 90° to the bone, have a smooth cut surface on the side of the wound with the obtuse angle, and a fractured bone on the side with the acute angle (Figure 10.20).[7] The fractured bone at the acute angle can have a flake or flakes of bone and the fractured bone underlying the wound can have large areas of bone broken away.[7,11] However, this finding is not universal as some hacking wounds will have acute angles without flaking of bone.[11] Cleavers produce cleaner wounds than axes, which have entrance defects often accompanied by chatter (multiple bone flakes) or fracture. Lynn and Fairgrieve found that axes produced an entry site as small as 1.7 mm in width, and opined that only a deep but very narrow entry site could be excluded as an axe in favor of a knife or scalpel.[11] Lynn and Hargrieve also found that fractures were commonly associated with axes and hatchet wounds.[11] In fleshed femora, the authors found curved transverse fractures most commonly, followed by spiral fractures. In fleshed fibulae, the authors saw a mixture of curve and straight transverse fractures.

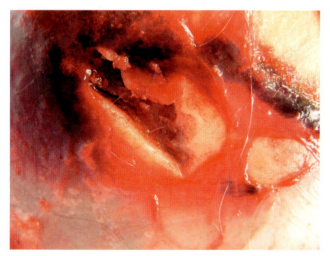

Figure 10.20. Non-perpendicular cut mark in the bone. On the left side of the image is the obtuse angle and on the right side is the acute angle, with flaking of the bone.

IDENTIFYING CLASS CHARACTERISTICS OF SHARP FORCE INJURIES IN THE BONE

Although analysis of sharp force injuries of the bone may not be able to determine the specific weapon used, through interpretation of class characteristics the general type of weapon used can potentially be determined.[9] In regard to analysis of knife cut wounds and saw marks of the bone, Symes et al. identified several important points: (1) cut mark analysis can yield information about at least the class characteristics of a blade; (2) non-mechanical saws, like mechanical saws, produce straight edges and smooth cut surfaces; (3) the bony defect produced by knives and saws are different in their appearance; and (4) sawing action with a sharp weapon does not necessarily destroy class or specific identifying features on the bone.[9]

To determine the class characteristics of a saw requires examination of the marks in the bone. Examination of features of the kerf and striae on the walls of the kerf can help identify a certain type of weapon as the causative agent. Repeated deep false start kerfs are more likely the result of a power saw than a manual saw.[9] A residual curved kerf floor can indicate a curved blade, such as with a circular saw or curved pruning saws.[9] While most saws have straight blades and will produce straight striae on the residual kerf walls, some saws have curved blades. Power circular saws, or those with a rigid circular blade will produce fixed-radius curvature striae, and the breakaway spur will be concave. In contrast, Gigli saws, or other flexible saws, produce non–fixed-radius striae and convex breakaway spurs.[10] While straight striations are most common, curved striations can indicate a flexible saw.[9]

The analysis of the features of the kerf may be used to identify the size, shape, set, and power of the saw.[9] The saw size is the size of the cut made by one individual saw tooth, or by multiple saw teeth acting in combination; and the number of teeth per inch.[9] The set of the saw blade indicates how the individual teeth of the blade are shaped (eg, are they bent to the left and right). If the teeth are bent left and right, the kerf created will be wider than the saw blade.[9] Examination of the kerf floor can reveal the set of the blade as well as the number of teeth per inch.[9] Examination of the kerf floor or kerf wall can also indicate polish, the amount of material waste, and the consistency of the cut and energy transfer, which are indicative of the saw's power (mechanized or manual), and examination of the kerf wall can indicate cut surface drift.[9] Uniformity of the cut can also indicate the power of the saw.[9] Distance between striae is not a sign of the number of teeth on a saw but instead the amount of force applied to the cut.[9] Regularly spaced striae can indicate a mechanized saw, while irregularly spaced, non-parallel striae that change direction can indicate a manual saw.[8,9]

> **PEARLS & PITFALLS**
>
> When a sharp force weapon damages the shaft of a long bone, the features described above are best identified; however, if the sharp force weapon injury involves the epiphysis, where spongy instead of cortical bone is found, the features described above are not identified (Figure 10.21).

OTHER FEATURES USED TO INTERPRET SHARP FORCE WOUND CHARACTERISTICS

The analysis of the features of the kerf may be used to identify the direction of the cut.[9] The direction of the saw cut has two components: direction of the blade stroke (direction of each stroke) and direction of saw progress, from initial contact with the bone to the terminal cut.[10] False start scratches, false start kerfs, or a breakaway spur (Figure 10.22) or notch indicates the direction of blade progress through the bone, while the direction of the cutting stroke is indicated by exit chipping. The breakaway spur is the projection of uncut bone at the terminal end of the cut, and its size can indicate the amount of force. For example, the heavy weight of a handheld circular saw or a chain saw will produce a large breakaway spur.[9] The exit chipping is most prominent on the side of the stroke emphasized by the

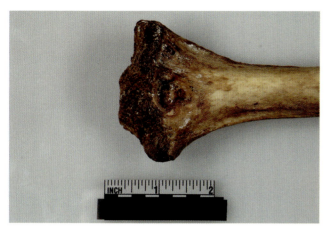

Figure 10.21. Cut mark at the epiphyseal end of the bone. The cut section involved the spongy bone and not the cortical bone, which does not produce the same findings on the bone as a cut mark on the thick cortical bone.

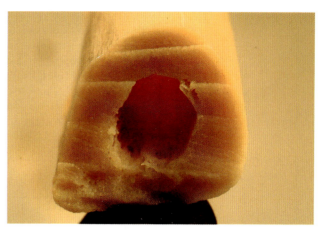

Figure 10.22. Breakaway spur. At the inferior edge of the cut mark is an irregular projection of bone, which is the breakaway spur. The size of the breakaway spur can help identify features of the saw used to cut the bone.

person using the saw (eg, emphasize of the push stroke, the cutting stroke for many saws, will produce chipping on the opposite side of the bone from the person using the saw). The passive stroke usually does not produce exit chipping.[9,10] Also, as they are indicative of the direction of travel of the blade, the residual striae on the kerf wall are oriented perpendicular to the kerf floor with cleavers, while the striae produced by saws and knives (with a cutting stroke) are oriented parallel to the kerf floor.[7] The documentation and subsequent analysis of the bony features of sharp force injuries on the bone are best done by a forensic anthropologist with specific training and experience in such injury patterns.

PEARLS & PITFALLS

While knives are the most common weapon used when a decedent sustains sharp force injuries, numerous other weapons can cause sharp force injuries, including stab wounds. These weapons include objects such as boat propellers, scissors (both open and closed), an ice pick, screwdrivers (both regular and Phillips), and arrows. Each can produce features different than other stab wounds, such as two blunt angles in a stab wound with closed scissors, although a regular screwdriver could produce a similar injury (Figure 10.23). Stab wounds with an ice pick could mimic gunshot wounds.

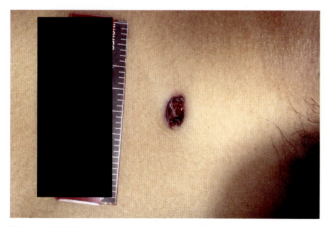

Figure 10.23. Stab wound with scissors. This stab wound was caused by closed scissors. Both angles are blunt. Just based upon the appearance of the wound, potentially a regular screwdriver or a small chisel could produce a similar wound.

> **PEARLS & PITFALLS**
>
> When examining the body of a decedent who died as the result of sharp force injuries, it is important to pay particular close attention to the hands. The identification of incised wounds or stab wounds of the hands can offer good support to help determine the manner of death. Injuries to the hands can occur when a decedent raises their hands to protect themself from the blows, but injuries to the hands can also occur when an attacker cuts themself by slipping on the blood-slicked weapon (Figure 10.24A and B).

NEAR MISSES

Near Miss #1: If a decedent is identified with a homicidal stab wound of the extremity with resultant fracture of the underlying bone, one question that the forensic pathologist may be asked during court proceedings is if the stab wound broke the bone, or if the stab wound resulted in the blade sticking in the bone, with a subsequent fall or other event breaking the bone. In the first case, the decedent would be unable to use their involved extremity effectively, whereas in the second case, the decedent would be able to use their involved extremity for some time after the infliction of the stab wound. Based solely upon the radiologic and gross examinations that are normally conducted with an autopsy, this question would be difficult to answer. However, removal of the bone with subsequent de-fleshing can provide features that may be able to answer that question (Figure 10.25A-F). The features of the humerus (no defect corresponding to the blade at the point of entry into the bone and a small rectangular defect at the point opposite entry, and from which the tip of the knife protruded) are consistent with the knife breaking the bone when it struck it.

Near Miss #2: This individual was alive at the time of a dog mauling, which was shown through the identification of bruises with evidence of hemorrhage. This injury was identified on the neck and could easily be interpreted as a stab wound (Figure 10.26).

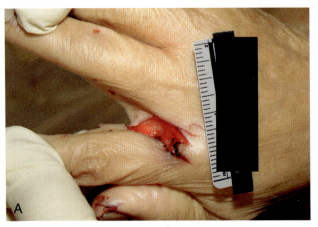
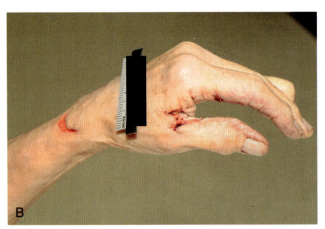

Figure 10.24. Defensive-type injuries of the upper extremities. In (**A** and **B**) are incised wounds of the hands and wrists, often involving the depths between two digits. The finding of defensive-type injuries on the hands can significantly assist with the determination of homicide vs suicide in a sharp force injuries related death, and, when in the depths between the fingers, could easily be covered with blood if the hands are not well cleaned and well inspected.

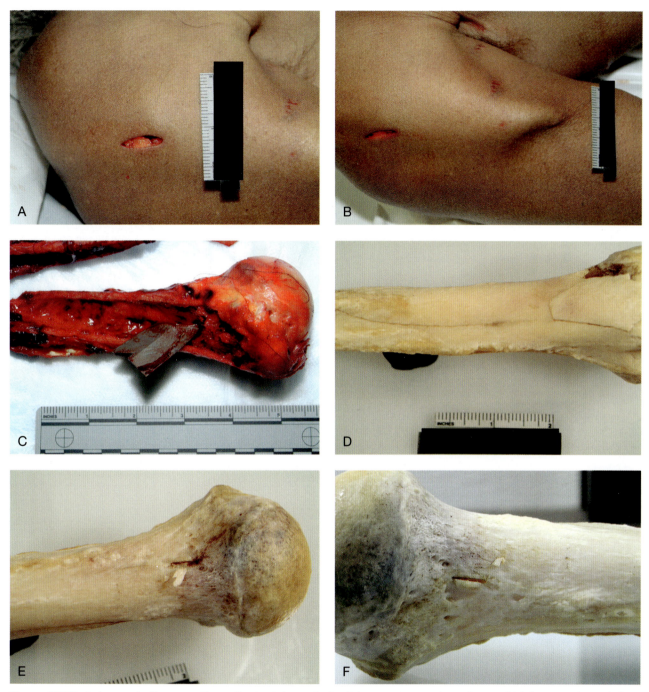

Figure 10.25. Stab wound of humerus. Externally, the right arm had a defect consistent with a stab wound (**A**); however, the underlying humerus was fractured (**B**), which could have created an open fracture, which could mimic a stab wound. A knife was embedded in the humerus (**C**). The humerus was removed at autopsy to potentially identify a pattern that might indicate how the fracture occurred. When the humerus was reconstructed, at the point where the knife entered the humerus, no slitlike defect matching the width of the knife was present (**D**). However, on the opposite side, there was a slitlike defect that matched the width of the knife at the tip (**E** and **F**).

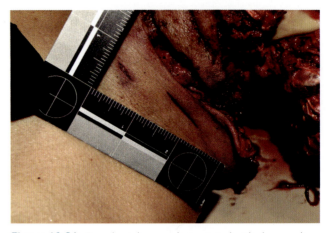

Figure 10.26. Pseudo-stab wound associated with dog mauling. The decedent was mauled by a dog. Contusions associated with the bite marks allowed for the determination that the decedent was alive at the time of the dog mauling. Adjacent to the defects of the neck created by the dog bites was a slitlike defect that could easily be misinterpreted as a stab wound (Figure 10.26).

References

1. Bolliger SA, Ruder TD, Ketterer T, Gläser N, Thali MJ, Ampanozi G. Comparison of stab wound probing versus radiological stab wound channel depiction with contrast medium. *Forensic Sci Int.* 2014;234:45-49.
2. Agarwal SS, Kumar L, Chavali KH, Mestri SC. Fatal venous air embolism following intravenous infusion. *J Forensic Sci.* 2009;54(3):682-684.
3. Banasr A, de la Grandmaison GL, Durigon M. Frequency of bone/cartilage lesions in stab and incised wounds fatalities. *Forensic Sci Int.* 2003;131(2-3):131-133.
4. Love JC, Derrick SM, Wiersema JM, Peters C. Validation of tool mark analysis of cut costal cartilage. *J Forensic Sci.* 2012;57(2):306-311.
5. Delabarde T, Cannet C, Raul JS, Géraut A, Taccoen M, Ludes B. Bone and soft tissue histology: a new approach to determine characteristics of offending instrument in sharp force injuries. *Int J Legal Med.* 2017;131(5):1313-1323.
6. deGruchy S, Rogers TL. Identifying chop marks on cremated bone: a preliminary study. *J Forensic Sci.* 2002;47(5):933-936.
7. Humphrey JH, Hutchinson DL. Macroscopic characteristics of hacking trauma. *J Forensic Sci.* 2001;46(2):228-233.
8. Komar DA, Buikstra JE. *Forensic Anthropology: Contemporary Theory and Practice.* Oxford University Press; 2008.
9. Symes SA, Chapman EN, Rainwater CW, et al. *Knife and Saw Toolmark Analysis in Bone: A Manual Designed for the Examination of Criminal Mutilation and Dismemberment.* US. Department of Justice; 2010. Award number 2005-IJ-CX-K016, Document number: 232864.
10. Symes SA, Berryman HE, Smith OC. Saw marks in bone: introduction and examination of residual kerf contour. In: Reichs KJ, ed. *Forensic Osteology: Advances in the Identification of Human Remains.* 2nd ed. Charles C. Thomas; 1998.
11. Lynn KS, Fairgrieve SI. Macroscopic analysis of axe and hatchet trauma in fleshed and defleshed mammalian long bones. *J Forensic Sci.* 2009;54(4):786-792.

FIREARM INJURY 11

CHAPTER OUTLINE

Introduction 292

Radiography 292
- Basics of Radiography in Firearm Injuries 292
- Specific Radiographic Findings Associated With Certain Types of Weapons 293

External Examination 299
- Overall Patterns of Injury to the Body 299

Interpretation of Gunshot Wound Patterns in the Skin 306
- Entrance Wounds for Handguns/Rifles 306
- Exit Wounds for Handguns/Rifles 310
- Features of Wound That Allow for General Determination of Range of Fire 316
- Special Types of Gunshot Wounds 325
  - Graze Wound 326
  - Tangential Wound 326
  - Superficial Perforating Wound 327
  - Re-Entrance Wound/Atypical Wound 327

Entrance and Exit Wounds for Shotguns and Relative Range of Fire 332
- Features of the Shotgun Wound That Allow for Determination of Relative Range of Fire 333

Internal Examination 337

Mechanism of Death in Gunshot Wounds 340

Composition of Projectiles 342

Manner of Death Determination With Gunshot Wounds 344

Near Misses 346

INTRODUCTION

Injuries from three main types of firearms are encountered by forensic pathologists: wounds caused by handguns, rifles, or shotguns. Other weapons, such as zip guns, are also rarely encountered.[1,2] Handguns can be small, medium, or large caliber, with 0.22, 0.38, and 0.45 caliber handguns respective examples of the three types. While some authors recommend describing handguns and rifles with their exact velocity,[3] for the purpose of basic review, rifles can be high-velocity/high-powered (eg, 30-06) or low-velocity/low-powered (eg, 0.22). Shotguns that are encountered are commonly 0.410 gauge, 12 gauge, and 20 gauge, and can shoot variable types of projectiles (eg, slugs, buckshot, and birdshot).

The overall evaluation for wounds sustained from each of the three types of weapons is similar, comprising radiography, external examination to (1) identify the wound itself, (2) distinguish entrance from exit, and (3) determine a relative range, and internal examination to identify the pathway of the projectile through the body, including direction of the projectile and organs injured. The interpretation of the pattern of the radiographic findings, the skin changes, and the injuries to the body allows the pathologist to identify the general weapon type, an entrance wound vs an exit wound, a relative range of fire, and the injuries caused. The term "relative range" is used in this chapter to indicate the general proximity of the weapon to the body (eg, contact or close) and not a specific range (eg, 6 inches or 2 feet). Interpretation of the overall pattern of autopsy findings in context with the scene investigation allows the pathologist to determine the cause and manner of death in individuals who have died as the result of a firearm injury.

As a component of the external examination, examination of the clothing and its collection for evidentiary purposes is performed and, as a component of the internal examination, the projectile and/or projectile fragments are recovered for evidentiary purposes.

CHECKLIST for Evaluation of a Firearm Injury (in addition to those for a general forensic autopsy)

- ☐ Radiographs of the body to identify projectiles and associated changes (eg, fractures, blood accumulation in body cavities).
- ☐ If requested by investigators or per office policy, collection of gunshot residue kit.
- ☐ Removal and examination of the clothing and retention as evidence when requested by investigators (or as per office policy).
- ☐ Examine the wounds to determine entrance and exit and relative range of the firearm injury based upon skin and other changes.
- ☐ Determine pathway of the projectile(s) through the body and identify the injuries caused.
- ☐ Collect projectile(s) both within the body and outside the body (ie, within the clothing).

RADIOGRAPHY

BASICS OF RADIOGRAPHY IN FIREARM INJURIES

Radiographs of the body of a decedent with a firearm injury serve several useful purposes: (1) potential identification of the weapon type, sometimes with very specific correlation (eg, one form of 0.25 ACP (Automatic Colt Pistol) ammunition, a Winchester Expanding Point); (2) identification of the location of the projectile to aid in recovery; (3) identification of injuries and other findings associated with the firearm wound, such as fractures, air embolus, pneumothorax, or hemothorax (Figure 11.1); and (4) potential assistance as to determination of the pathway of the projectile. For small-caliber handguns (eg, 0.22 and 0.25) and for some forms of larger-caliber projectiles (eg, wadcutter and semi-wadcutter), the projectile is often lead or lead with a copper gilding, with no separate copper jacket present. For larger-caliber weapons, the projectile most often consists of a lead core and a copper jacket. Copper and lead have two distinct appearances on a radiograph (Figure 11.2). Lead is more radio-dense than copper and thus will appear more white on a radiograph, whereas copper is less radio-dense than lead and will appear more transparent on a radiograph. If a copper jacket, specifically from the base of the projectile, is present, it should be recovered, as the copper jacket will have the rifling marks that will potentially allow a firearm examiner to match the projectile recovered from the body to the firearm that was used. If no copper jacket is present, then the lead or copper-gilded lead projectile will have the rifling marks.

SPECIFIC RADIOGRAPHIC FINDINGS ASSOCIATED WITH CERTAIN TYPES OF WEAPONS

Certain types of handgun/rifle ammunition and the three basic types of shotgun ammunition can each produce characteristic patterns on the radiograph. For shotguns, the three main types of ammunition are slugs, buckshot, and birdshot. A slug is one large projectile, which can fragment, and, on radiograph, will most characteristically have a C shape (Figure 11.3). Buckshot is large pellets, often present in multiples of three, with some newer ammunition having eight instead of nine pellets (Figure 11.4). Birdshot is smaller pellets than buckshot, with numerous tiny pellets present (Figure 11.5). High-powered rifles will most often produce a "lead snowstorm" pattern, with the projectile often partially breaking up into numerous tiny fragments but with a bulk of the projectile still usually contained within one fragment (Figure 11.6). Ratshot or snakeshot (essentially a small shotgun shell but fired by a handgun or rifle) will have numerous small pellets (Figure 11.7). A 0.25 ACP Winchester Expanding Point round will have a main projectile fragment, similar to a handgun or rifle projectile but also a single pellet (Figure 11.8). A Glaser round will have a main projectile fragment, which is a copper jacket, and numerous small pellets (Figure 11.9). Frangible projectiles will break up entirely or nearly entirely after entry into the body, with only those tiny fragments available for collection (Figures 11.10A-B and 11.10C-D). R.I.P. ammunition (Radically Invasive Projectile), termed a trocar round, manufactured by G2 Research and a Liberty Ammunition Civil Defense round each have a nose that breaks apart into several small fragments (Figure 11.11A and B), with each fragment becoming an independent projectile, and a base, which also continues to penetrate into the body.[4]

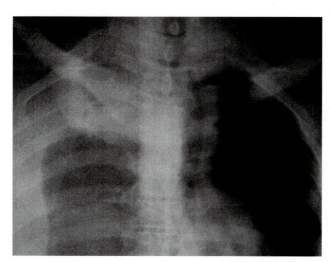

Figure 11.1. Radiograph of a decedent with a gunshot wound. The right pleural cavity is filled with blood (ie, a hemothorax) and the left pleural cavity is filled with air (ie, a pneumothorax), with both findings being caused by the gunshot wound. The trachea is deviated to the left side.

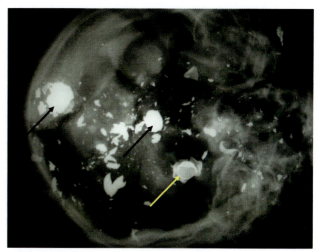

Figure 11.2. Radiograph of decedent with multiple gunshots. The lead core fragments (black arrows) are distinguishable from the copper jacket fragments (yellow arrow), with the copper jacket fragments being less radio-dense. Although all fragments of significant size should be recovered, it is most important to recover the copper jacket fragments as they will bear the rifling marks that will allow the firearm examiner to match the projectile(s) recovered from the body to the suspected weapon used. The fragment of most importance is the base of the projectile, as that is the fragment which will bear the rifling marks.

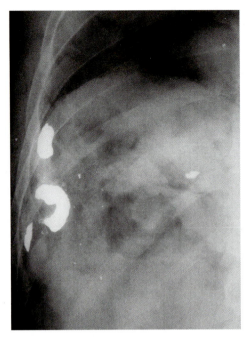

Figure 11.3. Radiograph of decedent shot with shotgun slug. A shotgun slug is fired as one large projectile, which can break into fragments while passing through the body. The most characteristic radiographic finding of a shotgun slug injury is a C-shaped fragment.

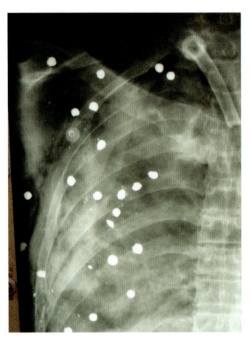

Figure 11.4. Radiograph of decedent shot with buckshot. Buckshot is similar to birdshot in that there are numerous pellets instead of a single projectile; however, the pellets are much larger and are often found in multiples of three, assuming that all fired pellets strike the decedent and can therefore all be identified at autopsy (ie, if any pellets in the group do not hit the decedent it would not be known exactly how many buckshot pellets were fired from the shell). Buckshot pellets vary from size 12, which is 0.24 inches each, to size 000, which is 0.36 inches each.

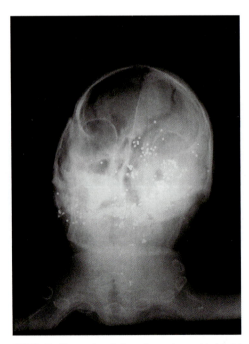

Figure 11.5. Radiograph of decedent shot with birdshot. The charge from the shotgun shell is composed of numerous tiny pellets, which range in size based upon the shotgun shell type. For birdshot, the pellets range from shot size 12, which is 0.05 inches each, to shot size BB, which is 0.180 inches each. Around 10 to 20 pellets should be recovered so that the ammunition type can be determined by the firearm examiner.

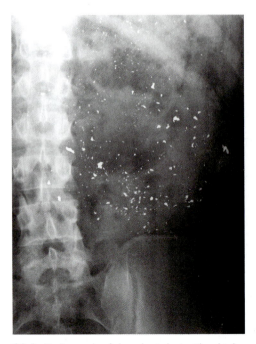

Figure 11.6. Radiograph of decedent shot with a high-powered rifle. With most high-powered rifle ammunition, a large fragment of the projectile with the base that has the rifling marks can be identified (although one is not visible in this radiograph); however, a lead snowstorm pattern is the characteristic feature of this weapon. The lead snowstorm pattern is created by a portion of the projectile breaking up into innumerable small fragments.

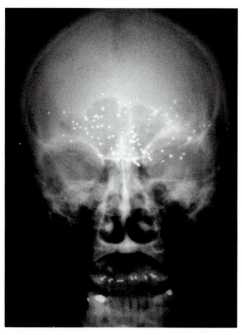

Figure 11.7. Radiograph of a decedent shot with snakeshot. Snakeshot or ratshot is a handgun or rifle type projectile filled with numerous tiny pellets, like a small shotgun shell. The appearance of the radiograph is similar to the radiograph of a decedent shot with birdshot from a shotgun; however, fewer pellets are present.

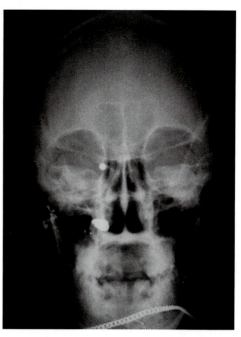

Figure 11.8. Radiograph of decedent shot with 0.25 ACP, Winchester Expanding Point ammunition. The projectile includes a lead core and a single large pellet. ACP, Automatic Colt Pistol.

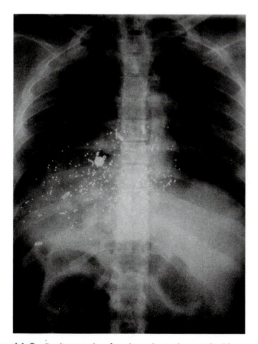

Figure 11.9. Radiograph of a decedent shot with Glaser round. The projectile consists of a hollow copper jacket filled with numerous tiny pellets and capped with a blue plastic cap. While the copper jacket portion and the pellets are visible on radiograph, the blue plastic cap will not be visible. Its presence must be suspected by the general appearance of the radiograph and then searched for and hopefully identified during the autopsy.

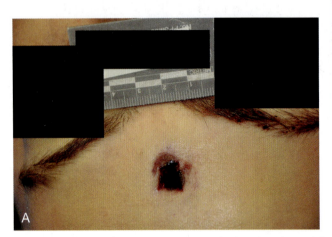
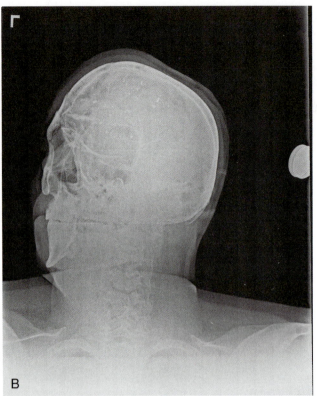

Figure 11.10A-B. Image and radiograph of a decedent shot with frangible ammunition. The decedent had a gunshot wound of the forehead (**A**). However, the frangible projectile fired from the 0.223 rifle completely broke up, leaving no fragment of significant size to recover (**B**). Encountering this form of ammunition can be disconcerting for the forensic pathologist, as the body will have an entrance wound and no exit wound, yet no large projectile fragment to recover. The numerous tiny fragments can be recovered as best as possible, but, with no base with rifling present to match to the suspected weapon, the evidentiary value is minimal.

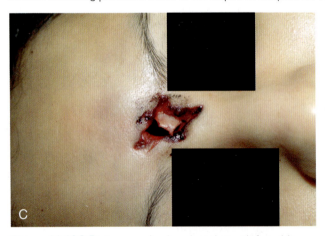
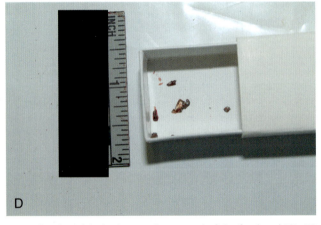

Figure 11.10C-D. Images of a decedent shot with frangible ammunition. The decedent had a gunshot wound of the forehead (**C**). (**D**) shows the fragments that were recovered during the autopsy, with no large fragment with rifling marks present.

FAQ: Should all decedents with a firearm injury have radiographs obtained?

Answer: Yes, radiographs can help identify the cause of the wound (ie, weapon type) and can help the pathologist locate the evidentiary material (ie, the projectile or projectile fragments). Even when an entrance wound and exit wound are both present, radiography should be performed, as important fragments of the projectile (eg, the copper jacket, if it has separated from the lead core, or a fragment of the copper jacket) may still remain in the body (Figure 11.12A and B). In addition to anterior-posterior radiographs, lateral radiographs can also be very useful in helping to pinpoint the location of the projectile in the body (Figure 11.13A and B). Also, in offices without access to a full-body radiography instrument, numerous radiographs can be printed and combined to produce an overall radiographic map of the body to help locate projectiles (Figure 11.14).

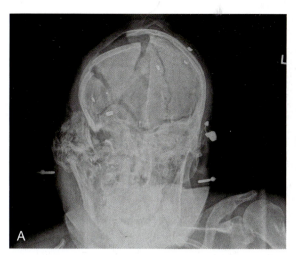
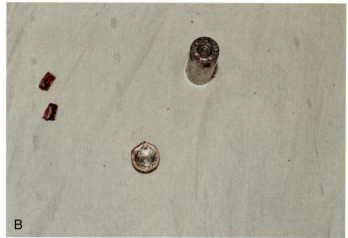

Figure 11.11. Radiograph of decedent shot with Liberty Ammunition Civil Defense round and image of cartridge and projectile recovery. The nose of the projectile is composed of numerous leaflets of copper jacket that break loose from the reminder of the projectile after penetration into the body, accounting for the numerous fragments on radiograph (**A**). The base of the projectile is a round disk. As best as possible, each fragment should be recovered; however, the base of the projectile has the rifling marks. In (**B**) are the fired cartridge case, the disklike base of the projectile, and two of the fragments of the copper jacket nose.

> **PEARLS & PITFALLS**
>
> It is best to x-ray a body with a known or suspected firearm(s) injury prior to removal of the clothing and even prior to removal of the body from the body bag. The projectile may have passed completely through the body but be caught up in the clothing (Figure 11.15A and B) or be loose in the body bag. If its presence is not identified prior to removal of the clothing, the projectile may be lost during removal of the clothing.

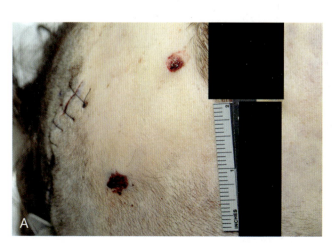
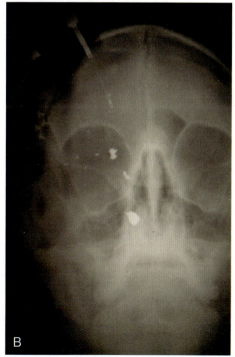

Figure 11.12. Image and radiograph of a decedent shot in the head. In (**A**), the scalp has both an entrance (the anteriorly located wound in the image) and an exit wound. When the projectile struck the cranium, it separated into a copper jacket and a lead core, with the lead core penetrating into the brain and the copper jacket exiting the scalp. (**B**) is a radiograph of the head revealing the fragments of the lead core of the projectile.

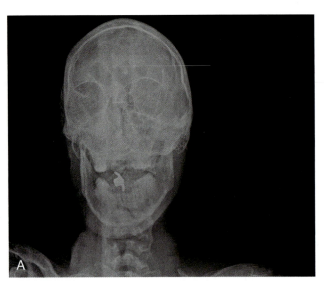 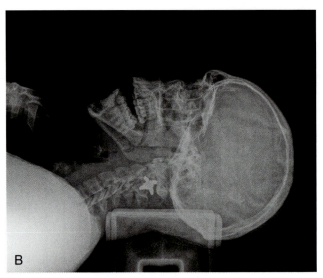

Figure 11.13. Radiographs of decedent with intra-oral gunshot wound, with projectile in neck. With an anterior-posterior oriented radiograph only, it is not possible to pinpoint the exact location of the projectile in the body (A); however, with a lateral image in combination with the anterior-posterior image, it is possible to pinpoint the location (B). Using a laterally oriented radiograph can save the forensic pathologist time and frustration by preventing searching for a projectile in the wrong location.

PEARLS & PITFALLS

While the copper and lead components of the projectile are easily identified on radiographs, other components of a projectile may not be apparent. The shot sleeve (or, shot cup) of a shotgun shell is made of plastic and the wadding can be made of a cardboard (Figure 11.16). The blue tip of a Glaser round and the plastic red tip found in a Hornaby Personal Defense Round will not show up on radiograph (Figure 11.17). In addition, some forms of projectiles (eg, aluminum) will not show up on a radiograph. Only a heightened level of suspicion, knowledge of the ammunition type, or some degree of thoroughness and/or luck during the dissection, all used in correlation with the autopsy findings, will allow for the identification and collection of these projectiles and projectile fragments. Another important and related consideration is that the jacket and core may separate and, if this situation is not recognized, one portion may not be recovered at autopsy. One clue that this has happened is that if only a lead core is recovered and that lead core does not have rifling marks then a jacket is most likely also present and should be searched for and recovered.

PEARLS & PITFALLS

General radiographs of the body, in addition to those in the vicinity of the wounds and the apparent pathway of the projectile, may be useful as they could help to identify a bullet embolus (Figure 11.18A and B), or another finding of interest (eg, an air embolus in the case of a gunshot wound of the neck (Figure 11.19A and B)). Bullet emboli can occur in a variety of circumstances, for example, entry into the heart or the aorta or another artery, with embolization to a distal location,[5-11] or entry into a vein, with subsequent embolization to heart or lung[12,13] or the arterial system through a patent foramen ovale.[14] In addition to embolization, aspiration of the projectile can also occur and projectiles can pass into the bladder.[15,16] Tandem projectiles can also occur (ie, two projectiles fired from one shot); thus, the decedent may have one entrance wound but two projectiles within the body. A similar situation could arise with overlapping gunshot wounds, in which the entrance of two separate gunshot wounds overlap, creating the appearance of a single entrance wound.

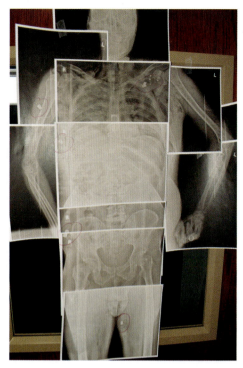

Figure 11.14. Radiographs of the decedent. Numerous radiographs of the decedent covering the majority or entirety of the body can be obtained, printed, and combined into one overall radiographic map of the body, which can help ensure all projectiles are recovered.

EXTERNAL EXAMINATION

OVERALL PATTERNS OF INJURY TO THE BODY

During the external examination, the pathologist will determine (1) whether wounds from a firearm injury are an entrance wound or an exit wound, and (2) a relative range of fire for the wound (ie, relative distance of the weapon from the body when it was fired [contact, close, etc.]). The actual distance of the weapon from the body is determined by the firearm examiner who test fires the weapon at sequential ranges and compares the distribution of gunpowder residue to that found on the body (if any). Cleaning the entrance and exit

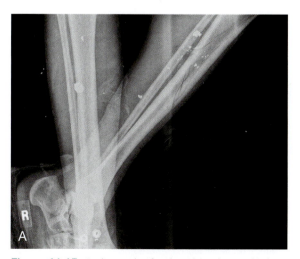
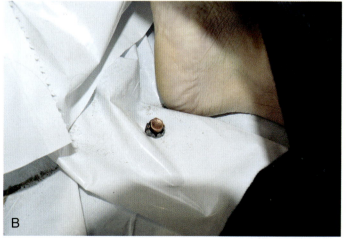

Figure 11.15. Radiograph of a decedent shot in the lower extremity and gross photograph of the clothing. When radiographs of the body were obtained, a projectile was identified that appeared to be in the right lower extremity (**A**). When the clothing was removed, the projectile was found within the clothing (**B**). If the presence of the projectile had not been known prior to removal of the clothing, the projectile may have been lost during the autopsy.

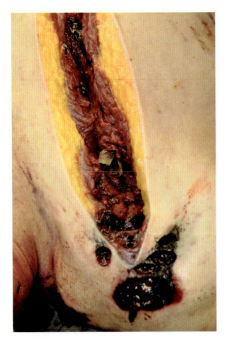

Figure 11.16. Decedent shot with a shotgun at a close range. Within the tissue is the plastic shot sleeve. The shot sleeve will not appear on radiograph so its presence must be suspected based upon the overall injury pattern to allow it to be identified during the autopsy. The shot sleeve can fragment and one or more of the plastic leaves may be separated from the main portion.

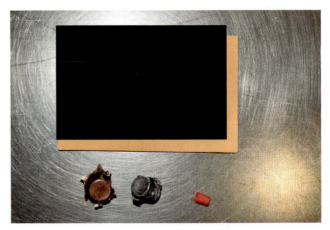

Figure 11.17. Decedent shot with type of ammunition with a plastic nose. In addition to the main projectile, with a copper jacket and a lead core, which separated in the body, at the tip of the projectile is a small rod of red plastic. This small rod of red plastic will not appear on a radiograph, but can be found at autopsy and would assist with identification of the ammunition type.

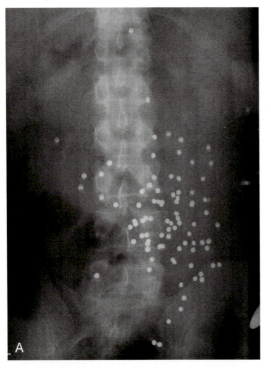
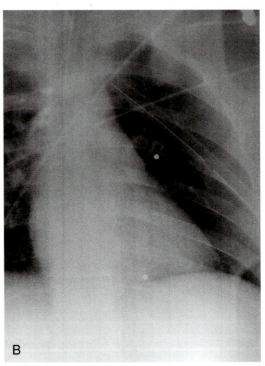

Figure 11.18. Radiographs of a decedent shot with birdshot. The main concentration of the pellets is centered on the abdomen (**A**); however, two pellets were found near the heart (**B**). They arrived at this location by penetrating into the vasculature and being carried by the flow of blood to their resting location (ie, a bullet embolus). Emboli can turn a non-lethal wound into a lethal wound. With a patent foramen ovale, a single pellet could enter the venous system, be carried to the right side of the heart, cross over into the left atrium, and embolize to a coronary artery or cerebral artery, causing death.

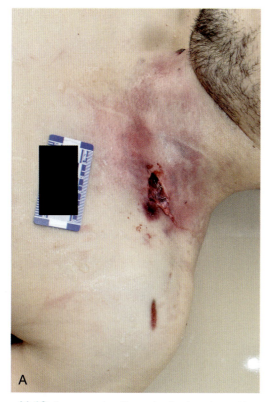
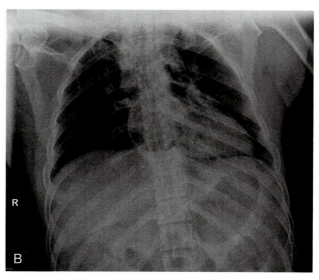

Figure 11.19. Image and radiograph of a decedent with a gunshot wound of the neck. (**A**) shows the gunshot wound of the neck. (**B**) is a radiograph of the chest, which reveals an air embolus. With a gunshot wound or stab/incised wound of the neck, obtaining a radiograph of the chest is useful as it may identify an air embolus.

wounds of extraneous blood is necessary prior to final examination of the defects, and will markedly improve one's ability to correctly examine the wound (Figure 11.20A and B). Given the tenacious nature of dried blood, care must be taken when removing that blood so as to prevent loss of important features (eg, soot on the skin). As such, certain techniques may help to preserve changes on the skin.[17]

The external examination can include evaluation of the clothing, which can potentially assist in determination of entrance vs exit and relative range for the wound. Sometimes soot

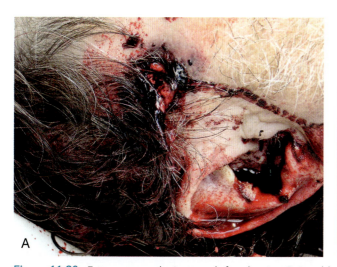
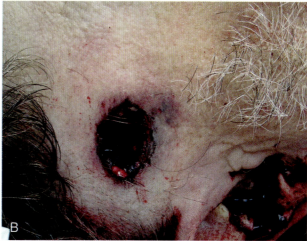

Figure 11.20. Entrance wound prior to and after cleaning. Being able to search for the patterns at the skin surface that allow for interpretation of entrance vs exit and relative range of fire depends upon sufficient preparation of the wound. (**A** and **B**) illustrate how features become much more apparent after the wound is cleaned. To best examine and subsequently photograph the wound for documentation purposes, blood (liquid, clotted, and dried) and scalp hair (or other body hair present) should be removed to provide for the best visualization of the gunshot wound. If determination of range is challenging, the hair that is shaved from around the wound can be retained for examination for gunshot residue by the firearm examiner.

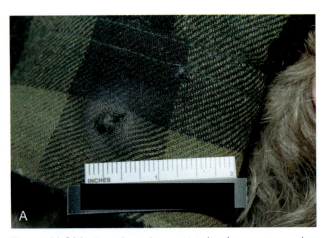

Figure 11.21A. Decedent who sustained a close range gunshot wound of the left upper extremity. Near the end of the shirt sleeve is an irregular circular defect in the clothing surrounded by a fine gray-black powder, which is soot.

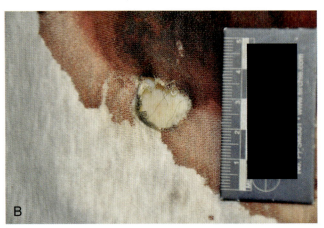

Figure 11.21B. Decedent who sustained a contact self-inflicted shotgun wound. The circular defect in the shirt has a rim of black, which is soot from the discharge of the shotgun. However, bullet wipe could appear very similar, rubbing off on the clothing at the very edge of the entrance defect.

or gunpowder will not be present on the skin surface around the wound, but will be present on the clothing; however, bullet wipe, from the material on the surface of the projectile rubbing off onto the clothing, can be present and must not be confused with soot, as bullet wipe would not be specific to a certain range of fire (Figure 11.21A and B).

By external examination, one common overall pattern is that of an extensively damaged head, with gaping lacerations of the scalp, complex and widespread fractures of the cranium, and avulsion of the brain from the cranial cavity (ie, the head is blown open). This pattern is produced most frequently by contact or intra-oral shotgun wounds or contact or intra-oral high-powered rifle wounds and is due to the expulsion of gas and smoke upon discharge of the weapon and the higher damaging capacity of these two weapons at a contact or intra-oral range (Figure 11.22). Even given the destruction of the head, the tissue can be re-approximated and the entrance defect identified (Figure 11.23A-D). Handguns and 0.22 caliber rifles would not normally produce such a wound (Figure 11.24). Thus, even the overall pattern of a firearm injury, without examining the specific details of the skin surface at the wounds, can guide a forensic pathologist toward the weapon type used in the death.

External examination of the body where the decedent has sustained a firearm injury also includes collection of evidence. Specific to a firearm injury is collection of the clothing, especially the clothing item(s) where the projectile passed through, and sampling the skin of the hands for gunshot residue.

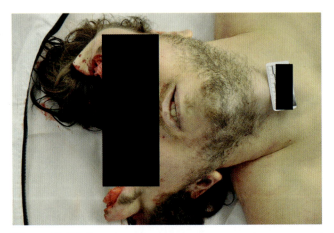

Figure 11.22. Decedent who sustained a contact shotgun wound of the head. The head is extensively damaged, with multiple lacerations of the scalp, extensive and comminuted fractures of the cranium, and avulsion of the brain.

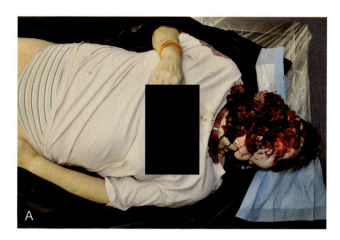
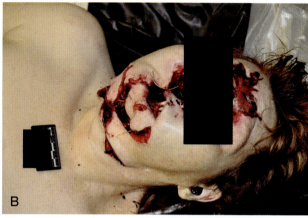
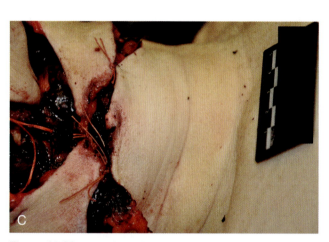
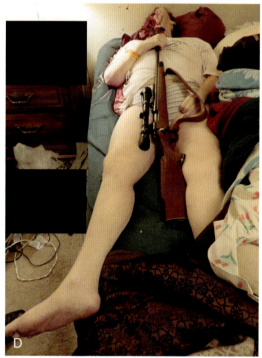

Figure 11.23. Decedent who shot themself with a high-powered rifle. Like a contact shotgun wound, the head is extensively damaged with multiple lacerations of the scalp and comminuted fractures of the cranium resulting in a near complete loss of the anterior portion of the head (**A**). As with a contact shotgun wound of the head, the tissue can be re-approximated (**B**) to help identify the entrance site (**C**). In this case, the entrance wound was at the chin. The marginal abrasion and some soot deposition are visible. While the entrance wound in such situations can essentially always be found, the exit wound may not be identified. Given the usual lack of abrasion ring or gunshot residue at the exit wound, the slitlike or stellate nature of an exit wound can easily be obscured by the other damage to the scalp. The scene photograph confirms the autopsy findings (**D**).

PEARLS & PITFALLS

While contact or intra-oral high-powered rifle wounds and contact or intra-oral shotgun wounds most often cause extensive damage to the head, with the scalp extensively lacerated, the cranium extensively fractured, and the brain often avulsed, and contact range or intra-oral handgun wounds most frequently do not cause nearly as extensive of damage, the head can be intact with a contact or intra-oral shotgun wound and can be extensively damaged (ie, with the cranial cavity open) with a contact or intra-oral handgun wound (Figure 11.25A and B).

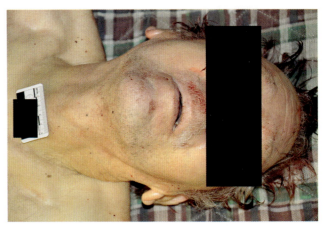

Figure 11.24. Decedent who sustained a contact gunshot wound of the head. In comparison to Figure 11.23A, this individual shot themselves with a handgun. Low-caliber weapons (eg, 0.22) will often only have an entrance wound, whereas high-caliber weapons (eg, a 9 mm) will often have an entrance and exit wound, but while they can have numerous fractures of the cranium, the overall general structure of the head itself is most often intact.

FAQ: Will gunshot residue testing help to distinguish a suicide from a homicide?

Answer: Gunshot residue testing will determine if an individual was in a gunshot environment and, given the firearm injury of the body, that fact is already known. Testing for gunshot residue is accomplished by using a small plastic device (a stub) with a sticky pad on one surface to sample the skin, touching the sticky pad against the skin repeatedly at various points on the dorsal and ventral surface of the hands to collect potential residue. This stub is then analyzed by a forensic science laboratory using a scanning electron microscope to look for primer particles (including barium, antimony, and lead). It is possible for an individual who is shot by another person to have gunshot residue on their hands, depending upon how close they were to the shooter, and it is possible for an individual who shot themselves to not have gunshot residue on their hands. Technically, gunshot residue testing could complicate an investigation. If gunshot residue testing is performed on an individual who by autopsy correlated with investigative findings is certainly a suicide, and that gunshot residue testing result is negative (ie, no gunshot residue is identified), family members, especially if they already suspect a homicide, may dispute the results of the investigation, and refuse to accept

---

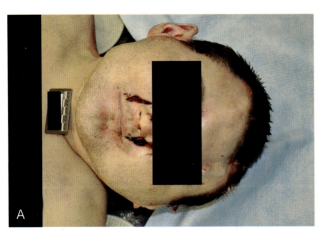
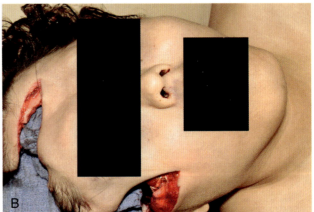

Figure 11.25. Decedents who sustained an intra-oral shotgun wound and a contact range 0.40 caliber handgun wound. In (**A**), although the weapon used was a shotgun, the head is relatively intact and the scalp is not widely lacerated; however, the cranium is extensively fractured. In (**B**), although the weapon used was a handgun, the head is extensively lacerated, the cranium markedly fractured, and the brain partially avulsed from the cranial cavity.

the determination of a suicide. Gunshot residue testing does have application in investigations however. If an individual reports that they were not at the location of the gunshot wound or were some distance from the weapon when it went off, they should not have gunshot residue on their hands. If that person is suspected to have caused the injury, collection of a gunshot residue kit from them may assist with the investigation. Gunshot residue kits most often contain three stubs: one for each hand and one for the forehead. While just using the hands after firing a weapon can remove gunshot residue from the skin, the forehead is less frequently touched, and gunshot residue deposited here can linger for a longer time period.

FAQ: In a body with an entrance wound but no exit wound, is a complete autopsy required to recover the projectile?

Answer: Whether a complete autopsy is performed to evaluate a firearm injury is dependent upon office policies, the forensic pathologist's experience, and the circumstances of the death. In some cases of suicide, a forensic pathologist may be comfortable with an external examination only with a perforating gunshot wound or with a partial autopsy for recovery of the projectile only for evidentiary purposes (ie, to potentially match to a weapon if ever needed). The two most difficult substances for the projectile to perforate are bone and skin, so often a projectile will become lodged just underneath the skin on the opposite side of the body from the entrance wound and can be recovered with an incision in the skin (Figure 11.26A-C).

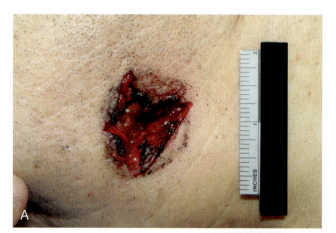
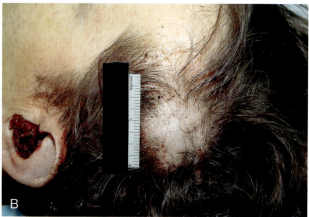
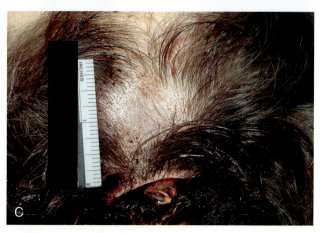

Figure 11.26. Recovery of projectile from underneath the skin. The individual sustained a contact range gunshot wound of the chin (**A**). The pathway of the projectile was from right to left, upward, and backward, with the projectile coming to rest just underneath the scalp in the left parietal region, noticeable as a bulge in the skin in (**B**) and revealed with an incision in the adjacent skin (**C**). Care should be taken to cut adjacent to the projectile and not over the projectile as, if the scalpel contacts the projectile, extraneous markings on the metal can be produced.

INTERPRETATION OF GUNSHOT WOUND PATTERNS IN THE SKIN

Introduction: While the radiography and overall appearance of the body may guide a forensic pathologist in their identification of a firearm injury as a cause of death, examination of the wound characteristics on the skin surface is vital to evaluation of the autopsy findings. With firearm injuries, once the location of the wound on the body has been determined, interpretation of the pattern of changes on the adjacent skin surface allows for determination of entrance wound vs exit wound and identification of features that will allow for a general determination of range of fire. The wounds are examined for the general shape of defect (eg, circular, stellate, slitlike), location on the body (with measurements from the top of the head or the sole of the foot to the wound, distance of the wound from the midline, and distance of the wound from the nearest fixed point (eg, a nipple) used to document the location of the wound), presence or absence of a marginal abrasion, the presence or absence of a muzzle abrasion, and presence or absence of soot or stippling (ie, soot, which is burned gunpowder, or stippling/powder tattooing, which is produced by unburned gunpowder striking the skin). In addition, carbon monoxide-induced discoloration of underlying musculature can assist in determination of a contact range firearm injury.

ENTRANCE WOUNDS FOR HANDGUNS/RIFLES

Pattern at autopsy: Classically, entrance wounds are a circular defect in the skin, which is usually completely surrounded by a rim of abrasion (ie, the marginal abrasion) (Figure 11.27). The circular defect is a permanent loss of tissue, with the tissue carried forward into the wound track and ejected backwards in the direction that the shot came from.[18] Soot will appear as a fine powder–like substance associated with the wound. Using soot to help determine range of fire will be discussed below, but the presence of soot at the skin defect assists in determination of entrance vs exit as well. Unburned gunpowder will strike the skin, sometimes embedding in the skin, producing a punctate, or dotlike, abrasion. This change is referred to as stippling or, with embedded gunpowder, powder tattooing. Like soot, using stippling to help determine range of fire will be discussed below, but the presence of stippling at the skin defect assists in determination of entrance vs exit as well. Of note, gunpowder residue can rarely be found at the exit[19] (Figure 11.28A and B). A muzzle abrasion will be a circular or semi-circular abrasion often slightly distant from the entrance defect and which surrounds or partially surrounds the wound (Figure 11.29A-D). A muzzle abrasion is characteristic of a contact entrance wound. Sometimes, specific details such as the sight at the end of the weapon or the recoil spring guide may create a more specific abrasion pattern (Figure 11.30A and B).

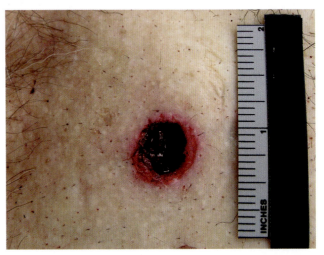

Figure 11.27. Entrance gunshot wound of the body. With a classic entrance-type gunshot wound, there is a central circular defect in the skin, which has a variably wide rim of marginal abrasion.

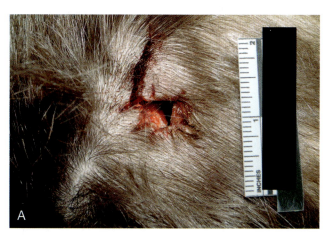
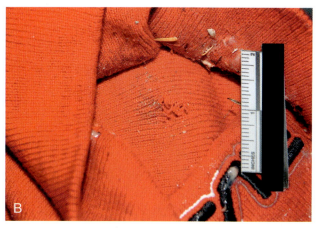

Figure 11.28. Exit gunshot wound with gunpowder. The decedent sustained a contact gunshot wound of the head, with the entrance a large gaping defect on the right side of the head, which was initially interpreted by the coroner as the exit. (**A**) shows the exit defect (with the hair unshaven in this image to preserve the gunpowder particles for photography). No marginal abrasion is present. (**B**) shows the inner surface of the snow-type cap the decedent was wearing with gunpowder being present.

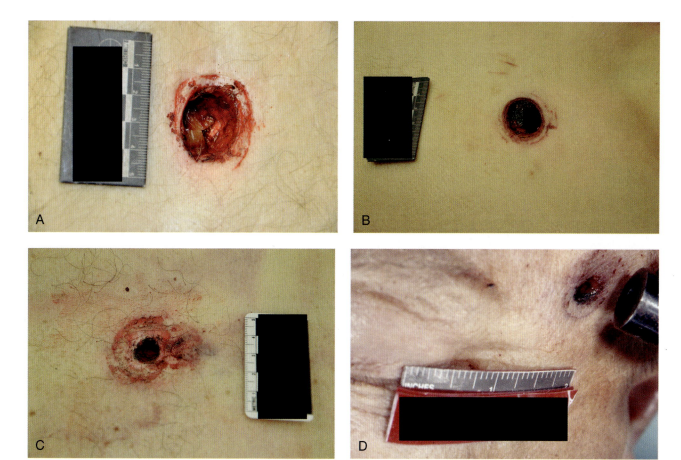

Figure 11.29. Entrance wound with muzzle abrasion. (**A**) is a contact shotgun wound of the chest with a muzzle abrasion, which is the nearly circumferential thin linear red discoloration on the skin just lateral to the wound. Other components of the end of the barrel such as the recoil spring guide or the gunsight can also leave an impression on the skin. (**B**) is a contact shotgun wound of the chest with a muzzle abrasion, but in which the sight impression is also present. (**C**) is a contact gunshot wound of the chest. The impression of the end of the firearm is present on the skin. (**D**) is an entrance gunshot wound with a muzzle abrasion. In this case, the impression of the end of the barrel is seen on the skin with soot on the skin as well. While images such as this with the causative weapon near the skin are good for demonstrative purposes, one must be careful that the weapon does not actually touch the skin, as that could allow for an argument of contamination of evidence.

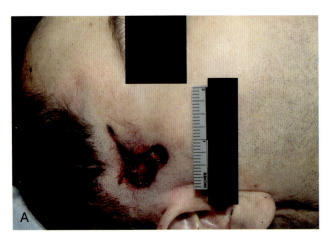 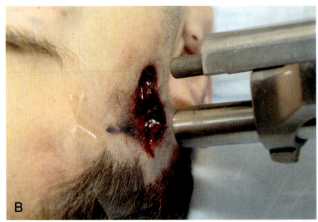

Figure 11.30. Entrance gunshot wound of the body with recoil spring guide injury. Although the recoil spring guide can cause a round abrasion on the skin adjacent to the entrance wound, in (A), it actually created a circular laceration adjacent to the gunshot wound, which, in combination with the marginal tear, caused the wound to appear larger. In (B), the weapon is compared to the entrance wound.

PEARLS & PITFALLS

When the projectile from a handgun or rifle enters the body perpendicular to the skin, the marginal abrasion will be a circumferential rim of uniform width; however, if the projectile enters the body at an angle, the marginal abrasion will be eccentric, wider in the direction from which the projectile entered the body (Figure 11.31). However, as the body at autopsy is usually not in the same position as the body when it was shot, caution must be used in interpreting an eccentric marginal abrasion. For example, a person who is moving when the projectile struck them may have skin folds that are different than when the body is being examined on a table at autopsy (Figure 11.32A and B).

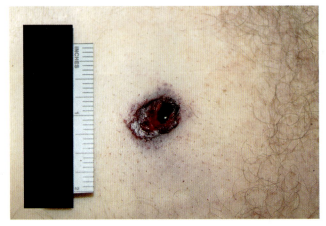

Figure 11.31. Entrance gunshot wound of the body with eccentric marginal abrasion. At 7 to 9 o'clock in the image, the marginal abrasion is much wider than elsewhere along the circumference of the wound. The projectile entered at an oblique angle to the skin, instead of perpendicular to the skin, entering from the side of the wider marginal abrasion.

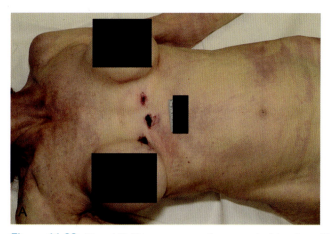 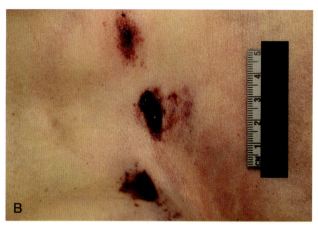

Figure 11.32. (**A** and **B**) Close range gunshot wound of the chest. This woman shot herself in the chest and the appearance of the wound illustrates the idea that the body at autopsy is not in the same position as when shot. There is a gunshot wound in the center of the chest and to each side, lateral and displaced from the entrance wound, are lesions of the skin and the medial surface of the right breast. Apparently, when the woman held the gun up to her chest, it compressed her skin and breasts together and more toward the center, allowing for the released hot gases to sear the skin.

FAQ: Can the caliber of the projectile be accurately estimated by the size of the entrance wound?

Answer: No, due to the elastic nature of the skin and variable anatomic properties of the target tissue the size of the entrance wound does not necessarily correspond to the caliber of the projectile[18]; however, the width of the abrasion ring can vary predictably with certain features of the weapon including projectile velocity.[20] In fact, even for gunshot wound defects in the bone, the size of the defect cannot reliably be used to predict the caliber of the projectile, although in any given case, certain calibers may be included or excluded.[21,22]

FAQ: Does surgical intervention block the ability to determine entrance wound and exit wound and relative range of fire?

Answer: While surgical intervention can obviously obscure features that allow for determination of entrance and exit wounds and relative range of fire, most often distinguishing features remain. For example, often when surgical intervention occurs, the fragment of cranium removed may be retained by the hospital and can be recovered from the hospital for examination. Also, even with surgical intervention, bony changes or presence of soot may remain, allowing for, in at least some cases, a proper evaluation of the gunshot wound as to entrance and exit, and relative range of fire.[23]

PEARLS & PITFALLS

Inexperienced observers often mistake entrance wounds for exit wounds based upon the size of the wound. A common misconception is that the exit wound is always larger than the entrance wound. While it is most often true for anything but contact range gunshot wounds of the head,[24] with contact gunshot wounds of the head, this is most often not true (Figure 11.33A-D). With a contact gunshot wound of the head, when the gases from the discharge of the weapon leave the barrel they enter the body and encounter the cranium, which forces the gases to extend laterally from the wound under the skin, which bulges the skin outward, causing it to tear. These tears can be quite extensive and make the entrance larger than the exit. Close re-approximation of the tips of the resultant skin tags allows for the identification of the entrance site, with the associated soot and marginal abrasion also being present. Also, examination of the underlying soft tissue and the dura and bone at the entrance defect will allow for the identification of soot as well as identification of a bevel.

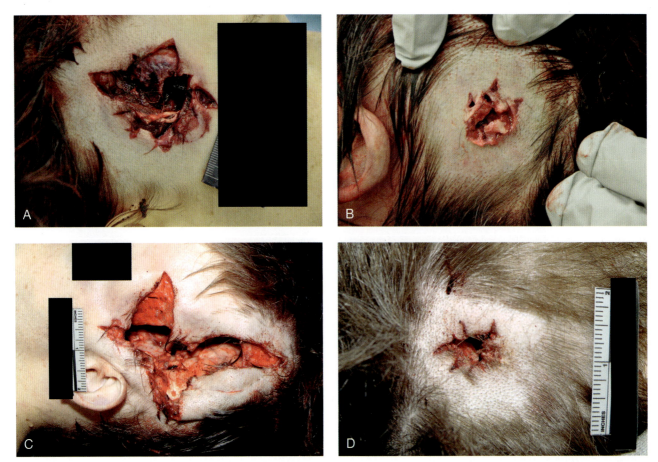

Figure 11.33. Two sets of entrance and exit gunshot wounds of the head. Images (**A** and **C**) are the entrances. One common misconception is that the exit wound is always larger than the entrance wound; however, with contact range gunshot wounds of the head, the entrance, due to marginal tears, is usually the larger of the two. In Image (**A**), the muzzle abrasion and recoil spring guide are faintly apparent as is soot. The tears are secondary to the contact nature of the wound in a portion of the body with underlying bone. With a contact gunshot wound, the hot air released along with the projectile enters the head, but, cannot penetrate deeper due to the presence of the cranium, and instead causes the skin to tent outward and tear, leading to a large wound. Re-approximation of the wound can identify a marginal abrasion and soot. In contrast, (**B** and **D**), which are the corresponding exits, have no marginal abrasions.

> **PEARLS & PITFALLS**
>
> Entrance wounds of certain portions of the body have a different appearance than the classic entrance wound described above. Entrance wounds on the palms of the hands or soles of the feet, given the presence of thick skin vs the normal thin skin, which covers the remainder of the body, have a different appearance (Figure 11.34); entrance wounds of the eye (Figure 11.35) and entrance wounds of the scrotum (Figure 11.36A and B) can be challenging to interpret.[25]

> **PEARLS & PITFALLS**
>
> Injuries other than gunshot wounds can potentially mimic a gunshot wound (Figures 11.37 and 11.38). A stab from an ice pick could mimic a 0.22 caliber wound. Open fractures can potentially also mimic a gunshot wound.[26]

EXIT WOUNDS FOR HANDGUNS/RIFLES

Pattern at autopsy: Classically, exit wounds are stellate or slitlike and have no rim of marginal abrasion (Figure 11.39A-C). There usually should be no soot or stippling on the skin surrounding an exit wound, although it is possible for soot and/or gunpowder to traverse the body from the entrance wound to the exit site. While exit wounds are most frequently slitlike or stellate, circular wounds are also possible (Figure 11.40A and B).

CHAPTER 11 FIREARM INJURY   311

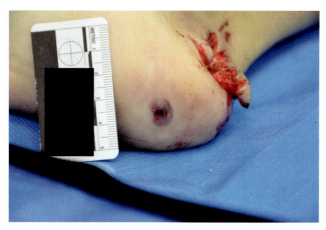

Figure 11.34. Decedent with a gunshot wound of the foot into the leg. The decedent was shot by her significant other. She apparently raised her right lower extremity between herself and him, and was shot in the sole of the foot. Unlike a typical entrance wound, there is no marginal abrasion. The thick skin of the sole of the foot (or palm of the hand) behaves differently than the thin skin covering the majority of the rest of the body.

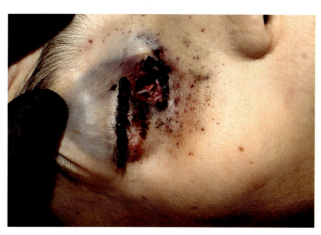

Figure 11.35. Decedent with close range gunshot wound of the right eye. While the presence of stippling/powder tattooing easily identifies the gunshot wound as an entrance, the typical features of an entrance gunshot wound (eg, the marginal abrasion) are not as apparent in the thin skin of the eyelid.

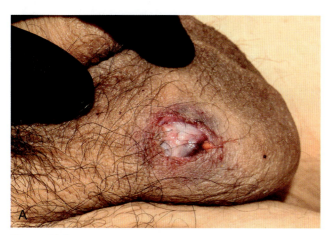

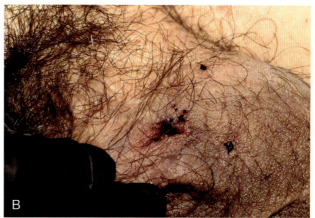

Figure 11.36. Gunshot wound of the scrotum. The decedent sustained a perforating gunshot wound of the scrotum. The entrance (**A**) and exit (**B**) can be difficult to distinguish. Often, to perforate the scrotum, the projectile will pass through one or both thighs, which can help to interpret the pathway through the scrotum.

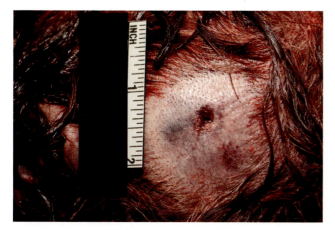

Figure 11.37. Decedent with gunshot wound mimic on back of head. On the posterior surface of head is a circular defect with a marginal abrasion, which mimics a small-caliber firearm injury such as a 0.22. However, there was no injury to the underlying cranium and a radiograph of the head revealed no projectile. The exact source of the injury is unknown, but is believed to have occurred during transport of the body to the morgue.

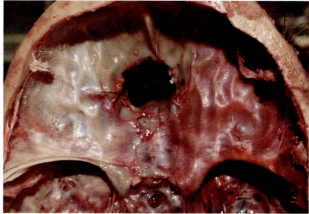

Figure 11.38. Cranial injury from farming accident. Although not on the external surface of the body, the round defect centered on the region of the cribriform fossa could mimic a firearm injury. The injury was caused during a farming accident, with an unspecified object on the vehicle driven into the cranium but not present at autopsy. If only skeletal remains had been recovered, the distinction from a gunshot wound could be more difficult.

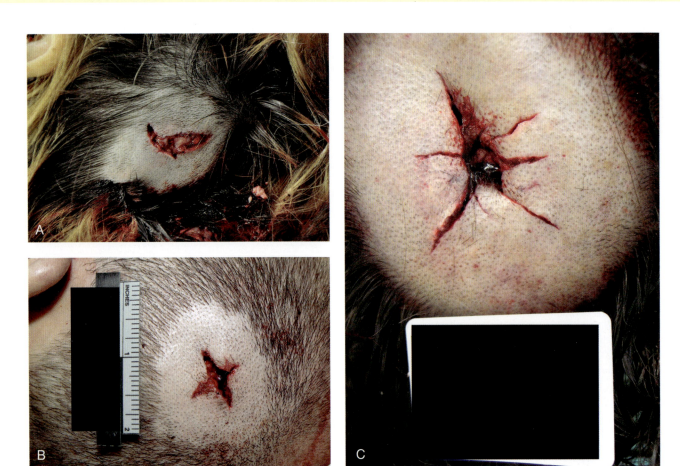

Figure 11.39. Exit wounds of the body. With a classic exit-type wound, there is usually no central defect in the skin and no marginal abrasion. Instead the wound has a slitlike (**A**) or stellate (**B** and **C**) appearance.

> **FAQ:** What do you do if the entrance and exit wounds are not distinguishable (ie, whether a wound is an entrance or an exit cannot be determined)?
>
> **Answer:** Features that may assist with the determination of entrance wound vs exit wound other than just the appearance of the wound in the skin are beveling of underlying bone, color of the underlying musculature, examination of the clothing, the appearance on radiography, and, when available, viewing a video of the incident. When the projectile strikes flat bone, such as the neurocranium, the sternum, a clavicle, a rib, or the pelvis, the defect in the bony surface on the side struck first is smaller than the defect in the surface where the projectile exits the bone. The overall defect in the bone is similar to the shape of a cone, with the narrow end being the point of entry into the bone and the wide end being the point of exit from the bone. At an entrance wound, the defect in the bone bevels inward (ie, internal beveling, which widens out toward the interior surface of the bone) and at the exit wound, the defect in the bone bevels outward (ie, external beveling, which widens out toward the exterior surface of the bone) (Figure 11.41A-H). The finding of even one fragment from the rim of the entrance wound with internal beveling when used in combination with the skin features can potentially help distinguish entrance from exit. Occasionally, external beveling can occur at an entrance wound and internal beveling can occur at the exit wound[27-30] and beveling can occur in the setting of injuries other than those that are firearm related as well.[31] For example, absent Wormian bones can potentially mimic a gunshot wound of the cranium.[32]

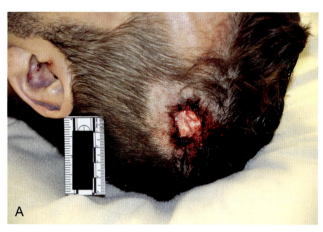 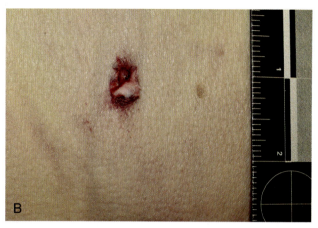

Figure 11.40. Exit wounds of the head and trunk. Exit woulds, while often slitlike or stellate, can have a variety of appearances, including more circular, with a permanent central region of tissue loss, similar to an entrance wound. These gunshot exit wounds of the head (**A**) and trunk (**B**) illustrate such a finding. Both gunshot wounds were found during separate autopsies.

With a contact gunshot wound, carbon monoxide staining (ie, a bright red discoloration) of the underlying musculature may be present due to binding of carbon monoxide from the gunshot wound with myoglobin or hemoglobin in the muscle (Figure 11.42). However, carbon monoxide-induced cherry red discoloration of the skeletal muscle has been identified at the exit wound in a reported case.[33]

Examination of the clothing for soot or gunpowder (informally by the forensic pathologist, or formally by the firearm examiner) may provide the answer as to whether a particular wound in the skin represents an entrance or an exit. And, while inversion of fibers at the point of entrance or eversion of fibers at the point of exit in the clothing is mentioned by some,[34] caution in the interpretation is advised. Projectile distribution on the radiograph or computed tomography (CT)/magnetic resonance imaging may help,[34-37] in that the fragments should spread outward from the entrance (Figures 11.43A and 11.43B). Review of the medical records may also assist in interpretation of firearm injuries after medical intervention has occurred, so as not to misinterpret medical intervention for an inflicted injury; however, clinical physicians are not accurate in determination of entrance and exit wounds of the body.[38] Videos of the incidence may also assist in distinguishing entrance from exit (Figure 11.44A-C).

PEARLS & PITFALLS

In the case of a shored (or supported) exit, a marginal abrasion will be present. A shored exit occurs when the skin at the exit site is against an object (eg, tight clothing) so that when the projectile impacts the undersurface of the skin and pushes it outward to create the exit, the skin impacts against the object against it, leading to abrasion of the margins of the exit wound. In a marginal abrasion created at the entrance of a projectile into the body, usually no residual epidermis is within the rim of abrasion; however, in a shored exit, islands of residual epidermis are often present. In addition, the marginal abrasion at an entrance wound often has a regular appearance, albeit which can be eccentric, whereas shored exit wounds tend to have a more irregular exit and the marginal abrasion tends to be lighter red in color. Distinguishing an entrance from a shored exit can be difficult for even an experienced forensic pathologist[39] (Figure 11.45A-K).

PEARLS & PITFALLS

When a projectile tangentially strikes the bone, a keyhole-type defect can be produced (Figure 11.46A-C). A keyhole defect will have both inward and outward bevel, inward bevel in the bone at the point the projectile was first in contact with and outward bevel in the bone at the point the projectile was last in contact with. While a keyhole defect is most commonly found at the entrance wound, keyhole defects have been reported at the exit wound.[40]

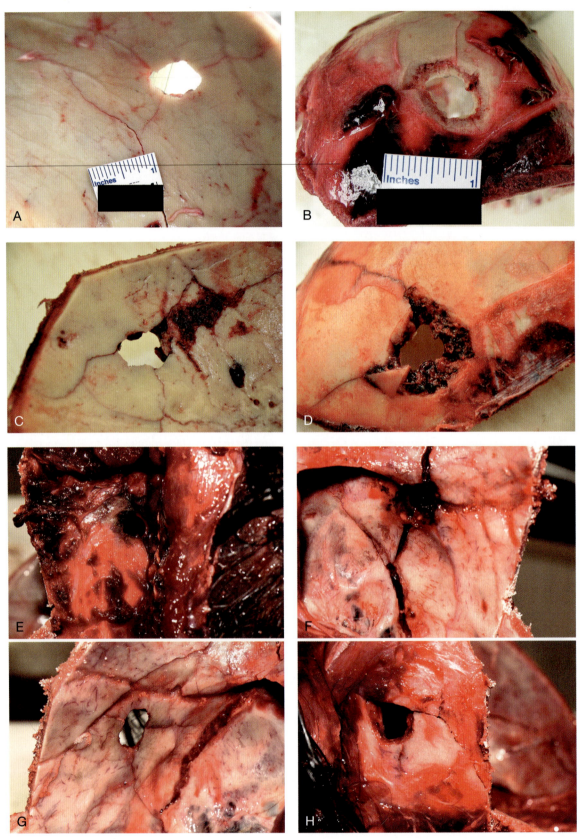

Figure 11.41. Examples of bevel in the cranium. (**A**) is the endocranial surface of an exit gunshot wound in the cranium. Note that the bone on the inner table extends all the way to the circular defect (ie, the defect has a punched out appearance). (**B**) is the ectocranial surface of the exit gunshot wound in (**A**). Note that the bone on the outer table of the cranium ends prior to the full thickness circular defect. This is outward bevel and is consistent with an exit wound. (**C**) is again the endocranial surface of an exit gunshot wound in the cranium, with (**D**) the corresponding ectocranial surface. Like (**A** and **B**), the bevel is outward, consistent with an exit wound. (**E-H**) are from a single gunshot wound. (**E** and **F**) show the defect in the bone at the entrance site, with inward bevel, and (**G** and **H**) show the defect in the bone at the exit site, with outward bevel.

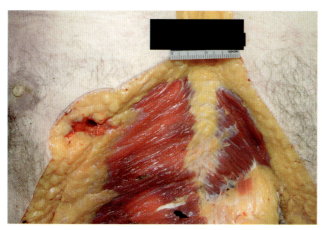

Figure 11.42. Contact gunshot wound of the body, with carbon monoxide staining of the underlying musculature. Carbon monoxide, which is released when a weapon fires, will, in a contact range wound, enter the body and bind to myoglobin and hemoglobin, which will give the musculature a more red or pink coloration. Some weapons, such as a 0.22 rifle, produce minimal soot, and identifying contact range gunshot wounds can be challenging; however, the carbon monoxide staining of the musculature can help.

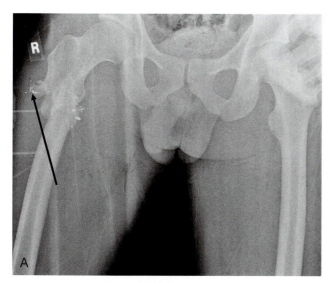

Figure 11.43A. Gunshot wound that struck the femur. At the point where the projectile first struck the femur are radio-dense fragments. Fragments are also present in the soft tissue on the lateral surface of the bone. In addition, the bone fractured and the bone fragments traveled in the same direction as the projectile and are seen in the soft tissue lateral to the femur on the left side of the radiograph (arrow).

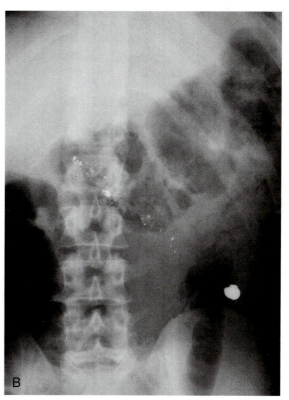

Figure 11.43B. Gunshot wound with pathway of projectile shown by fragments of the projectile. The projectile struck the vertebral column, which left a trail of tiny fragments that mark the pathway of the projectile. Since the projectile itself is present, the trail of projectile fragments can be used to determine the pathway.

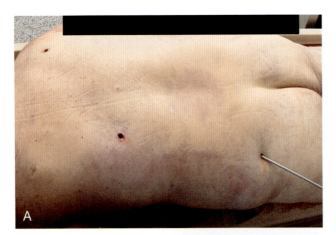
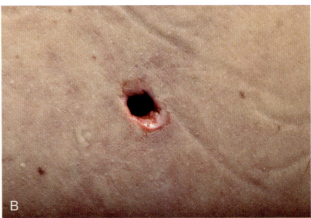
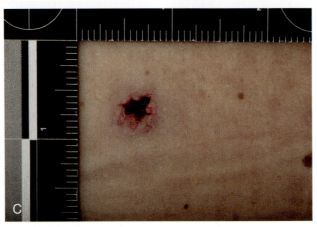

Figure 11.44. Gunshot wound of the body. This individual sustained multiple gunshot wounds. Two gunshot wounds, one representing entrance and one representing exit were present on the right side of the upper back and the left side of the middle of the back (**A**). The projectile pathway was between these two wounds, traveling roughly parallel to the vertebral column and just underneath the skin; however, both wounds are somewhat atypical. Viewing of a video of the incident showed the individual shot several times, and showed his body turning so his back was toward the shooters and falling forward bent at the hip, in which case his back would have been briefly parallel to the ground. From this video, (**B**) was determined to be the entrance wound and (**C**) was determined to be the exit.

KEY FEATURES to Evaluate to Distinguish an Entrance Wound From an Exit Wound

- Overall appearance of wound (circular vs slitlike or stellate)
- Presence or absence of soot
- Presence or absence of stippling/powder tattooing
- Presence or absence of marginal abrasion
- Presence or absence of muzzle abrasion
- Presence or absence of carbon monoxide staining of underlying musculature
- Inward or outward bevel in underlying bone

FEATURES OF WOUND THAT ALLOW FOR GENERAL DETERMINATION OF RANGE OF FIRE

Features of the wound that allow for general determination of range of fire are presence of soot either on the skin or within the depths of the wound and whether the soot on the skin easily wipes away or is associated with searing and is more adherent (Figure 11.47A-G), the presence of stippling/powder tattooing (Figure 11.48A-D), presence of a muzzle abrasion (Figure 11.49A and B), and carbon monoxide-related discoloration of the underlying musculature. DiMaio and Molina distinguish between a loose contact wound, which has a rim of soot that is easily wiped away and that occurs when the muzzle is loosely against the skin and a near-contact wound, which has a rim of soot that is associated with searing and is more tightly adherent to the skin and that occurs when the weapon is a short distance from the skin, but they indicate that there is overlap between loose contact and near contact wounds and that the distinction is not always possible.[41] DiMaio and Molina

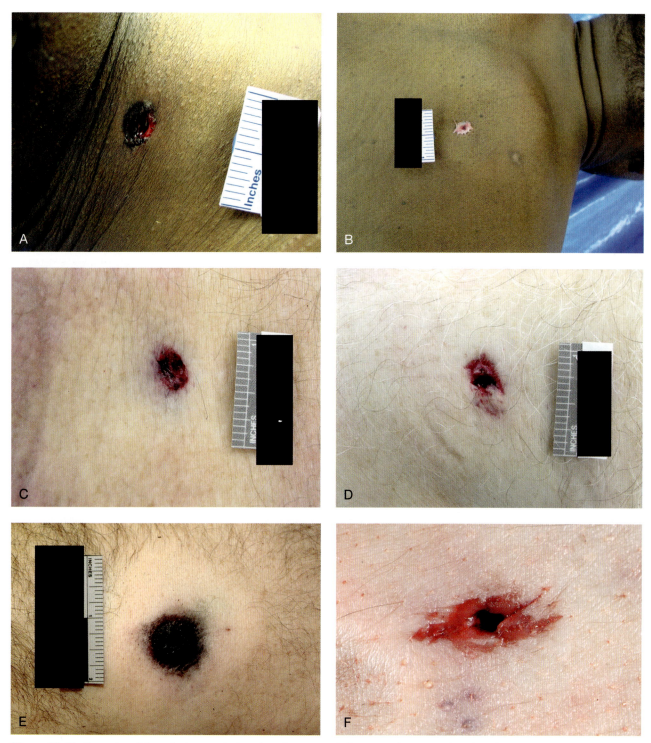

Figure 11.45. Examples of shored exit wounds. In a shored exit wound, there is an abrasion at the edge of the wound which can mimic the marginal abrasion normally found with an entrance wound. This occurs due to some object being against the skin at the exit site, thus, when the skin is pushed outward by the exiting projectile, the epidermis impacts that object, leading to an abrasion. Paired images (**A** and **B**), (**C** and **D**), and (**E** and **F**) are gunshot wounds illustrating both the entrance and exit wounds. (**A**, **C**, and **E**) are the entrance wounds with (**B**, **D**, and **F**) the corresponding shored exits. (**G-K**) are other examples of shored exit wounds, each with some amount of marginal abrasion.

Figure 11.45g-k (continued)

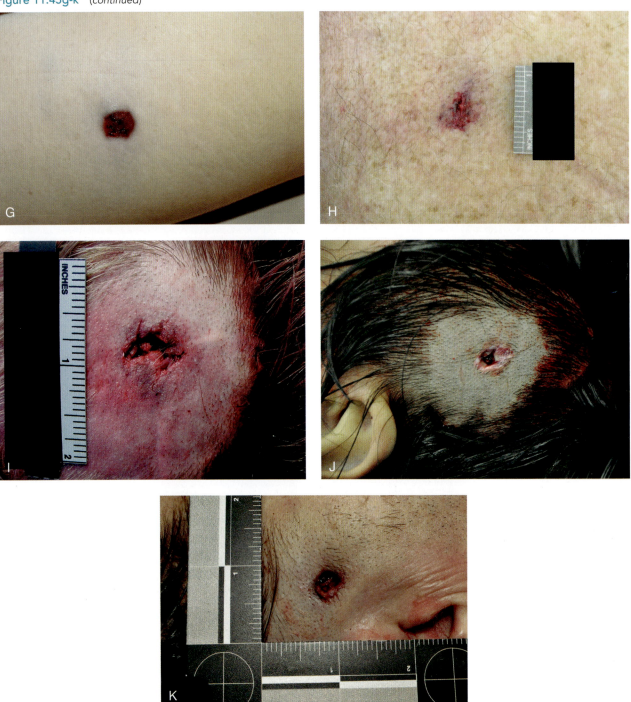

also prefer the term "powder tattooing" to describe the effect of unburned gunpowder on the skin, with the term "stippling" used as a more generic term for punctate red abrasions around the wound, which could describe the effect of unburned gunpowder or secondary objects such as glass fragments, whereas other authors, including Dolinak et al, prefer the term "stippling" to describe the effects of unburned gunpowder and the term "pseudo-stippling" to describe the effects of an intermediary object.[34,41] The determination of actual range of fire is done by the firearm examiner, who will test fire the suspected weapon and ammunition type and match the autopsy findings to those of the test firing results to determine a range of fire (ie, shooting the weapon at various ranges to determine how widespread the soot and stippling is at various ranges, and then comparing that distribution to the distribution found at autopsy on the skin around the wound); however, in

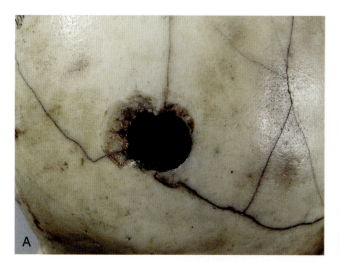
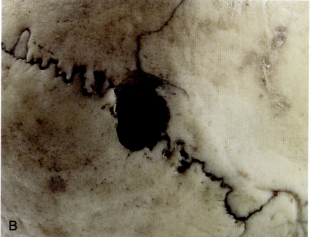
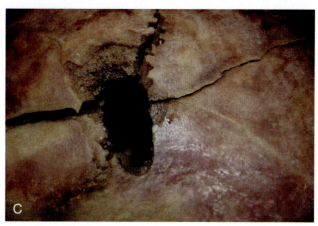

Figure 11.46. Examples of keyhole defects. In a keyhole defect, both inward (giving the surface a punched out appearance) and outward beveling of the bone occur at the same site. A keyhole defect is due to a projectile striking the bone in a tangential (ie, angled) manner. In (**A**), from 1 to 6 o'clock, the bony surface is punched out, whereas from 6 to 1 o'clock, there is an outward bevel. In (**B**), from 2 to 10 o'clock, the bony surface is punched out, whereas from 10 to 2 o'clock, there is outward bevel. In (**C**), from 3 to 9 o'clock, the bony surface is punched out, whereas from 9 to 3 o'clock, there is an outward bevel.

general, soot will mark the skin to around 6 to 8 inches from the weapon and stippling to 1 to 3 feet from the weapon.

Unfortunately, terminology used for the classification of gunshot wound ranges varies by author. Terms used include contact, tight contact or hard contact, loose contact, near contact, partial contact, close range, intermediate range, medium range, indeterminant range, and distant range (Table 11.1).[34,39,41-45] For the figure legends in this book, the terms contact and close (for wounds with soot and/or stippling) will be used.

KEY FEATURES to Help Determine a Relative Range of Fire
- Presence or absence of muzzle abrasion
- Presence or absence of carbon monoxide staining of underlying skeletal muscle
- Presence or absence of soot on the skin and/or within the depths of the wound
- Presence or absence of seared skin
- Presence or absence of stippling/gunpowder tattooing

SAMPLE NOTE

When documenting the distribution of soot and/or stippling around the periphery of an entrance gunshot wound, use a clock face. For example, "Surrounding the entrance wound is a rim of stippling which is 3/4 inch wide at 12 and 3 o'clock, and 1/8 inch wide at 6 and 9 o'clock."

SAMPLE NOTE

For classification of a gunshot wound in the summary section of the autopsy report, close range vs no evidence of close range may be best, as the terminology for various subcategories of close range varies from author to author; however, if features of a contact wound are present such as soot only at the rim and within the depths of the wound or the presence of a muzzle abrasion, the term "contact" could be applied. In the autopsy summary section, or at least in the description of the wound in the body of the autopsy report, a listing of the features of the gunshot wound that allows for the determination of a relative range of fire would be both useful and important (such as describing the presence or absence of soot and/or stippling and the presence or absence of muzzle abrasion and a description of whether the soot is easily removable). The determination of a distant range gunshot wound (ie, a wound with no evidence of closer range fire) should only be made if no intermediary object was present, which could have collected or blocked the soot or unburned gunpowder so it did not strike the skin. If no gunshot residue is present on the skin and no other features for determination of range are available, the range can be labeled as indeterminant, which does not preclude the possibility of an intermediary object.

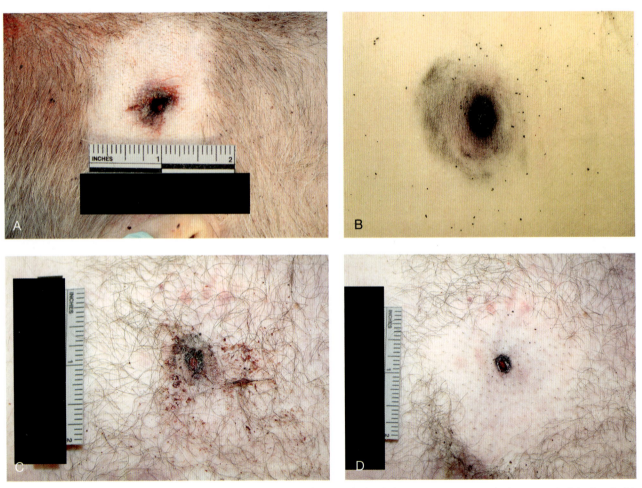

Figure 11.47. Soot deposition on the skin at the entrance wound. In (**A**), the body has a contact range gunshot wound of the head with soot at the rim of the entrance wound, but not on the surrounding skin. In (**B**), the body has a close range gunshot wound of the trunk, with a rim of soot on the surrounding skin. In addition, there are unburned gunpowder particles on the skin. In (**C** and **D**), the body has a close range gunshot wound of the trunk. In (**C**), prior to cleaning and shaving of the hair, a small rim of soot is present on the skin. In (**D**), after cleaning and shaving, the soot is no longer present (ie, easily wiped away). These images illustrate the importance of taking photographs of the entrance wound, especially when soot is identified, prior to cleaning as well as after, and the importance of a pathologist examining wounds prior to their being cleaned by an autopsy assistant.

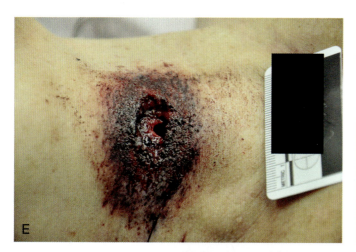
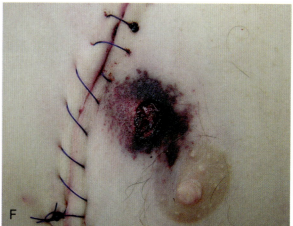
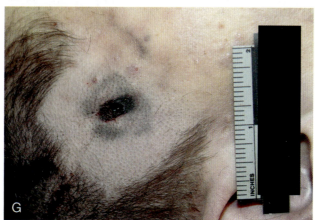

Figure 11.47 E-G. In (**E**), the body has a close range gunshot wound of the neck. The skin adjacent to the wound is seared, given it a rough texture, and the soot is more tightly adherent. In (**F**), the body has a close range gunshot wound of the chest, adjacent to the nipple, and has undergone medical intervention, presumably with cleaning of the wound. The rough irregular rim around the entrance wound illustrates the effects of searing on the skin. In (**G**), the body has a close range gunshot wound of the head. This gunshot wound illustrates the overlap between the loose contact and near contact described by DiMaio and Molina,[41] as there is a rim of soot immediately around the entrance, which is tightly adherent and a more peripheral rim of soot that is loosely adherent.

PEARLS & PITFALLS

Drying of the marginal abrasion can result in a black coloration, which can mimic soot and a contact gunshot wound (Figure 11.50A and B). In addition, there can be overlap between the marginal abrasion and a muzzle abrasion, and the muzzle abrasion can dry, mimicking a wider rim of soot than might actually have been present, confounding the determination by the firearm examiner (Figure 11.51A-D).

PEARLS & PITFALLS

Stippling/powder tattooing is produced by unburned gunpowder particles striking the skin, leaving punctate abrasions, with gunpowder sometimes embedded in the skin surface. Stippling/powder tattooing, as it is produced by gunpowder impacting the skin, tends to be regular in size, especially when ball gunpowder was used, with some slight variation in size occurring with flake gunpowder. Pseudo-stippling occurs when the projectile strikes an intermediary target (eg, a glass window) before hitting the victim, creating secondary projectiles (eg, fragments of glass). These secondary projectiles are often small and can produce punctate abrasions of the skin, similar to stippling (Figure 11.52A-D); however, in pseudo-stippling, there is more variation in size and shape of the punctate abrasions. Stippling due to unburned gunpowder striking the skin and pseudo-stippling due to secondary projectiles are not mutually exclusive, and it would be possible for a wound to have both.

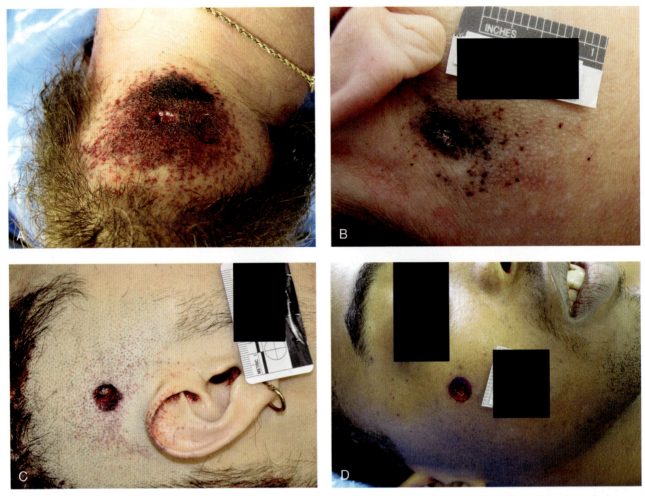

Figure 11.48. Stippling/powder-tattooing. In (A), the body has an entrance gunshot wound of the undersurface of the chin, which is surrounded by a dense rim of stippling. In (B), the body has a close range gunshot wound of the head just behind the ear. While there is a rim of soot, there is also stippling/powder-tattooing, with gunpowder loosely embedded in the skin. In (C), the body has a close range gunshot wound of the head. Compared to (A), the stippling around this wound is much finer in texture and as such more difficult to identify. In (D), the body has a close range gunshot wound of the cheek. Superior to the gunshot wound, adjacent to the right eye, is rare stippling. As stippling can indicate a distance of 1 to 3 feet, the identification of even rare stippling is important.

> **FAQ: Does decomposition preclude identification of entrance and exit wounds?**
>
> **Answer:** As long as the skin is intact, the entrance and exit wounds as well as their features for determination of range can often be identified[46,47] (Figure 11.53A-C). However, if the skin is not intact, the task becomes more difficult but not impossible if soot is present in the underlying soft tissue, or if the projectile passed through bone, which allows for a bevel pattern to develop.[48] However, in some cases of advanced decomposition, even with bone involvement, the entrance and exit wounds cannot be distinguished.[49,50]

SAMPLE NOTE: EXAMPLE OF GUNSHOT WOUND DESCRIPTION IN REPORT

"On the left side of the chest is a ½ inch circular entrance-type gunshot wound that is centered 13 inches below the top of the head, 3 inches to the left of midline, 1 inch superior to the left nipple and 2 inches medial to the left nipple. The wound has a circumferential 1/4 inch wide marginal abrasion. Circumferentially on the skin surface in a 1/2 inch wide rim from the edge of wound is soot. The width of the rim of soot is consistent circumferentially."

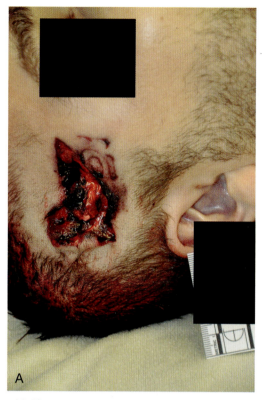
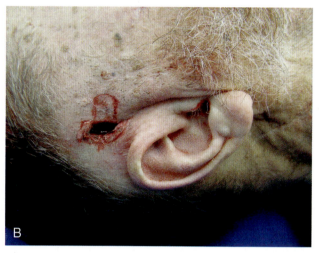

Figure 11.49. Muzzle abrasion at entrance wound. (**A** and **B**) both illustrate entrance gunshot wounds with a muzzle abrasion.

SAMPLE NOTE: EXAMPLE OF GUNSHOT WOUND DESCRIPTION IN REPORT

"In the left temporal region of the scalp is a 1/2 inch circular entrance-type gunshot wound that is centered 3 inches below the top of the head, 1 inch superior to the tragus of the left ear, and 1 inch anterior to the tragus of the left ear. At the edge of the gunshot wound is blackened discolored skin associated with a 1/8 inch wide circumferential marginal abrasion. At 1, 5, 6, and 9 o'clock are radiating tears, measuring 1/4, 1/2, 1/2, and 2 inches respectively."

FAQ: Should gunshot wound pathways be described with scientific terminology?

Answer: With forensic autopsies, especially those involving gunshot wounds, most commonly, non-physicians are the persons most likely to read the report. Front/back and up/down can be more familiar to these readers than anterior/posterior and superior/inferior.

SAMPLE NOTE: WORDING OF GUNSHOT WOUND FOR DEATH CERTIFICATE

"Gunshot wound of the head" vs "Perforating contact gunshot wound of the head." While both wordings are acceptable, it is good to remember that individuals who have a copy of the death certificate often will not have a copy of the autopsy report itself. Listing perforating (or penetrating, if the projectile only entered the head but did not exit) contact gunshot wound of the head as the cause of death provides more information.

TABLE 11.1: Terminology Used for the Classification of Gunshot Wound Ranges

	Fisher	DiMaio	Dolinak	Knight	Spitz	Wetli	Mason
Contact						Muzzle abrasion, ejector rod abrasion; gunshot residue	Muzzle abrasion
Tight contact/ hard contact	Muzzle abrasion, powder residue deep in wound	Powder residue deep in wound; searing and powder blackening at edge	On head, radiating lacerations				
Loose contact	Powder residue on skin and in depths	Soot in band around edge that can be wiped away		Soot in immediate vicinity of wound			
Near contact		Rim of soot and seared blackened skin; soot cannot be wiped away				Circular band of charred skin and gunshot residue; residue on skin	Muzzle abrasion
Near (loose) contact			Searing of skin, giving black discoloration; soot on skin				
Close	Cutaneous tattooing or stippling from particulate powder	Contact, near contact, and intermediate range wounds are considered together as close range		Soot and powder tattooing	Gunsmoke deposited on skin	Soot on skin around wound that is easily wiped away	Soot on skin
Intermediate		Powder tattooing (not stippling); can have soot	Stippling from un-burned gunpowder			Stippling; soot can be present	
Medium							Powder tattooing (grains embedded); stippling (impact marks)
Distant	None of above	Not possible to accurately determine			No gunsmoke deposited on skin		

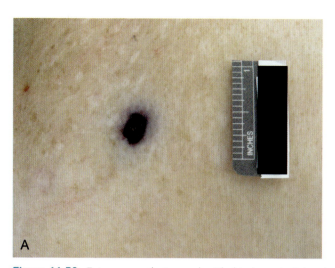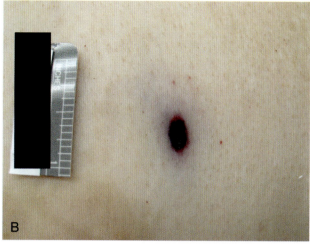

Figure 11.50. Entrance gunshot wounds with dried marginal abrasions. In both (**A** and **b**), the individuals were shot from a distance (which was determined based upon the scene investigation). Both entrance wounds have marginal abrasions, which have dried, giving them a dark coloration, which can mimic soot. Close inspection of the wound including with a dissecting-type microscope detailed examination of the underlying soft tissue (as, with a contact wound, should have soot if it is not present on the skin, or carbon monoxide discoloration), and examination of the clothing can help determine the true nature of the wound.

SPECIAL TYPES OF GUNSHOT WOUNDS

Introduction: To describe some gunshot wounds, specific terms are used, including shored exit, graze wound, tangential wound, superficial perforating wound, and re-entrance. Each has some features different from the classic entrance or exit wound described above. While

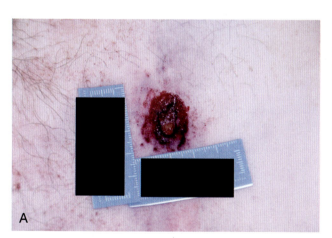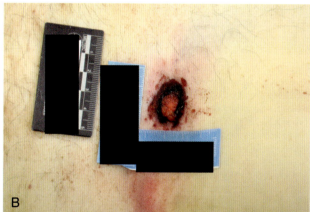
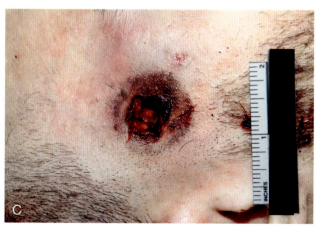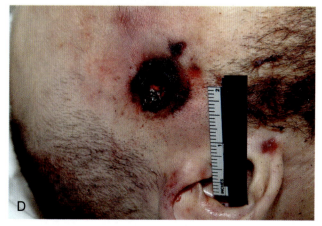

Figure 11.51. Decedents with firearm injury illustrating drying of the marginal abrasion/muzzle abrasion. In (**A** and **B**), the body has both a pre-autopsy photograph of the wound taken by investigators (**A**) and an autopsy photograph of the same wound (**B**) illustrating the effect of drying on the marginal abrasion/muzzle abrasion, producing a discoloration which can mimic soot. In (**C** and **D**), both autopsy photographs, but with time between the two photographs, (**C**) illustrates a muzzle abrasion, with some embedded soot, but (**D**) illustrates the same wound at a later time, with drying of the muzzle abrasion, mimicking a more dense rim of soot around the wound.

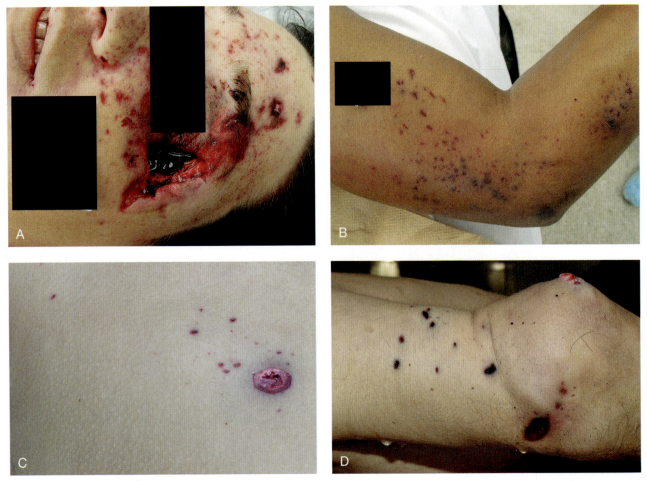

Figure 11.52. Pseudo-stippling on the skin. In (**A**), the decedent was shot through a door. The projectile mushroomed causing an atypical entrance wound at the lateral corner of the left eye. While the skin of the face surrounding the entrance has numerous abrasions, these abrasions are all quite variable in size and shape and were produced from secondary projectiles caused by the bullet striking the door first. In (**B**), the decedent was shot through a glass window. When the window broke, secondary projectiles (ie, fragments of glass) were propelled forward and struck the decedent. The punctate abrasions are similar to stippling/powder tattooing; however, there is significant variation in size and shape, and no embedded powder grains. In (**C**), the decedent has an entrance gunshot wound with a circumferential marginal abrasion but surrounding the skin are several punctate abrasions. The abrasions vary in size and shape and were created by secondary projectiles, from an object interposed between the shooter and the victim. In (**D**), the decedent has an entrance and exit gunshot wound of the knee. The numerous abrasions of the legs are pseudo-stippling due to an interposed target.

DiMaio and Molina separate between graze wound, tangential wound, and superficial perforating wound, other authors overlap the terminology.[41] The descriptions below are made using DiMaio and Molina's terminology.

Description: A shored exit occurs when there is a marginal abrasion at the exit wound (Figure 11.54A-C). The cause is often tight clothing or some other object abutting against the skin at the site of the exit wound, such that when the skin bulges outward at the exit it strikes the adjacent object, leaving a marginal abrasion.[51] The marginal abrasion of a shored exit wound is usually less regular and lighter red in color than a marginal abrasion on a typical entrance wound, and may have residual islands of epidermis within its confines but can still present a challenge to the observer.

Graze Wound

Description: A graze gunshot wound is essentially a wide linear abrasion of the skin, as the projectile does not or just barely perforates through the epidermis into the underlying subcutaneous tissue (Figure 11.55A and B).

Tangential Wound

Description: A tangential wound is essentially a laceration of the skin, where the projectile creates one continuous linear defect from the point it first contacts the skin, which will often

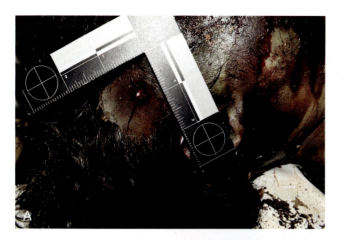
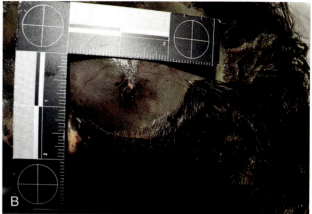
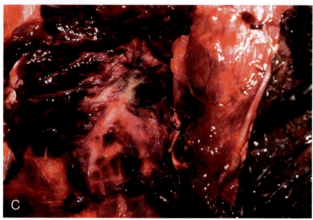

Figure 11.53. Entrance and exit gunshot wound in a decomposed body. Although the entrance (**A**) and exit (**B**) are difficult to distinguish, the presence of soot (**C**) on the bone underlying the entrance (as well as inward bevel at the entrance and outward bevel at the exit) confirmed the pathway of the projectile.

have a marginal abrasion, to the point where it loses contact with the skin (Figure 11.56). While some authors separate graze and tangential wounds,[41] other authors use the terms more interchangeably, with a graze wound describing both.[34,39]

> **PEARLS & PITFALLS**
>
> The skin tags in a tangential wound will point in the direction that the projectile was fired from (i.e., "points toward the weapon") (Figure 11.57A-C). Close examination of one end of the defect will also often reveal a marginal abrasion, which was the point of first contact of the projectile. If there is an underlying fracture of the cranium, it may have a keyhole-type defect.

Superficial Perforating Wound

Description: A superficial perforating wound is a wound that has a distinct entrance wound and exit wound but which only perforates the skin and underlying soft tissue (Figure 11.58).

Re-Entrance Wound/Atypical Wound

Description: A re-entrance wound occurs when the projectile passes through one part of the body (eg, the upper extremity) and re-enters another part of the body (eg, the chest), or when the projectile passes through another object prior to striking the decedent (eg, a window). The re-entrance wound produced is often atypical. The atypical features can be a wider and more irregular marginal abrasion or non-circular shape of the entrance wound or

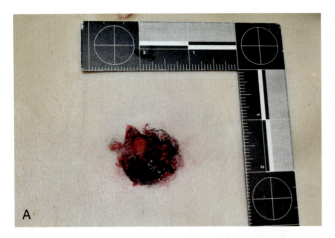
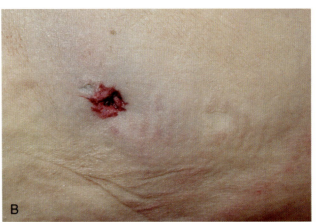
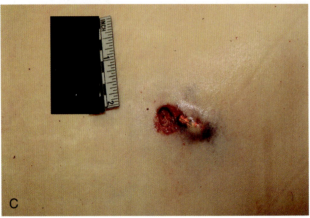

Figure 11.54. Shored exit wounds. The decedent in (**A** and **B**) died from the result of a single self-inflicted gunshot wound of the trunk. (**A**) is the entrance wound on the anterior surface of the trunk, with soot visible at edge. (**B**) is the exit wound on the posterior surface of the trunk. Note the abrasion at the margin of the exit wound, which mimics the marginal abrasion seen with entrance wounds. In (**C**), there is an exit wound with the projectile adjacent and just underneath the skin. From 2 to 6 o'clock is an eccentric abrasion ring. Based upon the angle at which the projectile exited the body, it created a marginal abrasion, which would, if the projectile were not in place, mimic an entrance wound with an eccentric marginal abrasion.

both (Figure 11.59A-G). The underlying reason for the atypical appearance of the wound is that the projectile, having struck another object prior to entering the body, will have become deformed or will have had its stable rotation disrupted, causing it to strike the body not in the usual fashion (eg, the projectile might strike the body sideways instead of tip first). An atypical entrance wound may be misinterpreted as a form of injury other than a gunshot wound.[52]

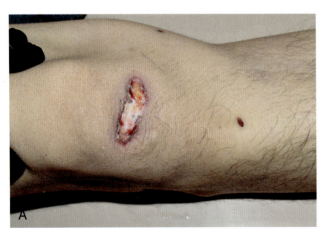
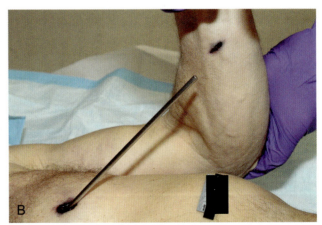

Figure 11.55. Graze entrance wounds. (**A**) is a graze wound of the right knee, with the projectile essentially just scraping away the epidermis and superficial dermis. While skin tags on a tangential wound can assist in determining the direction of fire, given the superficial nature of the wounds such as the one in the image, the edges can easily not develop sufficient skin tags to determine the pathway of the projectile, or the edges can dry, which also hinders interpretation. (**B**) is a graze wound of the left forearm, with subsequent entry of the projectile into the chest.

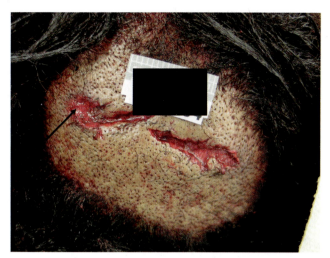

Figure 11.56. Tangential wound. This individual was shot multiple times. One of the gunshot wounds produced a tangential wound of the top of the head. Compared to a graze wound, the wound is deeper into the dermis, in this case, extending to the cranium. The pathway of the projectile was, in the image, left to right, which can be determined by examining the skin tags (see text and Figure 11.57A-C). At the arrow is a marginal abrasion.

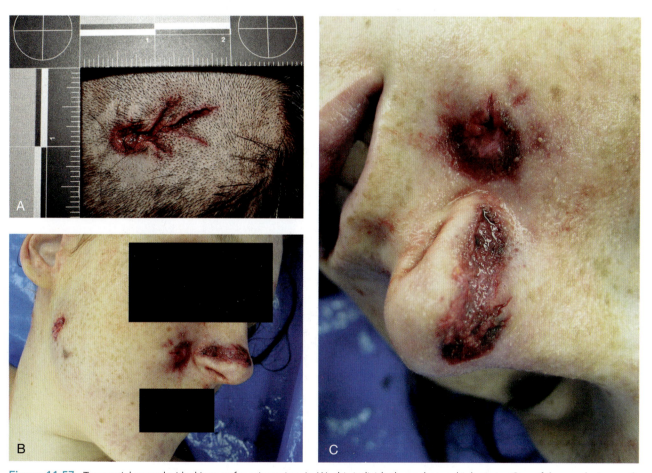

Figure 11.57. Tangential wound with skin tags for orientation. In (A), this individual was shot multiple times. One of the gunshot wounds produced a tangential wound of the top of the head. At the left side of the wound in the image is a marginal abrasion. The skin tags point to the left, which is the direction the projectile came from. The pathway of the projectile is left to right in the image. In (B and C), the individual sustained multiple gunshot wounds. The wound in the images was not lethal but illustrates several features of gunshot wounds. In (B) is a graze wound/tangential gunshot wound of the nose, with the entrance at the medial portion of the right cheek having a wide marginal abrasion from 12 to 6 o'clock and with the exit wound on the lateral surface of the right cheek having no marginal abrasion. (C) is a close-up of the wounds of the nose and cheek, with the wound of the nose having skin tags that point in the direction the projectile came from.

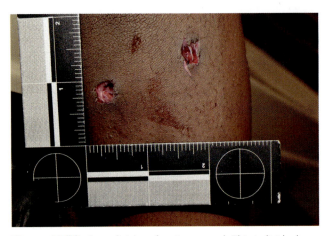

Figure 11.58. Superficial perforating wound. This individual was shot multiple times. One of the wounds of the extremities was a superficial perforating wound. On the left side of the image is the entrance wound, with a marginal abrasion. On the right side of the image is the exit wound, with no marginal abrasion. Unlike graze wounds or tangential wounds, the projectile perforated the skin and soft tissue of the body, with no communication on the skin surface between the two points; however, the projectile only perforates skin and subcutaneous tissue, not penetrating deeper into the body.

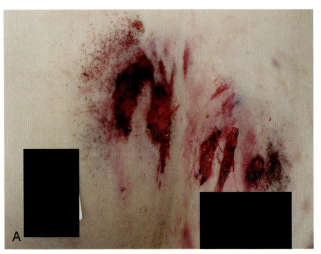

Figure 11.59A. Re-entrance wounds of the breast. This woman was shot at a close range through the breast. The round defect on the right side of the image is the entrance wound, with soot on the skin to the right. The projectile perforated the skin and soft tissue at the inferior aspect of the breast (ie, the two elongated defects in the middle of the image), and re-entered the trunk at the left side of the image, which is a more irregular defect, with an abrasion to the left, which likely resulted from the skin above being forced against the skin below, and stippling to the left of the abrasion. The wound also again illustrates how at the time of autopsy the orientation of the skin is not the same as when the decedent was shot. In this case, on the autopsy table, the breast does not rest against the body in the same fashion as it would when the decedent was standing or sitting, at the time they were shot.

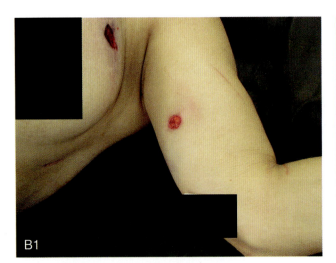

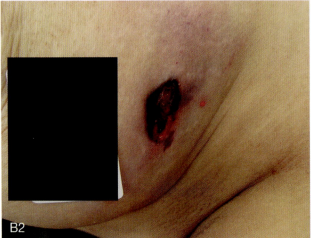

Figure 11.59B1-B2. Re-entrance wound of the chest. The decedent was shot through the left upper extremity and that projectile then re-entered the chest at the upper border of the left breast. In (**B1**) can be seen the exit on the medial surface of the left arm and the re-entrance in the chest. (**B2**) is a close-up of the re-entrance in the chest. Instead of a round circular defect, the wound is more oval and irregular, and the marginal abrasion is also more irregular than if the projectile had not passed through the left arm first. Most ammunition types encountered by forensic pathologists will expand/mushroom after making contact with the body, which serves to dissipate all of the kinetic energy of the projectile into the body, causing more injury.

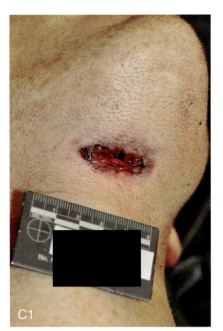 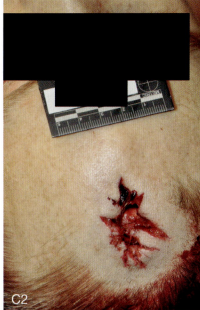 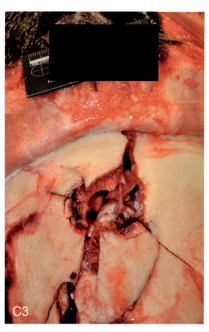

Figure 11.59C1-C3. Atypical entrance wound. Although re-entrance of the projectile can and often does produce an atypical entrance wound, sometimes entrance wounds may just appear atypical. In (**C1**) is an elongated entrance wound of the undersurface of the chin, with soot at the margin. (**C2**) is the corresponding exit wound, which has a typical stellate appearance. (**C3**) is the outward bevel present at the exit wound. Given that the individual's neck was most likely flexed at the time of the gunshot wound, the folding of the skin could alter the wound created by entrance of the projectile.

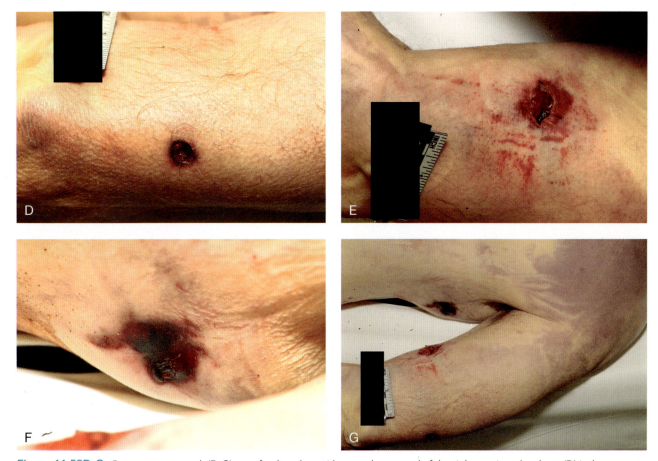

Figure 11.59D-G. Re-entrance wound. (**D-G**) are of a decedent with a gunshot wound of the right arm into the chest. (**D**) is the entrance wound in the lateral surface of the right arm. The wound is circular with a uniform marginal abrasion. (**E**) is the exit wound from the medial surface of the right arm. The wound is irregular in shape, with an irregular in width marginal abrasion. This is a shored exit, caused by the arm being against the chest. (**F**) is the re-entrance wound, with the defect non-uniformly surrounded by an irregular wide and large marginal abrasion, which resulted most likely from the projectile having mushroomed upon impact with the arm, and due to impact of the skin of the medial surface of the arm against the chest. (**G**) is an overall photo of the three defects.

> **PEARLS & PITFALLS**
>
> The presence of an atypical entrance wound often indicates that an intermediary target was present (ie, an object between the shooter and the decedent, which can include the decedent themself, in the case of a re-entrance wound). When there is an intermediary target, it is possible for a fragment of that object to be carried forward with the projectile and into the body.[53] This fragment of the object may assist in re-constructing the events of the shooting.[54]

> **PEARLS & PITFALLS**
>
> If the projectile is more superficially located in the body in comparison to its degree of deformation (eg, if the projectile is flattened but only perforated the skin of the abdomen and penetrated into the liver), consider a ricochet or intermediary target (Figure 11.60A-C).[34]

ENTRANCE AND EXIT WOUNDS FOR SHOTGUNS AND RELATIVE RANGE OF FIRE

Entrance wounds for shotguns: While shotgun entrance wounds can have the same features described above for handguns/rifles (eg, marginal abrasion and soot/stippling), the nature of most shotgun projectiles, specifically buckshot and birdshot, allows for other patterns to be present at the entrance wound, which are discussed below under determination of relative range.

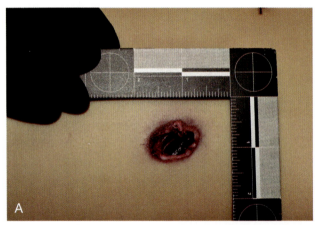
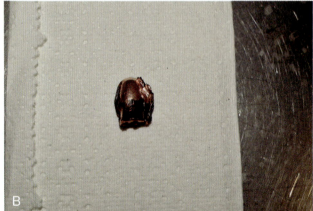
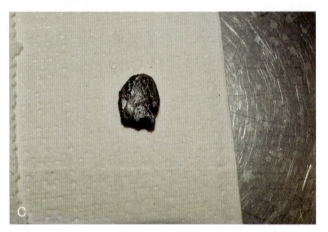

Figure 11.60. Decedent with gunshot wound following ricochet. (**A**) is the gunshot entrance wound on the trunk, which, for the caliber of projectile used, appeared larger than expected. The projectile did not strike any bone, but only penetrated into the abdominal cavity a short distance. The projectile, when recovered, was a flattened copper-jacketed lead core projectile (**B** and **C**), which is consistent with a ricochet.

Exit wounds for shotguns: The pellets, whether buckshot or birdshot, most often do not exit, although buckshot, given the large mass of each projectile, may be more likely to exit (Figure 11.61), and birdshot, when shot through a thin portion of the body (eg, the hand), could also exit.

FEATURES OF THE SHOTGUN WOUND THAT ALLOW FOR DETERMINATION OF RELATIVE RANGE OF FIRE

While a shotgun wound can be associated with both soot and stippling similar to a handgun or rifle wound, the nature of shotgun shells loaded with birdshot or buckshot allows for additional findings that allow for determination of range of fire beyond that for which stippling is normally present. When a shotgun shell with birdshot or buckshot is discharged, a mass of pellets and the shot sleeve (or shot cup)/wadding exit the barrel. At first, the mass of pellets will be tightly packed together and create a single round defect in the skin (Figure 11.62). As the pellets at the edge of the mass start to separate, the edge of the wound will be scalloped (Figure 11.63). Then, at a farther distance, individual pellets will separate from the central mass, creating satellite perforations near the edge of the main defect in the skin (Figure 11.64), and ultimately, no mass of pellets is present and only individual perforations will be present (Figure 11.65). In addition, the wadding/shot sleeve can strike the body and/or lodge within the entrance wound (Figure 11.66), or strike the skin at another point, leading to an abrasion (Figure 11.67A-D). Some shotgun shells contain tiny white particles which act as a filler among the shot pellets. This filler material can strike the skin or deposit within the wound (Figure 11.68). When individuals are shot multiple times with a shotgun, multiple appearances are, of course, possible (Figure 11.69). Given the variable nature of shotgun barrels, in that there are those with full choke or modified choke, or those that are sawed off or not sawed off, each of which could affect the spread of the pellets after leaving the barrel, the range of fire is best determined by a firearm examiner; however, the general knowledge of the pattern produced by the pellets as described above would allow a forensic pathologists to give investigators a general idea of how close the shot was fired at.

SAMPLE NOTE: SHOTGUN WOUND RANGE

Determination of range of fire of a shotgun wound is very difficult at the time of autopsy due to a variety of factors including tangenital wounds and incomplete patterns of spread represented on the body (eg, not all birdshot or buckshot pellets struck the skin, so the true distribution of the pellets is unknown). Determination of range of fire of a shotgun wound is best left to the firearm examiner; however, the pathologist can assist in the most accurate determination by extensively photographing the wound and obtaining complete measurements of the injuries in the skin.

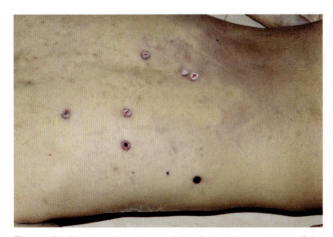

Figure 11.61. Decedent shot with buckshot. The entrance of the buckshot was in the back. On the right side of the chest were exit defects and also projectiles just underneath the skin. Some of the buckshot only penetrated into the body; whereas some of the buckshot perforated the body, with one pellet identified in the clothing.

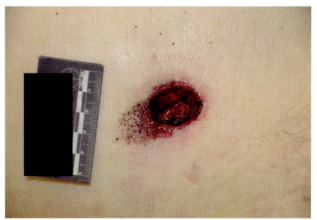

Figure 11.62. Circular shotgun wound entrance. When the charge of pellets that exits the barrel immediately or nearly immediately comes into contact with the skin, the resulting defect will be round, as the pellets all struck the skin in one cohesive mass, mimicking a large projectile. The soot present at 7 to 8 o'clock in the image resulted from a slight gap in the seal between the barrel and the skin which allowed some soot to escape and deposit on the skin.

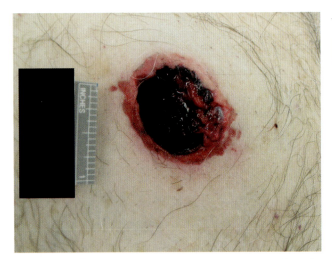

Figure 11.63. Scalloped shotgun wound entrance. When the charge of pellets that exits the barrel travels a short distance prior to striking the skin or travels through clothing, the mass of pellets is allowed to separate slightly, which will give the edge of the wound a scalloped appearance.

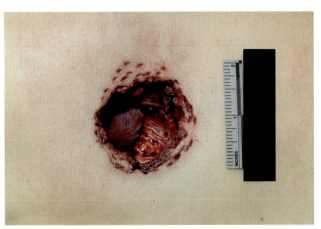

Figure 11.64. Shotgun wound created by central mass of pellets with satellite perforations. As the charge of pellets continues to distance from the end of the barrel, some pellets break away from the central mass and will produce satellite perforations at the periphery of a large defect created by the bulk of the pellets still within a central mass. Examination of the wound in the image reveals soot. This wound was essentially a contact range gunshot through clothing. Passing through the clothing allowed for the slight dispersion of pellets.

FAQ: With the extensive destruction of the head that occurs with high-velocity rifle wounds or contact range shotgun wounds, can an entrance and exit always be identified?

Answer: Yes and no; while close inspection of the edges of the wound and re-approximation of skin edges should allow for the identification of the entrance site (Figure 11.70A-C), the exit site may not be identified.

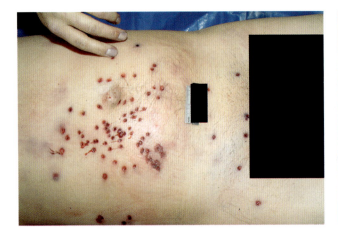

Figure 11.65. Shotgun wound created by individual pellet perforations only. Once the central mass of pellets has entirely dispersed, only single individual defects from each pellet will be identified.

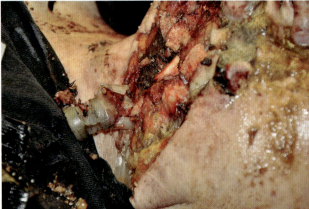

Figure 11.66. Wadding lodged in body. This individual was shot multiple times with both birdshot and buckshot. When the body was first viewed, one shot sleeve was partially entangled in the disrupted tissue at the left side of the jaw.

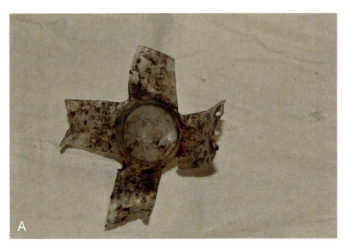

Figure 11.67A. Representative fired shot sleeve. This shot sleeve, fired from a 12 gauge shotgun, has opened up, with the four wings forming a plus sign. A 0.410 shell has a shot sleeve with only three wings.

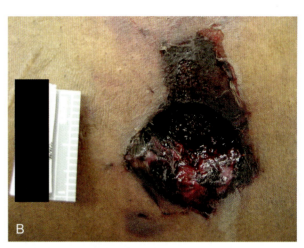

Figure 11.67B. Wadding strike against the skin. When the shot sleeve passes through the air, the wings of the shot sleeve will open. The rectangular abrasion at 12 o'clock in the image is from a wing of the shot sleeve striking the skin.

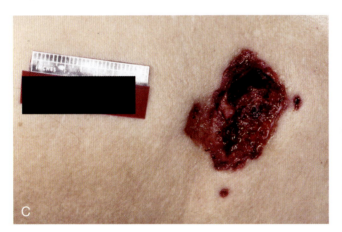

Figure 11.67C. Wadding strike against the skin. At 12 o'clock, 6 o'clock, and 9 o'clock, and faintly at 3 o'clock are rectangular abrasions, consistent with the wings of the shot sleeve. At 3 and 6 o'clock are satellite perforations.

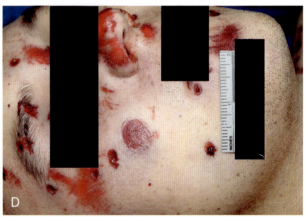

Figure 11.67D. Wadding strike against the skin. On the right cheek is a round abrasion, which is from the base of the shot sleeve impacting the skin (arrow). There are pellet perforations of the right eyelids, the right cheek, and the peri-oral region. The decedent has abrasions of the nose and chin that occurred after they collapsed from the shotgun wounds.

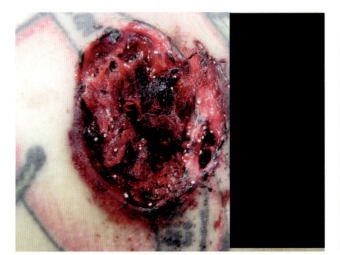

Figure 11.68. Scalloped shotgun wound with filler material. Contained within some shotgun shells are tiny white plastic pellets, which are filler material. These pellets can be found in closer range shotgun wounds.

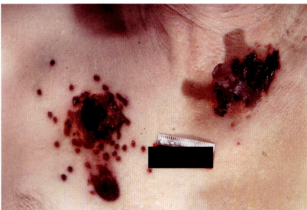

Figure 11.69. Individual shot multiple times with a shotgun. The defect on the left side of the image has a central defect with numerous satellite perforations. Inferior to the wound is a round abrasion. This resulted from the base of the shot sleeve impacting the skin. The defect on the right side of the image has a shot sleeve embedded within the wound. Based solely upon this image, the shot that caused the wound on the left side of the image was fired at a greater distance than the shot that caused the wound on the right side of the image.

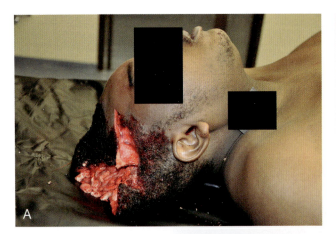
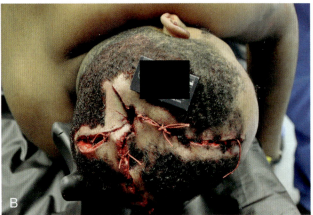
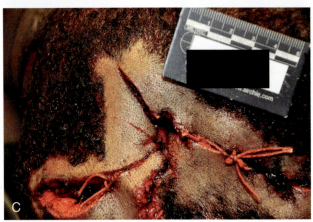

Figure 11.70. Extensively damaged head with identification of entrance wound. When a pathologist is confronted with a gaping defect of the head (**A**), finding the entrance wound can appear daunting; however, re-approximation of the wound edges (**B**) will usually always reveal the entrance wound (**C**). There is a marginal abrasion, with soot at the edge of the wound.

SAMPLE NOTE: WORDING CAUSE OF DEATH FOR HANDGUN/RIFLE WOUND VS SHOTGUN WOUNDS

In general, gunshot wounds are considering those caused by a handgun or rifle, and shotgun wounds are those caused by shotguns. If an individual dies from a self-inflicted wound of the head caused by a handgun or rifle, the death certificate is usually certified as "Contact gunshot wound of the head" or "Gunshot wound of the head." If the individual dies from a self-inflicted wound of the head by a shotgun, the death certificate is usually certified as "Contact shotgun wound of the head" or "Shotgun wound of the head."

SAMPLE NOTE: WORDING CAUSE OF DEATH FOR MULTIPLE GUNSHOT WOUNDS

If an individual dies from multiple gunshot wounds, the certifier can attempt to distinguish the most immediately lethal gunshot wound as the cause of death and list other gunshot wounds as contributory. For example, the cause of death is certified as "Gunshot wound of the head" in part I, and "Gunshot wounds of the extremities" are listed as contributory causes of death in part II. However, lumping everything together as "Multiple gunshot wounds" is often preferred, with a distinction of which gunshot wound(s) was/were most likely the lethal injury discussed with the family or in court as the question arises.

INTERNAL EXAMINATION

One important concept in understanding the pattern of injuries in the internal organs is the concept of a temporary cavity and a permanent cavity.[55] The permanent cavity is created by the actual passage of the projectile, and is the damage created when the projectile impacts tissue. Projectiles that deform (eg, hollow-point projectiles) and projectiles that are yawing (ie, rotating off their axis of flight) create a wider permanent cavity.[3] Also, fragmentation of the projectile will contribute to a larger permanent cavity, with the secondary projectiles expanding the size of the permanent cavity.[3]

The temporary cavity is a wider zone of potential injury created by the transfer of kinetic energy to the tissue and can cause injury distal to the pathway of the projectile.[56,57] The temporary cavity is created by tissue at the edge of the permanent cavity being pushed away from the projectile.[3] Non-elastic tissues such as liver or bone are at greater risk for damage from the temporary cavity than elastic tissues such as muscle, bowel, and lung.[3] This temporary cavity can also briefly expand the brain, leading to temporary herniation and resultant contusions (eg, of the uncus or cerebellar tonsils) (Figure 11.71A and B). Figure 11.72 illustrates the effects of a temporary cavity. The temporary cavity can stretch and tear tissue.

For handguns and rifles, the amount of damage done by the projectile is determined by its kinetic energy ($KE = 1/2\ mv^2$), the type of projectile (eg, full metal-jacketed projectile vs hollow point), the bullet caliber and mass, the organ system struck, and the tendency for the bullet to lose speed and to tumble.[24] A high-velocity rifle will have more kinetic energy and can potentially cause more damage than a handgun, which have lower velocities; however, if a full metal-jacketed projectile is used, the bullet may pass entirely through the body, without imparting all of its kinetic energy to the tissue, whereas with an expanding projectile, such as a hollow point, the entirety of the projectile's kinetic energy will be imparted to the body, causing more damage. Also, an expanded bullet will create a larger permanent cavity. Both rifle wounds and contact shotgun wounds can cause extensive damage, whereas, contact range handgun wounds, even if a large caliber (eg, 0.38), can cause less extensive damage. Powder gases from contact wounds can contribute to injury and, with wounds of the head, can contribute to fracturing of the cranium, with fractures of the cranium due to the temporary cavity being rare[3] (Figure 11.73).

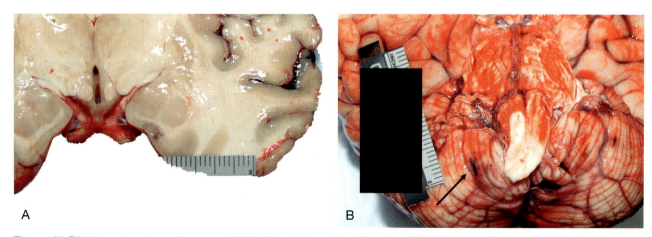

Figure 11.71. Contusions in gunshot wound of the head. This individual sustained a contact gunshot wound of the head, with the projectile passing through the cerebral hemisphere, and not affecting the hippocampus or cerebellum. When the brain expanded with the wound, the unci and cerebellar tonsils briefly herniated, producing herniation contusions (**A** and **B** respectively, with arrow for tonsillar herniations).

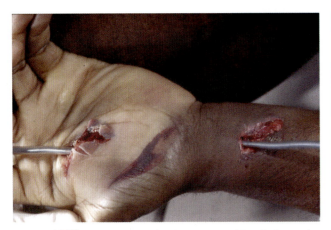 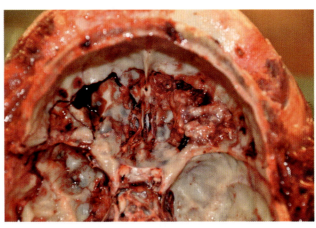

Figure 11.72. Gunshot wound of the wrist and hand. The probe passes from the entrance wound at the wrist to the exit wound on the hand. In between, there is hemorrhage underlying an intact epidermis. When the temporary cavity expanded this region, it tore tissue leading to hemorrhage. The area of the hemorrhage between the entrance and exit wounds is not directly in the pathway of the projectile. (Courtesy of Hamo Muergerditchian.)

Figure 11.73. Fracture of orbital plates, not in pathway of projectile. This individual sustained a contact gunshot wound of the right side of the head, with the projectile passing upward and backward, but not through the orbital plates. The fracture of the orbital plates most likely resulted from powder gases, unless within a few centimeters of the wound track, in which case the temporary cavity could contribute.

> **FAQ:** In a decedent with multiple gunshot wounds, can the pathway of each projectile be accurately determined prior to internal examination and, if not, can the pathway always be determined after internal examination?
>
> **Answer:** While the possible pathway of the projectile(s) should at least be considered during the external examination following radiography, opening the body and documenting the injuries to the internal organs is necessary for determination of the actual pathway of the projectile, and often, the perceived pathways of the projectiles based upon the external examination are modified greatly by the internal examination. With multiple gunshot wounds that have intersecting pathways, accurate determination of the pathway for each projectile may not be possible in any given autopsy.

SAMPLE NOTE: DOCUMENTING INTERMINGLED PATHWAYS OF PROJECTILES

In the body of the report, when there is an overlap between projectile pathways, the report can be written such as to account for that. The report can separate out two (or more) gunshot wounds as to their entrances but can list shared injuries in a single paragraph and assign exits to the shared list of injuries and not to the entrance wounds themselves.

PEARLS & PITFALLS

Photographs displaying a probe to demonstrate the pathway of the projectile can be useful to the pathologist when they write their autopsy report, law enforcement when conducting their investigation, and attorneys when trying the case in court (Figure 11.74).

PEARLS & PITFALLS

Documenting an intra-oral gunshot wound can be difficult, especially since rigor mortis is most often present and renders opening the mouth a physical challenge, with the potential for damaging the teeth if done incorrectly. Removal of the neck organs, including the tongue, allows for better access to the area for photography; however, it is still often necessary to take more than one photograph until a good image is obtained.

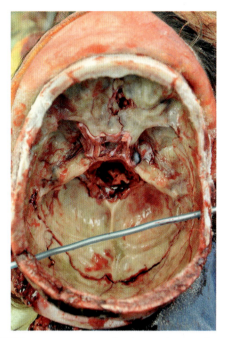

Figure 11.74. Documentation of pathway of projectile with probe. A probe can most often easily be placed between the entrance and exit wounds. This provides a nice visual representation of the pathway of the projectile, for use by the pathologist in writing their report or in explaining the injuries to other parties.

> **PEARLS & PITFALLS**
>
> Microscopic examination of the skin or soft tissue at the entrance wound or from the soft tissue underlying an entrance wound can, in the case of a contact gunshot wound, be used to help identify soot (Figure 11.75A and B), although separation of soot from bullet wipe on microscopic examination is problematic. Bullet wipe should only be present at the rim of the defect (ie, where the projectile contacted the soft tissue) and not on the soft tissue adjacent to the wound margin. In addition, it is possible to collect a cytologic specimen from the projectile and, using microscopic examination, potentially help determine what organs the projectile passed through.

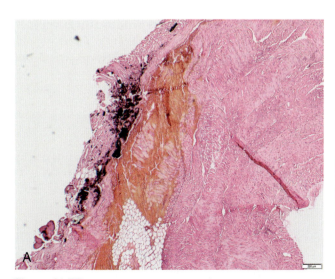
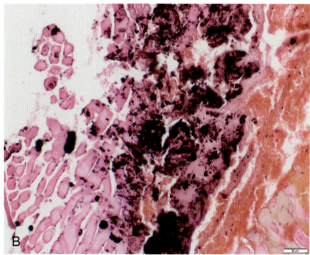

Figure 11.75. Microscopic examination for soot. Microscopic examination of the edge of the wound can assist in the identification and documentation of soot (**A** and **B**). This can be particularly useful in decomposed individuals or when drying to the edge of the wound has created artifact appearing as soot (hematoxylin and eosin, low power and high power).

PEARLS & PITFALLS

When an individual with a firearm injury is autopsied and blood is removed from a body cavity, that blood should be retained until all projectiles are accounted for; either that or strained or otherwise examined in a fashion to ensure no projectile is present before the blood is discarded The same is true for any disaster pouch or other body bag in which the body is received. Accounting for all projectiles can involve additional radiographs of removed organs, removed clothing, and other items.

PEARLS & PITFALLS

While in almost all circumstances, for each entrance, there should be an exit wound, or, if no corresponding exit is present, the projectile should be found within the body, in the case of frangible bullets, after entrance of the projectile into the body, it can fragment to such a degree that no large projectile fragment is identifiable, and, on rare occasions, the pathways for two entrances can merge, leading to a single exit.[58]

PEARLS & PITFALLS

Close inspection of the inner surface of the cranium can help identify an impact site. When projectiles impact the cranium, they often do not have enough energy to fracture through the bone and will instead tumble along the surface and come to final rest at a point some distance from where they impacted the cranium. Using the final resting point of the projectile in the determination of pathway may lead to a marked misrepresentation of the pathway of the projectile, whereas using the impact site, if one is present, should allow for the best determination of the pathway of the projectile (Figure 11.76A and B).

MECHANISM OF DEATH IN GUNSHOT WOUNDS

Lethal firearm injuries produce a variety of physiologic changes, which can lead to a relatively immediate death or a more delayed death. A delayed death can occur minutes to hours following the gunshot wound or days to months to years following the injury (Figure 11.77A-G). During a death investigation, a delayed death due to a gunshot wound is always important to consider in certain individuals as, if missed, the manner of death may be miscertified as natural, instead of as homicide, suicide, or accident. For example, if

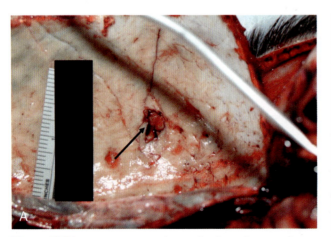
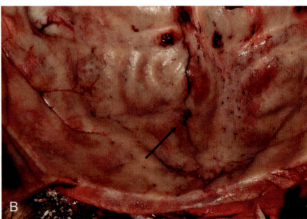

Figure 11.76. Impact site on endocranial surface of cranium from gunshot wound. Both (**A** and **B**) illustrate an impact site on the endocranial surface from a gunshot wound (arrow in each image), with both images coming from separate autopsies. The identification of an impact site can assist in a more accurate determination of the pathway of the projectile in gunshot wounds in which the projectile does not perforate the cranium.

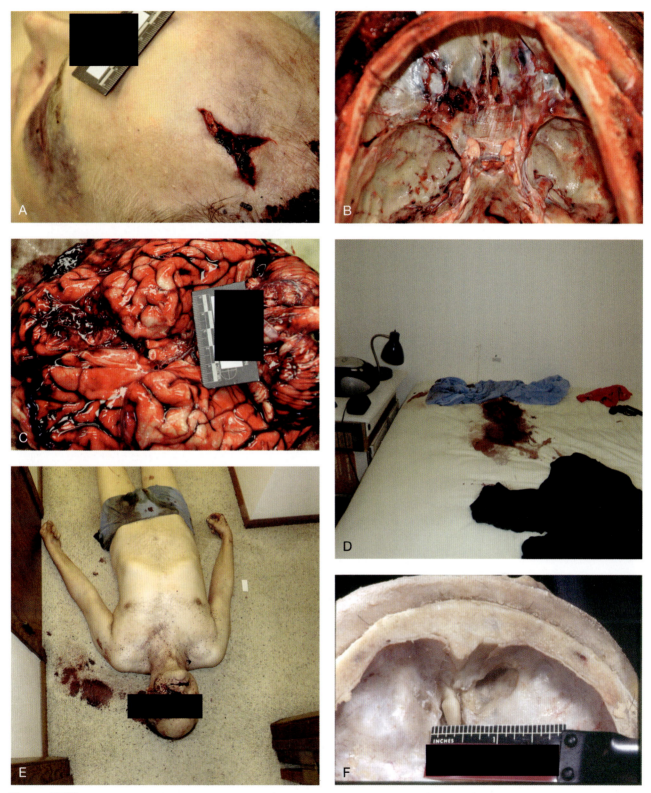

Figure 11.77. Delayed deaths from gunshot wounds of the head. In (A-E), this individual survived for a short period of time after a self-inflicted gunshot wound of the head. (A) is the exit wound, with the pathway of the projectile being mostly upward through the anterior portion of the head. The projectile entered the cranial cavity through the floor of the left anterior cranial fossa (B) and perforated the left frontal lobe of the brain (C). The decedent shot himself while lying in bed (D), following which he got up and walked out into the hallway, where he collapsed and was subsequently found (E). In (F and G), this individual was shot by another person 10+ years prior to his date of death. The previous gunshot wound created a fistula between a cranial sinus and his cranial cavity (F).

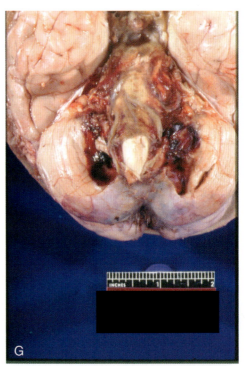

Figure 11.77. He developed sinusitis many years later, leading to meningitis and a cerebral abscess (**G**), and his death. The death certificate was initially signed by the clinical physician with meningitis as the cause of death, with gunshot wound of the head as a contributory condition, and the manner of death was natural. This certification was flagged by the Bureau of Vital Statistics, and referred to the medical examiner's office, with an autopsy subsequently performed.

a 40-year-old man dies due to pneumonia secondary to quadriplegia, it is possible that his quadriplegia is due to a gunshot wound.

While common mechanisms for immediate or relatively immediate death following a gunshot wound could include damage to the brainstem and exsanguination, other less common mechanisms can include tension pneumothorax, tension pneumocephalus,[59] air embolus,[60-63] indirect damage to the spinal cord, development of a subdural hemorrhage,[64,65] aortic dissection,[66] or fat embolus.[67] Meningitis can also occur relatively acutely following the gunshot wound.[68] In addition, gunshot wounds can cause acute ischemia due to inducing arterial vasospasm, which could produce downstream effects in an individual who survives for some period of time after the wound was incurred.[69]

Common mechanisms for a significantly delayed death following a gunshot wound could include sepsis, pneumonia, seizure disorder, and pulmonary thromboembolism. Sepsis can develop due to perforation of the gastrointestinal tract or just the gunshot wound itself as all gunshot wounds are contaminated with bacteria.[3] Other less common mechanisms that could result in a significantly delayed death include atrio-esophageal or arteriovenous fistula and intracranial aneurysm.[70-72]

> **PEARLS & PITFALLS**
>
> Gunshot wounds of the heart, aorta, and even the head may not be immediately incapacitating, and individuals are capable of purposeful movement for some period of time after the injury occurred[73-78] and can even survive the event.[77,79,80]

COMPOSITION OF PROJECTILES

As forensic pathologists will be collecting projectiles as evidence, it is important to understand the basic composition of a projectile. In general, most handgun and rifle projectiles are a lead core with a copper jacket, although other types of jacket are possible. The jacket will have rifling marks from the barrel of the weapon, and examination of these rifling marks will potentially allow the firearm examiner to match the projectile found in the body to a weapon recovered and suspected to have been used in the death. The jacket will have both lands and grooves, from the rifling in the barrel, that can allow for an estimation of firearm type. However, the rifle barrel also produces microscopic scratches on the jacket, and this pattern can potentially be matched to the specific weapon that fired it (Figure 11.78). When the jacket is recovered from the body, care must be taken to not introduce additional damage to the surface; therefore, a metal instrument should not be used, and instead plastic forceps or fingers are best to handle the jacket so as to prevent damage and potentially obscuring of rifling marks. On radiographs, a copper jacket can be distinguished from a lead core based upon its radiodensity. The copper jacket is less radio-dense. Smaller-caliber projectiles, especially 0.22 caliber, often do not have a distinct copper jacket but may instead have a copper gild or simply be lead (Figure 11.79). Some forms of larger-caliber projectiles, such as wadcutter and semi-wadcutter, do not have a copper jacket (Figure 11.80). With shotgun wounds, the projectile will be either a slug, buckshot, or birdshot. In addition, if the range is close enough, the shot sleeve (ie, a plastic shot cup with three [0.410] or four [12, 20 gauge] petals) will be present (Figure 11.81). Some plastic shot cups produced by some manufacturers will have more than three or four petals. The wadding can be a component of the shot sleeve or separate.

> **FAQ:** If an individual is shot with a shotgun, do all the pellets need to be recovered?
>
> **Answer:** If the shotgun shell contained birdshot, only 10 to 20 representative pellets must be recovered, along with the wadding/shot sleeve (or shot cup) if present. In recovering birdshot pellets, recovery of intact pellets to enable accurate weight and diameter determination is most important (ie, five undamaged pellets are more useful to determine the ammunition type than 20 flattened pellets). If the individual was shot with buckshot, all pellets need to be recovered. The entry defect for a buckshot pellet and the entry defect for a handgun or rifle projectile can appear similar, and, on radiograph, a mushroomed smaller-caliber projectile and a deformed buckshot pellet could easily be confused. Therefore, recovery of all buckshot pellets is necessary to ensure that the individual was not shot with a shotgun with buckshot as well as a handgun or rifle.

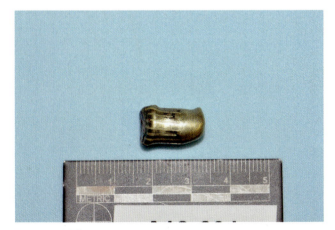

Figure 11.78. Copper-jacketed projectile recovered from body. The jacket has large striations at the left side, which are lands and grooves. The pattern of lands and grooves can assist in identification of ammunition type (eg, Winchester vs Remington); however, microscopic examination reveals tiny grooves secondary to imperfections in the barrel, which will allow the firearm examiner to match the projectile recovered from the body to the weapon suspected of having fired it. Care must be taken at autopsy not to damage the projectile, so use gloved fingers or plastic forceps to retrieve the projectile and not metal forceps so as not to damage the rifling marks.

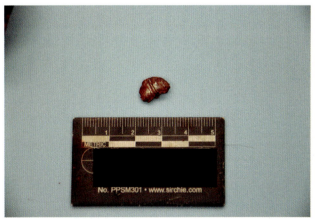

Figure 11.79. Lead projectile. Low caliber projectiles, such as a .22, are often only a lead projectile with no copper jacket, although some will be copper gilded. The lead projectile in these cases will bear the rifling marks.

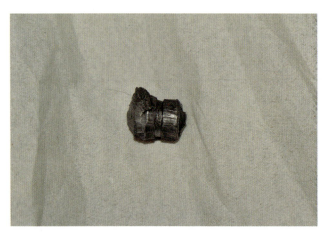

Figure 11.80. Lead projectile. Not a 0.22 caliber projectile, but a larger-caliber projectile. Wadcutter and semi-wadcutter projectiles do not have a copper jacket.

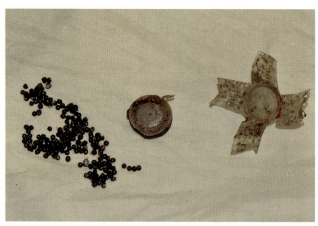

Figure 11.81. Shotgun pellets, wadding, and shot sleeve. From left to right in the image are birdshot pellets, wadding, and the plastic shot sleeve.

MANNER OF DEATH DETERMINATION WITH GUNSHOT WOUNDS

With a firearm injury, depending upon the circumstances, four manners of death are possible: homicide, suicide, accident, and undetermined. Accidental firearm injuries are rare, and often represent a concealed suicide. Copeland and Dobi-Babic and Katalinic discuss features of accidental gunshot wounds.[81,82] With the vast majority of firearm injuries, the manner of death is homicide or suicide; however, distinguishing between the two can be difficult. Other than a confirmed distant range gunshot wound (ie, with no soot on the clothing or skin, no intermediary object, and no other evidence of a closer range fire) and without a mechanism for doing so at the scene (ie, it is possible for an individual to set up a mechanism for causing a self-inflicted distant gunshot wound,[83] any other range can be encountered both as a homicide and as a suicide. Also, the location of a gunshot wound cannot, by itself, distinguish between a homicide and a suicide. A gunshot wound of the back of the trunk or back of the head can be the result of a suicide.[84,85] While contact range gunshot wounds are the most common range encountered with gunshot wound suicides, close range gunshot wounds (with soot and stippling, or just stippling) of the face or scalp can still occur from suicidal actions[86] (Figure 11.82A and B). To assist in the determination

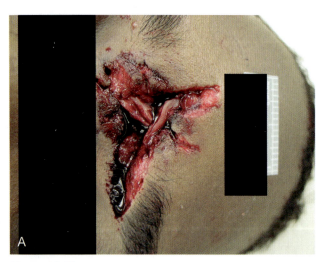
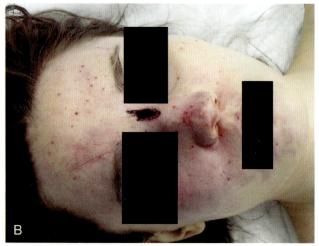

Figure 11.82. Homicide (contact of forehead) vs Suicide (with stippling). In (A), the decedent sustained a contact gunshot wound of the glabella region, which produced radiating tears characteristic of a contact wound. The wound was inflicted by another person. In (B), the decedent sustained a self-inflicted gunshot wound of the face, similar in region to (A) for comparison. This individual shot themself while holding the weapon at arm's length to look down the barrel of the weapon as it fired. Because the weapon was a distance from the body, only stippling is present. These two images illustrate how range of fire alone is an inadequate predictor of manner of death.

of homicide vs suicide, Cave et al. introduced a method for obtaining a likelihood ratio using various features of a gunshot wound to predict homicide vs suicide.[87]

Determination of manner of death is based upon the scene investigation in combination with the autopsy findings. Additional findings, other than just the gunshot wound, may be identified at autopsy that would help support either homicide or suicide as a manner of death and should be searched for. For example, if an individual has a gunshot wound of the hand in addition to a lethal gunshot wound of another region of the body, that the individual held their hand between them and their attacker is most likely, and would support the manner as homicide (Figure 11.83). When individuals shoot themself, they may hold the weapon with one hand or with two. When holding a handgun or rifle with a second hand, soot can deposit on the non-firing hand, from the muzzle or from the gap in revolvers (Figure 11.84A and B). Another deposit that can be found on the hands is a rust-colored discoloration, which indicates that the barrel of the weapon was against the skin for a prolonged period of time (Figure 11.85). When an individual uses an intra-oral site for the gunshot wound, they will often seal their lips around the barrel. When the weapon discharges, the gases released by the weapon will expand the mouth with no release, which can cause tears at the corners of the mouth and in a peri-oral distribution on the face (Figure 11.86). While grouped parallel scars on the extremities, both upper and lower, do not necessarily indicate the current gunshot wound was suicidal in origin, the scars do indicate past episodes of self-harm, which can add support to a determination of suicide (Figure 11.87A and B).

> **PEARLS & PITFALLS**
>
> Manner of death determinations of suicide can be the most controversial cases that a forensic pathologist will have, with families adamantly opposed to the death being a suicide. Having as much information as possible from the investigation and autopsy to support the manner of death as suicide is the best method to diffuse this disbelief.

> **FAQ:** Is the finding of a weapon at a distance from the body necessarily indicative of a homicide?
>
> **Answer:** No, individuals can easily throw a weapon after they have fired it.[88] Also, the individual can stagger and fall backward from a weapon, or after the shot has been fired, the weapon can tumble and end up some distance from the body.

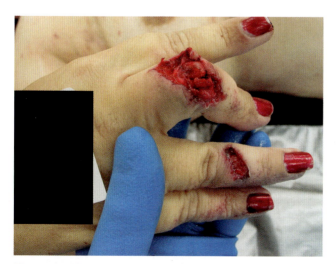

Figure 11.83. Defensive type injuries of the hands. As with sharp force and blunt force injuries, a person being shot by another person can interpose their extremities, often upper extremities, but lower extremities are also possible, between themselves and their attacker. This type of injury is consistent with the decedent defending themselves, and would help establish homicide as the manner of death.

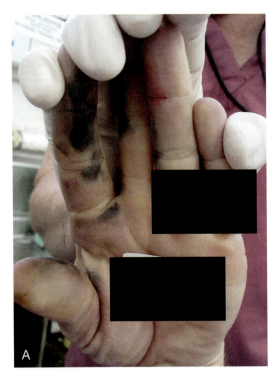

Figure 11.84A. Soot on the hand. If an individual holds a weapon with their second hand, such as for stabilization against their body while they fire the weapon, soot can be deposited on the hand being used to stabilize the weapon. Finding such soot on the hand helps support suicide as a manner of death, unless the individual was grabbing that weapon that was held by their attacker as that weapon was fired.

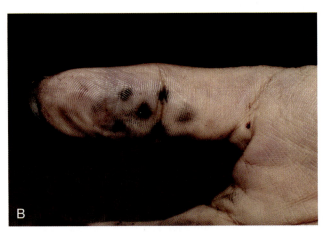

Figure 11.84B. Soot on hand. Soot deposited on the hands from holding the weapon can sometimes have a specific pattern. The evenly dispersed dots of soot on the hands are consistent with a muzzle flash suppressor on a rifle.

SAMPLE NOTES: DOCUMENTING A GUNSHOT WOUND

I. Contact gunshot wound of the head:
   A. Entrance: near the center of the forehead is a 1/2 inch entrance-type gunshot wound that is centered 2 inches below the top of the head and 1 inch to the left of midline. There is a circumferential marginal abrasion, which is up to 1/8 inch wide from 12 to 6 o'clock and up to 3/16 inch wide from 6 to 12 o'clock. On the skin around the wound is a rim of stippling, which is overall 3 × 2 inches in size.
   B. Injuries: the projectile perforated the skin of the forehead, the left side of the frontal bone, with inward beveling, 1/2 inch in width on the inner surface of the bone, the left frontal lobe of the brain, the left temporal lobe of the brain, the left temporal bone, and exited.
   C. Projectile recovery: within the left temporal lobe is recovered a fragment of copper jacket.
   D. Exit: on the left side of the head, posterior to the left ear, is a 3/4 inch exit-type stellate gunshot wound that is centered 3 inches below the top of the head, 1 inch posterior to the tragus of the left ear, and 2 inches superior to the tragus of the left ear.
   E. Associated findings: the left upper eyelid is hemorrhagic. There is patchy subgaleal hemorrhage, most prominent at the entrance and exit defects. The brain has patchy subarachnoid hemorrhage and a patchy thin subdural hemorrhage. Along the wound track are punctate hemorrhages of the cerebral parenchyma.
   F. Pathway of the projectile: right to left, front to back, and slightly downward.

These injuries, having been once described, will not be repeated.

NEAR MISSES

Near miss #1: Interpreting the skin changes at the entrance wound alone as to the presence of soot or stippling/powder tattooing without considering clothing that might not have been received with the body but was worn by the decedent at the time of the firearm

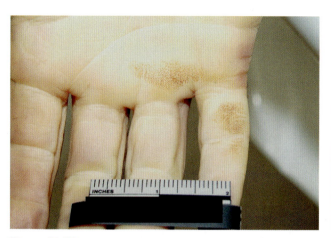

Figure 11.85. Rust colored deposit on hand. When the hand has been in contact with the barrel of a weapon for a prolonged period, a rust-colored discoloration of the skin can occur.

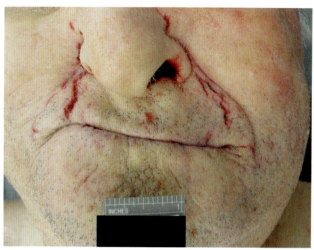

Figure 11.86. Oral stretch marks. When a decedent shoots themself in the mouth, they will most often have their lips sealed around the barrel. When the hot air and gases from the gunshot enter the mouth, they cannot exit, leading to over-expansion of the mouth which can produce stretch-type tears of the peri-orbital region, and even full-thickness tears of the lips.

injury can lead to misinterpretation of range. Figure 11.88A-C illustrates how clothing can block the deposition of soot on the skin and the ability of unburned gunpowder to create stippling. If the individual in Figure 11.88A-C had been wearing a solid shirt instead of a jersey, and if the gunshot wound to the neck had been lower, and if the clothing had been removed prior to the autopsy examination, no soot or stippling would have been identified, and the two wounds could have been misinterpreted as distant range gunshot wounds.

Near miss #2: Firearms injury and other injury types (eg, blunt and/or sharp force injuries) can be admixed and potentially misinterpreted. The individual in Figure 11.89A and B was both beaten and shot.

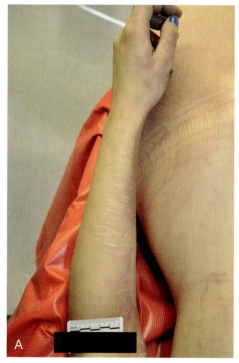
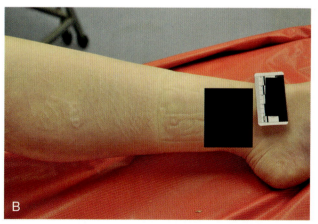

Figure 11.87. (**A** and **B**) Scars on extremities. In cases of suicide, examination of the body may provide other evidence of self-harm. Parallel linear scars on the extremities are indicative of past incidents of self-harm and can help support a current determination of a manner of suicide.

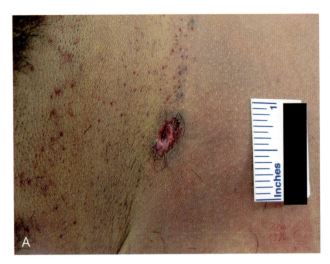
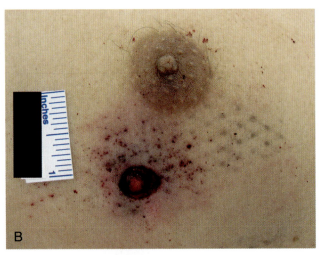
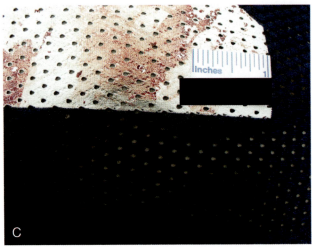

Figure 11.88. Clothing obstructing gunshot residue from striking the skin. This individual was shot twice. (A) is an entrance wound just at the junction between the neck and the back. Notice that to the left of the wound (which would be toward the head) there is stippling on the skin, but to the right of wound, there is no stippling on the skin. (B) is an entrance wound of the chest near the nipple. Around the wound are numerous same size and spaced circular collections of soot. (C) is the clothing the decedent was wearing—a jersey. On the anterior surface in the image can be seen soot. While the jersey blocked some soot, other soot entered through the holes and marked the skin as in (B). On the back, above the collar line, unburned gunpowder reached the skin, causing stippling, but below the collar line, the shirt blocked gunpowder from reaching the skin. If the shirt had been solid, instead of a jersey, and if the gunshot wound of the neck and back junction had been lower, neither soot nor stippling would have been found. This case illustrates the importance of not using the lack of soot or stippling as a sole criterion for a distant range gunshot wound.

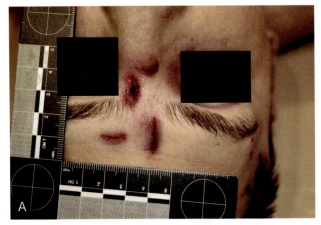
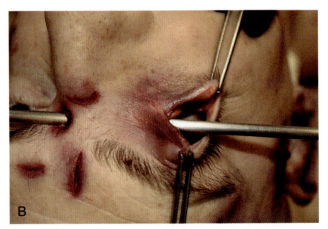

Figure 11.89. Blunt force injuries and gunshot wound of the forehead and bridge of nose. Examination of the bridge of the nose and forehead revealed what were initially interpreted as a patch of lacerations (A); however, a radiograph of the head revealed a projectile fragment at this site. Re-examination of the wounds revealed that one of the lacerations was actually an entrance gunshot wound with a marginal abrasion, with the exit wound located at the medial corner of the right eye. A probe illustrates the pathway of the projectile (B).

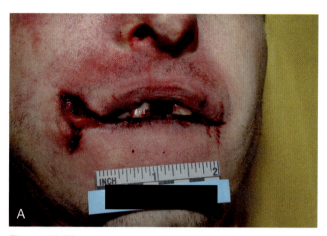
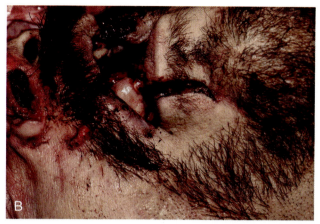

Figure 11.90. Oral and peri-oral tears. In (**A**), the injuries were associated with an intra-oral gunshot wound; whereas in (**B**), the injuries were associated with a train accident, with no evidence of a firearm injury from scene investigation or autopsy examination.

Near miss #3: While self-inflicted intra-oral rifle and shotgun wounds of the head frequently have oral and peri-oral tears in the skin, including up to full thickness tears of the lips (Figure 11.90A), a similar pattern of injury can be found in other circumstances. The decedent in Figure 11.90B was found on train tracks. Initial observation at autopsy identified oral and peri-oral tears. Despite extensive dissection, no definitive evidence of a gunshot wound or shotgun wound was identified, and radiography revealed no metallic fragments. Scene investigation did not identify a firearm. Review of the train videos, because of the incident occurring at night, were not informative, as it could not be determined whether the decedent was alive or dead at the time the train hit them.

Near miss #4: The individual in Figure 11.91A and B was shot multiple times with shotguns, both with buckshot and birdshot. The face had numerous punctate red lesions, which could be misinterpreted as birdshot, since birdshot loaded shells were used during the shooting incident; however, the lesions were actually stippling related to a close range shotgun wound.

Near miss #5: Incomplete radiography of the body can allow for projectiles to be missed. While many offices have access to a full-body scanner, which can produce a 3D radiograph of the entire body, and/or a CT scanner, many offices do not. If a radiograph does not include all areas of interest, a projectile may be missed. For example, if the projectile is just underneath the skin of the chest, but the radiograph does not include that

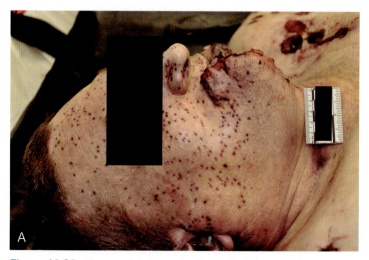
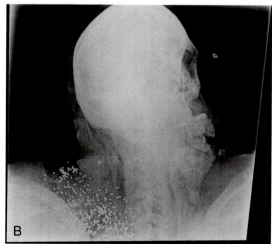

Figure 11.91. Photo and radiograph of individual shot with shotguns. (**A**) shows the face with numerous punctate red discolorations of the face, which could, in the context of the other injuries be interpreted as birdshot pellet entrances from a more distant range shotgun wound, in which the pellets had time to disperse completely from the central mass. (**B**) shows a radiograph of the head and upper chest. While there is a mass of birdshot pellets on the right side of the chest from another wound, there are no corresponding pellets in the head. The punctate red lesions on the face are stippling associated with a close range shotgun wound.

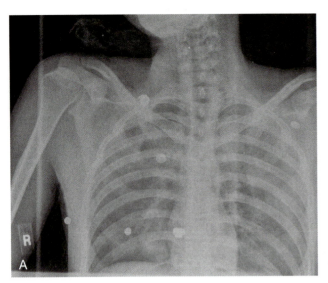 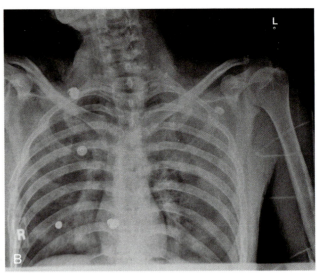

Figure 11.92. Radiographs of a decedent who was shot multiple times, both with buckshot and handgun projectiles. One radiograph (**A**) reveals a buckshot pellet that was immediately underneath the skin on the right side of the chest inferior to the axilla; however, radiograph (**B**), which during the course of the autopsy was actually taken first, does not include the very edge of the body and thus does not reveal the projectile. These two images illustrate the importance of complete coverage of the body by radiography when searching for projectiles.

area, the projectile may be missed (Figure 11.92A and B). Also, on a 2D radiograph, it is possible for projectiles and projectile fragments to overlap, and although one is recovered, the second one may be missed (Figure 11.93). Also, metallic objects in and on the clothing or associated with medical intervention can overlap a projectile, obscuring it on the radiograph.

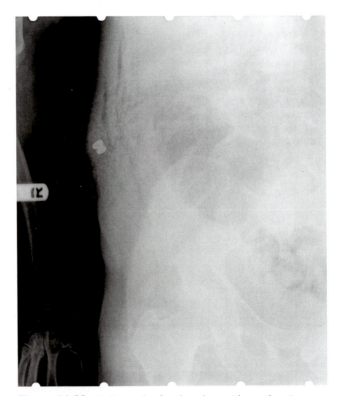

Figure 11.93. Radiograph of a decedent with overlapping projectiles. In the radiograph, two projectiles overlap but do not completely obscure each other; however, the image should represent how it is possible for one projectile to completely overlap another projectile, appearing as only one projectile on the radiograph. Use of two views (eg, anterior-posterior and lateral) or use of a device capable of producing a 3D radiograph would, obviously, automatically correct for this possible problem.

Near miss #6: It is not uncommon to encounter a retained projectile (ie, from a gunshot or shotgun wound that occurred previous to the decedent's terminal event) (Figure 11.94). This retained projectile should be recovered to confirm its identification. Retained projectiles can be difficult to find via dissection, as they are often contained within a fibrous coat and there is no associated hemorrhage. A retained birdshot pellet or BB from a previous gunshot wound, when present in the radiograph with a typical handgun projectile, could mimic a 0.25 ACP (Figure 11.95A-C).

Near miss #7: In suicidal gunshot wounds, while the temple, mouth, chin, and chest are common locations for the entrance,[89] the external ear canal (almost completely invisible to external examination), vagina, and anus are rare but potential locations for an entrance wound[90] (Figure 11.96A-D). In the same context, while projectiles most commonly exit the body through the skin, it is possible for the projectile to exit through the mouth, anus, or another naturally occurring orifice (Figure 11.97).

Near miss #8: To correctly interpret bevel in the bone, the entire circumference of the defect is required. If only half of the defect in the bone were available for interpretation, a keyhole defect in the bone could be misinterpreted as an exit defect (Figure 11.98).

Near miss #9: While it could appear that an individual with a firearm injury would not be missed at autopsy, such is not the case. With later stages of decomposition or with other significant injuries (eg, a person shot and then run over by a vehicle), gunshot wounds can be missed at autopsy. An index of suspicion based upon the scene investigation or additional imaging can help ensure that these cases are not missed.[91,92]

Near miss #10: Cast projectiles are sometimes encountered. Because of their elongated form and cannelures for lubricants, they are easily identified on radiographs.[93]

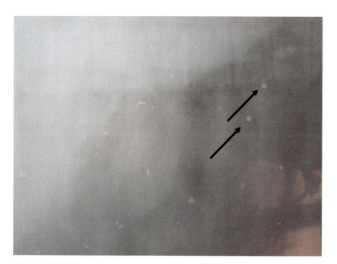

Figure 11.94. Radiograph of a decedent who was shot with a high-powered rifle. The radiograph reveals the characteristic lead snow storm pattern of a high-powered rifle, with the projectile at least partially breaking up into innumerable tiny fragments, but at the arrows are two round radio-dense objects. The round appearance of the radio-dense objects would not be compatible with a fragmenting high-powered rifle projectile, as the fragments so produced are irregular in size and shape and would not be essentially perfectly round. The individual had been previously shot with birdshot and had retained pellets. Any retained pellets/projectiles will be identified on radiographs and should be removed at autopsy to confirm their origin and retained.

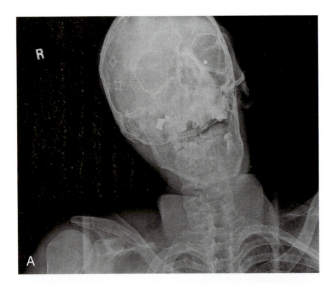
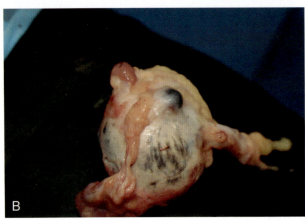
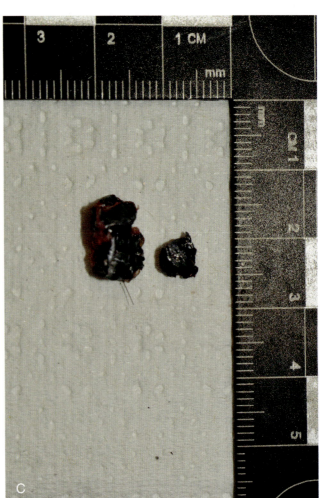

Figure 11.95. Radiograph and images of decedent shot with handgun, with retained projectile. (**A**) is radiograph, which revealed a single pellet near the left eye and projectile fragments and appeared as 0.25 ACP ammunition. The pellet actually was a retained BB (**B**) in a fibrous capsule at the edge of the left eye. (**C**) is of the projectile fragments recovered.

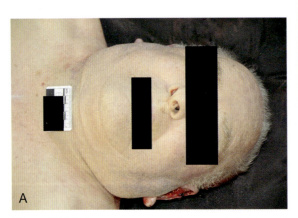
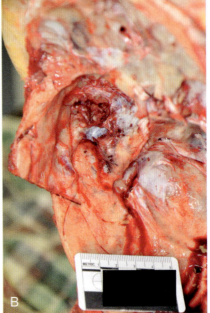

Figure 11.96. Decedent with gunshot wound of the ear. An autopsy was conducted on an individual who sustained a suicidal gunshot wound. Initially, blood was found in the left ear, but no entrance was identified upon external examination of the body including the head (**A**). The entrance was presumed to be intra-oral, with blood in the left ear being from basilar skull fractures, a common injury sequence pattern seen with gunshot wounds of the head. Upon removal of the brain, a defect was found in the left petrous ridge, which was the entry point of the projectile into the cranial cavity (**B**). Externally, no gunshot wound of the left ear was easily apparent (**C**) as the barrel of the weapon had been placed deep into the external ear canal. The pathway of the projectile is illustrated in (**D**).

Figure 11.96c-d (continued)

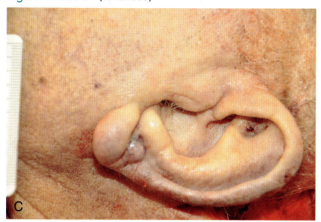

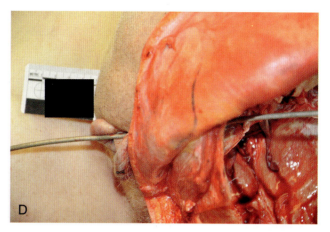

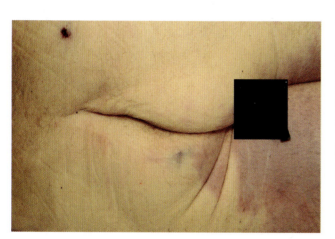

Figure 11.97. Near anal exit of projectile. Just lateral to the gluteal cleft at the left buttock is an ill-defined blue-purple contusion, underlying which was the projectile in the soft tissue. While the projectile did not actually exit through the anus, its proximity to the anus illustrates how such an event could occur.

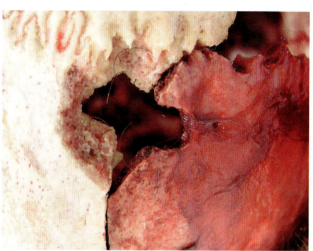

Figure 11.98. Example of a keyhole defect in the bone to illustrate that both sides of the defect are needed for proper interpretation. The image represents the re-approximation of two fragments of bone that encompassed the entrance wound. The fragment to the right side has a punched out appearance and the fragment to the left has a beveled appearance. When viewed together, the keyhole nature of the wound is apparent, and keyhole defects essentially always represent an entrance wound; however, if only the bone fragment on the left side of the image were examined (ie, the fragment with the outward bevel), the wound could easily be misinterpreted as an exit wound.

References

1. Cunliffe CH, Denton JS. An atypical gunshot wound from a home-made zip gun—the value of a thorough scene investigation. *J Forensic Sci*. 2008;53(1):216-218.
2. Hiss J, Shoshani E, Zaitsew K, Giverts P, Kahana T. Self inflicted gunshot wound caused by a home-made gun—medico-legal and ballistic examination. *J Clin Forensic Med*. 2003;10(3):165-168.
3. Fackler ML. Gunshot wound review. *Ann Emerg Med*. 1996;28(2):194-203.
4. Ditkofsky N, Maresky HS, Steenburg S. Radically invasive projectiles-first reports and imaging features of this new and dangerous bullet. *Emerg Radiol*. 2020;27(4):393-397.
5. Biswas S, Cadot H, Abrol S. Gunshot wound of the thoracic aorta with right popliteal artery embolization: a case report of bullet embolism with review of relevant literature. *Case Rep Emerg Med*. 2013;2013:198617. doi:10.1155/2013/198617.
6. Burihan E, Pepe EV, Miranda FJr. Bullet embolism following gunshot wound of the chest. Case report and review of the literature. *J Cardiovasc Surg*. 1980;21(6):711-716.

7. Painter MW, Britt LG. Distal bullet embolism after gunshot wound of the chest: a case report. *Am Surg*. 1971;37(2):106-108.
8. Saltzstein EC, Freeark RJ. Bullet embolism to the right axillary artery following gunshot wound of the heart. *Ann Surg*. 1963;158(1): 65-69.
9. Shen P, Mirzayan R, Jain T, McPherson J, Cornwell EEIII. Gunshot wound to the thoracic aorta with peripheral arterial bullet embolization: case report and literature review. *J Trauma*. 1998;44(2):394-397.
10. Ward PA, Suzuki A. Gunshot wound of the heart with peripheral embolization. A case report with review of literature. *J Thorac Cardiovasc Surg*. 1974;68(3):440-446.
11. Ward RJ, Nealon TF Jr, Bregman D. Gunshot wound of the brachiocephalic artery with peripheral bullet embolization. *N Y State J Med*. 1984;84(11):543-544.
12. Duke E, Peterson AA, Erly WK. Migrating bullet: a case of a bullet embolism to the pulmonary artery with secondary pulmonary infarction after gunshot wound to the left globe. *J Emerg Trauma Shock*. 2014;7(1):38-40.
13. Lanzi GL, Rehm CG, Baldino WA. Bullet embolus to the heart following gunshot wound of the mandible: a case report. *J Oral Maxillofac Surg*. 1992;50(2):179-180.
14. Duerr S, Cocco T. Gunshot wound of the abdomen with cerebral embolization. *J Trauma*. 1977;17(2):155-157.
15. Hammoudeh ZS. Mandibular gunshot wound with bullet aspiration. *J Craniofac Surg*. 2012;23(6):e540-e541.
16. Marantidis J, Biggs G. Migrated bullet in the bladder presenting 18 years after a gunshot wound. *Urol Case Rep*. 2020;28:101016.
17. Copeland AR. An improved method of gunshot wound examination. *J Forensic Sci*. 1981 26(3): 552-553.
18. Grosse Perdekamp M, Vennemann B, Mattern D, Serr A, Pollak S. Tissue defect at the gunshot entrance wound: what happens to the skin. *Int J Legal Med*. 2005;119(4):217-222.
19. Lieske K, Janssen W, Kulle KJ. Intensive gunshot residues at the exit wound: an examination using a head model. *Int J Legal Med*. 1991;104(4):235-238.
20. Randall B, Jaqua R. Gunshot entrance wound abrasion ring width as a function of projectile diameter and velocity. *J Forensic Sci*. 1991;36(1):138-144.
21. Berryman HE. A systematic approach to the interpretation of gunshot wound trauma to the cranium. *Forensic Sci Int*. 2019;301:306-317.
22. Berryman HE, Smith OC, Symes SA. Diameter of cranial gunshot wounds as a function of bullet caliber. *J Forensic Sci*. 1995;40(5):751-754.
23. Prahlow JA, Barnard JJ. Contact gunshot wound of the head: diagnosis after surgical debridement of the wound. *J Clin Forensic Med*. 1999;6(3):156-158.
24. Santucci RA, Chang YJ. Ballistics for physicians: myths about wound ballistics and gunshot injuries. *J Urol*. 2004;171(4):1408-1414.
25. Ben Simon GJ, Moisseiev J, Rosen N, Alhalel A. Gunshot wound to the eye and orbit: a descriptive case series and literature review. *J Trauma*. 2011;71(3):771-778, discussion 778.
26. Paranitharan P, Parai JL, Pollanen MS. Pseudo-gunshot wound injury from perforating rib fracture: a cautionary case report. *Forensic Sci Med Pathol*. 2008;4(2):113-115.
27. Baik S. External beveling of an entrance gunshot wound to the skull. *Am J Forensic Med Pathol*. 1993;14(1):89.
28. Baik SO, Uku JM, Sikirica M. A case of external beveling with an entrance gunshot wound to the skull made by a small caliber rifle bullet. *Am J Forensic Med Pathol*. 1991;12(4):334-336.
29. Bhoopat T. A case of internal beveling with an exit gunshot wound to the skull. *Forensic Sci Int*. 1995;71(2):97-101.
30. Lantz PE. An atypical, indeterminate-range, cranial gunshot wound of entrance resembling an exit wound. *Am J Forensic Med Pathol*. 1994;15(1):5-9.
31. Delannoy Y, Colard T, Becart A, Tournel G, Gosset D, Hedouin V. Typical external skull beveling wound unlinked with a gunshot. *Forensic Sci Int*. 2013;226(1-3):e4-e8.
32. Machado MP, Simoes MP, Gamba Td O, et al. A wormian bone, mimicking an entry gunshot wound of the skull, in an anthropological specimen. *J Forensic Sci*. 2016;61(3):855-857.
33. Bogdanović M, Atanasijević T, Popović V, Durmić T, Radnić B. Gunshot suicide: cherry-red discoloration of the temporal muscle beneath the exit wound. *Am J Forensic Med Pathol*. 2019;40(2):147-149.

34. Dolinak D, Matshes E, Lew E. *Forensic Pathology: Principles and Practice*: Elsevier Academic Press; 2005.
35. Gascho D, Bolliger SA, Thali MJ, Tappero C. Postmortem computed tomography and magnetic resonance imaging of an abdominal gunshot wound. *Am J Forensic Med Pathol*. 2020;41(2):119-123.
36. Harcke HT, Levy AD, Abbott RM, et al. Autopsy radiography: digital radiographs (DR) vs multi-detector computed tomography (MDCT) in high-velocity gunshot-wound victims. *Am J Forensic Med Pathol*. 2007;28(1):13-19.
37. Levy AD, Abbott RM, Mallak CT, et al. Virtual autopsy: preliminary experience in high-velocity gunshot wound victims. *Radiology*. 2006;240(2):522-528.
38. Shuman M, Wright RK. Evaluation of clinician accuracy in describing gunshot wound injuries. *J Forensic Sci*. 1999;44(2):339-342.
39. Spitz WU, Diaz FJ. *Spitz and Fisher's Medicolegal Investigation of Death*. 5th ed. Charles C. Thomas; 2020.
40. Dixon DS. Exit keyhole lesion and direction of fire in a gunshot wound of the skull. *J Forensic Sci*. 1984;29(1):336-339.
41. DiMaio VJM, Molina DK. *DiMaio's Forensic Pathology*. 3rd ed. CRC Press; 2022.
42. Fisher RS, Petty CS. *Forensic Pathology: A Handbook for Pathologists*. National Institute of Law Enforcement and Criminal Justice, Law Enforcement Assistance Administration, US Department of Justice (Grant to College of American Pathologists, NI 71-118G); 1977.
43. Wetli C, Mittelman RE, Rao VJ. *An Atlas of Forensic Pathology*. ASCP Press; 1999.
44. Saukko P, Knight B. *Knight's Forensic Pathology*. CRC Press; 2016.
45. Mason JK, Purdue BN, eds. *Pathology of Trauma*. 3rd ed. Arnold; 2000.
46. MacAulay LE, Barr DG, Strongman DB. Effects of decomposition on gunshot wound characteristics: under moderate temperatures with insect activity. *J Forensic Sci*. 2009;54(2):443-447.
47. MacAulay LE, Barr DG, Strongman DB. Effects of decomposition on gunshot wound characteristics: under cold temperatures with no insect activity. *J Forensic Sci*. 2009;54(2):448-451.
48. Harada K, Kuroda R, Nakajima M, Takizawa A, Yoshida K.. An autopsy case of a decomposed body with keyhole gunshot wound and secondary skull fractures. *Leg Med*. 2012;14(5):255-257.
49. Mohd Nor F, Das S. Gunshot wound in skeletonised human remains with partial adipocere formation. *J Forensic Leg Med*. 2012;19(1):42-45.
50. Kobayashi M, Sakurada K, Nakajima M, et al. A "keyhole lesion" gunshot wound in an adipocere case. *Leg Med*. 1999;1(3):170-173.
51. Aguilar JC. Shored gunshot wound of exit. A phenomenon with identity crisis. *Am J Forensic Med Pathol*. 1983;4(3):199-204.
52. Shaqiri E, Xhemali B, Ismaili Z, Sinamati A, Vyshka G. An unusual lethal gunshot wound to the head. *Med Leg J*. 2017;85(1):51-54.
53. Jones AM. An unusual atypical gunshot wound. A coin as an intermediate target. *Am J Forensic Med Pathol*. 1987;8(4):338-341.
54. Smędra A, Sidelnik P, Goryca W, Berent J. Gunshot wound in an 18-year-old woman, inflicted with a hunting weapon through an obstacle (mobile phone): reconstruction of events. *Am J Forensic Med Pathol*. 2017;38(3):249-253.
55. Holt GR, Kostohryz GJr. Wound ballistics of gunshot injuries to the head and neck. *Arch Otolaryngol*. 1983;109(5):313-318.
56. Klein Y, Shatz DV, Bejarano PA. Blast-induced colon perforation secondary to civilian gunshot wound. *Eur J Trauma Emerg Surg*. 2007;33(3):298-300.
57. Torba M, Gjata A, Rulli F, Kajo I, Ceka S, Mici A. Blunt abdominal trauma following gunshot wound case report and literature review. *Ann Ital Chir*. 2018;7:S2239253X1802830X.
58. Hiss J, Kahana T. Confusing exit gunshot wound–"two for the price of one." *Int J Legal Med*. 2002;116(1):47-49.
59. Wang A, Solli E, Carberry N, Hillard V, Tandon A. Delayed tension pneumocephalus following gunshot wound to the head: a case report and review of the literature. *Case Rep Surg*. 2016;2016:7534571.
60. Ellis GR, Brown JR. Massive air embolism due to gunshot wound. *J Am Med Assoc*. 1964;189:953-955.
61. Temlett J, Byard RW. Air embolism: an unusual cause of delayed death following gunshot wound to the chest. *Med Sci Law*. 2011;51(1):56-57.

62. Smith JMIII, Richardson JD, Grover FL, Arom KV, Webb GE, Trinkle JK. Fatal air embolism following gunshot wound of the lung. *J Thorac Cardiovasc Surg.* 1976;72(2):296-298.
63. Platz E. Tangential gunshot wound to the chest causing venous air embolism: a case report and review. *J Emerg Med.* 2011;41(2):e25-e29.
64. Demontis R, d'Aloja E, Manieli C, et al. Case report of sudden death after a gunshot wound to the C2 vertebral bone without direct spinal cord injury: histopathological analysis of spinal-medullary junction. *Forensic Sci Int.* 2019;301:e49-e54.
65. Stone JL, Ladenheim E, Wilkinson SB, Cybulski GR, Oldershaw JB. Hematoma in the posterior fossa secondary to a tangential gunshot wound of the occiput: case report and discussion. *Neurosurgery.* 1991;28(4):603-605; discussion 605-606.
66. Domingo E, Levy D, Iosovich S. Atypical presentation of aortic dissection secondary to a gunshot wound. *Emerg Med J.* 2006;23(6):e38.
67. Kralovec ME, Houdek MT, Martin JR, Morrey ME, Cross WWIII. Atypical presentation of fat embolism syndrome after gunshot wound to the foot. *Am J Orthop.* 2015;44(3):E71-E74.
68. Spitz DJ, Ouban A. Meningitis following gunshot wound of the neck. *J Forensic Sci.* 2003;48(6):1369-1370.
69. Goerlich CE, Challa AB, Malas MM. Acute limb ischemia from gunshot wound secondary to arterial vasospasm. *J Vasc Surg Cases Innov Tech.* 2019;5(2):99-103.
70. Bliznak J, Ramsey JD. Atrio-esophageal fistula secondary to gunshot wound of the chest. *Mil Med.* 1971;136(6):584-585.
71. Capanna AH. Traumatic intracranial aneurysm and Gradenigo's syndrome secondary to gunshot wound. *Surg Neurol.* 1984;22(3):263-266.
72. Forbes HW, Thompson CQ, Smith JW. Mesenteric arteriovenous fistula after a gunshot wound. *J Trauma.* 1969;9(9):806-811.
73. Aesch B, Lefrancq T, Destrieux C, Saint-Martin P. Fatal gunshot wound to the head with lack of immediate incapacitation. *Am J Forensic Med Pathol.* 2014;35(2):86-88.
74. Juvin P, Brion F, Teissiere F, Durigon M. Prolonged activity after an ultimately fatal gunshot wound to the heart: case report. *Am J Forensic Med Pathol.* 1999;20(1):10-12.
75. Kline DG, LeBlanc HJ. Survival following gunshot wound of the pons: neuroanatomic considerations. Case report. *J Neurosurg.* 1971;35(3):342-347.
76. Levy V, Rao VJ. Survival time in gunshot and stab wound victims. *Am J Forensic Med Pathol.* 1988;9(3):215-217.
77. Rudich MD, Rowland MC, Seibel RW, Border J. Survival following a gunshot wound of the abdominal aorta and inferior vena cava. *J Trauma.* 1978;18(7):548-549.
78. Love CR, Evans SS. Gunshot wound of the abdominal aorta and anoxic cardiac arrest: report of a survival. *Ann Surg.* 1963;158(1):131-132.
79. Mehta AI, Bagley CA. Gunshot wound to the clivus. *Br J Neurosurg.* 2011;25(1):136-137.
80. Winter B. Through and through gunshot wound of the heart with recovery. *J Am Med Assoc.* 1968;204(4):337-338.
81. Copeland AR. Accidental death by gunshot wound—fact or fiction. *Forensic Sci Int.* 1984;26(1):25-32.
82. Dobi-Babić R, Katalinić S. Death due to accidentally self-inflicted gunshot wound. *Croat Med J.* 2001;42(5):576-578.
83. Gips H, Yannai U, Hiss J. Self-inflicted gunshot wound mimicking assault: a rare variant of factitious disorder. *J Forensic Leg Med.* 2007;14(5):293-296.
84. Hirsch CS, Adelson L. A suicidal gunshot wound of the back. *J Forensic Sci.* 1976;21(3):659-666.
85. Zugibe FT, Costello JT, Breithhaupt MK. Gunshot wound to the back of the head—self defence vs homicide. *J Forensic Sci Soc.* 1989;29(4):255-259.
86. Pawsey SC, Wilson CG, Gunther WM, Fantaskey AP. Suicide by close-range gunshot wound to the bridge of the nose. *J Forensic Sci.* 2020;65(3):984-986.
87. Cave R, DiMaio VJ, Molina DK. Homicide or suicide? Gunshot wound interpretation: a Bayesian approach. *Am J Forensic Med Pathol.* 2014;35(2):118-123.
88. Zech WD, Kneubuhl B, Thali M, Bolliger S. Pistol thrown to the ground by shooter after fatal self inflicted gunshot wound to the chest. *J Forensic Leg Med.* 2011;18(2):88-90.

89. Nikolić S, Zivković V, Babić D, Juković F. Suicidal single gunshot injury to the head: differences in site of entrance wound and direction of the bullet path between right- and left-handed—an autopsy study. *Am J Forensic Med Pathol*. 2012;33(1):43-46.
90. Prahlow JA. Suicide by intrarectal gunshot wound. *Am J Forensic Med Pathol*. 1998;19(4):356-361.
91. Ampanozi G, Schwendener N, Krauskopf A, Thali MJ, Bartsch C. Incidental occult gunshot wound detected by postmortem computed tomography. *Forensic Sci Med Pathol*. 2013;9(1):68-72.
92. Atkins J, Piazza D, Pierce J. Overlooked gunshot wound in a motor vehicle accident victim: clinical and legal risks. *J Emerg Nurs*. 1988;14(3):142-144.
93. DiMaio. *Gunshot Wounds*. 2nd ed. CRC Press; 1999.

FIRE DEATHS 12

CHAPTER OUTLINE

Introduction 360

Features of Thermal Injury 365

Description of Flash Fire 367

Autopsy Features of Fire Deaths 368

Heat-Related Fractures 371

Explosion-Related Deaths 374

Near Misses 375

INTRODUCTION

Fire deaths are frequently encountered by forensic pathologists. Common situations in which fire deaths occur include house fires and fires following a motor vehicle accident. While many bodies found after a fire often have a charred external surface with relative preservation of the internal body cavities and organs, the exact condition of any body found after a fire can be highly variable, from the body being completely intact and just coated with some soot, to the body being only represented by calcine fragments of bone. Important to always consider is that bodies found after a fire may have a variety of causes of death and a variety of manners of death, with natural, accident, suicide, homicide, or undetermined all being possible. Because of this variation, each autopsy performed on a body found after a fire can be very different in its approach; however, the three most important questions that are required to be answered when a body is found after a fire are, (1) Who is the individual? (2) Was the individual alive at the time of the fire? and (3) What are the cause and manner of death?

For the first question, it is important to understand the range of methods available to make an identification, as, depending upon the condition of the body after the fire, any one of several identification methods may be necessary to develop a positive identification for any given death. For example, for an individual with soot on the skin, the circumstances of the death (eg, apartment found in) and visual comparison of the face to an identification photo may be enough; whereas, if the remains are essentially only calcine bone, identifying the individual would require finding residual DNA in a surviving tooth or the fortunate presence of orthopedic hardware (Figure 12.1). For the second question, the presence of blood to enable testing for carboxyhemoglobin (COHb) is required for definitive confirmation of life at the time of the fire, unless scene investigation otherwise provides an answer (eg, there is evidence at the scene that the decedent moved around the house after the fire was started). For the third question, it is important to understand the patterns of findings that thermal injuries can cause so as to not misinterpret them as antemortem injuries.

As described above, the extent of postmortem thermal injuries varies greatly, with the appearance of the body of individuals being found after a house fire varying from being essentially undamaged by the fire, and with only a thin layer of soot on the body, to bodies that are essentially cremated, with only some bone fragments recovered after the fire (Figure 12.2A and B). Because of this fact, the investigation of fire deaths varies greatly from case to case in the approach used by a forensic pathologist.

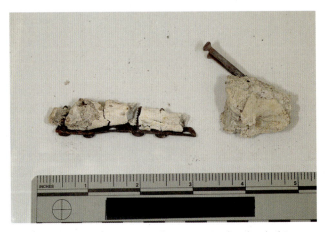

Figure 12.1. Orthopedic hardware in cremated remains. In the distal tibia were two orthopedic screws and the distal fibula has a plate with screws. These fragments found among the cremated remains could be matched to antemortem skeletal images of the decedent.

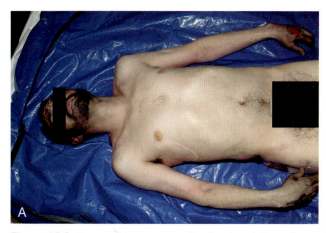
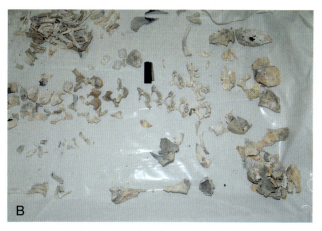

Figure 12.2. Range of appearance of bodies found after a fire. In (**A**), the decedent has soot on their face (comment: clothing has been removed) and some skin slippage on the face and hands, which would have been exposed to the heat, but is otherwise intact and easily able to be examined for injuries. In (**B**), the skeletal remains were found after a house fire. While cremation of the body is rare in house fires or vehicle fires, it does occur. In some cases, the only human remains present after a house fire or vehicle fire will be calcine bone fragments.

PEARLS & PITFALLS

While rare, bodies found after a fire can be reduced to only fragments of skeletal remains with or without some attached soft tissue. The removal of these fragments of bone from the death scene, if just done with the purpose of collecting the bone fragments, can result in a loss of information (Figure 12.3A-D). The presence of a forensic anthropologist assisting in such a recovery can not only assist in identification of all skeletal remains but also assist in establishing a context for the body itself (ie, the position of the bone fragments may say something about the body itself, but this context is lost if the fragments are not collected in an organized fashion).

Key questions to answer when investigating a fire death
- Who is the individual?
- Was the individual alive at the time of the fire?
- What are the cause and manner of death?

CHECKLIST for Fire Deaths (in addition to the steps in a standard autopsy)
- ☐ Examination of the airway and gastrointestinal tract for soot
- ☐ Collection of blood for COHb analysis
- ☐ Unless the skin is intact, x-ray the body to search for projectiles or other foreign objects, such as orthopedic hardware, which could aid in identification.
- ☐ Collection of clothing for analysis for accelerants

PEARLS & PITFALLS

It must always be remembered that a fire is not infrequently started to conceal a crime (Figure 12.4). A fire may also be started to ensure a suicide (ie, an individual can first set their house on fire and then hang or shoot themself, with the idea that the fire will complete the act, if the asphyxia, gunshot wound, or other mechanism does not).

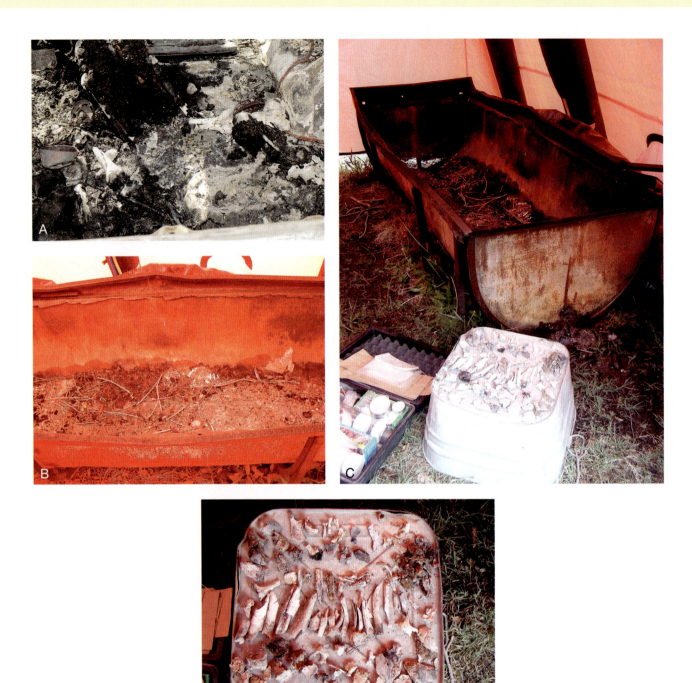

Figure 12.3. Importance of position of fragments of bone after fire. In (**A**), the body was cremated by the fire and fragments of skeletal elements were found. In this instance, the bones were recovered by law enforcement and any information based upon the location of the bone fragments was lost. (**B-D**) illustrate a burn container into which a man placed his significant other after shooting her with a shotgun ((**B** and **C**); the over-saturation with orange is due to the tent placed over the site for privacy and lack of compensation when shooting the digital image). During the burning process, the contents in the container were stirred. Although law enforcement had removed some skeletal fragments from the container (**D**), a forensic pathologist with anthropology experience was able to remove the remaining fragments from the burn container and identify their location within the burn container, which confirmed the history, in that fragments of bone were not found in anatomic location (eg, with fragments of the cranium found scattered throughout and sometimes adjacent to fragments of the distal lower extremities), which would have been consistent with the perpetrator mixing the contents of the container during the burning process.

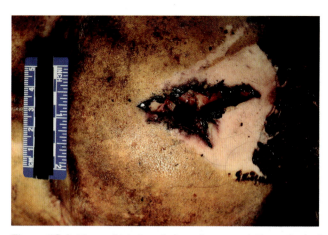

Figure 12.4. Thermal injuries after gunshot wound. The individual in Figure 12.4 shot their family, including wife and children, and set fire to their house prior to shooting himself. The amount of thermal injury to the bodies was minimal, with only soot on the face of the decedent visible in the photo; however, the bodies could have been more completely consumed.

FAQ: How can it be determined at autopsy whether an individual was alive at the time of the fire?

Answer: At autopsy, soot can be found in the oral cavity (eg, on the tongue), in the larynx, or on the tracheal or bronchial mucosa. The amount of soot present in the airway can be variable, from a diffuse layer of black discoloration to wispy strands of black carbonaceous material (Figure 12.5A-E). Microscopic examination of the airway can assist in the identification of soot (Figure 12.5F). Soot can also be identified in the gastrointestinal tract in individuals who were alive during the time of the fire. In addition to checking the airway and gastrointestinal tract for soot, testing of the blood will reveal an elevated level of COHb. However, the findings of soot in the trachea or soot in the gastrointestinal tract are not always present in any given body where the death occurred after the fire began. In their study, Gerling et al. found that of 85 decedents who all died due to a fire, only 28.2% had all three findings: evidence of inhalation of soot, swallowing of soot, and an elevated COHb.[1] Of the three, the presence of an elevated concentration of hemoglobin is the most vital and most objective finding to confirm the individual was alive at the time of the fire. While the coloration of the skin and blood (Figure 12.5G and H) can suggest an elevated concentration of COHb in the blood, laboratory confirmation is necessary.

PEARLS & PITFALLS

Identification of soot in the airways does not necessarily correlate with the presence of COHb in the blood. Gerling et al. found that around 70% of decedents with elevated COHb had evidence of aspirated soot; however, three individuals had evidence of inhaled soot but did not have elevated COHb concentrations.[1]

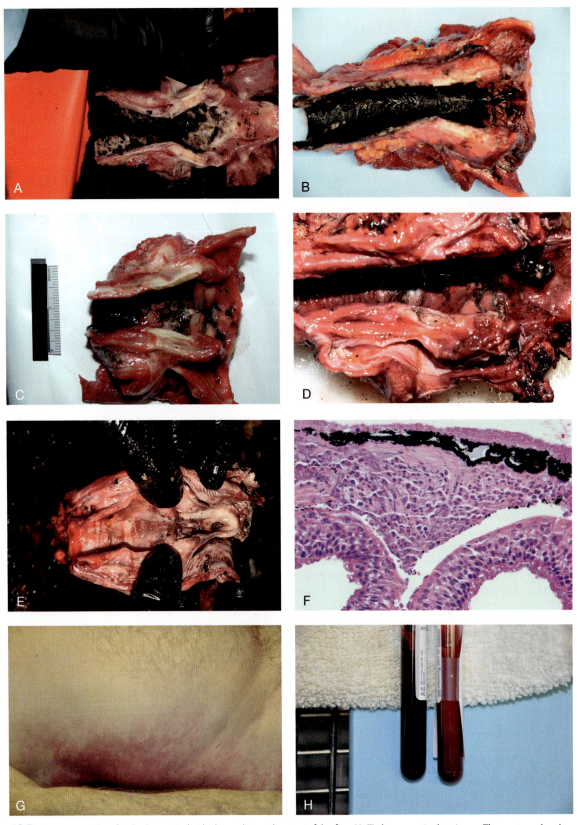

Figure 12.5. Features to identify whether an individual was alive at the time of the fire. (**A-E**) show soot in the airway. The soot can be dense (**A-C**) or more dispersed, wispy, or minimal in amount (**D** and **E**). If the neck and trachea are open to the outside due to thermal injury of the overlying skin and soft tissue, interpretation of soot in the airway must be done with caution, as charred residue from the outer surface of the body could enter the airway. In addition, thermal injury could contribute to blackening of the airway mucosa. If confirmation of the presence of soot is required, a microscopic section of the tracheal mucosa can be obtained (**F**). For individuals exposed to carbon monoxide, the lividity will often be more light red in color (**G**) as will the skeletal muscles and the blood in the body (**H**). (**H**) is blood from the two autopsies. The blood on the right is from an individual who died in a house fire, whereas the blood on the left is from a non-fire and non-carbon monoxide related death.

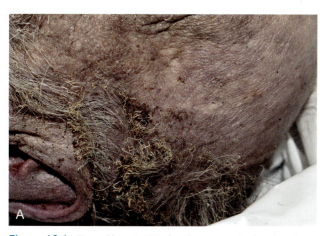 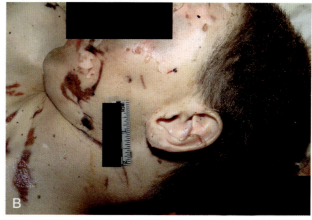

Figure 12.6. Singed hair. In (**A**), the changes in the hair (ie, the more tightly curly yellow appearance of the ends of the hair) are secondary to thermal injury. In (**B**), the hair has similar changes, but the face also has numerous areas of skin slippage, which was from a flash fire.

FEATURES OF THERMAL INJURY

While the presence of soot in the airways or digestive tract and the presence of an elevated concentration of COHb in the blood can be used to determine that an individual was alive at the time of the fire, these findings are from inhalation and swallowing of the smoky air and not from exposure to the fire itself. They would confirm smoke inhalation but not thermal injuries. Bohnert et al. list gross and microscopic findings associated with exposure to heat.[2] Gross findings include singed hair (Figure 12.6A and B), crow's feet (ie, contracted linear regions of skin at the lateral margins of the eyes), burn blisters (with a neutrophilic reaction), patchy detachment of mucosa of pharynx or epiglottis, and edema of the epiglottis. Microscopic findings can include vesicular detachment of the mucosa in the trachea and bronchi and hyperemia and edema. The importance of thermal injury in the cause of death can vary greatly depending upon the nature of the fire. In a house fire, smoke inhalation and not thermal injury are more likely to be the cause of death, whereas in a flash fire, the direct effects of the thermal injuries are more likely to be the cause of death.

SAMPLE NOTES: CERTIFICATION OF CAUSE OF DEATH IN INDIVIDUAL WHO DIED IN HOUSE FIRE

If the body has minimal to no burns and evidence of the individual having been alive at the time of the fire through an elevated concentration of COHb, the cause of death could be certified as "Smoke inhalation." If the individual has thermal injuries and evidence of the individual having been alive at the time of the fire, the cause of death could be certified as "Smoke inhalation and thermal injuries." While it is often impossible to determine whether the individual was dead or alive at the time they were exposed to the flames and heat, it is also often impossible to determine that the individual was not alive at the time they were exposed to the flames and heat, so certifying the cause of death as both conditions is more academically honest. If the individual has evidence of exposure to flames, but no elevation, or only a minimally elevated concentration of COHb, the cause of death could be certified as "Thermal injuries."

PEARLS & PITFALLS

When an extensively charred body is being examined at autopsy, it is a mistake to assume that no blood is present or that all blood present is heat coagulated. Even in situations where most of the body is absent due to thermal injury, dissection of the remaining tissue may reveal a preserved pocket of liquid blood (Figure 12.7A-C).

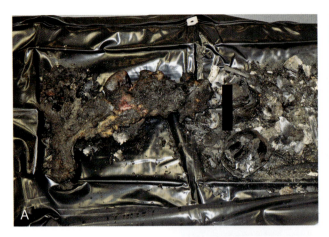
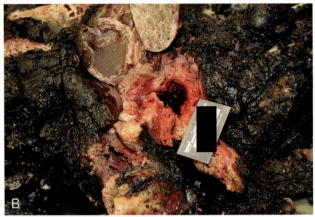
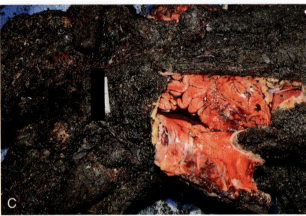

Figure 12.7. Identification of liquid blood in a markedly thermal injured body. In (**A** and **B**), the individual's body was found after a house fire. Despite the marked thermal damage (**A**), a pocket of liquid blood was identified that could be used for carboxyhemoglobin testing (**B**). In (**C**), the cut-down on the femoral region in a markedly thermally injured body revealed liquid blood.

FAQ: What is a lethal concentration of COHb?

Answer: COHb can be detected in the blood in smokers and in individuals who were involved with a fire, and of course, individuals involved with a fire can be smokers. The two general types of fires that occur are those due to inflammable liquid and those which are due to smoldering fires. Rogde and Olving in a review of 286 fire deaths found that COHb concentrations varied from 0 to >45% in victims of fires, and considered a sublethal concentration of COHb as <50%.[3] In their study, Rogde and Olving found that nearly 80% of victims of a smoldering fire (n = 130) had HbCO concentrations of >45%, but only 30% of victims of a fire due to an inflammable liquid (n = 49) had a COHb concentration of >45%.[3] In five cases where an individual was doused with gasoline and set on fire, Gerling et al. did not find evidence of soot aspiration, soot swallowing, or elevated blood COHb concentration, which would also support that in victims of flash fires, the COHb is most frequently lower than that in house fires or minimally or not detectable in the blood.[1] In their study, the source of the fire was not always known, and considering all fire deaths (n = 286), 70% had a COHb concentration >45%. Hirsch et al. also failed to identify COHb elevations in the victims of flash fires that they studied.[4]

While COHb is not normally found in healthy individuals, it can be identified in those individuals who smoke; however, such smoking derived concentrations only reach a certain level. If the concentration of COHb in smokers is above 10% to 13%, it is indicative of the person being alive during the fire. In contrast, essentially any elevation in concentration of COHb in a non-smoker is indicative of that person being alive during the fire. In part, the concentration of COHb required to cause death depends upon the characteristics of the individual in the fire. People with significant underlying natural disease (eg, congestive heart failure or emphysema) can succumb to a lower concentration of COHb than a healthy individual with no comorbidities. However, Rogde and Olving found no difference in COHb concentrations based upon age or sex alone.[3] Gerling et al. also observed no association between age and COHb concentrations in the victims of fires.[1] Also, as described above, some types of fire deaths such as flash fires are associated with a lower concentration of COHb than typical house fires or even the absence of COHb and with these flash fires the mechanism of death may be different (eg, thermal-induced injury to the airway instead of simply carbon monoxide poisoning).[4]

Another important consideration regarding COHb testing is that some labs will often just report <10% and not give an exact measurement; however, the exact number may be important. For example, a 5% COHb concentration in a non-smoker means that the person was alive at the time of the fire, which can be very useful information in any given case. If a more specific number is required than <10%, send the blood out to another laboratory for additional testing.

DESCRIPTION OF FLASH FIRE

A flash fire could occur for a variety of reasons, which include ignition of a flammable liquid, such as in the driver of a gasoline truck that is involved in an accident, with the truck subsequently catching fire. Flash fires can occur on a less significant of a scale as well, for example, a cook in a kitchen who sets fire to grease which flashes in their face (Figure 12.8A) or an individual who is on oxygen therapy, and smokes while on the oxygen (Figure 12.8B). While individuals in a flash fire can have no COHb in their blood, with the mechanism of death likely related to the effects of the fire on the airway, overlap with types of fire deaths occur, and bodies found after a flash fire can certainly have an elevated concentration of COHb.

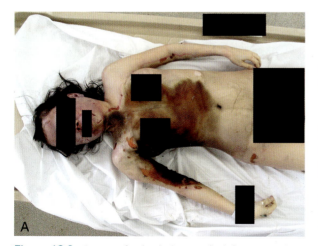 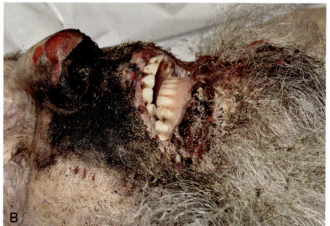

Figure 12.8. Causes of a death due to a flash fire. In (**A**), the decedent was working in a kitchen when a grease fire was set off in her face. The degree of body surface area damaged by the fire combined with the carboxyhemoglobin concentration was insignificant to explain her death. (**B**), the decedent was smoking while on home oxygen. The flames caused thermal injury around his face, and the concentration of carboxyhemoglobin was not significantly elevated. In this situation, the stress of the burns combined with underlying natural disease can contribute to his death.

> **PEARLS & PITFALLS**
>
> Other than COHb, other inhaled components in a fire may contribute to the cause of death. Ferrari and Giannuzzi studied 32 of 33 inmates who died as the result of a polyurethane mattress fire in a prison.[5] They found that a majority of the inmates had COHb concentrations that would be considered non-lethal, with the concentrations varying from 10% to 43%. However, a majority of the decedents had hydrogen cyanide concentrations of >1 mg/L. The authors also indicated that the temperature of the fire created by the burning polyurethane mattresses and pillows, which was >400 °C, may have depleted the level of oxygen in the area, which could have contributed to the death of the inmates. Gerling et al. based upon their review of the literature indicate that while cyanide poisoning can be a component of fire deaths, in the majority of their cases, unless there were extenuating circumstances as to a source for the cyanide, the COHb will be elevated comparatively with the cyanide (ie, in individuals with elevated concentrations of cyanide a comparatively equally elevated concentration of COHb will also be found).[1] However, it is possible that the two components (COHb and cyanide) could act synergistically. Gasoline as a component of the inhaled substance could also contribute to the cause of death.[6]

AUTOPSY FEATURES OF FIRE DEATHS

While the appearance of the body can vary greatly between any two given cases of thermal injuries, certain features are common. Often the skin will be absent exposing charred skeletal muscle; however, the underlying organs and body cavities frequently are minimal damaged, easily allowing for the identification of traumatic injuries (Figure 12.9A and B). Because of the charred skeletal muscle, the extremities will often develop contractures at the elbows, wrists, knees, and ankles, leading to the characteristic pugilistic posture associated with fire deaths (Figure 12.9C-E). The pugilistic posture is caused by contraction of skeletal muscles due to dehydration and protein denaturation as a result of the fire. The flexors are stronger muscles, which are bulkier, and therefore contract more than the extensors, leading to flexion in the extremities.[7] Associated with the contractions, fractures of the distal forearms and distal legs often occur.

Of course, when a body is recovered after a fire, it is also often not intact. Because of thermal injuries, the body cavities can be breached, which can lead to expulsion of the intestine and charring of internal organs (Figure 12.9F and G). Quite frequently, the top of the head will be absent exposing the brain (Figure 12.9H-K). Associated with charring of the head can be an artifactual epidural hemorrhage, potentially from bone marrow extruding from the cranium with the high heat (Figure 12.9L and M). Gerling et al. found an epidural hemorrhage in 16 of 60 cases with extensive charring.[1] However, a subdural or subarachnoid hemorrhage would not be an artifact of thermal injury and would indicate an antemortem pathologic condition. In addition to an epidural hemorrhage, thermal damage can cause swelling of the brain, which could mimic edema (Figure 12.9N and O).

Gerling et al. proposed three grades of thermal injury, with grade A being little soft tissue loss, with possible rupture of the abdominal wall; grade B being moderate soft tissue loss, including exposure of the pleural and/or peritoneal cavities, but with an intact head; and grade C involving soft tissue loss and including exposure of the cranial cavity.[1]

SAMPLE NOTES: DESCRIPTION OF BODY FOUND AFTER FIRE

The body has full-thickness thermal injuries involving the head, trunk, and both the upper and lower extremities, with exposure of the underlying skeletal muscle, with some preservation of the skin of the back and posterior surface of the thighs. The top of the cranium is absent exposing the brain, with the edges of the residual cranium charred. The upper extremities are contracted at the wrists and elbows with fracture of the distal aspect of the bones of the forearms. The lower extremities are contracted at the knees and ankles.

> **PEARLS & PITFALLS**
>
> While protrusion of the tongue is a common finding at autopsy of burned bodies, in their review of 61 cases, Bohnert and Hejna found no correlation between incidence of tongue protrusion or no tongue protrusion based upon the individual being alive or dead at the time of the fire nor of the degree of thermal injury, from unburned to charring.[8]

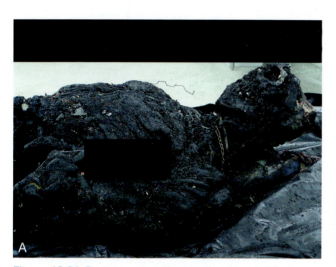
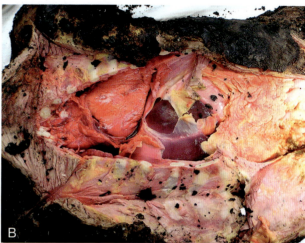

Figure 12.9A-B. Comparison of external and internal findings in a charred body. While the possible range of findings that a thermally damaged body might exhibit is fairly extensive, most frequently, bodies recovered from after a fire will have a charred external surface (**A**), but will have preservation or at least relative preservation of the internal organs and body cavities (**B**).

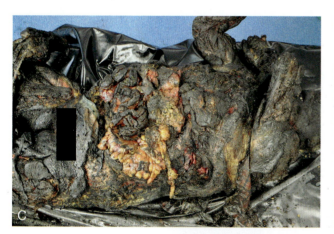
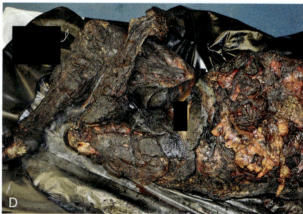
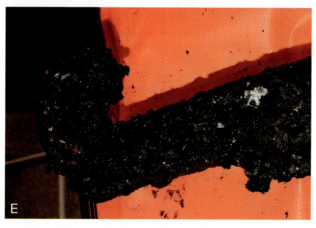

Figure 12.9C-E. Pugilistic posture. In (**C** and **D**), the entire body is illustrated and contracture can be identified at elbows, wrists, knees, and ankles. In (**E**), a close-up view of the wrist and forearm illustrates the contraction.

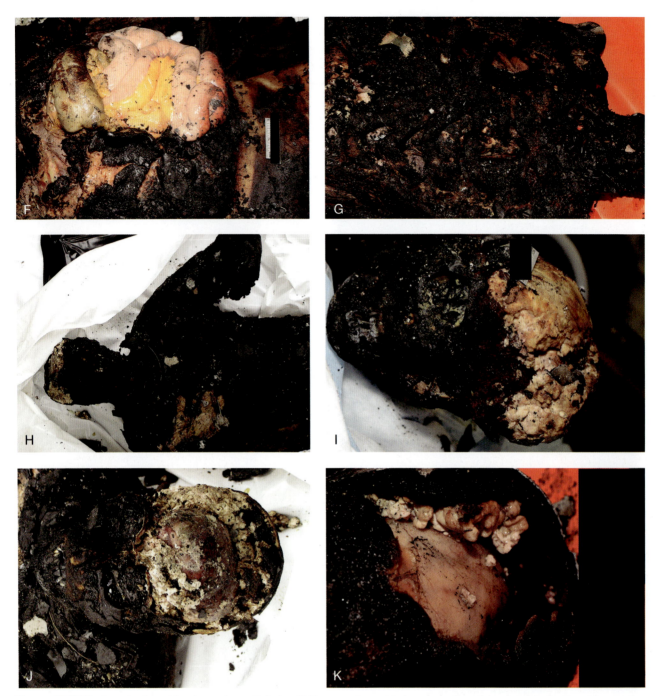

Figure 12.9F-K. Open body cavities due to thermal injuries. (F) illustrates thermal-induced opening of the abdominal cavity with extrusion of a segment of small intestine. Since the small intestine is not charred, the rupture of the abdominal wall occurred after the fire subsided and was not actively burning this region of the body otherwise, the small intestine would also be charred. (G) illustrates a chest with essential absence of soft tissue between the ribs exposing the lungs and heart to the fire. (H-K) illustrate the loss of the top of the cranium that frequently occurs with thermal injury. (H) is an overall view, which also provides a good illustration of pugilistic posture. (I and J) provide a closer view of the top of the head with the absence of the cranium, exposing the brain. (I) also has a thermal-induced epidural hemorrhage in the frontal region. (K) illustrates a loss of the superior portion of the cranium, with contraction of the dura, causing extrusion of cerebral parenchyma.

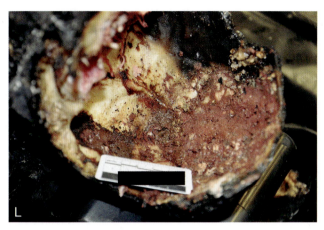 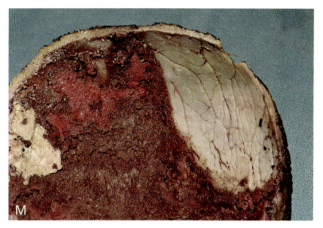

Figure 12.9L-M. Thermal-induced epidural hemorrhage. (L) (in situ) and (M) (calotte removed) reveal a thermal-induced epidural hemorrhage. The hemorrhage often appears more light red (ie, a more cooked appearance).

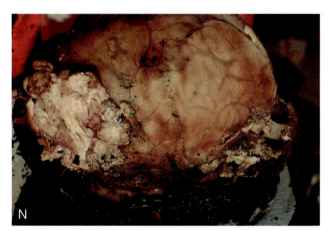 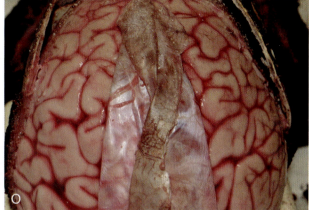

Figure 12.9N-O. Mimic of cerebral edema. Thermal injury can contract the dura, causing it to shrink against the cerebral parenchyma, which can lead to expulsion of the cerebral parenchyma as in (N), but it can also flatten the cerebral surface. In addition, expansion of fluid in the brain secondary to the heat can cause swelling of the brain and also contribute to mimicking cerebral edema (O).

HEAT-RELATED FRACTURES

Five types of fractures occur as the result of heat: longitudinal, curved transverse (ie, thumbnail) (Figure 12.10A), straight transverse, delamination, and patina. While the first three are descriptive of the shape of the fracture, delamination is separation of the cortical from the cancellous bone and patina fractures appear like flaking paint at the epiphyses.[9,10] Delamination of the outer table of bone in the skull can obscure normal features of traumatic injuries, such as beveling in a gunshot wound.[11] However, deGruchy and Rogers tested the effects of an outdoor fire contained within a steel container on the appearance of pig bones subjected to blows with edged weapons and found that the characteristics of hacking trauma on the bones were not altered, with the exception of the rough area at the acute angle (the point of exit of the weapon from the bone), which was increased in size when burnt.[10] Hermann and Bennett also found that sharp force trauma, including Stryker saw and knife cutmarks, remained visible on the skeletal elements following burning.[9] Pope and Smith found that features of sharp force injury in bone were retained throughout all stages of burning.[11]

In regard to fractures of the cranium, Hammarlebiod et al. indicate that heat-related fractures occur through the dipole, parallel to the cortex of the bone, producing separation of the external and internal tables of the cranium, whereas traumatic fractures are perpendicular through the bone.[12] Pope and Smith indicate that in the skull, only trauma-induced

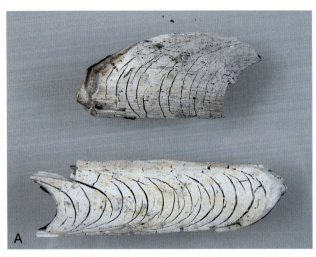
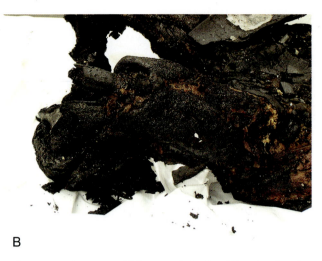

Figure 12.10. Thermal-induced fractures. The bones in (A) exhibit curved transverse fractures, which can assist in identifying the direction of fire involvement of the skeletal muscle.[14] The fractured femur in (B) is near the knee, which would undergo contraction and potential fracture of the bone, and the bone itself is charred. While each fracture must be carefully evaluated, the features of this fracture are consistent with being thermal injury induced.

> **FAQ:** How can fractures that occurred prior to the fire be distinguished from those that occurred due to the fire?
>
> **Answer:** While in some situations, the cause of the fracture is easily apparent (Figure 12.10B), in any given case, distinguishing traumatic fractures from thermal related fractures can be difficult[7]; however, even so, distinguishing between perimortem fractures and postmortem fractures (thermal-induced fractures) can be vital. If the fractures occurred prior to the fire they are most likely related to the cause of death, whereas those occurring due to the fire are most likely just an artifact of the fire itself.

fractures will radiate into unburned bone.[11] As the mechanism of fracture including the location of the fracture is often different between fractures of the cranium induced by thermal injury and those fractures caused by gunshot wounds or other traumatic event, with thermal injury affecting the skull cap first, and as the base of the cranium is protected for some time in a fire, Bohnert et al. indicate that fractures of the base of the cranium in a body found after a fire are consistent with the fracture being present prior to the thermal injury, unless another event superimposed, such as an object falling during the fire and striking the head (Figure 12.11).[13] Other features that may help distinguish trauma-induced fractures of the skull from heat-induced fractures of the skull include (1) blackened and eroded margins in trauma-induced fractures, (2) fractures originating from calcine bone in heat-induced trauma, and (3) reconstruction of the skull revealing different colors and therefore different thermal environments indicates trauma-induced fractures.[11] If the bone is found in fragments (eg, a cremated or semi-cremated body) try to identify two fragments that share a fracture line. If the two fragments have a similar appearance, the fracture was likely thermally induced; however, if the two fragments are different in appearance (eg, one is more blackened and one is more calcine), this would indicate that the two fragments were separate at the time they were burned, each sustaining different effects from the fire, and that the fracture occurred before the body was burned (Figure 12.12). Thus, the heat-related fractures can be realigned more effectively.[11] The same concept could be applied to post-cranial skeletal elements to determine whether a particular fracture occurred before or as a result of the fire.

In regard to fractures of the extremities, Symes et al. describe patterns of thermal injuries that occur in the body based upon contracture at the joints, the effects of joint shielding, and exposure of certain bones as closer to the skin surface.[14] Thermal injuries of the long bones are usually bilateral and symmetric whereas trauma induced fractures are usually

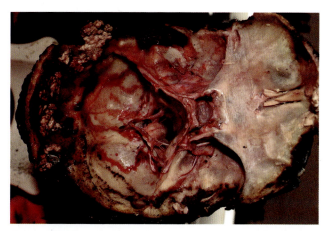

Figure 12.11. Intact base of the cranium. Although the superior portion of the cranium is often damaged by postmortem thermal injury and absent at the time of the autopsy, the base of the cranium is fairly resilient to thermal injury and can maintain its integrity for a longer period. In Figure 12.11, the cranium had extensive thermal-mediated destruction; however, the base of the cranium was intact. A fracture in the base of this cranium would be a result of injury sustained before the fire, or, if scene investigation reveals it, blunt force injury sustained during or after the fire, such as with collapse of the structure (comment: no fracture is present in the image; the purpose of the image is to illustrate the resilience of the base of the cranium to thermal injury, and its potential use to identify antemortem trauma in thermally damaged human remains).

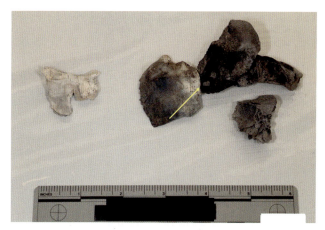

Figure 12.12. Fracture match. The decedent in Figure 12.12 was shot with a shotgun and then their body burned. Two fragments of the cranium that shared a fracture line were identified. If the fracture was secondary to the fire, the appearance of the bone on each side of the fracture line should be similar; however, in this case, the two bone fragments appeared different (arrow), consistent with the two fragments having been exposed to the burn differently, consistent with them having been fractured prior to the fire.

asymmetrical. Sites of trauma are exposed to the effects of thermal injury because of the disruption of the overlying skin and soft tissue and thus will not necessarily have a symmetrical pattern.[11] Symes et al. provide diagrams indicating the distribution of thermal injuries of the bones.[14] Hammarlebiod et al. indicate that fractures of the long bones that occur due to a fire have a beveled end, which has been described as a "flute-mouth piece."[12] The morphology of the fracture margin and discoloration of the fracture surface and margin may also help distinguish fractures due to a fire from fractures occurring prior to the fire.[14,15]

PEARLS & PITFALLS

Although open skulls at autopsy in a fire death have been associated with heat effects on a non-injured skull (ie, without a defect to vent pressure, the cranium will fragment), significantly damaged skulls can also result from collapse of building material during or following the fire or postmortem handling of the burned bone following the fire.[11] Therefore, when a fire involves a structure, that secondary damage occurred to the body due to collapse of the structure must always be considered. In addition to fractures of the cranium, collapse of the structure on the body could obviously involve other bones of the body as well. Scene investigation would be important in the accurate determination of the nature of the injuries to the body in such a situation. Pope and Smith stressed the importance of recovery technique when dealing with burned cranial bone to best preserve evidence of traumatic injury in the bone.[11]

PEARLS & PITFALLS

When a fire-related death is suspicious for being secondary to arson or for an attempt to conceal a homicide, collection of clothing to analyze for accelerants would be helpful in the investigation. In situations where arson or a concealed homicide is suspected, communication with the fire investigator can provide very useful information in the final determination of cause and manner of death.

> **PEARLS & PITFALLS**
>
> In a fire death, it is possible for some areas of the body to be unaffected or less affected by the thermal effects than other portions of the body. The site of these relatively uninvolved areas of the body may provide context to help interpret the scene investigation and autopsy findings. For example, if a body is found after a vehicle fire, with the fire the result of an accident, sparing of the skin of the neck from thermal injuries likely indicates that the decedent's head was compressed against their chest, protecting the skin, and that the cause of death may be traumatic asphyxia, and not thermal injuries (Figure 12.13A and B).

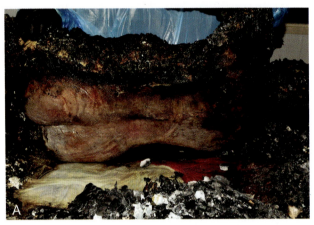 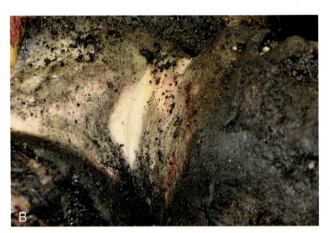

Figure 12.13. Focal preservation of skin. In (**A**), the anterior portion of the body is charred, with skeletal muscle exposed; however, the skin of the back is relatively intact, indicating this portion of the body was protected from thermal injury during the fire. In (**B**), the decedent was found in a vehicle after a fire. The intact region of skin on the neck is consistent with the chin being against the chest. Carboxyhemoglobin testing would confirm whether the COHb was significantly elevated, or whether the cause of death was likely traumatic asphyxia.

EXPLOSION-RELATED DEATHS

As part of a fire, or separate from a fire with potentially no thermal component, explosion-related deaths can occur. Explosions can occur for four main reasons: occupational accidents, miscellaneous accidents (eg, an explosion in a house heated with propane or natural gas), suicide, and terrorist activity.[16] The cause of death in explosions can include direct injuries to internal organs from the blast, secondary shrapnel from the explosion, extensive burns (if the explosion involves a significant amount of inflammable liquid or gas), and mass movement of the body induced by the blast.[16,17]

Key internal findings in explosion-related deaths[16,17]

- Tympanic membrane rupture
- Bilateral hemorrhages of the vocal folds
- Bilateral fractures of the laryngeal skeleton, including the hyoid bone
- Ruptures of the trachea and lungs, with airways containing blood or a blood-tinged foam
- If no rupture of the lungs, hyperinflation and/or lung contusions
- Aortic laceration
- Avulsion of the heart
- Intestinal perforations

NEAR MISSES

Near Miss #1: Although the finding of a body after a house fire and with autopsy revealing neither soot in the airway or gastrointestinal tract nor COHb in the blood is highly suspicious for a homicide, with the decedent killed prior to the start of the fire, the individual could have started a fire and then committed suicide, or it is also possible that following a natural death, a house fire just happened to start. In both of these situations, the decedent would have no evidence of being alive at the time of the fire (Figure 12.14).

Near Miss #2: The decedent was involved in a vehicular accident, following which a fire occurred. In such a situation, survival time after the point of impact is often important for insurance policies and subsequent civil litigation that can result from the accident. Whether or the individual was alive at the time of the fire is an important determination, and just accepting that a charred body was alive at the time of the fire is never acceptable without confirmatory or exclusionary information (Figure 12.15A-C).

Near Miss #3: While carbon monoxide exposure typically produces a cherry red discoloration of the lividity of the skin, the presence of purple lividity does not rule out carbon monoxide exposure (Figure 12.16). Unfortunately, since older individuals with underlying co-morbidities can succumb to carbon monoxide before younger healthier individuals, and because older individuals due to their underlying co-morbidities may not be autopsied, carbon monoxide deaths can easily be missed and a hazardous living condition not identified, until, unfortunately, a second (or more) death in the household or living area occurs that necessitates an autopsy, allowing for the identification of the carbon monoxide threat. Doing routine carbon monoxide testing on individuals found in vehicles or in a house can catch these cases.

Near Miss #4: Even though a body may be damaged in a fire, the epidural hemorrhage present may be an actual traumatic epidural hemorrhage and not a thermal-induced epidural hemorrhage. Also, subdural hemorrhage and subarachnoid hemorrhage are not caused by postmortem thermal injury, and, if present, represent trauma that occurred before the fire (Figure 12.17A-E).

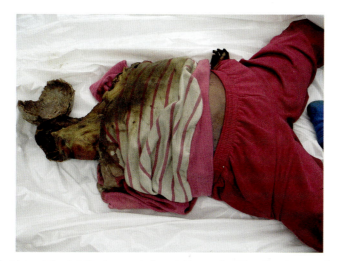

Figure 12.14. Natural death in background of partial house fire. The decedent was found in a house with evidence of significant postmortem animal activity, with her dogs having consumed much of the upper 1/3 of her body. Neither investigation nor autopsy identified any traumatic injury. Scene investigation did reveal a small portion of the house where a fire had started, but subsequently burned itself out, before expanding and consuming the house. However, if the fire had done so, presuming it occurred after the death of the individual and not before, scene investigation would have found a deceased body after a fire and autopsy would not have confirmed that the person was alive at the time of the fire nor that there were significant injuries. The cause and manner of death would likely both have been recorded as undetermined, or with the manner as homicide, and the cause of death unknown.

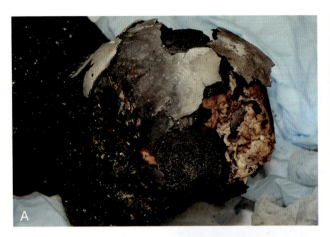
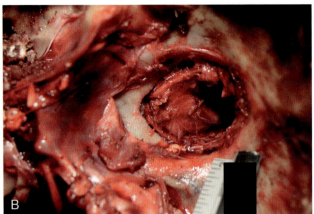
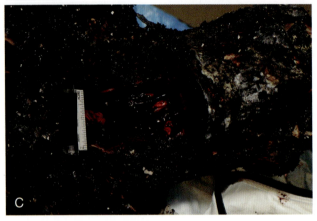

Figure 12.15. Vehicular fire after accident. (**A**) illustrates the typical delamination of the cranium secondary to thermal injury that can occur, with a small thermal-induced epidural hemorrhage in the frontal region. The findings are not consistent with pre-fire injury. However, with removal of the brain from the cranial cavity, a fracture at the foramen magnum was identified (**B**), which was associated with hemorrhage in the anterior neck (**C**). The individual died with the accident, and was not alive during the fire.

Near Miss #5: The presence of soot in the airway as a marker for the decedent being alive prior to the fire must be confirmed with testing for COHb in the blood. The determination of whether an individual was alive or not at the time of the fire should not be determined based upon the presence of soot in the airway alone. The decedent in the image had a 1% COHb concentration (with normal results often listed as <1%) (Figure 12.18).

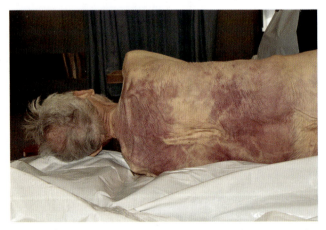

Figure 12.16. Purple lividity with carbon monoxide exposure. This individual was found in a house fire, and was undamaged by the fire. The lividity is purple; however, carbon monoxide testing revealed a concentration of 36%. The higher the concentration, the greater the likelihood of red lividity.

Near Miss #6: When a body has extensive thermal injuries rendering examination of the skin impossible, full body radiographs are appropriate to examine for the possibility of projectiles or other foreign objects, including orthopedic hardware, which may potentially be used for identification of the decedent. Occasionally, depending upon the circumstances of the fire or the body retrieval, metallic fragments or metal objects not in their normal orientation can be identified on the radiographs, and potentially confused for a projectile (Figure 12.19). If the identification of what the metallic object represents cannot be made based only on the radiograph, it is best to isolate the object from the body and visually inspect the fragment to potentially determine its origin and whether it is of value in the investigation.

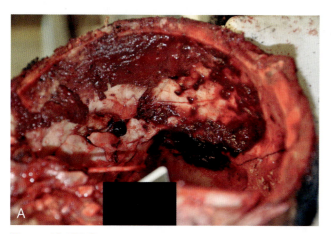
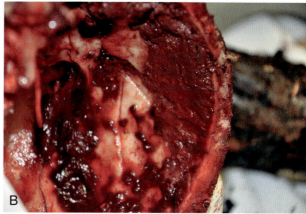

Figure 12.17A-B. Traumatic epidural in decedent found after fire. This individual was in a vehicle accident with a subsequent fire. At autopsy, there was an epidural hemorrhage (**A**); however, close examination of the cranium revealed a fracture at the right petrous ridge (**B**).

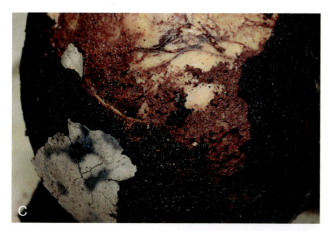
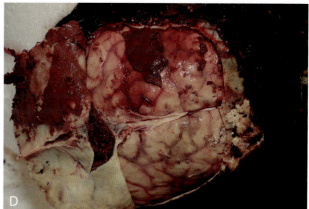
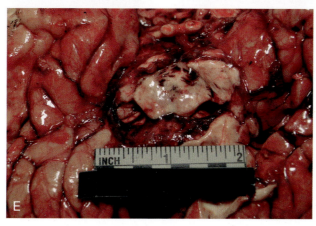

Figure 12.17C-E. Traumatic subdural hemorrhage with subsequent fire. (**C**) reveals thermal injury to the cranium with delamination of the cranial bones and a thermal-induced epidural hemorrhage. (**D**) reveals a cranium with thermal injury; however, with reflection of the dura, a subdural hemorrhage is identified, which is not a thermal artifact. (**E**) reveals punctate hemorrhage in the brainstem, which confirms the traumatic nature of the death.

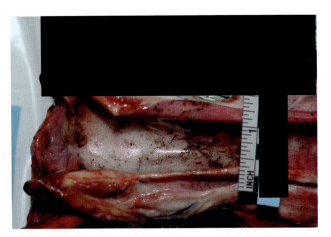

Figure 12.18. Apparent soot in the trachea. In this individual whose body was found after a house fire, examination of the trachea revealed fine strands of black material on the mucosa, which can be interpreted as soot; however, the carboxyhemoglobin concentration was 1%, indicating most like that the decedent was not alive during the fire for any length of time.

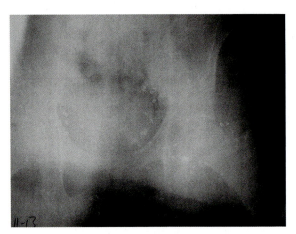

Figure 12.19. Numerous metallic fragments associated with body. The radiograph revealed numerous metallic fragments, which, at first glance, could be interpreted as possible birdshot pellets from a shotgun wound; however, closer inspection revealed that they were the metal components of a zipper, which had locally scattered when the clothing was consumed by the fire.

References

1. Gerling I, Meissner C, Reiter A, Oehmichen M. Death from thermal effects and burns. *Forensic Sci Int.* 2001;115(1-2):33-41.
2. Bohnert M, Werner CR, Pollak S. Problems associated with the diagnosis of vitality in burned bodies. *Forensic Sci Int.* 2003;135(3):197-205.
3. Rogde S, Olving JH. Characteristics of fire victims in different sorts of fires. *Forensic Sci Int.* 1996;77(1-2):93-99.
4. Hirsch CS, Bost RO, Gerber SR, Cowan ME, Adelson L, Sunshine I. Carboxyhemoglobin concentrations in flash fire victims: report of six simultaneous fire fatalities without elevated carboxyhemoglobin. *Am J Clin Pathol.* 1977;68(3):317-320.
5. Ferrari LA, Giannuzzi L. Assessment of carboxyhemoglobin, hydrogen cyanide, and methemoglobin in fire victims: a novel approach. *Forensic Sci Int.* 2015;256:46-52.
6. Martinez MA, Ballesteros S. Suicidal inhalation of motorbike exhaust: adding new data to the literature about the contribution of gasoline in the cause of death. *J Anal Toxic.* 2006;30(9):697-702.
7. Ubelaker DH. The forensic evaluation of burned skeletal remains: a synthesis. *Forensic Sci Int.* 2009;183(1-3):1-5.
8. Bohnert M, Hejna P. Tongue protrusion in burned bodies. *Int J Legal Med.* 2016;130(5):1253-1255.
9. Herrmann NP, Bennett JL. The differentiation of traumatic and heat-related fractures in burned bone. *J Forensic Sci.* 1999;44(3):461-469.
10. deGruchy S, Rogers TL. Identifying chop marks on cremated bone: a preliminary study. *J Forensic Sci.* 2002;47(5):933-936.
11. Pope EJ, Smith OC. Identification of traumatic injury in burned cranial bone: an experimental approach. *J Forensic Sci.* 2004;49(3):431-440.
12. Hammarledbiod S, Farrugia A, Bierry G, et al. Thermal bone injuries: postmortem computed tomography findings in 25 cases. *Int J Legal Med.* 2022;136:219-227.
13. Bohnert M, Rost T, Faller-Marquardt M, Ropohl D, Pollak S. Fractures of the base of the skull in charred bodies—postmortem heat injuries or signs of mechanical traumatisation? *Forensic Sci Int.* 1997;87(1):55-62.
14. Symes SA, L'Abbe EN, Pokines JT, et al. Thermal alteration in bone. In: Pokines JT, Symes SA, eds. *Manual of Forensic Taphonomy.* CRC Press; 2014.
15. Krap T, Krap T, Duijst W, Aalders MCG, Oostra RJ. Mechanical or thermal damage: differentiating between underlying mechanisms as a cause of bone fractures. *Int J Legal Med.* 2022;136(4):1133-1148.
16. Rajs J, Moberg B, Olsson JE. Explosion-related deaths in Sweden-A forensic-pathologic and criminalistic study. *Forensic Sci Int.* 1987;34(1-2):1-15.
17. Galante N, Franceschetti L, Del Sordo S, Casali MB, Genovese U. Explosion-related deaths: an overview on forensic evaluation and implications. *Forensic Sci Med Pathol.* 2021;17(3):437-448.

CHILD ABUSE 13

CHAPTER OUTLINE

Introduction   380

Features of Subdural Hemorrhage   383

Features of Retinal Hemorrhages   386

Other Features in the Eye: Retinoschisis   389

Differential Diagnosis of Subdural and Retinal Hemorrhages   389

Differential Diagnoses: Glutaric Aciduria Type I and Galactosemia   389

Differential Diagnosis: Congenital Heart Disease, Meningitis, and Leukemia   389

Differential Diagnosis: Menkes Disease   390

Differential Diagnosis: Neurosurgical Complications and Traumatic Labor   391

Differential Diagnosis: Aneurysms   391

Differential Diagnosis: Hypernatremia   392

Differential Diagnosis: Coagulation Disorders   392

Differential Diagnosis: Accidental Injury   393

Other Important Topics With Regard to Inflicted Head Trauma in Infants   395
- Rib Fractures   395
- Falls   401
- Apparent Life-Threatening Event   403

Alternative Theories as to the Causation of Findings Associated With Abusive Head Trauma   403

Other Features of Child Abuse   406
- Fractures   406
- Bruising and Lacerations   408
- Burns   411
- Malnourishment and Dehydration   412

Near Misses   412

INTRODUCTION

Fatal child abuse can take many forms but usually falls under the categories of inflicted trauma (due to one event or due to multiple events over time) or neglect, which can lead to malnourishment and dehydration. Sexual trauma can be a component of fatal inflicted trauma and both fatal inflicted trauma and evidence of neglect can be present at the same time. While fatal inflicted trauma of infants and children can include the same types of injuries seen in other age groups including blunt force injuries (eg, laceration of liver from kick to abdomen), sharp force injuries, and gunshot wounds (Figures 13.1 and 13.2), inflicted trauma in infants also includes fatal head injuries of a type not usually seen in other age groups, that is, that due to shaking or shaking with impact. Caffey originally described the features associated with whiplash-shaking as chronic subdural hematomas, retinal hemorrhage, metaphyseal fractures, and potential for permanent brain damage.[1] Duhaime listed retinal hemorrhage, subarachnoid or subdural hemorrhage (or both), cranial contusions, skull fracture, white matter tears, and diffuse brain swelling as features of the condition, with not all findings in each case they reported.[2] The key findings of this form of inflicted head injury in infants have also been described as intracranial hemorrhage, retinal hemorrhage, and acute encephalopathy,[3] widespread bilateral retinal hemorrhages and large macular folds, thin-film subdural hemorrhage, and encephalopathy,[4] and subdural hemorrhage, retinal hemorrhage, brain parenchymal injuries, and rib fractures, with three of the four having a high positive predictive value.[5]

> **FAQ:** Is the diagnosis at autopsy of inflicted head injury/abusive head trauma in infants as simple as identifying subdural hemorrhage, retinal hemorrhages, and evidence of encephalopathy?
>
> **Answer:** No, definitely not, although these three findings are commonly present in cases of inflicted head injury in infants, other conditions, including even natural diseases, can be a cause of these findings as well, which the pathologist must rule out before making their final determination.
>
> **FAQ:** What is shaken baby syndrome?
>
> **Answer:** The term "shaken baby syndrome" is used to describe infants with a characteristic group of findings, which most commonly includes subdural hemorrhage, retinal hemorrhages, and encephalopathy, and has been used in the medical literature for decades (with a PubMed search in August 2022 finding 965 citations using "Shaken Baby Syndrome" with many in 2022). Caffey originally used the term "whiplash

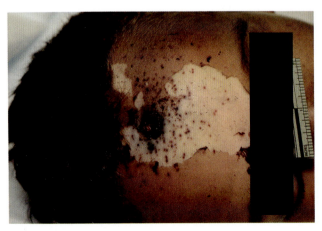

Figure 13.1. Close-range gunshot wound of the forehead. This child was shot in the forehead by their father. Present around the gunshot wound is powder tattooing.

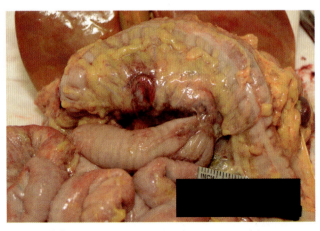

Figure 13.2. Peritonitis due to blunt force injuries of the pancreas. This young child was kicked in the abdomen by their mother's boyfriend, and subsequently developed pancreatitis and peritonitis.

shaking," acknowledging the indirect acceleration-deceleration forces that play the role in development of the injuries, and later the term "whiplash shaken infant syndrome,"[1,6] with Duhaime apparently introducing "shaken baby syndrome."[2] However, the existence of shaken baby syndrome is debated in the forensic community, specifically, whether or not shaking alone or shaking combined with impact would cause the pathologic findings associated with shaken baby syndrome.[7] To be clear, that the features are associated with abusive head trauma is not debated, but instead the physical mechanism by which those injuries occur (ie, shaking, or shaking with impact) is the subject of debate in the forensic community. In support of shaking alone as a cause of death, Gill et al published "Fatal head injury in children younger than 2 years in New York City and an overview of the Shaken Baby Syndrome," and the conclusion of the abstract stated, "We describe a subset of fatal, nonaccidental head injury deaths in infants without an impact to the head. The autopsy findings and circumstances are diagnostic of a nonimpact, shaking mechanism as the cause of death."[8]

CHECKLIST of Procedures for Evaluation of Suspicious Infant Death
- Completion of sudden unexpected infant death investigation (SUIDI) form with scene photography including doll reenactment by investigators
- Full-body radiography
- Reflection of scalp and examination for foci of subgaleal hemorrhage
- Examination of brain, spinal cord, and dura after formalin fixation
- Removal of eyes and orbital tissue, followed by fixation and examination
- Removal of cervical segment of vertebral column in total for examination of dorsal root ganglia and spinal nerves and roots, or examination of the structures in situ
- Back dissection, including extremities
- Even with radiography performed, consider in situ dissection of long bones of extremities
- Examination of ribs after removal of pleura
- Blood spot card for genetic testing

PEARLS & PITFALLS

If during the investigation a caregiver offers an accident as the cause of an infant's injuries, the investigator should collect as much information as possible regarding that accident, including measurements (eg, distance from bed where the infant was said to have rolled from to the floor where they were said to have landed) and photographs. In addition, the caregiver may, with handling of a doll, be able to recreate the accident for the investigators. Such information can be useful in helping to confirming or refute whether the autopsy findings could be caused by the event described.

CHECKLIST of Findings to Examine for in the Evaluation of a Suspicious Infant Death
- Abrasions, contusions, and lacerations of the scalp and of the body, noting the distribution of bruises and checking for patterned injuries
- Subgaleal hemorrhage, which can indicate an impact site
- Cranial fractures
- Intracranial hemorrhage, most specifically subdural hemorrhage
- Retinal hemorrhages
- Hemorrhage within the dorsal root ganglia and spinal nerves
- Rib fractures
- Other fractures

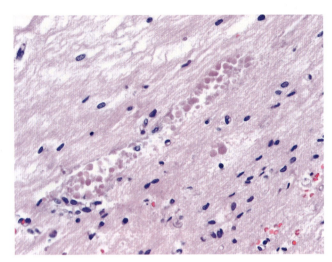

Figure 13.3. Axonal spheroids in infant who died from abusive head trauma. Focally, in the image is a cluster of axonal spheroids (hematoxylin and eosin, high power).

FAQ: What is the pathologic mechanism of death in inflicted head injury in infants?

Answer: The exact mechanism of death in inflicted head injury in infants is debated; however, whether the cause is diffuse axonal injury (DAI),[9] injury to the brain stem and/or cervical spinal cord,[10] or global ischemic injury resulting from a combination of subdural hemorrhage, vasospasm, and trauma-induced respiratory and/or circulatory failure[11] or a combination of two or more of these mechanisms is more academic than relevant in the determination of cause and manner of death. The finding of DAI is consistent with abusive head trauma when there is no competing severe trauma (eg, car accident), but DAI is not commonly found in abusive head trauma[12] (Figure 13.3). In addition to the primary effects of the injury, secondary effects including ischemic injury and edema, depending upon the time frame between injury and death, will develop. Figure 13.4A and B is from a child who survived an episode of abusive head trauma, dying 10 years later. With cerebral edema, diastatic fractures can occur (Figure 13.5A-C).

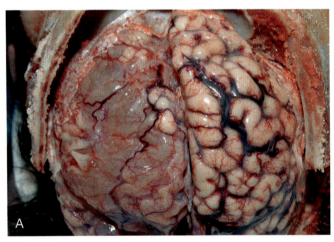
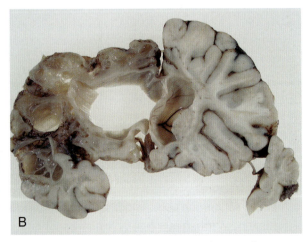

Figure 13.4. Child who survived for 10 years after episode of abusive head trauma. In situ, the left cerebral hemisphere can be seen to be almost completely cystic (**A**). A cross section of the brain (**B**) confirms the cystic appearance of the cerebral parenchyma. Although the mechanism can be multifactorial, with a significant ischemic component likely, the images serve to illustrate how the damage induced by the abusive head trauma is not just confined to the dura and retina.

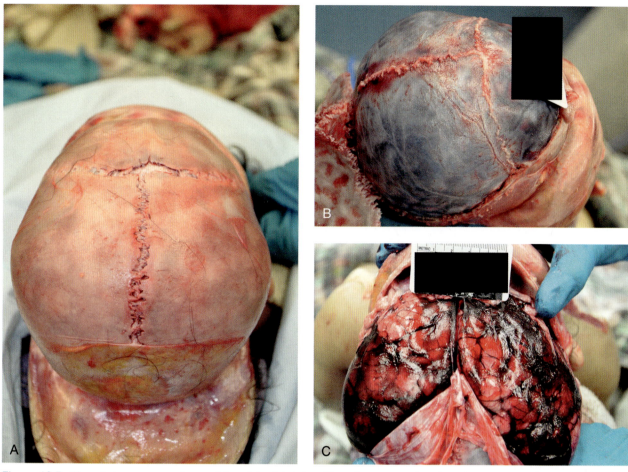

Figure 13.5. Diastatic fracture secondary to delayed death in infant. This infant sustained a subarachnoid hemorrhage and subsequently developed cerebral edema and died several days after the event. Autopsy and investigation were unable to definitively determine the nature of the hemorrhage. (**A**) illustrates the diastatic fracture which developed. (**B**) shows the intact dura overlying the brain, which was meticulously prepared by the autopsy assistant. Reflection of the dura reveals mostly diffuse subarachnoid hemorrhage (**C**).

> **PEARLS & PITFALLS**
>
> Reflection of the scalp can show focal subgaleal hemorrhage (Figure 13.6A-C), which can indicate an impact site. The scalp overlying a subgaleal hemorrhage may not exhibit any blunt force injuries, such as an abrasion or contusion; however, it is useful to shave the region, and, if necessary, to shave the entire scalp searching for such injuries. The lack of an impact site, as evidenced by no focal subgaleal hemorrhage, does not mean that an impact did not occur. If the infant's head was impacted against a broad and/or soft object, such as a bed mattress, there may be no subgaleal hemorrhage at the impact site.

FEATURES OF SUBDURAL HEMORRHAGE

There are two basic forms of subdural hemorrhage that could be identified in an infant: thin-film and space-occupying. A thin-film subdural hemorrhage (Figure 13.7A-E) is a thin layer of red blood cells, perhaps only a millimeter or two thick, which can be on the dura or the cerebral surface often at the cerebral convexities and which occurs as the result of inertial rotational motion tearing bridging veins.[13] This thin-film subdural hemorrhage is admixed with cerebral spinal fluid and can be termed an infantile subdural hemorrhage.[14] A thin-film subdural hemorrhage represents a diffuse injury.[13] Commonly associated with the thin-film subdural hemorrhage is subarachnoid hemorrhage. A space-occupying subdural hemorrhage (Figure 13.8A and B) is one that forms a mass lesion between the dura and the adjacent cerebral hemisphere and is usually more of a focal injury and should be viewed with more caution when assessing for the presence of inflicted

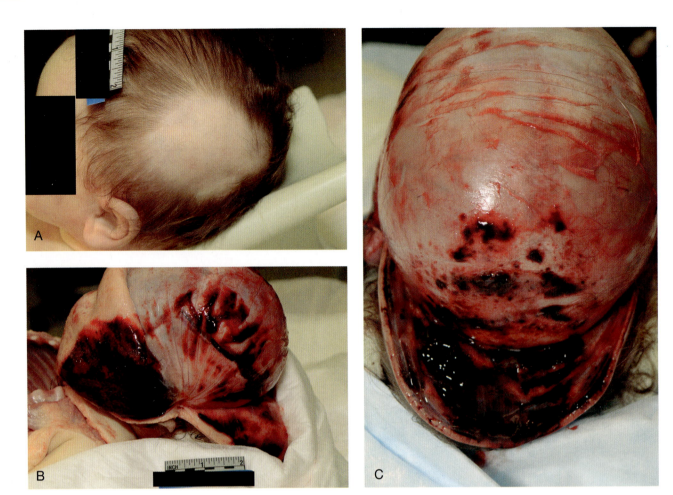

Figure 13.6. Impact site. While the overlying skin can have no evidence of injury (**A**), the reflected scalp can show focal hemorrhage (**B**), which can help identify the impact site. In (**C**), this infant was forcefully impacted backward, hitting their head against an object.

head injury.[4,13] A space-occupying subdural hemorrhage could be the result of a fall (ie, a mechanism that produces a focal injury). The presence of a space-occupying subdural hemorrhage does not exclude inflicted trauma as the cause of death; however, given that a space-occupying subdural is more consistent with a focal lesion, and could be the result of an accident, caution in interpretation is important.

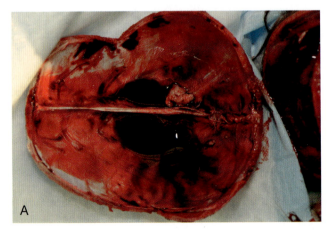

Figure 13.7A. Thin-film subdural hemorrhage. The top of the cranium, which has been resected, is still lined by the dura, and on the undersurface of the dura is a thin layer of blood. Adjacent to the falx cerebri are pools of blood, which is an artifact of removal of opening the cranium. As artifact can occur, the pathologist should always witness the cut cranium on an infant being retracted to assess for hemorrhage at that time.

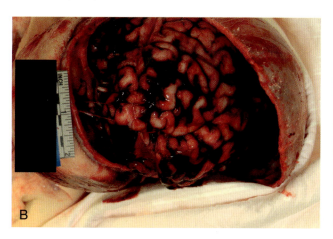
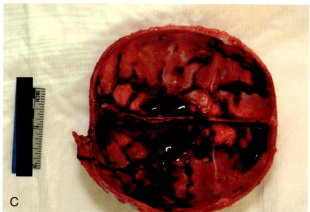
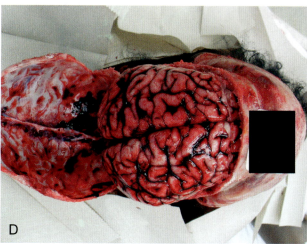

Figure 13.7B-D. Thin-film subdural hemorrhage and subarachnoid hemorrhage. In (B), the top of the cranium has been partially retracted, revealing the thin film of subdural hemorrhage on the undersurface of the dura and the relatively diffuse subarachnoid hemorrhage on the surface of the brain. In (C), the top of the cranium, which has been resected, is still lined by the dura, and on the undersurface of the dura is a thin layer of blood. In a separate autopsy from (B) and (C), (D) also shows a thin film of subdural hemorrhage on the undersurface of the dura and the relatively diffuse subarachnoid hemorrhage on the surface of the brain.

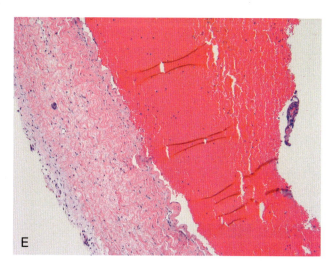

Figure 13.7E. Infant subdural hemorrhage. The image shows an acute subdural hemorrhage, with no evidence of organization (hematoxylin and eosin, medium power).

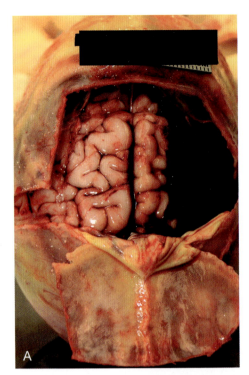 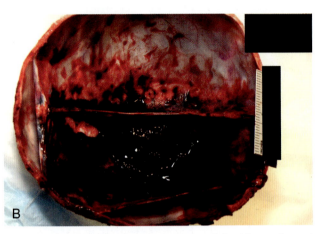

Figure 13.8. Space-occupying subdural hemorrhage. In (**A**), on the right side of the cranial cavity is a subdural hemorrhage. In (**B**), the resected top portion of the cranium has a clot of blood on one side, but minimal on the opposite site. A space-occupying subdural hemorrhage would create a mass effect and can lead to a midline shift, unlike a thin-film subdural hemorrhage, which, on its own, would not.

FAQ: What is the difference between a focal injury and a diffuse injury?

Answer: A focal injury is an injury where the primary damage is due to impact or force involving a single localized area of the head. When a child falls and hits their head, the damage occurs at the point of impact, with the remainder of the brain spared, or relatively spared, of any traumatic injury, even though secondary changes may later occur that diffusely affect the brain, such as cerebral edema. A diffuse injury is an injury where the primary damage is due to force involving a broad (ie, diffuse) area, with essentially the entire brain involved. When a child is shaken, or shaken with impact, rotational acceleration of the brain occurs. As with focal injury, in a diffuse injury secondary pathologic changes can occur, which overlap the primary pathologic changes (eg, in an infant with traumatic diffuse axonal injury due to abusive head trauma, secondary ischemic axonal injury can develop).

PEARLS & PITFALLS

Unless an infant or child has had recent surgery involving the posterior fossa or has comminuted fractures of the occipital bone, a spinal subdural hemorrhage is highly suggestive of abusive head trauma.[15]

FEATURES OF RETINAL HEMORRHAGES

Importance: In their study of 110 children aged 15 months or younger, Binenbaum et al, who did not exclude children with a coagulopathy, found that retinal hemorrhages are highly associated with abusive head trauma, and as the severity of the retinal hemorrhages increases, the likelihood of abuse increases.[16] Gilliland et al opined that "In the absence of a verifiable history of a severe head injury or life-threatening central nervous system disease, retinal and ocular hemorrhages were diagnostic of child abuse."[17]

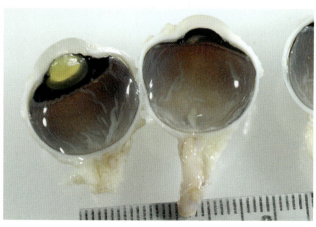

Figure 13.9. Eyes photographed on light stand. Using the light stand allowed for light to be directed into the depths of the bisected eyes, allowing for good illumination of the retina. In this case, no retinal hemorrhages were present. The same thing can be accomplished with a penlight, or similar light source.

PEARLS & PITFALLS

Photographically documenting retinal hemorrhages can be challenging. If the eyes are merely cross-sectioned and photographed, the retina is usually not illuminated adequately to see the interior. Two methods for good photographic documentation of the retinal hemorrhages are by directing light (eg, with a penlight) onto the inner surface of the retina, or by backlighting the retina (Figures 13.9-13.10A and B).

Location: In regard to retinal hemorrhages and inflicted injury vs other causes, Bechtel et al said, "Thus, it is not the presence of retinal hemorrhages but the location and number of them that are most helpful in distinguishing accidental from inflicted head trauma."[18] Franzco and Kelly reviewed the literature regarding retinal hemorrhages and found that in inflicted head trauma, retinal hemorrhages are most often too numerous to count, in multiple layers of the retina, and extend to the periphery (Figure 13.11A and B).[19] There are several types of retinal hemorrhage, depending upon the location of the hemorrhage in the eye or the layers of the retina: intravitreal, preretinal, intraretinal, subretinal, and subretinal pigment epithelium (Figure 13.12A-C).[20] Intravitreal hemorrhages are within

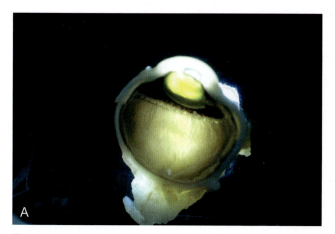
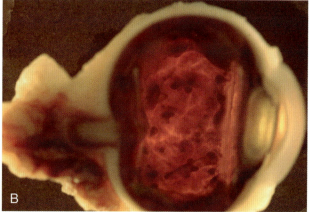

Figure 13.10. Backlit sectioned eyes. Another method to demonstrate the presence of retinal hemorrhages is to backlight the eyes (ie, place a light source on the side of the eye opposite the camera). A headlamp is a simple and low cost way to accomplish this. (**A**) is a backlit eye with no retinal hemorrhages for comparison. (**B**) is a backlit eye with extensive retinal hemorrhages, which extend to the ora serrata, and involve essentially the entire retina.

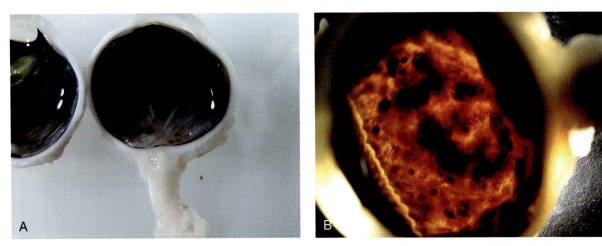

Figure 13.11. Distribution of retinal hemorrhages. In (**A**), the bisected eye has retinal hemorrhages, and, although a few are present anterior and near the ora serrata, most are present at the posterior pole (ie,. around the optic disc). In (**B**), the retinal hemorrhages are florid, present throughout most of the retina, and to the ora serrata.

the vitreous fluid. Preretinal hemorrhages are just beneath the internal limiting membrane. Intraretinal hemorrhages are hemorrhages within the retina itself, and can be superficial or deep, depending upon the layer of the retina involved. Subretinal hemorrhages are between the rods and cones, and the pigmented epithelial layer. And subretinal pigment epithelium or choroidal hemorrhages are deep to the pigmented epithelium.[20]

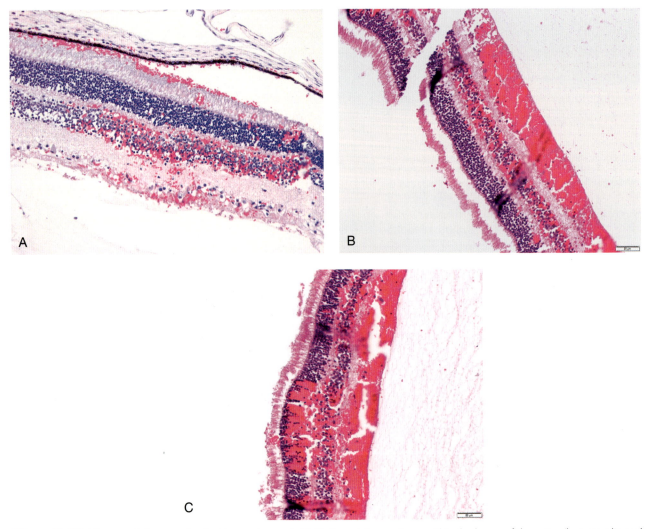

Figure 13.12. Microscopic images of retinal hemorrhages. In (**A-C**), there is hemorrhage within the layers of the retina (hematoxylin and eosin, medium power all images).

OTHER FEATURES IN THE EYE: RETINOSCHISIS

Rao et al describe retinoschisis at autopsy as cavities between the internal limiting membrane and the nerve fiber layer of the retina producing a domelike lesion.[21] Franzco and Kelly describe that retinoschisis is characteristic of, but not entirely specific for, abuse (being seen in crush injuries and other severe injuries).[19]

> **PEARLS & PITFALLS**
>
> Optic nerve sheath hemorrhage, which is frequently associated with retinal hemorrhage, is not by itself specific for child abuse (Figure 13.13A and B).[22]

DIFFERENTIAL DIAGNOSIS OF SUBDURAL AND RETINAL HEMORRHAGES

In the evaluation of subdural and retinal hemorrhages in infants, a lengthy differential diagnosis must be considered as the list of conditions causing both subdural and retinal hemorrhages in infants is fairly long (Tables 13.1 and 13.2).[23-26] In addition, Hymel et al provide an extensive list of conditions in the differential diagnosis of abusive head injury.[27]

DIFFERENTIAL DIAGNOSES: GLUTARIC ACIDURIA TYPE I AND GALACTOSEMIA

How to distinguish from abusive head injury: Both of these conditions are routinely screened for in the neonatal period and results should be available in the hospital records. However, retaining a blood spot card at autopsy for future genetic testing is a useful step, as some infants may not have had pre-natal screening performed. Children with glutaric aciduria type I typically present between the ages of 6 and 18 months of age with dystonia and strokelike episodes, which are triggered by fever and infection.[28] On magnetic resonance imaging, children will have widening of Sylvian fissures, widened mesencephalic cisterns, and expanded subarachnoid spaces at anterior tips of temporal lobes.[28]

DIFFERENTIAL DIAGNOSIS: CONGENITAL HEART DISEASE, MENINGITIS, AND LEUKEMIA

How to distinguish from abusive head injury: Each of these conditions in the differential diagnosis should be identifiable in the medical record, at autopsy (congenital heart disease, meningitis), or by microscopic examination (meningitis, leukemia) (Figure 13.14A and B).

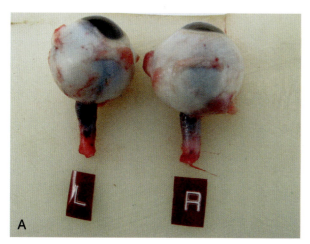

Figure 13.13A. Eyes and optic nerves. There is bilateral hemorrhage of the optic nerve sheath.

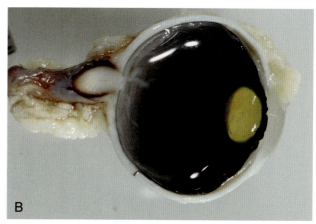

Figure 13.13B. Optic nerve sheath hemorrhage. This bisected eye has hemorrhage in the optic nerve sheath; however, there are no retinal hemorrhages. Optic nerve sheath hemorrhage can occur in a variety of circumstances and is not, by itself, indicative of trauma.

TABLE 13.1: Causes of Subdural Hemorrhage in Infants/Children

Intentional injury
Non-intentional injury (ie, accidents)
Coagulation and hematological disorders (leukemia, sickle cell anemia, disseminated intravascular coagulation (DIC), hemophilia, von Willebrand disease, hemorrhagic disease of the newborn, idiopathic thromobocytopenic purpura)
Glutaric aciduria
Galactosemia
Hypernatremia
Iatrogenic (neurosurgical complications, traumatic labor)
Aneurysms
Arachnoid cysts
Meningitis
Congenital heart disease
Menkes syndrome
Brain tumors

Based upon Kemp AM. Investigating subdural haemorrhage in infants. *Arch Dis Child.* 2002;86(2):98-102 and Lo WD, Lee J, Rusin J, Perkins E, Roach ES. Intracranial hemorrhage in children: an evolving spectrum. *Arch Neurol.* 2008;65(12):1629-1633.

DIFFERENTIAL DIAGNOSIS: MENKES DISEASE[28]

How to distinguish from abusive head injury: Children with Menkes disease can develop subdural hemorrhage and metaphyseal fractures; however, they also have hair dysmorphisms (short, sparse, coarse and lightly pigmented hair) and facial dysmorphisms (including sagging cheeks), bladder diverticula, wormian bones, skin laxity, pectus excavatum, and flaring of anterior rib ends.

TABLE 13.2: Causes of Retinal Hemorrhage in Infants/Children

Inflicted injury
Accidental injury
Hypertension and increased intracranial pressure
Coagulation disorders
Meningitis
Vasculitis
Aneurysm
Retinal disease
Carbon monoxide poisoning
Anemia
Hypoxia
Glutaric aciduria
Osteogenesis imperfecta
Retinopathy of prematurity
Hypernatremia
Birth
Leukemia

Based upon Levin AV. Retinal hemorrhages: advances in understanding. *Pediatr Clin North Am.* 2009;56(2):333-344 and Kaur B, Taylor D. Retinal haemorrhages. *Arch Dis Child.* 1990;65(12):1369-1372.

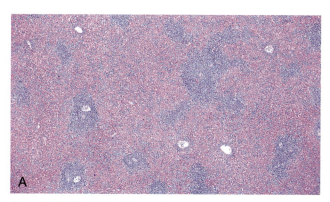 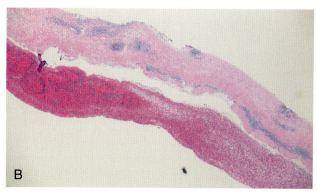

Figure 13.14. Subdural hemorrhage due to B-cell acute lymphoblastic leukemia. This infant was brought unresponsive to the hospital after a period of illness at home, but was unable to be resuscitated. An autopsy revealed a bilateral subdural hemorrhage. The neoplastic leukemic cells were present in the liver (**A**) and the dura adjacent to the hemorrhage (**B**) (both images, hematoxylin and eosin, low power).

DIFFERENTIAL DIAGNOSIS: NEUROSURGICAL COMPLICATIONS AND TRAUMATIC LABOR

How to distinguish from abusive head injury: Both of these conditions should be able to be determined by review of medical records.

DIFFERENTIAL DIAGNOSIS: ANEURYSMS

How to distinguish from abusive head injury: As aneurysms have the potential to cause subdural and retinal hemorrhages and mimic abusive head injury, and because they can be small, potentially causing difficulty in finding the lesion, a more extensive discussion of this condition is below.

Incidence of aneurysm: Elgamal et al in their review of the literature indicated that only 85 cases of cerebral aneurysms occurring in the 1st year of life had been reported in the medical literature, and that 63 of them presented with a subarachnoid hemorrhage.[29] Plunkett, in his reported case of a 7-month-old male who died as the result of a ruptured berry aneurysm, stated, "Sudden death caused by rupture of a cerebral aneurysm has not been previously described in an infant."[30] This statement by the author of the case report likely represents the forensic context and not the clinical context, as children with a ruptured aneurysm are more likely to present to the hospital. Infants and children with a ruptured berry aneurysm would likely have a period of unconsciousness and coma, which would be recognized by caregivers and for which treatment would be sought. The infant would be less likely to present with sudden death. Prahlow et al presented a 3.5-year-old child who died as the result of a ruptured berry aneurysm, and also described that scenario as rare.[31]

Presentation of aneurysm: Most infants with a ruptured cerebral aneurysm will present with subarachnoid hemorrhage and most will survive. Garg et al reported 62 pediatric patients, under the age of 18 years, with intracranial aneurysms, with 58% (n = 36) having subarachnoid hemorrhage on presentation and only one having subdural hemorrhage.[32] Koroknay-Pal et al reported 114 pediatric patients with intracranial aneurysms, aged 3 months to 18 years, with 89 patients presenting with subarachnoid hemorrhage.[33] Pasqualin et al reported 38 pediatric patients with intracranial aneurysms, 36 presenting with subarachnoid hemorrhage.[34] Aryan et al reported 50 pediatric patients with intracranial aneurysms, with subarachnoid hemorrhage being the most common presenting feature, with only one death occurring.[35] Related to subarachnoid hemorrhage due to intracranial aneurysms would be the possible presence of a subdural hemorrhage, due to rupture of the subarachnoid hemorrhage through the arachnoid mater and into this region. However, based upon their review of the literature, Marbacher et al found that the incidence of subdural hemorrhage combined with subarachnoid hemorrhage in patients with a ruptured cerebral aneurysm was between 0.5% and 10%.[36]

Location of aneurysms: Buis et al reviewed the literature in children under 1 year of age and found that aneurysms were nearly three times more commonly found in the middle cerebral artery than other vessels.[37]

Size of aneurysm: The size of an aneurysm is important, as, although with a subarachnoid hemorrhage due to a ruptured berry aneurysm, the aneurysm is essentially always identified; very small aneurysms could still potentially be missed at autopsy. Buis et al found that the mean aneurysm size in infants and children was 1.8 cm (+/− 1.4 cm), with a range of 0.1 to 9.0 cm, median of 1.5 cm.[37] Ferrante et al reported that 13 of 56 aneurysms in their study were small (<1 cm).[38] Koroknay-Pal et al reported 114 pediatric patients with intracranial aneurysms; the mean size of ruptured aneurysms was 0.9 cm, with a range of 0.2 to 5.0 cm.[33]

KEY FEATURES to Help Distinguish a Cerebral Aneurysm From Abusive Head Trauma

- Cerebral aneurysms are extremely rare in the infant population.
- Almost all cerebral aneurysms are of a size that would be identified at autopsy.
- Cerebral aneurysms are almost always a cause of only subarachnoid hemorrhage and not subdural hemorrhage.

> **FAQ:** Does intracranial hemorrhage and Terson syndrome cause retinal hemorrhages?
>
> **Answer:** Also of importance in regards to intracranial aneurysms is the association of subarachnoid hemorrhage and retinal hemorrhages. Neß et al reviewed 74 patients with subarachnoid hemorrhage, with 28 patients having retinal hemorrhages, 45% with bilateral involvement.[39] Stiebel-Kalish et al found intraocular hemorrhages in 19 of 70 patients with a subarachnoid hemorrhage due to a cerebral aneurysm. Of hemorrhage found in 30 eyes total, 14 was vitreous, 12 was subhyaloid, and 4 had retinal hemorrhages.[40] Bhardwaj et al describe a 7-month-old with subarachnoid hemorrhage (right side) and right-sided subdural hemorrhage, and intraparenchymal hematoma due to a complex 5 to 6 mm aneurysm in the right Sylvian fissure, associated with 1 to 2 cm of midline shift, who suddenly became floppy and apneic at home and had extensive preretinal and intraretinal hemorrhages in the right eye, with the left eye appearing normal.[41] Stiebel-Kalish et al describe that Terson syndrome is actually vitreous hemorrhage in association with subarachnoid hemorrhage, but that many authors have considered all forms of intraocular hemorrhage occurring in association with subarachnoid hemorrhage to be Terson syndrome.[40]

DIFFERENTIAL DIAGNOSIS: HYPERNATREMIA

How to distinguish from abusive head injury: Although case reports exist of hypernatraemia causing intracranial and retinal hemorrhages,[42,43] this association has been called into question,[44,45] and the hypernatremia is likely due to the intracranial hemorrhage and not the reverse.

DIFFERENTIAL DIAGNOSIS: COAGULATION DISORDERS

How to distinguish from abusive head injury: Coagulation disorders can be associated with easier bleeding and are often impossible to identify postmortem. Rutty et al used PIVKA II, which tests factor II function, and found abnormalities in patients on warfarin and with hemolytic disease of the newborn, and, as such, PIVKA II testing may be useful in the identification of some coagulation abnormalities postmortem.[46] Among coagulation disorders, von Willebrand disease (vWD) is a consideration as a cause of both a subdural hemorrhage and retinal hemorrhages.[47,48] Stray-Pederson et al reported an 11-month-old girl with a massive subdural hemorrhage (note: not thin and diffuse) and retinal hemorrhages, who had a minor fall, and was later diagnosed with type I vWD. The girl made a full recovery.[48] The author's last sentence stated, "Without the full triad of subdural hematoma, retinal hemorrhages and encephalopathy, the conclusion that observed injuries are caused by shaking must be made with great caution." Laposata and Laposata describe two infants with subdural and retinal hemorrhages due to vWD; as with the case described above, both infants recovered.[47] With both these cases, the infants developed larger subdural hemorrhages (ie, space-occupying) and survived, because there was no underlying injury to the brain, such as there is with abusive head trauma. With a coagulation disorder, an infant could be expected to bleed more easily following more minor trauma; however, the mechanism of death would be through the formation of a large, space-occupying subdural hemorrhage, which then puts pressure on the brain because of the confined space within the skull.

> **PEARLS & PITFALLS**
>
> When a suspicious infant death is investigated where the infant was brought to the hospital prior to final declaration of death, contact the hospital to determine if any blood drawn during that time is available. This antemortem hospital blood, if drawn into the proper types of tubes, could be used for coagulation studies, if such studies were not performed during the time of medical intervention.

> **PEARLS & PITFALLS**
>
> Hemorrhagic disease of the newborn, which is due to insufficient amounts of vitamin K-dependent coagulation factors, can also occur in older infants due to insufficient levels of vitamin K in maternal breast milk, and can be found anywhere from 1 week to 6 months after birth. This deficiency of vitamin K can lead to intracranial hemorrhage (ie, late-type VKDB (vitamin K deficiency bleeding) and can mimic abusive head injury.[49]

DIFFERENTIAL DIAGNOSIS: ACCIDENTAL INJURY

How to distinguish from abusive head injury: According to Case,[50,51] infants who die from injuries sustained in an accidental short fall would characteristically have a bruise or laceration of the scalp, a skull fracture, and an epidural hemorrhage, or rarely a space-occupying subdural hemorrhage. As described by Case, the injuries sustained in a fall would be focal, while the finding of a small thin subdural hemorrhage and retinal hemorrhages, with no skull fracture, is indicative of a diffuse injury (as might be expected in an infant who is shaken, with or without impact).[7,50,51] In addition, studies comparing fatal inflicted head injuries and fatal accidents have been done. Vinchon et al compared the findings in 45 cases of confessed inflicted head injury and 39 cases of accidental trauma occurring in a public place and found that if the child had a subdural hemorrhage, diffuse retinal hemorrhage, and no scalp swelling, in their study population, the only possibility was inflicted trauma.[52]

> **FAQ:** Can retinal hemorrhages occur in a short fall or accidental injury?
>
> **Answer:** Yes, in an article by Christian et al, the authors reported that they found retinal hemorrhages in 3 of 1617 children admitted to the hospital with head injuries, and in all three, the retinal hemorrhages were confined to the posterior pole of the retina.[53] Vinchon et al reviewed 44 cases of abuse and 35 cases of accidental head injuries. They found retinal hemorrhages in 56.8% of the abuse cases and in 6 of 35 accidents. In 5 of 6 accident victims with retinal hemorrhages, the retinal hemorrhages were described as mild, with mild defined as illustrated. In only 1 of 35 accident victims was severe retinal hemorrhages identified and, in this case, they were due to facial trauma.[52] Levin describes that retinal hemorrhages in non-inflicted injury situations are usually few in number and confined to the posterior pole.[25]

PEARLS & PITFALLS

While a broad differential diagnosis must always be carefully considered, no unexpected death of an infant where a subdural hemorrhage and a retinal hemorrhage were identified at autopsy should ever be certified as to the cause of death without considering abusive head trauma.

SAMPLE NOTE

If autopsy identifies a group of findings that the forensic pathologist determines are from non-accidental origin, the cause of death can be certified in variety of ways. Although the term "Shaken baby syndrome" could be used as the cause of death for the death certificate, this term implies a knowledge of the mechanism by which the injuries occurred, and could be difficult to defend later in court, especially if the accused individual offers another mechanism for the injuries. While the term "Abusive head trauma" or "Inflicted head trauma" have been used in place of shaken baby syndrome in the medical literature,[5] for death certification, these terms are also not necessarily ideal as they have a subjective connotation. "Craniocerebral trauma" or "Craniocerebrocervical trauma" is an objective way to certify the cause of death, with no regard to mechanism or intent. "Blunt force injuries of the head" or "Blunt force injuries of the head and neck" would also be an objective way to certify the cause of death.

FAQ: Can the time of abusive head injury be determined based upon the symptomatology reported?

Answer: Talbert opined that given the proposed mechanical nature of shaken baby syndrome (ie, shearing of axons), that immediate disruption of cortical function would occur, resulting in a coma, and no lucid interval.[54] Crying would constitute a lucid interval. In 36 children who were victims of homicide reviewed by Reichard et al likely only one with a Glasgow Coma Scale of 9 would have been potentially capable of crying.[55] Arbogast et al reviewed 314 fatally injured children, with injuries both inflicted in some and due to accidents in others, and found that of children less than 11 months of age who died of inflicted injury a Glasgow Coma Scale consistent with a lucid interval was possible (around 10%-15%),[56] and thus, after sustaining fatal abusive head injuries, an infant might be able to cry; however, regardless, their behavior would not be normal after the injury.

PEARLS & PITFALLS

When performing an autopsy on an infant who is believed to have died from inflicted injury, or in an infant whose death is highly suspicious for being from inflicted injury, removal of the neck and examination of the dorsal root ganglia and spinal nerves/roots for hemorrhage very useful adjunct procedure (Figure 13.15A-C). Matshes et al reviewed 35 deaths and saw such dorsal root ganglia and adjacent nerve hemorrhage (Figure 13.16A-K) only in infants who died as the result of blunt force injuries, either accidentally or intentionally inflicted, and the authors opined that the mechanism of injury is hyperextension or flexion.[10] The authors did identify hemorrhage in the dorsal root ganglia in one child who died under unknown circumstances; however, it cannot be excluded that this child died from blunt force injuries, likely inflicted, as no history of an accident was given. Peterson et al described how to perform this removal, without removing the cervical vertebral column.[57] Brennan et al also described dorsal root ganglia hemorrhage in children who died from abusive trauma.[58]

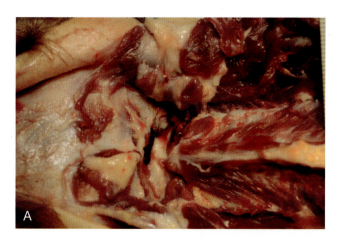
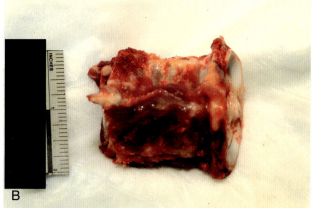
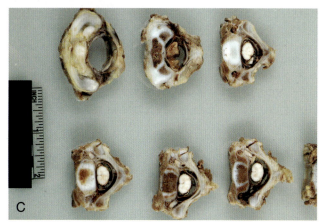

Figure 13.15. Neck dissection for evaluation of infant trauma. Examination of the dorsal root ganglia and spinal nerves in the neck of an infant who has most likely died from inflicted trauma or who is suspected of having died from inflicted trauma can provide very useful information in the evaluation of the autopsy findings. The cervical portion of the vertebral column is exposed (**A**), resected (**B**), fixed in formalin, and sectioned (**C**). This procedure will allow for direct examination of the dorsal root ganglia and spinal nerves. Using wooden dowels, the head/neck junction can be re-formed.

PEARLS & PITFALLS

Parenchymal contusions, which occur in children under similar circumstances as those that cause coup and contre-coup contusions in adults, are much more commonly associated with accidental rather than abusive trauma.[12] Parenchymal contusions do not occur in infants less than 5 months of age; however, these infants can get parenchymal clefts (ie, parenchymal lacerations, subcortical clefts, contusional tears, gliding contusions), which are blood-filled cavities in the subcortical white matter that are >5 mm in size and are strongly associated with abusive head trauma (Figure 13.17A-C). They commonly occur in the frontal, temporal and occipital lobes.[12] The mechanism for formation potentially is due to the nature of the infant head (smooth cranial floors, gelatinlike white matter, and open sutures) providing a differential vs white and gray matter allowing for easier separation with trauma.[12]

OTHER IMPORTANT TOPICS WITH REGARD TO INFLICTED HEAD TRAUMA IN INFANTS

RIB FRACTURES

Introduction: As rib fractures are commonly associated with abusive head trauma, a thorough discussion of their features is warranted. The location of rib fractures (anterior, lateral, or posterior) is very important information as posterior rib fractures are strongly associated with inflicted trauma; however, rib fractures at any location can be related to inflicted trauma.

Location of rib fractures: Numerous authors have described the association of posterior rib fractures with abuse (Figure 13.18A-D). Thomas in a review of 25 infants with rib fractures (out of 10,000 with chest radiographs) indicated that most infants with non-accidental injury had posterior rib fractures.[59] Smith et al described four case reports with costovertebral rib fractures occurring in association with abuse.[60] Carter and McCormick presented four cases of child abuse, one of which was identified by four posterior rib fractures on the left side of the chest.[61] Smeets et al present one abused child with posterior rib fractures.[62] Ng and Hall identified posterior rib fractures in two infants who sustained non-accidental injury.[63] Barsness et al found 130 posterior fractures, 107 lateral fractures, and 66 anterior fractures in their non-accidental injury group, and, in comparison, two posterior fractures, 30 lateral fractures, and one anterior fracture in their accidental group.[64] Hansen et al reviewed 21 cases of child abuse, with a mean age of 4 months, and between all 21 cases, identified a total of 85 rib fractures. The mean number of rib fractures per child was 4 (with a range of 1-15), and 38% of the fractures were posterior, 48% were lateral, and only 8% were anterolateral or anterior in location.[65]

However, not all studies or reviews link posterior rib fractures so highly with abuse. Bulloch et al found that 5 of 7 non-abused infants had posterior rib fractures and 20 of 32 abused infants had posterior rib fractures. The difference was not significant, with a *P*-value of >.05. The accidental causes of the posterior rib fractures included a motor vehicle accident, a fall downstairs in the hands of an adult, and an adult falling on an infant.[66] Cadzow and Armstrong found 9 rib fractures that were accidentally inflicted, and 92 that occurred secondary to abuse. In the accidental group, 5 of the 9 fractures were posterior, and in the abused group, 39 of 92 fractures were posterior. The difference was not statistically significant.[67] Clouse and Lantz described posterior rib fractures due to cardiopulmonary resuscitation (CPR) in four hospitalized neonates or infants; however, this report is only an abstract presented at a meeting.[68]

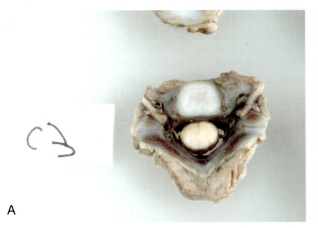
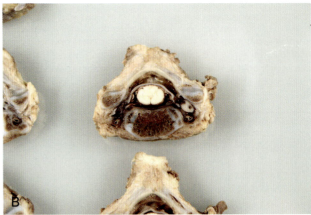
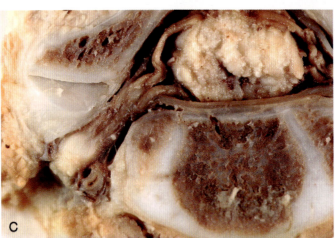

Figure 13.16A-C. Dorsal root ganglia and spinal nerves. (**A**) is a normal cross section for comparison. The dorsal root ganglia and spinal nerves will appear white or tan-white. With blood within the dorsal root ganglia, the hemorrhage can appear focal (**B**) or more diffuse (**C**).

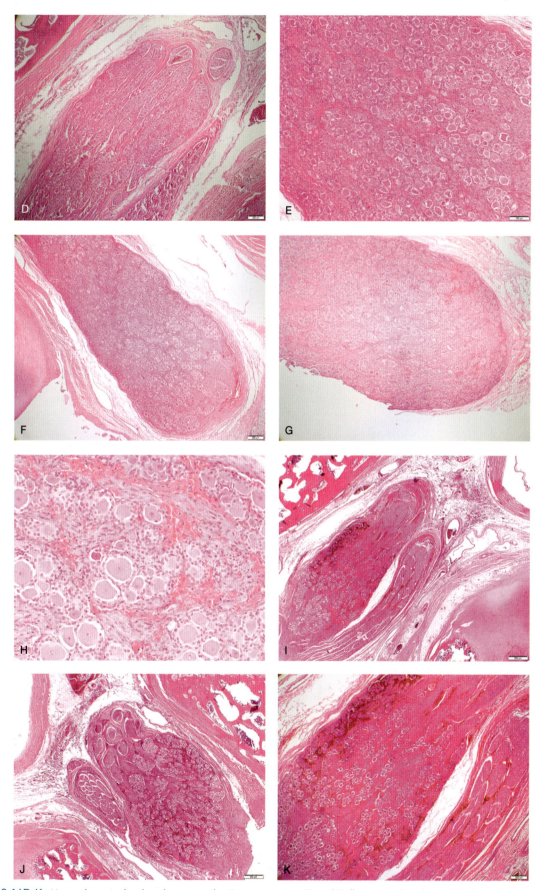

Figure 13.16D-K. Hemorrhage in the dorsal root ganglia. For comparison, (D and E) illustrate a dorsal root ganglion with no hemorrhage. (F) shows a dorsal root ganglion with very minimal hemorrhage. (G and H) have a dorsal root ganglion with focal hemorrhage involving only a small area of the ganglion. (I-K) reveal extensive hemorrhage within the dorsal root ganglion, involving nearly all of the structure (hematoxylin and eosin, all low power, except (H), which is high power).

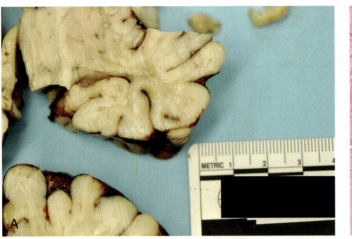
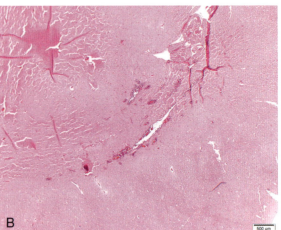
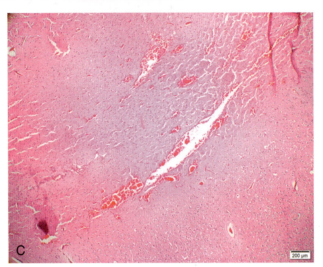

Figure 13.17. Parenchymal cleft. In Image (**A**), the temporal lobe has a linear split in the white matter, which, by microscopic examination (**B** and **C**), was a cleft in the white matter filled with red blood cells. Although uncommonly identified in the brain of infants who have sustained abusive head trauma, they are very characteristic for the condition (hematoxylin and eosin, low power).

> **PEARLS & PITFALLS**
> Posterior rib fractures in infants are highly suggestive of inflicted injury; however, in any given case, the history by caregivers must be compared to the injuries identified at autopsy as not every instance of posterior rib fractures is due to inflicted trauma.

> **FAQ:** Are rib fractures associated with CPR?
>
> **Answer:** Feldman et al reviewed radiographs from 113 living children, 41 victims of child abuse, 50 who had received CPR, and 22 who had incidental rib fractures (ie, found during investigation for another medical condition), and 29 infants had rib fractures, 14 of these infants were victims of abuse. Other causes of rib fractures were motor vehicle accidents, rickets or osteoporosis, surgery, and osteogenesis imperfecta.[69] Feldman et al opined that "children's ribs are rarely, if ever, fractured by resuscitation, but frequently fractured by child abuse."[69] Radiographs, however, are not the most accurate method to identify rib fractures.[70] Ryan et al reviewed 153 infants who died of non-traumatic causes and had undergone CPR, with none having rib fractures detected at autopsy.[71] Maguire et al reviewed studies of rib fractures and CPR in infants less than 18 months of age. Of 923 children represented, three had anterior rib fractures due to CPR. Importantly, Maguire et al acknowledged that subtle rib fractures may be missed on postmortem

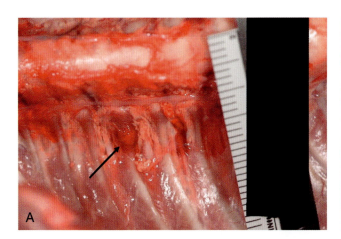
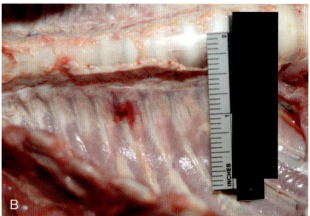
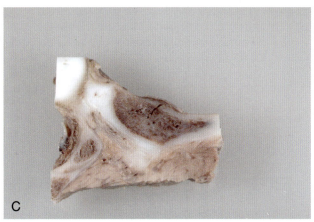

Figure 13.18A-C. Posterior rib fracture. In (**A**), the uncleaned version with the pleura still intact reveals a focal area of hemorrhage in the rib adjacent to the vertebral column (arrow). In (**B**), the pleura has been removed and the area cleaned, which clearly reveals the fracture and adjacent hemorrhage. In (**C**), a cross section of the fixed and resected rib, there is an acute fracture superimposed on a more remote fracture, which is undergoing repair.

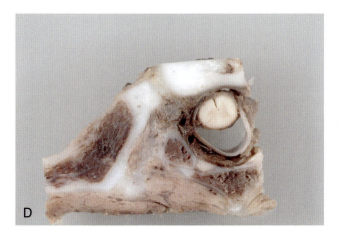

Figure 13.18D. Posterior rib fracture. Compared to the fracture in Figure 13.18A-C, this fracture is much more subtle, and is in the organizational phase, with no acute component.

examination if the parietal pleura is not reflected.[72] Matshes and Lew reviewed 382 infants who died from non-traumatic causes and had CPR, and found no rib fractures. Matshes and Lew reported that "dissection and visual inspection, rib cage palpation, stripping of the parietal pleura, and liberal use of radiography" were used to identify rib fractures, but that "it is conceivable that small, undisplaced perimortem fractures without localized hemorrhage were, on rare occasions, overlooked."[73] However, Dolinak reviewed 70 consecutive autopsies on infants aged 2 weeks to 8 months who had undergone CPR, and found recent anterolateral rib fractures in 8 of the 70, and in 7 of the 8 children, there were multiple rib fractures, from 2 to 10 per infant. No posterior rib fractures were identified associated with CPR. In reference to other articles citing a lack of rib fractures due to CPR identified at autopsy, Dolinak stated, "In these articles, it is not clear how actively the presence of rib fractures was pursued and whether or not the parietal pleura was stripped to optimize the detection of more subtle rib fractures"[74] (Figure 13.19A and B). Other recent publications have also identified rib fractures in infants associated with CPR. Weber et al identified 25 infants (from a sample of 546) who were found at autopsy to have rib fractures. In seven infants, with recent anterolateral fractures, the cause was determined to be CPR.[75]

The method by which resuscitation is conducted on an infant can impact whether or not rib fractures may occur. In the past, infant CPR was performed exclusively by placing the infant on the responder's forearm, or a hard surface, and compressing the chest with two fingers; however, relatively recent changes involve holding the infant with both hands and compressing the chest with two thumbs. Although Matshes and Lew did not identify any posterior rib fractures,[76] Worn and Jones stated, "The TT [two-thumb] method bears a striking resemblance to the method commonly believed by authors to be attributable to abusive compression or shaking of an infant."[77] Menegazzi discuss the two-thumb technique and that without lateral chest support, there is an increased risk of fracture.[78] Reyes et al reviewed 571 autopsied infants, age newborn to 6 months, and found rib fractures in 19, all of them of the anterior or lateral segment of the rib. Of the 19 who had rib fractures, 15 had postmortem radiography, and fractures were only seen in four infants, reinforcing the inadequacy of radiography in detecting acute rib fractures.[79] Reyes et al noted that the frequency of acute rib fractures identified at autopsy had increased since the mid-2006 (around the time when two-thumb CPR was first instituted), and that their study reinforced the idea that anterior and antero-lateral rib fractures can occur as a result of CPR and are not necessarily indicative of abuse.[79] Of course, although two-thumb CPR may contribute to infant rib fractures, poorly performed two-finger CPR, or adult-type CPR (with the hands), may also subject the ribs to abnormal stress.

PEARLS & PITFALLS

Microscopic examination of the rib head can reveal small fractures (Figure 13.20A-C). These fractures, when >1 mm in size, are statistically significantly associated with child abuse homicides and infant deaths that at autopsy combined with investigation were suspicious, but with a definitive determination of homicide not made.[80]

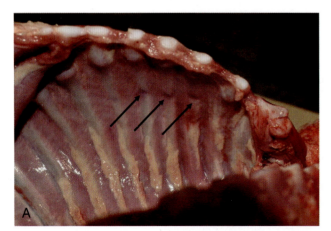
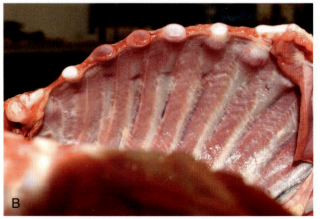

Figure 13.19. (A and B) CPR-related rib fractures. At the anterior portion of the ribs on both sides of the chest are subtle linear red discolorations (arrows), which is hemorrhage within the fracture line, but with essentially no hemorrhage spilling into the surrounding soft tissue. Removal of the pleura facilitates identification of these fractures; however, close examination is still required, and these fractures can easily be missed. Anterior rib fractures are not specific to CPR and can occur as a result of inflicted injury as well. CPR, cardiopulmonary resuscitation.

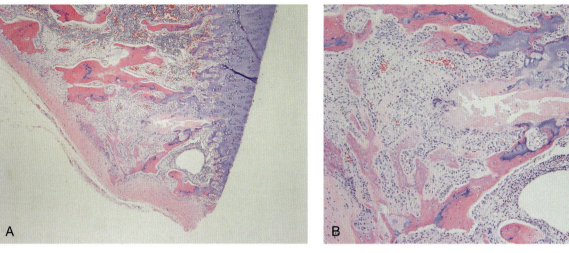
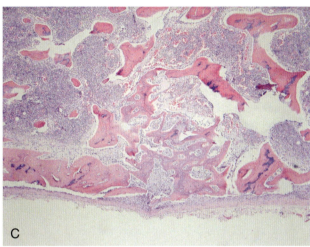

Figure 13.20. Microscopic rib fractures at the rib head in infants. (**A**) shows a low power view of the rib head and a fracture. (**B**) shows a higher power view of this same region of a rib, but in a different infant, with the fracture appearing as the cleft with the acellular amorphous eosinophilic material lining it with adjacent woven bone. (**C**) shows healing fracture composed of just woven bone (hematoxylin and eosin, low power A and C, high power B).

FALLS

Introduction: Falls are commonly reported by caregivers as the mechanism by which features that are consistent with inflicted head trauma occurred.

> **FAQ:** How common are short falls?
>
> **Answer:** Warrington et al who followed 14,541 pregnancies with questionnaires asked mothers at 6 months after the delivery how many had had infants who sustained an accidental fall. The mothers reported 3357 falls for 2554 infants (including 1117 from a bed, 203 from arms, and 43 from a changing unit). In only 437 cases was an injury sustained. Of these injuries, 244 were only bruises, 18 children were admitted to a hospital, and there were no deaths.[81] In another study of 11 newborn infants who fell while in the hospital (onto vinyl tile upon concrete) with 10 of 11 newborns having less than 3 feet falls, 8 newborns had no clinical findings, 1 had a bruise, and 1 had swelling of the scalp. None had a subdural hemorrhage and none died.[82] Haney et al, through questionnaires asked of parents, found that of 307 children, 122 fell from a height before the age of 2 years, and of 209 falls total reported, only two resulted in concussions (the most serious injury reported). Haney et al concluded that "A history of a short fall in a seriously injured child should raise the suspicion for child abuse."[83]

FAQ: Can a short fall cause death?

Answer: Chadwick et al reviewed three public injury databases and the medical literature, and found, in California, only 6 deaths from falls less than 4.7 feet among children <5 years of age, or 0.48 cases per 1 million children.[84] Helfer et al reported that in 246 children, aged 5 years or less, who fell from bed, three sustained skull fractures, and none had damage to the brain or spinal cord.[85] Tarantino et al reviewed 167 infants (aged less than or equal to 10 months), who presented to the emergency room with a history of a short (<4 feet) vertical fall. Twelve sustained skull fractures and only two sustained intracranial hemorrhage, with these two found to be the victims of child abuse confirmed through multi-disciplinary investigation and re-canting of the original story by caretakers. Tarantino et al concluded that "No child sustained significant intracranial injury from a short vertical fall, and no child sustained multiple significant injuries or visceral injuries from a short vertical fall."[86] Hall et al reported 44 children who died from falls, with 18 dying from falls of less than or equal to 3 feet. The authors did not separate out each of their cases, but said, of those who died primarily from head injury, 19 had mass lesions (ie, space-occupying), 7 had edema and subarachnoid hemorrhage, and 5 had extensive lacerations, with skull fractures present in 42%, 71%, and 100% of the groups, respectively.[87]

Reiber reviewed three infants who fell 10 to 25 feet, all had multiple fractures, two had space-occupying subdural hemorrhages requiring evacuation and the remaining child had multiple cerebral (brain) lacerations. Reiber also reviewed 19 children who died from reported 1 to 5 foot falls. Fourteen were homicides (identified through autopsy findings and investigation, including inconsistent stories and confessions), three were undetermined (with one having evidence of battering), and only two were apparently genuine accidents—one with an acute subdural hemorrhage with severe brain swelling, and the second had an acute left subdural hemorrhage. Of the 15 cases in Reiber with falls onto a carpeted surface, only 1 had a skull fracture. In concluding, Reiber states, "The conclusion that appears best at this time, with our current state of information, is that, while children on occasion suffer fatal injury from short falls, such events are an extreme rarity. Major injuries nearly always result from major impacts and serious falls."[88]

Plunkett reviewed the U.S. Consumer Product Safety Commission database for head injury associated with playground equipment from 1-1-88 to 6-30-99 and identified 18 deaths. No children were under 12 months of age. Of the 18 cases, 6 were not autopsied, and in 6 the incident was unwitnessed. Eight had (by description) a space-occupying subdural or epidural hemorrhage, four had coup–contrecoup lesions consistent with the provided history, two had severe cerebral edema associated with no or a small subdural hemorrhage and no skull fracture, and one had carotid artery occlusion and subsequent infarcts. Of the remaining three, one had complex skull fractures and very likely was crushed by a parent during a fall, one child had acute cerebral edema associated with a small subdural hemorrhage, but no fracture, and with extensive bilateral retinal hemorrhages (with the descriptive term extensive for the retinal hemorrhages not defined), and the final child was a 20-month-old who fell off a jungle gym and hit a pole, causing a depressed skull fracture (4 mm depression; size of fracture overall unlisted), and had extensive bilateral retinal and preretinal hemorrhage (once again, with the descriptive term extensive for the retinal hemorrhages not defined). Plunkett indicates the distance from the platform to the support post that the decedent struck was 42 in, but does not list the height of the decedent.[89]

John et al identified a subset of children aged <6 years with a subdural hemorrhage and retinal hemorrhages occurring with no history of trauma, or the history of a short fall, and concluded that "…when a young child (particularly an infant younger than 6 months) presents with traumatic intracranial pathology and either no history of trauma or a history of a minor fall, it must be seriously considered that the history is false."[90]

APPARENT LIFE-THREATENING EVENT

Introduction: Associated with inflicted head injury, caregivers will often describe choking, difficulty breathing, cyanosis, and/or apnea, which is a set of symptoms that is very similar to that for an apparent life-threatening event (ALTE), which has been described as "an episode that is frightening to the observer and that is characterized by some combination of apnoea (central or occasionally obstructive), colour change (usually cyanotic or pallid but occasionally erythematous or plethoric), marked change in muscle tone (usually marked limpness), choking or 'gagging.'"[91]

Incidence and Mechanism: McGovern and Smith found that the incidence of ALTE was 0.6/1000 live-born infants, and that the most common underlying causes were gastroesophageal reflux disease (GERD) (31% of cases), seizure (11% of cases), and lower respiratory tract infection (8% of cases). In 23% of cases, the underlying cause was unknown. Only five deaths were reported (0.8% of children); of these five infants, two died with severe GERD while sleeping and three had rare congenital metabolic disorders.[91] In their review of 563 children with an ALTE, Parker and Pitetti only found three deaths (0.5% of children), one of which was due to child abuse and the other two were due to sudden infant death syndrome (SIDS).[92]

> **FAQ:** Is ALTE associated with retinal hemorrhages?
>
> **Answer:** At least two authors have studied this association. Curcoy et al reviewed 108 children with ALTE, none of whom were found to have retinal hemorrhages. The authors estimated the chance of retinal hemorrhages occurring as a result of an ALTE alone at 0.028.[93] Pitetti et al reviewed 73 children who presented with an ALTE and had a fundoscopic examination to check for retinal hemorrhages. Only one child was found to have retinal hemorrhages, and this child was subsequently determined to have been the victim of child abuse.[94] Choudhary et al discuss the refutation of this hypothesis.[5]

ALTERNATIVE THEORIES AS TO THE CAUSATION OF FINDINGS ASSOCIATED WITH ABUSIVE HEAD TRAUMA

Introduction: Child abuse homicides will be some of the most contentious cases that a forensic pathologist will face in court, with the defense team often calling expert witnesses to refute the findings of the autopsy pathologist, assuming that the manner of death was determined by the autopsy pathologist to be homicide. Choudhary (2018) state, "…the courtroom has become a forum for speculative theories that cannot be reconciled with generally accepted medical literature," with these alternative theories including cerebral sinovenous thrombosis, hypoxic-ischemic injury, dysphagic choking/vomiting, and rebleeding of a birth-related subdural hemorrhage.[5] Counter-arguments against such opinions must be considered whenever an autopsy for a suspicious infant death is performed, as the pathologist will very likely have to defend their final determination against those offered by other expert witnesses. Other authors also provide evidence against alternative opinions.[12,14] However, while the findings of a thin-film subdural hemorrhage associated with bilateral retinal hemorrhages and an acute encephalopathy are consistent with inflicted head injury, to assume that these findings are not of another origin is a major error. The differential diagnoses of subdural and retinal hemorrhages in an infant must always be considered and causes other than inflicted injury ruled out before determining that the manner of death is homicide. A meticulous and thorough approach to infant autopsies and a dutiful consideration of other causes prior to a final determination of cause and manner of death will help support the forensic pathologist's decision and refute alternative theories as to the cause of the autopsy findings. Hymel et al provide an extensive list of conditions in the differential diagnosis of abusive head injury, and refutations of some alternative theories as to the cause of the findings in abusive head injury.[27]

FAQ: Are the findings of subdural hemorrhage, retinal hemorrhage and encephalopathy routinely accepted as being commonly associated with abusive head injury?

Answer: In one article, two doctors presented opposing opinions to the statement, "The triad of retinal hemorrhage, subdural hemorrhage and encephalopathy in an infant unassociated with evidence of physical injury is not the result of shaking, but is most likely to have been caused by a natural disease."[95] One doctor answered the statement, "Yes" and addressed four concerns with the concept that shaking causes that triad, which can be summarized as (1) no one had, at that time, witnessed a shaking death, (2) confessions to shaking deaths by the perpetrator are not accurate, (3) no biomechanical evidence to support shaking as a cause of death exists (ie, the author opined that research to that point had not determined that shaking could cause the degree of trauma necessary to kill an infant), and (4) the anatomy does not support the pathologic findings (ie, tearing of bridging veins leading to thin-film subdural hemorrhage). However, not having an event witnessed is insufficient reason to not accept its validity and many fatal incidents of violent deaths, especially intimate-type violent deaths, such as strangulation, stabbings, and fatal child abuse, and smothering, often involve only two people: the perpetrator and the victim. A confession is a witnessed account of the events, and thus, many shaking episodes have been witnessed, by the perpetrator. While confessions can be coerced or given incorrectly (ie, confessing to something that the person does not realize the implications of their confession), to maintain that all confessions of shaking an infant resulting in death are coerced or otherwise incorrect is not tenable. Some biomechanical testing available at that time did support that shaking could potentially lead to focal axonal injury, tearing of bridging veins, and development of subdural hemorrhage.[96] And the author described that bridging veins carry large volumes of blood, which, based upon their size and the fact they are venous, and not arterial, does not seem accurate.

FAQ: How common are birth-related retinal and subdural hemorrhages and can such subdural hemorrhages re-bleed at a later time?

Answer: Retinal hemorrhages are found in up to 40% of vaginally-delivered infants and subdural hemorrhages are found in up to 45% of term infants. Hayashi et al discussed the association of subdural and retinal hemorrhages with vaginal deliveries, specifically those with a breech presentation or requiring forceps or suction, and causing tearing of a bridging vein.[97] Hymel et al suggest that re-bleeding into such a subdural hemorrhage would most likely be microscopic and inconsequential, unless induced by re-injury.[27]

FAQ: What is Valsalva retinopathy?

Answer: Duane described Valsalva hemorrhagic retinopathy as preretinal hemorrhages due to the Valsalva maneuver, which is any rise in intrathoracic or intra-abdominal pressure against a closed glottis, such as can occur in coughing, vomiting, or straining at stool, among other activities.[98] In regard to the Valsalva manuever causing retinal hemorrhages in infants, Herr et al reviewed 100 infants with pyloric stenosis, a condition known for its association with vomiting due to obstruction of the outflow of the stomach, and found no retinal hemorrhages; however, the duration between emesis and examination in their study was between 1 and 120 days with a median of 9.5 days.[99]

FAQ: Does hypoxia, brain swelling, and raised central venous pressure cause subdural and retinal hemorrhages?

Answer: Geddes et al opined that severe hypoxia, brain swelling, and raised central venous pressure would produce a thin-film subdural hemorrhage.[100] Geddes et al's hypothesis would not explain subarachnoid hemorrhage, which often accompanies subdural hemorrhage in inflicted head trauma, as the subdural hemorrhage

Geddes refers to would derive from blood leaking into the subdural space and would have to pass through the arachnoid mater to produce a subarachnoid hemorrhage. Also, in refutation of the Geddes et al hypothesis, other authors[101] have failed to find an association between hypoxia and macroscopic subdural hemorrhage. Choudhary et al also discuss the refutation of this hypothesis.[5]

FAQ: What is paroxysmal coughing and what is its association with infant subdural and retinal hemorrhages?

Answer: Geddes and Talbert opined that paroxysmal coughing could cause retinal hemorrhages and subdural hemorrhage based upon a computer model of a 3-month-old infant.[102] Geddes and Talbert indicate that "Paroxysmal coughs are in effect very high pressure Valsalva manoeuvers—indeed, if reflex laryngeal closure takes precedence, coughs will be replaced by Valsalvas, which have a well-established association with retinal haemorrhage." The authors describe an association between pertussis infection and subdural hemorrhage and conjunctival and periorbital petechiae to support their theory, as pertussis infections can cause paroxysmal coughing.[102] However, in 1992 and 1993, there were around 10,000 cases of pertussis reported in the United States and, in the same time frame, only 23 deaths.[103] Lack and Kozakewich chart 16 autopsied cases of fatal pertussis, and, in the "Autopsy Findings" column, subdural hemorrhage is not listed once, which would not support the idea that paroxysmal coughing does cause subdural hemorrhage.[104] Oates list paroxysmal coughing as a false mimic of abusive head trauma.[12] Choudhary et al also discuss the refutation of this hypothesis.[5]

FAQ: What is dysphagic choking and what is its association with infant subdural and retinal hemorrhages?

Answer: Barnes et al presented the death of a 4.5-month-old male, which they attribute to a dysphagic choking-type of ALTE; however, in their abstract, they state, "Although NAI [non-accidental injury] could not be ruled out…" In support of their case, Barnes et al cite Geddes and Talbert,[102] which, as described above, lacks substantiated support. Also, in the case presented by Barnes et al, there were two acute posterolateral rib fractures, which they attribute to CPR. However, posterior rib fractures are strongly associated with child abuse in the medical literature.[105] Oates lists dysphagic choking as a false mimic of abusive head trauma.[12] Choudhary et al also discuss the refutation of this hypothesis.[5]

FAQ: Is benign enlargement of subarachnoid space a risk factor for subdural hemorrhage?

Answer: Kleinman stated, "given that SDH is rare with minor injury and that prominent CSF spaces are common in normal infants, the view that enlarged CSF spaces predispose to SDH does not have a firm scientific basis."[106] Care does indicate that it is possible that a spontaneous non-traumatic subdural hemorrhage could arise in the setting of benign enlargement of subarachnoid space but that any child in which subdural hemorrhage arises should be fully evaluated for the potential etiologies with abusive head trauma considered.[107]

FAQ: Can a sagittal sinus thrombus lead to subdural hemorrhage, retinal hemorrhages, and infant death?

Answer: While sagittal sinus thrombosis has been proposed as a mechanism for causing subdural hemorrhage, with back pressure from the thrombus opined to lead to rupture of bridging veins, clinical reports do not support such a conclusion.[5] A sagittal sinus thrombus can lead to bilateral cortical infarcts but has not been reported in the clinical literature to be associated with subdural hemorrhage and sudden collapse of a child, and is instead often secondary to another disease process.[5]

> **FAQ:** Is hypermobile Ehlers-Danlos syndrome a risk factor for multiple fractures?
>
> **Answer:** Children with hypermobile Ehlers-Danlos syndrome tend to develop fractures after they become ambulatory and develop fractures in the same scenarios as children without hypermobile Ehlers-Danlos syndrome. That hypermobile Ehlers-Danlos syndrome is a risk factor for increased risk for fracture is not generally accepted.[28]

OTHER FEATURES OF CHILD ABUSE

Introduction: In the evaluation of a child abuse homicide, or a potential child abuse homicide, it is important to gather as much information as possible to support one's conclusion. Other features to be discussed include fractures other than rib fractures, bruising, burns, and malnourishment and dehydration.

FRACTURES

> **PEARLS & PITFALLS**
>
> When determining whether or not a particular fracture is due to abusive injury or accidental injury, each situation needs to be evaluated based upon the entirety of the circumstances and not just the fracture itself. While certain types of fractures have a higher or lower association with abusive injury, there are no absolutes. For example, Hobbs indicates that multiple or wide complex skull fractures are associated with abuse[108]; however, Maguire indicates that complex, multiple, diastatic, and depressed fractures have conflicting data as to their abusive vs accidental origin.[109] However, the key features listed below at least provide an initial guide when evaluating fractures.

KEY FEATURES of Fractures Associated With Child Abuse[108]
- One fracture with multiple bruises
- Metaphyseal or epiphyseal fractures
- Rib fractures
- Multiple or wide complex skull fractures (Figure 13.21)
- Scapula fractures
- Sternal fractures
- Multiple fractures, and fractures of different ages (Figure 13.22)
- Formation of new periosteal bone
- Skull fracture associated with intracranial injury

KEY FEATURES of Fractures Associated With Non-Inflicted Injury[108,109]
- Single fractures
- Linear, narrow parietal skull fractures (Figure 13.23)
- Fractures of shaft of long bone (unless child is <15 years of age)
- Clavicle fractures

KEY FEATURES of Fractures Associated With Child Abuse[106]
- **High specificity:** classic metaphyseal lesion (also referred to as corner fracture and bucket handle fracture based upon the radiographic view), posterior rib fractures, scapular fractures, spinous process fractures, sternal fractures
- **Moderate specificity:** multiple, bilateral fractures; fractures of different ages, epiphyseal separations, vertebral body fractures, digital fractures, complex skull fractures
- **Low specificity:** subperiosteal new bone formation, clavicular fractures, long bone shaft fractures, linear skull fracture

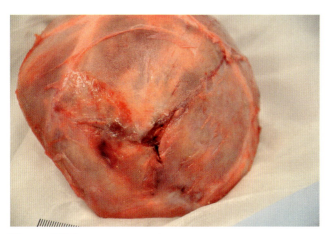

Figure 13.21. Complex skull fracture. In the parietal region is a stellate fracture with focal slight depression and with a focally wide fracture margin. This fracture was the result of inflicted trauma.

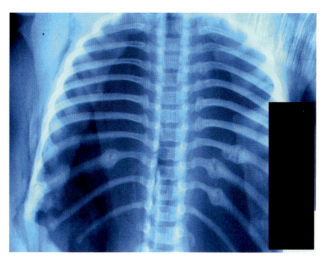

Figure 13.22. Multiple remote rib fractures. This infant had multiple remote rib fractures, as exhibited by the callus formation, with the fractures having a posterior location.

PEARLS & PITFALLS

When evaluating fractures, Hobbs describes other factors to consider: (1) that a cranial fracture may instead be a variant suture, mimicking a fracture (Figure 13.24), (2) that the fracture may be birth-related (such as of clavicle or humerus), and (3) that underlying natural disease such as osteogenesis imperfecta, rickets, prematurity, disuse osteoporosis, copper deficiency, Caffey disease, and osteomyelitis may have contributed to the development of the fracture.[108]

PEARLS & PITFALLS

With multiple fractures, the diagnosis of osteogenesis imperfecta should be considered. Features often seen with osteogenesis imperfecta include blue sclerae, osteopenia and wormian bones, and few fractures (only 10% of affected children have more than three fractures), and not posterior rib fractures or classic metaphyseal lesions. A pathologist can order genetic testing for mutations in COL1A1 and COL1A2.[28]

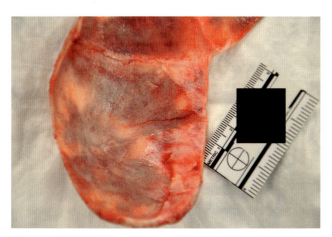

Figure 13.23. Linear skull fracture. By itself, this is a linear skull fracture, which is more consistent with an accidental injury; however, this linear fracture was identified on the side of the cranium opposite the fracture in Figure 13.21, and thus occurred in the context of abusive head trauma.

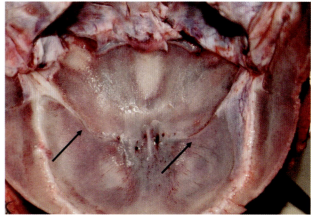

Figure 13.24. Mendosal sutures in the posterior cranial fossa are common incidental findings in infant deaths (arrows), but which can be misinterpreted as bilateral linear fractures.

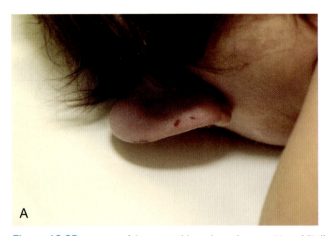
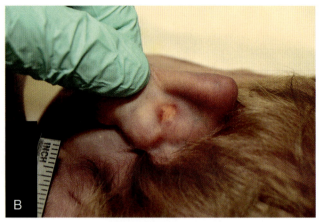

Figure 13.25. Injuries of the ears. Although not bruises, (**A** and **B**) illustrate injuries of the ear, which are, in this case, abrasions. Abrasions of the ear would be more likely abusive than accidental in origin.

BRUISING AND LACERATIONS

> **PEARLS & PITFALLS**
>
> The distribution of the bruising can help with the determination of its origin.[109] In premobile infants, any bruising is suspicious. Bruising, if present on an infant <4 months of age, or on a <4-year-old child on the torso, ears or neck, are consistent with non-accidental trauma.[109] Accidental bruises usually involve the knees and shins in mobile infants and the face, buttocks, and back of head in older children. Abusive bruising tends to involve the ears (Figure 13.25A and B), cheeks, neck, extremities (Figure 13.26), and genitalia (Figure 13.27), and is often associated with petechiae.[109] Patterned injuries would be rare in an accident and are always concerning for an abusive injury unless otherwise adequately explained (Figure 13.28). Resolving bruises can be very subtle, even with a back dissection. Iron stains can help highlight hemosiderin in these regions (Figure 13.29A-C). A quick and easy way to document site of origin for soft tissue taken to document the site of hemorrhage is to take a photo of the location along with the cassette that will be used to process the specimen (Figure 13.30). With bruising, mimics must be considered, including dermal melanosis (Figure 13.31A-C), bleeding disorders, vasculitis, Henoch-Schönlein purpura, hemangioma (Figure 13.32A and B), and others.[110]

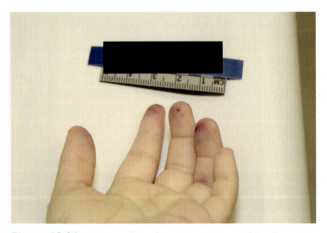

Figure 13.26. Bruises of the fingertips. Bruises of the fingertips are more likely abusive in origin (eg, may be due to pinching of the fingertips) than accidental in origin. In this image, the bruises are associated with petechiae.

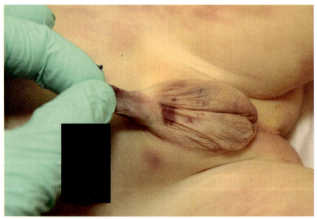

Figure 13.27. Bruises and abrasions of the genitalia. The scrotum at the base of the penis has abrasions and contusions, which are most consistent with being abusive in origin.

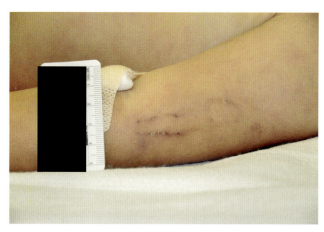

Figure 13.28. Patterned abrasion. Patterned abrasion on the upper extremity of an infant who died under suspicious circumstances. The object causing the patterned injury was not identified.

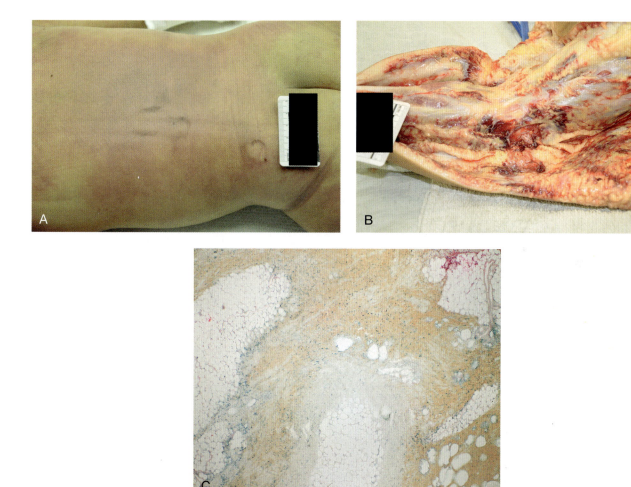

Figure 13.29. Infant with multiple remote bruises. This infant sustained multiple blunt force injuries of varying ages. Image **A** illustrates changes in the skin on the back. Image **B** illustrates underlying changes in the subcutaneous tissue. Image **C** is an iron stain of one region which was sampled microscopically, which shows abundant iron deposition (Prussian blue, low power).

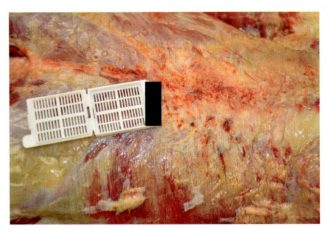

Figure 13.30. Use of cassette to document location of tissue sample. A quick and easy way to easily document the location from which tissue samples were obtained is to place the cassette (with number or lettering identifying it) adjacent to the region sampled and photograph the cassette. The same procedure works well with the brain.

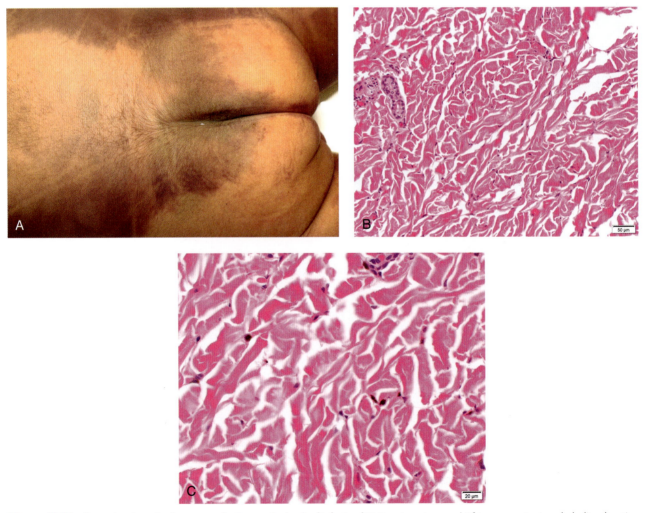

Figure 13.31. Dermal melanosis. A common finding on the back of infants of Native American and African ancestry is a dark discoloration of the skin just superior to the gluteal cleft, although they can be located anywhere along the back. These discolorations are due to dermal pigment collections, but can be misinterpreted as trauma. (**A**) is the typical gross appearance, while (**B** and **C**) illustrate the microscopic appearance (hematoxylin and eosin, medium and high power.)

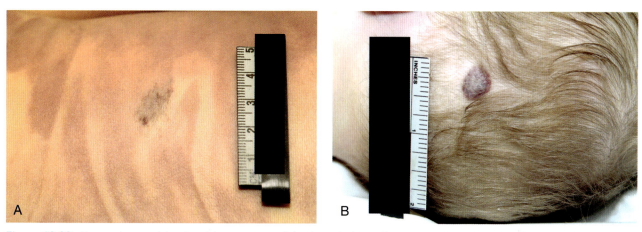

Figure 13.32. Hemangiomas of the skin. A hemangioma of the skin, which, in infants and children, are most often capillary, can mimic a contusion (**A** and **B**).

> **PEARLS & PITFALLS**
>
> While injuries of the frenulum have usually been associated with non-accidental injury (Figure 13.33), Maguire indicates that a torn frenulum can occur accidentally, but the incident is usually known, as the child will have bloody discharge from the mouth, and most likely seek care from a parent.[109]

BURNS

> **PEARLS & PITFALLS**
>
> The distribution of burns/scalds can help with the determination of its origin.[109] Accidental scalds occur when the infant/child pulls something onto themself and so involve the upper limb, face, anterior trunk, and neck. Accidental scalds/burns tend to be asymmetric with irregular edges and an irregular burn depth. Abusive burns/scalds tend to involve the lower limbs, perineum/buttocks, and can have a glove and stocking pattern. The burns/scalds tend to have clear limits, a consistent burn depth, and are symmetrical. With burns/scalds, mimics must be considered including bullous impetigo, staphylococcal scalded skin syndrome, erysipelas, diaper dermatitis, Stevens-Johnson syndrome, and others.[110]

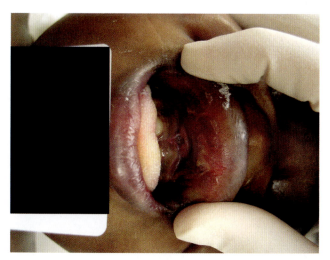

Figure 13.33. Laceration of the frenulum. The frenulum has a split lined with ill-defined yellow discoloration. This infant survived for some period of time after the injury. While once always considered to be indicative of abusive injury (eg, forceful closing of the mouth, pushing the lips against the teeth), a laceration of the frenulum can occur as the result of an accident.

MALNOURISHMENT AND DEHYDRATION

> **PEARLS & PITFALLS**
>
> To help diagnose malnourishment and dehydration at autopsy, use photographs, examine the skin and soft tissue assessing for skin turgor (Figure 13.34), take measurements and compare to known standards, and test vitreous electrolytes and assess for dehydration.

NEAR MISSES

Near Miss #1: Although injuries of the face in a pre-mobile or mobile infant are concerning for abuse, other conditions must be considered. Figure 13.35 illustrates ill-defined abrasions of the cheek and peri-orbital region that, based upon investigation combined with the autopsy findings, were determined to be non-suspicious in origin, and were most likely secondary to resuscitation attempts by an untrained individual.

Near Miss #2 (Figure 13.36A-D): An infant was found under suspicious circumstances. At autopsy, a widely spaced linear fracture in the left parietal bone was identified (Figure 13.36A), which could be interpreted as being from a fall; however, a thin subdural hemorrhage and diffuse subarachnoid hemorrhage was present (Figure 13.36B), which is consistent with a diffuse injury and not a focal impact. In addition, there was hemorrhage in the dorsal root ganglia (Figure 13.36C). Finally, mendosal sutures were present (Figure 13.36D), which could have been misinterpreted as bilateral linear fractures. The autopsy findings in combination with the investigation were consistent with abusive head trauma.

Near Miss #3 (Figure 13.37A-G): An infant died under suspicious circumstances. At autopsy, a thin-film subdural hemorrhage was identified (Figure 13.37A). The blood pooled next to the falx cerebri is artifact from removal of the top of the cranium. It could be argued that the thin film on the undersurface of the dura is artifact also; however, on the undersurface of the dura adjacent to the falx cerebri was slightly raised collections of hemorrhage (Figure 13.37B), which was definitely subdural hemorrhage. Reflection of the scalp revealed no foci of subgaleal hemorrhage (Figure 13.37C). Examination of the eyes revealed no retinal hemorrhage on either side (Figure 13.37D). The cervical portion of the vertebral column was removed to examine the dorsal root ganglia and spinal nerves and roots. Other than some peri-vascular hemorrhage around the vertebral artery, no other significant foci of hemorrhage were identified (Figure 13.37E). A back dissection revealed no hemorrhage (Figure 13.37F and G). The autopsy in combination with the scene investigation, while suspicious for abusive head trauma, could not identify substantial evidence to support that conclusion and both the cause and manner of death were ruled undetermined.

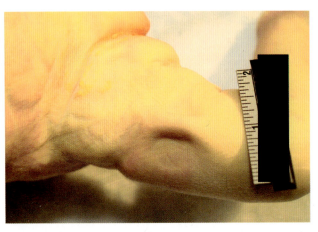

Figure 13.34. Skin tenting. While not absolute, tenting and a doughy texture of the skin and subcutaneous soft tissue are associated with dehydration. Vitreous electrolyte testing can help identify dehydration.

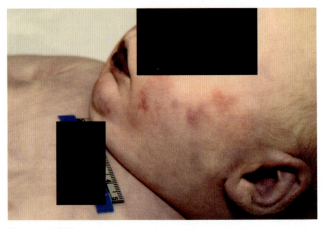

Figure 13.35. Abrasions of cheek. Abrasions of cheek may be associated with cardiopulmonary resuscitation and do not necessarily indicate trauma occurred.

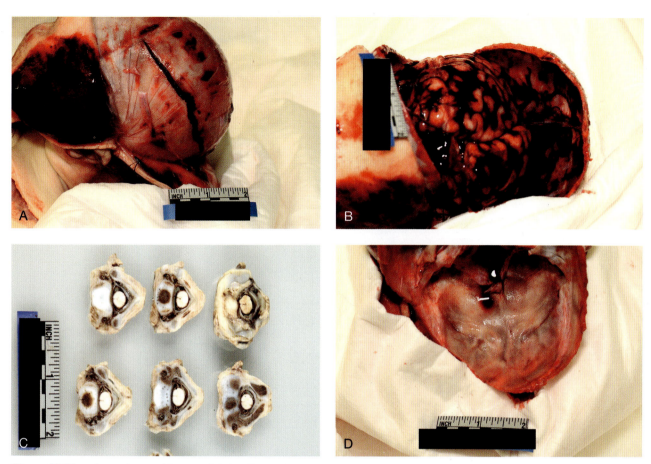

Figure 13.36. Infant with cranial fracture, subdural hemorrhage, dorsal root ganglia hemorrhage, and mendosal sutures. A widely spaced linear fracture is in the left parietal bone (**A**). A thin subdural hemorrhage and diffuse subarachnoid hemorrhage was present (**B**). There was hemorrhage in the dorsal root ganglia (**C**). Mendosal sutures were present (**D**).

Near Miss #4 (Figure 13.38A and B): While injuries of the genitalia are suspicious for inflicted trauma, diaper rash, as in present in Figure 13.38A and B, can be misinterpreted as trauma.

Near Miss #5 (Figure 13.39A and B): Contusions are oftentimes vague and ill-defined and difficult to identify on the surface of the skin; however, even a small contusion in certain regions of the body can be a significant finding. In Figure 13.39A, this infant has a faint discoloration of the left labia majora. Sectioning of that region revealed hemorrhage in the underlying subcutaneous tissue (Figure 13.39B). As contusions of the genitalia are very concerning for abuse, especially in a pre-mobile or mobile infant, identification and documentation of such a lesion can be very important.

Near Miss #6 (Figure 13.40A and B): This young child was brought to the emergency room after becoming unresponsive at home. She had been feeling ill for a few days, and had within the same time frame been brought to the emergency room to evaluate her illness, with no specific diagnosis having been made. With the terminal hospitalization, she had a computed tomography scan of the head, which revealed a hemorrhage, and the presumptive diagnosis of child abuse was made. An autopsy was performed, which revealed the intracerebral hemorrhage (Figure 13.40A) to be a septic embolic event related to endocarditis of the mitral valve (Figure 13.40B). No evidence of abuse was identified at the time of autopsy.

Near Miss #7 (Figure 13.41A and B): At the distal femur is a fracture (Figure 13.41A and B). Unfortunately, the pathologist missed this fracture on review of the radiographs and no further evaluation of the fracture was done.

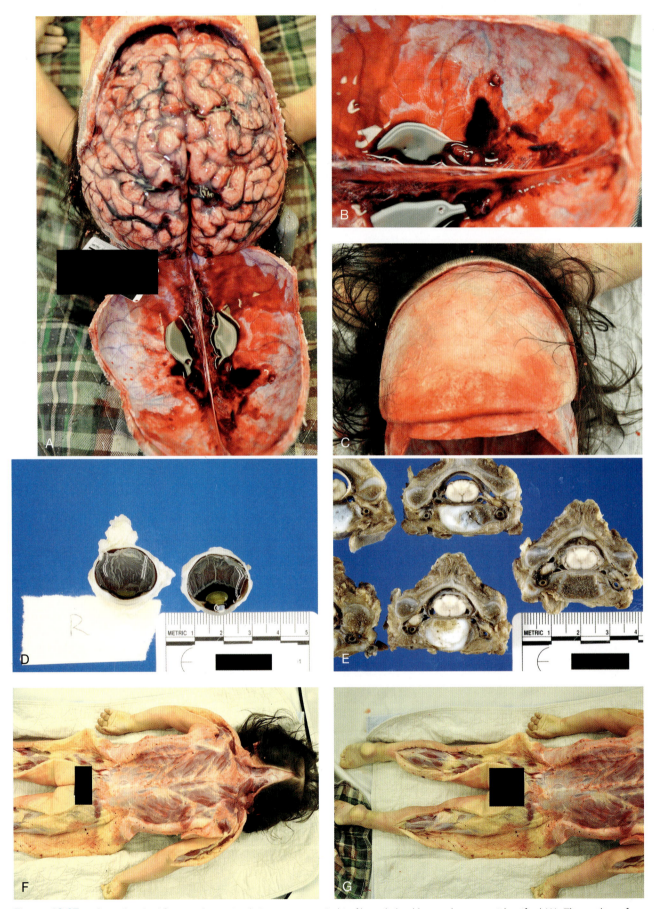

Figure 13.37. Infant who died from undetermined circumstances. A thin-film subdural hemorrhage was identified (**A**). The undersurface of the dura adjacent to the falx cerebri had a slightly raised collection of hemorrhage (**B**). No foci of subgaleal hemorrhage were present (**C**). No retinal hemorrhage was present (**D**). Other than some peri-vascular hemorrhage around the vertebral artery, no other significant foci of hemorrhage were identified in the cervical segment of the vertebral column (**E**). A back dissection revealed no hemorrhage (**F** and **G**).

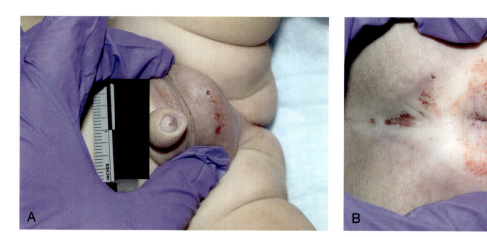

Figure 13.38. Diaper rash. While injuries of the genitalia are suspicious for inflicted trauma, diaper rash (**A** and **B**) can mimic trauma.

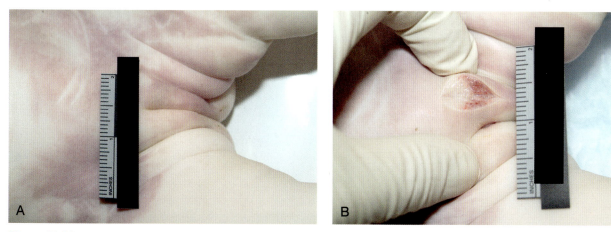

Figure 13.39. Contusion of the female genitalia. In (**A**), there is a faint discoloration of the left labia majora. Sectioning of that region revealed hemorrhage in the underlying subcutaneous tissue (**B**).

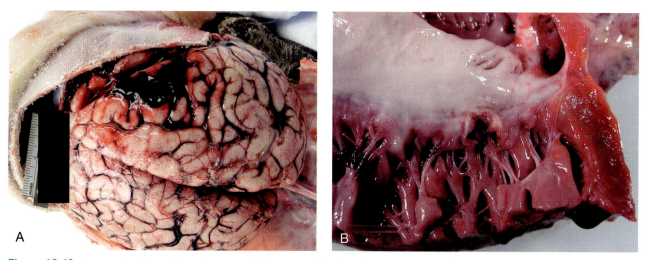

Figure 13.40. Intracerebral hemorrhage in young child associated with endocarditis. This young child had an intracerebral hemorrhage (**A**) due to septic embolic event related to endocarditis of the mitral valve (**B**).

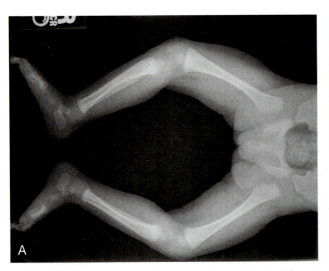 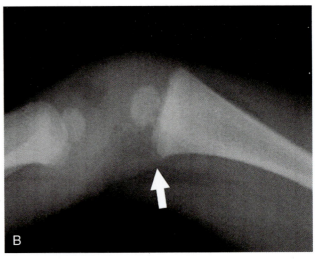

Figure 13.41. Distal femoral fracture in infant. At the distal femur is a fracture (**A** and **B**).

Near Miss #8 The investigation of child abuse homicides is very challenging, and forensic pathologists are often required to defend their conclusions in court against one or more expert witnesses hired by the defense. One effective way to do this is by using the medical literature to support autopsy conclusions. Each pathologist should develop and maintain a reference library of articles and books related to child abuse. Numerous excellent articles regarding this topic were cited in the chapter. Additional useful articles the authors have utilized are listed in the reference section.[111-141]

References

1. Caffey J. On the theory and practice of shaking infants. Its potential residual effects of permanent brain damage and mental retardation. *Am J Dis Child.* 1972;124(2):161-169.
2. Duhaime AC, Gennarelli TA, Thibault LE, Bruce DA, Margulies SS, Wiser R. The shaken baby syndrome: a clinical, pathological, and biomechanical study. *J Neurosurg.* 1987;66(3):409-415.
3. Krous HF, Byard RW. Controversies in pediatric forensic pathology. *Forensic Sci Med Pathol.* 2005;1:9-18.
4. Royal College of Pathologists. *Report of a Meeting on the Pathology of Traumatic Head Injury in Children. Meeting at 2 Carlton House Terrance, London SW1Y 5AF*; December 10, 2009.
5. Choudhary AK, Servaes S, Slovis TL, et al. Consensus statement on abusive head trauma in infants and young children. *Pediatr Radiol* 2018;48(8):1048-1065.
6. Caffey J. The whiplash shaken infant syndrome: manual shaking by the extremities with whiplash-induced intra-cranial and intraocular bleedings, linked with residual permanent brain damage and mental retardation. *Pediatrics.* 1974;54(4):396-403.
7. Case ME, DiMaio VJ. *Controversies in forensic pathology: abusive head trauma and the question of shaking as a mechanism of injury.* Abstract presented at: *Annual Meeting of the National Association of Medical Examiners; August 8th, 2011; Holland-American Alaskan Cruise.* 2011.
8. Gill JR, Goldfeder LB, Armbrustmacher V, Coleman A, Mena H, Hirsch CS. Fatal head injury in children younger than 2 years in New York city and an overview of the shaken baby syndrome. *Arch Pathol Lab Med.* 2009;133(4):619-627.
9. Dolinak D, Reichard R. An overview of inflicted head injury in infants and young children, with a review of β-amyloid precursor protein immunohistochemistry. *Arch Pathol Lab Med.* 2006;130(5):712-717.
10. Matshes EW, Evans RM, Pinckard JK, et al. Shaken infants die of neck trauma, not of brain trauma. *Acad For Path.* 2011(1):82-91.
11. Oehmichen M, Schleiss D, Pedal I, Saternus KS, Gerling I, Meissner C. Shaken baby syndrome: re-examination of diffuse axonal injury as cause of death. *Acta Neuropathol.* 2008;116(3):317-329.
12. Oates AJ, Sidpra J, Mankad K. Parenchymal brain injuries in abusive head trauma. *Pediatr Radiol.* 2021;51(6):898-910.

13. Case ME. Distinguishing accidental from inflicted head trauma at autopsy. *Pediatr Radiol*. 2014;44(suppl 4):S632-S640.
14. Vinchon M, Noule N, Karnoub MA. The legal challenges to the diagnosis of shaken baby syndrome or how to counter 12 common fake news. *Childs Nerv Syst*. 2022;38(1):133-145.
15. Garcia-Pires F, Jayappa S, Desai S, Ramakrishnaiah RH, Choudhary AK. Spinal subdural hemorrhage in abusive head trauma: a pictorial review. *Pediatr Radiol*. 2021;51(6):980-990.
16. Binenbaum G, Mirza-George N, Christian CW, Forbes BJ. Odds of abuse associated with retinal hemorrhages in children suspected of child abuse. *J AAPOS*. 2009;13(3):268-272.
17. Gilliland MGF, Luckenbach MW, Chenier TC. Systemic and ocular findings in 169 prospectively studied child deaths: retinal hemorrhages usually mean child abuse. *Forensic Sci Int*. 1994;68(2):117-132.
18. Bechtel K, Stoessel K, Leventhal JM, et al. Characteristics that distinguish accidental from abusive injury in hospitalized young children with head trauma. *An Pediatr*. 2004;114(1):165-168.
19. Franzco ALV, Kelly P. Retinal hemorrhages in inflicted traumatic brain injury: the ophthalmologist in court. *Clin Experiment Ophthalmol*. 2010;38:521-532.
20. Aryan HE, Ghosheh FR, Jandial R, Levy ML. Retinal hemorrhage and pediatric brain injury: etiology and review of the literature. *J Clin Neurosci*. 2005;12(6):624-631.
21. Rao N, Smith RE, Choi JH, Xu XH, Kornblum RN. Autopsy findings in the eyes of fourteen fatally abused children. *Forensic Sci Int*. 1988;39(3):293-299.
22. Leeuw MD, Beuls E, Jorens PG, Parizel P, Jacobs W. The optic nerve sheath hemorrhage is a non-specific finding in cases of suspected child abuse. *J Forensic Leg Med*. 2015;36:43-48.
23. Kemp AM. Investigating subdural haemorrhage in infants. *Arch Dis Child*. 2002;86(2):98-102.
24. Lo WD, Lee J, Rusin J, Perkins E, Roach ES. Intracranial hemorrhage in children: an evolving spectrum. *Arch Neurol*. 2008;65(12):1629-1633.
25. Levin AV. Retinal hemorrhages: advances in understanding. *Pediatr Clin North Am*. 2009;56(2):333-344.
26. Kaur B, Taylor D. Retinal haemorrhages. *Arch Dis Child*. 1990;65(12):1369-1372.
27. Hymel KP, Jenny C, Block RW. Intracranial hemorrhage and rebleeding in suspected victims of abusive head trauma: addressing the forensic controversies. *Child Maltreat*. 2002;7(4):329-348.
28. Shur NE, Summerlin ML, McIntosh BJ, Shalaby-Rana E, Hinds TS. Genetic causes of fractures and subdural hematomas: fact versus fiction. *Pediatr Radiol*. 2021;51(6):1029-1043.
29. Elgamal EA, Murshid WR, Abu-Rahma HM, Samir D. Aneurysmal subarachnoid hemorrhage in the first year of life: case report and review of the literature. *Childs Nerv Syst*. 2004;20(7):489-493.
30. Plunkett J. Sudden death in an infant caused by rupture of a basilar artery aneurysm. *Am J Forensic Med Pathol*. 1999;20(2):211-214.
31. Prahlow JA, Rushing EJ, Barnard JJ. Death due to a ruptured berry aneurysm in a 3.5-year-old child. *Am J Forensic Med Pathol*. 1998;19(4):391-394.
32. Garg K, Singh PK, Sharma BS, et al. Pediatric intracranial aneurysms-our experience and review of literature. *Childs Nerv Syst*. 2014;30(5):873-883.
33. Koroknay-Pal P, Lehto H, Niemela M, Kivisaari R, Hernesniemi J. Long-term outcome of 114 children with cerebral aneurysms. *J Neurosurg Pediatr*. 2012;9(6):636-645.
34. Pasqualin A, Mazza C, Cavazzani P, Scienza R, DaPian R. Intracranial aneurysms and subarachnoid hemorrhage in children and adolescents. *Childs Nerv Syst*. 1986;2(4):185-190.
35. Aryan HE, Giannotta SL, Fukushima T, Park MS, Ozgur BM, Levy ML. Aneurysms in children: review of 15 years experience. *J Clin Neurosci*. 2006;13(2):188-192.
36. Marbacher S, Tomasi O, Fandino J. Management of patients presenting with acute subdural hematoma due to ruptured intracranial aneurysm. *Int J Vasc Med*. 2012;2012:753596. doi 10.1155/2012/753596.
37. Buis DR, van Ouwerkerk WJR, Takahata H, Vandertop WP. Intracranial aneurysms in children under 1 year of age: a systematic review of the literature. *Childs Nerv Syst*. 2006;22(11):1395-1409.
38. Ferrante L, Fortuna A, Celli P, Santoro A, Fraioli B. Intracranial arterial aneurysms in early childhood. *Surg Neurol*. 1988;29(1):39-56.
39. Neß T, Janknecht P, Berghorn C. Frequency of ocular hemorrhages in patients with subarachnoid hemorrhage. *Graefes Arch Clin Exp Ophthalmol*. 2005;243:859-862.
40. Stiebel-Kalish H, Turtel LS, Kupersmith MJ. The natural history of nontraumatic subarachnoid hemorrhage-related intraocular hemorrhages. *Retina* 2004;24(1):36-40.

41. Bhardwaj G, Jacobs MB, Moran KT, Tan K. Terson syndrome with ipsilateral severe hemorrhagic retinopathy in a 7-month-old child. *J AAPOS*. 2010;14(5):441-443.
42. Roberton NRC, Howat P. Hypernatraemia as a cause of intracranial haemorrhage. *Arch Dis Child*. 1975;50(12):938-942.
43. Fenton S, Murray D, Thornton P, Kennedy S, O'Keefe M. Bilateral massive retinal hemorrhages in a 6-month-old infant: a diagnostic dilemma. *Arch Ophthalmol*. 1999;117(10):1432-1434.
44. Handy TC, Hanzlick R, Shields LB, Reichard R, Goudy S. Hypernatremia and subdural hematoma in the pediatric age group: is there a causal relationship? *J Forensic Sci*. 1999;44(6):1114-1118.
45. Ali SA, Jaspan T, Marenah C, Vyas H. Does hypernatremia cause subdural hematoma in children? Two case reports and a meta-analysis of the literature. *Am J Forensic Med Pathol*. 2012;33(2):132-136.
46. Rutty GN, Woolley A, Brookfield C, Shepherd F, Kitchen S. The PIVKA II Test: the first reliable coagulation test for autopsy investigations. *Int J Legal Med*. 2003;117(3):143-148.
47. Laposata ME, Laposata M. Children with signs of abuse: when it is not child abuse? *Am J Clin Pathol*. 2005;123(suppl l):S119-S124.
48. Stray-Pedersen A, Omland S, Nedregaard B, Klevberg S, Rognum TO. An infant wit subdural hematoma and retinal hemorrhages: does von Willebrand disease explain the findings? *Forensic Sci Med Pathol*. 2011;7(1):37-41.
49. Cekinmez M, Cemil T, Cekinmez EK, Altinörs N. Intracranial hemorrhages due to late-type vitamin K deficiency bleeding. *Childs Nerv Syst*. 2008;24(7):821-825.
50. Case ME. Accidental traumatic head injury in infants and young children. *Brain Pathol*. 2008;18(4):583-589.
51. Case ME. Inflicted traumatic brain injury in infants and young children. *Brain Pathol*. 2008;18(4):571-582.
52. Vinchon M, DeFoort-Dhellemmes S, Desurmont M, Delestret I. Confessed abuse versus witnessed accidents in infants: comparison of clinical, radiological, and ophthalmological data in corroborated cases. *Childs Nerv Syst*. 2010;26(5):637-645.
53. Christian CW, Taylor AA, Hertle RW, Duhaime AC. Retinal hemorrhages caused by accidental household trauma. *J Pediatr*. 1999;135(1):125-127.
54. Talbert D. The nature of shaken baby syndrome injuries and the significance of a "Lucid interval." *Med Hypotheses*. 2008;71(1):117-121.
55. Reichard RR, White CL, Hladik CL, Dolinak D. Beta-amyloid precursor protein staining of nonaccidental central nervous system injury in pediatric autopsies. *J Neurotrauma*. 2003;20(4):347-355.
56. Arbogast KB, Margulies SS, Christian CW. Initial neurologic presentation in young children sustaining inflicted and unintentional fatal head injuries. *Pediatrics*. 2005;116(1):180-184.
57. Peterson JEG, Love JC, Pinto DC, Wolf DA, Sandberg G. A novel method for removing a spinal cord with attached cervical ganglia from a pediatric decedent. *J Forensic Sci*. 2016;61(1):241-244.
58. Brennan LK, Rubin D, Christian CW, Duhaime AC, Mirchandani HG, Rorke-Adams LB. Neck injuries in young pediatric homicide victims. *J Neurosurg Pediatr*. 2009;3:232-239.
59. Thomas PS. Rib fractures in infancy. *Ann Radiol*. 1977;20(1):115-122.
60. Smith FW, Gilday DL, Ash JM, Green MD. Unsuspected costo-vertebral fractures demonstrated by bone scanning in the child abuse syndrome. *Pediatr Radiol*. 1980;10(2):103-106.
61. Carter JE, McCormick AQ. Whiplash shaking syndrome: retinal hemorrhages and computerized axial tomography of the brain. *Child Abuse Negl*. 1983;7(3):279-286.
62. Smeets AJ, Robben SG, Meradji M. Sonographically detected costo-chondral dislocation in an abused child. A new sonographic sign to the radiological spectrum of child abuse. *Pediatr Radiol*. 1990;20(7):566-567.
63. Ng CS, Hall CM. Costochondral junction fractures and intra-abdominal trauma in non-accidental injury (child abuse). *Pediatr Radiol*. 1998;28(9):671-676.
64. Barsness KA, Cha ES, Bensard DD, et al. The positive predictive value of rib fractures as an indicator of nonaccidental trauma in children. *J Trauma*. 2003;54(6):1107-1110.
65. Hansen KK, Prince JS, Nixon GW. Oblique chest views as a routine part of skeletal surveys performed for possible physical abuse—is this practice worthwhile? *Child Abuse Negl*. **2008;32(1):155-159.**

66. Bulloch B, Schubert CJ, Brophy PD, Johnson N, Reed MH, Shapiro RA. Cause and clinical characteristics of rib fractures in infants. *Pediatrics*. 2000;105(4):E48.
67. Cadzow SP, Armstrong KL. Rib fractures in infants: red alert! The clinical features, investigations and child protection outcomes. *J Paediatr Child Health*. 2000;36(4):322-326.
68. Clouse JR, Lantz PE. Posterior rib fractures in infants associated with cardiopulmonary resuscitation. Annual Meeting of the American Academy of Forensic Sciences; 2008; Washington, DC.
69. Feldman KW, Brewer DK. Child abuse, cardiopulmonary resuscitation, and rib fractures. *Pediatrics*. 1984;73(3):339-342.
70. Marine MB, Forbes-Amrhein MM. Fractures of child abuse. *Pediatr Radiol*. 2021;51(6):1003-1013.
71. Ryan MP, Young SJ, Wells DL. Do resuscitation attempts in children who die, cause injury? *Emerg Med J*. 2003;20(1):10-12.
72. Maguire S, Mann M, John N, et al. Does cardiopulmonary resuscitation cause rib fractures in children? A systematic review. *Child Abuse Negl*. 2006;30(7):739-751.
73. Matshes EW, Lew EO. Do resuscitation-related injuries kill infants and children? *Am J Forensic Med Pathol*. 2010;31(2):178-185.
74. Dolinak D. Rib fractures in infants due to cardiopulmonary resuscitation efforts. *Am J Forensic Med Pathol*. 2007;28(2):107-110.
75. Weber MA, Risdon RA, Offiah AC, Malone M, Sebire NJ. Rib fractures identified at postmortem examination in sudden unexpected deaths in infancy (SUDI). *Forensic Sci Int*. 2009;189(1-3):75-81.
76. Matshes EW, Lew EO. Two-handed cardiopulmonary resuscitation can cause rib fractures in infants. *Am J Forensic Med Pathol*. 2010;31(4):303-307.
77. Worn MJ, Jones MD. Rib fractures in infancy: establishing the mechanisms of cause from the injuries—a literature review. *Med Sci Law*. 2007;47(3):200-212.
78. Menegazzi JJ. Infant chest compression depth needs further evaluation. *Resuscitation*. 2011;82(10):1362.
79. Reyes JA, Somers GR, Taylor GP, Chiasson DA. Increased incidence of CPR-related rib fractures in infants—is it related to changes in CPR technique? *Resuscitation*. 2011;82(5):545-548.
80. Kemp WL. Microscopic examination of rib heads: a useful adjunct in the investigation of infant deaths. PhD dissertation. University of Montana:3024; 2014.
81. Warrington SA, Wright CM; ALSPAC Study Team. Accidents and resulting injuries in premobile infants: data from the ALSPAC study. *Arch Dis Child*. 2001;85(2):104-107.
82. Ruddick C, Platt MW, Lazaro C. Head Trauma outcomes of verifiable falls in newborn babies. *Arch Dis Child Fetal Neonatal*. 2010;95(2):F144-F145.
83. Haney SB, Starling SP, Heisler KW, Okwara L. Characteristics of falls and risk of injury in children younger than 2 years. *Pediatr Emerg Care*. 2010;26(12):914-918.
84. Chadwick DL, Bertocci G, Castillo E, et al. Annual Risk of death resulting from short falls among young children: less than 1 in 1 million. *An Pediatr*. 2008;121(6):1213-1224.
85. Helfer RE, Slovis TL, Black M. Injuries resulting when small children fall out of bed. *Pediatrics*. 1977;60(4):533-535.
86. Tarantino CA, Dowd MD, Murdock TC. Short vertical falls in infants. *Pediatr Emerg Care*. 1999;15(1):5-8.
87. Hall JR, Reyes HM, Horvat M, Meller JL, Stein R. The mortality of childhood falls. *J Trauma*. 1989;29(9):1273-1275.
88. Reiber GD. Fatal falls in childhood: how far must children fall to sustain fatal head injury? Report of cases and review of the literature. *Am J Forensic Med Pathol*. 1993;14(3):201-207.
89. Plunkett J. Fatal pediatric head injuries caused by short-distance falls. *Am J Forensic Med Pathol*. 2001;22(1):1-12.
90. John SM, Kelly P, Vincent A. Patterns of structural head injury in children younger than 3 years: a ten-year review of 519 patients. *J Trauma Acute Care Surg*. 2013;74(1):276-281.
91. McGovern MC, Smith MBH. Causes of apparent life threatening events in infants: a systematic review. *Arch Dis Child*. 2004;89(11):1043-1048.
92. Parker K, Pitetti R. Mortality and child abuse in children presenting with apparent life-threatening events. *Pediatr Emerg Care*. 2011;27(7):591-595.

93. Curcoy AI, Trenchs V, Morales M, Serra A, Pou J. Retinal hemorrhages and apparent life-threatening events. *Pediatr Emerg Care*. 2010;26(2):118-120.
94. Pitetti RD, Maffei F, Chang K, Hickey R, Berger R, Pierce MC. Prevalence of retinal hemorrhages and child abuse in children who present with an apparent life-threatening event. *Pediatrics*. 2002;110(3):557-562.
95. Squier W. The triad of retinal haemorrhage, subdural haemorrhage and encephalopathy in an infant unassociated with evidence of physical injury is not the result of shaking, but is most likely to have been caused by a natural disease: Yes. *J Prim Health Care*. 2011;3(2):159-161.
96. Couper Z, Albermani F. Mechanical response of infant brain to manually inflicted shaking. *Proc Inst Mech Eng H*. 2010;224(1):1-15.
97. Hayashi T, Hashimoto T, Fukuda S, Ohshima Y, Moritaka K. Neonatal subdural hematoma secondary to birth injury. Clinical analysis of 48 survivors. *Childs Nerv Syst*. 1987;3(1):23-29.
98. Duane TD. Valsalva hemorrhagic retinopathy. *Trans Am Ophthal Soc*. 1972;70:298-313.
99. Herr S, Pierce MC, Berger RP, Ford H, Pitetti RD. Does Valsalva retinopathy occur in infants? An initial investigation in infants with vomiting caused by pyloric stenosis. *Pediatrics*. 2004;113(6):1658-1661.
100. Geddes JF, Tasker RC, Hackshaw AK, et al. Dural haemorrhage in non-traumatic infant deaths: does it explain the bleeding in "shaken baby syndrome." *Neuropathol App Neurobiol*. 2003;29(1):14-22.
101. Byard RW, Blumbergs P, Rutty G, Sperhake J, Banner J, Krous HF. Lack of evidence for a causal relationship between hypoxic-ischemic encephalopathy and subdural hemorrhage in fetal life, infancy, and early childhood. *Pediatr Dev Pathol*. 2007;10(5):348-350.
102. Geddes JF, Talbert DG. Paroxysmal coughing, subdural and retinal bleeding: a computer modelling approach. *Neuropathol App Neurobiol*. 2006;32(6):625-634.
103. Wortis N, Strebel PM, Wharton M, et al. Pertussis deaths: report of 23 cases in the United States, 1992 and 1993. *Pediatrics*. 1996;97(5):607-612.
104. Lack EE, Kozakewich HPW. Whooping cough (pertussis). In: Connor DH, Chandler FW, Manz HJ, Schwartz DA, Lack EE, eds. *Pathology of Infectious Diseases*. Appleton y Lange; 1997.
105. Barnes PD, Galaznik J, Gardner H, Shuman M. Infant acute life-threatening event dysphagic choking versus nonaccidental injury. *Sem Pediatr Neurol*. 2010;17(1):7-11.
106. Kleinman PK. *Diagnostic Imaging of Child Abuse*. 2nd ed. Mosby; 1998.
107. Care MM. Macrocephaly and subdural collections. *Pediatr Radiol*. 2021;51(6):891-897.
108. Hobbs CJ. ABC of child abuse. Fractures. *BMJ*. 1989;298(6679):1015-1018.
109. Maguire S. Which injuries may indicate child abuse? *Arch Dis Child Educ Pract Ed*. 2010;95(6):170-177. doi: 10.1136/adc.2009.170431.
110. Kos L, Shwayder T. Cutaneous manifestations of child abuse. *Pediatr Dermatol*. 2006;23(4):311-320.
111. Benseler S, Schneider R. Central nervous system vasculitis in children. *Curr Opin Rheumatol*. 2004;16(1):43-50.
112. Betz P, Liebhardt E. Rib fractures in children—resuscitation or child abuse? *Int J Legal Med*. 1994;106(4):215-218.
113. Betz P, Puschel K, Miltner E, Lignitz E, Eisenmenger W. Morphometrical analysis of retinal hemorrhages in the shaken baby syndrome. *Sci Int*. 1996;78(1):71-80.
114. Bilginer B, Onal MB, Oguz K, Akalan N. Arachnoid cyst associated with subdural hematoma: report of three cases and review of the literature. *Childs Nerv Syst*. 2009;25(1):119-124.
115. Breysem L, Loyen S, Boets A, Proesmans M, De Boeck K, Smet MH. Pediatric emergencies: thoracic emergencies. *Eur Radiol*. 2002;12(12):2849-2865.
116. Bush CM, Jones JS, Cohle SD, Johnson H. Pediatric injuries from cardiopulmonary resuscitation. *Ann Emerg Med*. 1996;28(1):40-44.
117. Cameron JM, Rae LJ. *Atlas of the Battered Child Syndrome*. Churchill Livingstone; 1975:90.
118. Cutter C. *A Treatise on Anatomy, Physiology, and hygiene*. J.B. Lippincott Co; 1852:462.
119. deRooij NK, Linn FHH, van der Plas JA, Algra A, Rinkel GJE. Incidence of subarachnoid haemorrhage: a systematic review with emphasis on region, age, gender and time trends. *J Neurol Neurosurg Psychiatry*. 2007;78(12):1365-1372.

120. Dolinak D, Matshes E. Child abuse. In: Dolinak D, Matshes E, Lew E, eds. *Forensic Pathology: Principles and Practice*. Elsevier Press; 2005:369-412.

121. Emerson MV, Jakobs E, Green WR. Ocular autopsy and histopathologic features of child abuse. *Ophthalmology*. 2007;114(7):1384-1394.

122. Galloway A. Fractures patterns and skeletal morphology: the axial skeleton. In: Galloway A, ed. *Broken Bones: An Anthropological Analysis of blunt Force Trauma*. Charles C. Thomas; 1999:81-112.

123. Gayle MO, Kissoon N, Hered RW, Harwood-Nuss A. Retinal hemorrhage in the young child: a review of etiology, predisposed conditions, and clinical implications. *J Emerg Med*. 1995;13(2):233-239.

124. Gerber P, Coffman K. Nonaccidental head trauma in infants. *Childs Nerv Syst*. 2007;23(5):499-507.

125. Gnanaraj L, Gilliland MGF, Yahya RR, et al. Ocular manifestations of crush head injury in children. *Eye*. 2007;21(1):5-10.

126. Hanzlick R, Hunsaker JC, Davis GJ. *A Guide for Manner of Death Classification*. 1st ed. National Association of Medical Examiners; 2002.

127. Ildan F, Cetinalp E, Bağdatoğlu H, Boyar B, Uzuneyuoglu Z. Arachnoid cyst with traumatic intracystic hemorrhage unassociated with subdural hematoma. *Neurosurg Rev*. 1994;17(3):229-232.

128. Jaspan T. Current controversies in the interpretation of non-accidental head injury. *Pediatr Radiol*. 2008;38(suppl 3):S378-S387.

129. Katz JS, Oluigbo CO, Wilkinson CC, McNatt S, Handler MH. Prevalence of cervical spine injury in infants with head trauma. *J Neurosurg Pediatr*. 2010;5:470-473.

130. Knight B. *Forensic Pathology*. Arnold; 1996:636.

131. Kogutt MS, Swischuk LE, Fagan CJ. Patterns of injury and significance of uncommon fractures in the battered child syndrome. *Am J Roentgenol Radium Ther Nucl Med*. 1974;121(1):143-149.

132. Krings T, Geibprasert S, terBrugge KG. Pathomechanisms and treatment of pediatric aneurysms. *Childs Nerv Syst*. 2010;26(10):1309-1318.

133. Krishna H, Wani AA, Behari S, Banerji D, Chhabra DK, Jain VK. Intracranial aneurysms in patients 18 years of age or under, are they different from aneurysms in adult population? *Acta Neurochir*. 2005;147(5):469-476; discussion 476.

134. Lee CH, Han IS, Lee JY, et al. Analysis of a bleeding mechanism in patients with the sylvian arachnoid cyst using a finite element model. *Childs Nerv Syst*. 2014;30(6):1029-1036.

135. Liu Z, Xu P, Li Q, Liu H, Chen N, Xu J. Arachnoid cysts with subdural hematoma or intracystic hemorrhage in children. *Pediatr Emerg Care*. 2014;30(5):345-351.

136. Pagana KD, Pagana TJ. *Mosby's Diagnostic and Laboratory Test Reference*. 10th ed. Elsevier Mosby; 2011:1130.

137. Silverman FN. Radiologic aspects of the battered child syndrome. In: Helfer RE, Kempe CH, eds. *The Battered Child*. 2nd ed. University of Chicago Press; 1974:41-60.

138. Spevak MR, Kleinman PK, Belanger PL, Primack C, Richmond JM. Cardiopulmonary resuscitation and rib fractures in infants. A postmortem radiologic-pathologic study. *JAMA*. 1994;272(8):617-618.

139. Vinchon M, Defoort-Dhellemmes S, Desurmont M, Dhellemmes P. Accidental and nonaccidental head injuries in infants: a prospective study. *J Neurosurg*. 2005;102(4 suppl l):380-384.

140. Willman KY, Bank DE, Senac M, Chadwick DL. Restricting the time of injury in fatal inflicted head injuries. *Child Abuse Neg*. 1997;21(10):929-940.

141. Yokota A, Kajiwara H, Matsuoka S, Kohchi M, Matsukado Y. Subarachnoid hemorrhage from brain tumors in childhood. *Childs Nerv Syst*. 1987;3(2):65-69.

ENVIRONMENTAL DEATHS 14

CHAPTER OUTLINE

Introduction 424

Hyperthermia 424
- Introduction 424
- Clinical Features of Heat Stroke 424
- Pattern at Autopsy 424

Hypothermia 426
- Introduction 426
- Pattern at Autopsy 426

Autopsy Findings Associated With Hypothermia 429
- Wischnewski Spots 429
  - Gross Appearance 429
  - Microscopic Appearance 429
  - Other Associations 429
  - Important Points 429
- Frost Erythema 429
  - Gross Appearance 429
  - Microscopic Appearance 430
- Subnuclear Vacuolization of the Proximal Convoluted Tubular Epithelial Cells 430
  - Gross Appearance 430
  - Microscopic Appearance 430
- Vacuolation of Pancreatic Adenoid Cells 430
  - Microscopic Appearance 430
  - Other Associations 430

Description of Snow Immersion 430

Bodies Found in the Water 430
- Did the Decedent Drown? 430
- What Environmental and Human Factors Were Involved? 431
- Postmortem Artifacts Associated With Bodies Found in the Water 432

Scuba Diving-Related Deaths 432
- Causes of Death Associated With Scuba Diving 432
- How to Test for Gas Embolism and Barotrauma in a Scuba-Related Death 433

Electrocution 434
- Introduction 434
- Gross Appearance 434
- Microscopic Appearance 434

Dog Attacks 434
- Introduction 434
- Autopsy Findings Associated With Fatal Dog Attack 435

Snake Bite 436
- Introduction 436
- Pathologic Features of Pit Viper Injury 436
- Clinical Features of Pit Viper Injury 436
- Pathologic Features of Recluse Bite 436
- Clinical Features of Recluse Bite 436

Spider Bite 437

Other Forms of Animal Attack Encountered by Forensic Pathologists 437

High-Altitude Pulmonary Edema/High-Altitude Cerebral Edema 437
- Features of High-Altitude Cerebral Edema 437
- Features of High-Altitude Pulmonary Edema 437
- Autopsy Findings in High-Altitude Pulmonary Edema 437

Near Misses 438

INTRODUCTION

The term "environmental deaths" encompasses deaths that are associated with an environmental factor and will include discussion of death due to temperature extremes (both hot and cold), but also death due to exposure to environmental dangers such as water and high altitude, and death due to exposure to various dangerous creatures in the environment including large animals, insects, and snakes. As electrocutions can occur outdoors (such as lightning or exposure to power lines), this type of death is also discussed below.

HYPERTHERMIA

INTRODUCTION

Deaths due to hyperthermia can occur secondary to environmental extremes in temperature but also due to endogenous causes of hyperthermia (eg, malignant hyperthermia[1]). The definitive postmortem diagnosis of hyperthermia is problematic, as the autopsy findings are non-specific. To diagnosis hyperthermia as the cause of death requires knowledge of the environment the decedent was found in (eg, what was the outside temperature, what was the inside temperature if they were found indoors, and did the decedent have appropriate cooling mechanisms available to them, such as a functioning air conditioner) and knowledge of particular susceptibilities of the decedent for a heat-related death (eg, underlying medical co-morbidities) as well as the autopsy findings, which, in the case of hyperthermia, are best at ruling out another cause of death. If knowledge of the decedent's terminal behavior, including signs and symptoms, are available, this too can assist with the diagnosis of fatal hyperthermia. The clinical correlate of an exogenous hyperthermia death is heat stroke.

CLINICAL FEATURES OF HEAT STROKE

The clinical diagnosis of heat stroke requires two findings: a body core temperature of 40 °C or more (104 °F) and knowledge that the individual manifested a central nervous system dysfunction, which can include delirium, seizures, or coma.[2] Other features of heat stroke can include lack of sweating, nausea and vomiting, tachycardia, and hypotension.[2] Heat stroke can result in the death of the patient. While an autopsy cannot identify any of the clinical features of hyperthermia other than the elevated body temperature, scene investigation, including interviewing of witnesses who saw decedent prior to their death, could be useful to elucidate such terminal event history about the decedent.

PATTERN AT AUTOPSY

If the body is found soon enough after the time of death, a measurement of the body temperature may assist in the diagnosis of hyperthermia as the cause of death, with the caveat that elevated environmental temperature is not the only reason for an individual to have an elevated body temperature and the body temperature at the time the body is found may not be representative of the body temperature when the death occurred. Based upon the circumstances of the decedent's collapse, the body temperature may rise significantly after death (eg, if the decedent collapsed adjacent to a fireplace or other source of heat).

The autopsy features of hyperthermia are non-specific and may include congestion and edema, cerebral and/or pulmonary edema, right ventricular cardiac dilation, intrathoracic petechiae, subendocardial hemorrhage (Figure 14.1), and necrosis of the liver.[3,4] If the individual survives in the hot environment for a long enough period of time prior to their collapse, dehydration may occur and vitreous electrolyte analysis combined with physical examination may provide the cause of death. Autopsy findings of dehydration include sunken eyes, sticky serosal surfaces, decreased skin turgor (which can also occur secondary

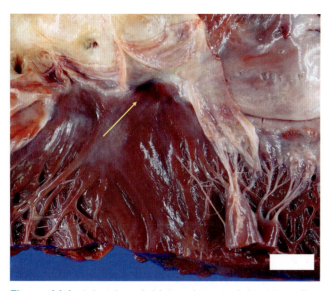

Figure 14.1. Subendocardial hemorrhage in the aortic outflow tract. Subjacent to the aortic valve is subendocardial hemorrhage (arrow). While subendocardial hemorrhage is associated with hyperthermia, the finding is non-specific and can be seen in a range of other conditions.

to loss of skin elasticity), dark urine, and constipation.[5] While tenting of the skin upon palpation with failure of a quick return to a normal texture after palpation has ended is consistent with dehydration and decreased skin turgor, with time spent in a cooler, the skin and subcutaneous tissue can take on a doughy texture and, with palpation, can tent and likewise fail to quickly return to normal texture.

KEY FEATURES to Identify Individuals at Risk for Heat Stroke[2,6]
- History of high environmental temperatures and humidity
- Demographics: elderly and infants
- Socio-economic: poor individuals and those without access to air conditioning or who are socially isolated
- Chronic alcoholics
- Obesity
- Medical history: dementia, cardiac disease, chronic obstructive pulmonary disease, other chronic disease processes, use of psychiatric medications and diuretics
- Heavy exertion in a hot environment

SAMPLE NOTE: HOW TO CERTIFY THE CAUSE OF DEATH IN AN INDIVIDUAL WHO DIES DUE TO EXOGENOUS HYPERTHERMIA

The cause of death could be worded in several ways: hyperthermia (which is technically non-specific as the hyperthermia can be due to environmental exposure or due to endogenous heat production), exogenous hyperthermia (which some individuals reading the death certification may not understand), environmental hyperthermia (which is specific as to the etiology, and with a wording that most people should understand), or complications of heat stroke, using the clinical term for the condition. If the decedent has underlying natural disease, as will often be the case, these disease processes can be listed in the other significant conditions section of the death certificate.

SAMPLE NOTE: HOW TO CERTIFY THE CAUSE AND MANNER DEATH OF AN INFANT OR CHILD LEFT INSIDE A CAR[3]

If an infant or child is left inside a hot car and dies, the cause of death may be certified as hyperthermia, given that neither investigation nor autopsy reveals any other findings to suggest another cause of death. The manner of death could be considered accident or homicide, with the distinction to be possibly determined by factors such as the length of time the infant or child was in the vehicle, the actions of the caregiver in the intervening time, and underlying reason why the infant or child was left in the vehicle (eg, Was the infant or child known to be left in the vehicle by the caregiver or unknown to be in the vehicle?).[3] The distinction between an accident and a homicide as to the manner of death in such a case could depend upon the specifics of the investigation, the education and experience of the forensic pathologist, and office policies.

HYPOTHERMIA

INTRODUCTION

Deaths due to hypothermia occur secondary to prolonged exposure to low environmental temperatures. The postmortem diagnosis of hypothermia is challenging, as the autopsy findings are considered non-specific, although compared to hyperthermia, the findings are somewhat more unique. To diagnose hypothermia as the cause of death, a forensic pathologist requires knowledge of the environment the decedent was in (eg, What was the outside temperature? What was the inside temperature if the decedent was found indoors? and Did the decedent have an appropriate heating mechanism available to them, such as a functioning furnace?) and knowledge of particular susceptibilities of the decedent for a cold-related death (eg, old age, underlying medical co-morbidities, intoxication) as well as the autopsy findings.

PEARLS & PITFALLS

The National Oceanic and Atmospheric Administration website (www.noaa.gov) is an excellent resource for recent temperatures. Since autopsy reports are often completed months after the actual autopsy, obtaining the necessary weather information during the initial investigation is useful to ensure that the information is available at a later time.

PATTERN AT AUTOPSY

While hypothermia, like hyperthermia, is a diagnosis of exclusion in which other causes of death must be ruled out at autopsy, individuals who die from hypothermia often have one or more pathologic findings, including bright-red lividity (Figure 14.2A); frost erythema (Figure 14.2B-D), which is red discoloration of the knees; Wischnewski spots (Figure 14.2E-H); abrasions of the knees and ankles; abrasions of the dorsal surface of the hands (Figure 14.2I); and, at scene investigation, evidence of pathologic undressing (Figure 14.2J). Because of the abrasions of the hands and knees and because of the delayed manner of hypothermia deaths, blood can easily be identified at the scene but is not necessarily indicative of suspicious trauma. By microscopic examination, in addition to confirming the above gross findings, subnuclear vacuolation of the proximal convoluted tubular epithelial cells can also be identified (Figure 14.2K). Like the kidney, fatty degeneration can occur in the myocardium but must be distinguished from lipofuscin deposition.[7]

Turk et al. indicate that a decreased rectal temperature that is out of proportion to other postmortem changes can also assist with the diagnosis of fatal hypothermia.[8] This finding must be interpreted with caution; however, if the body is cooler than might be expected, this observation would support hypothermia as the cause of death. Pancreatic hemorrhage is associated with hypothermia but is a rare finding. Preuss et al identified gross hemorrhage in only five of 143 cases of hypothermia.[9] They concluded that given the unclear distinction between the amount of hemorrhage and inflammation present in both the hypothermia cases and the control cases that these findings are unreliable signs of hypothermia. Hemorrhage into the synovial membranes and synovial fluid, hemorrhages into large muscles (eg, iliopsoas), black esophagus, and vacuolization of liver, adrenal, and pituitary cells are also associated with hypothermia.[10]

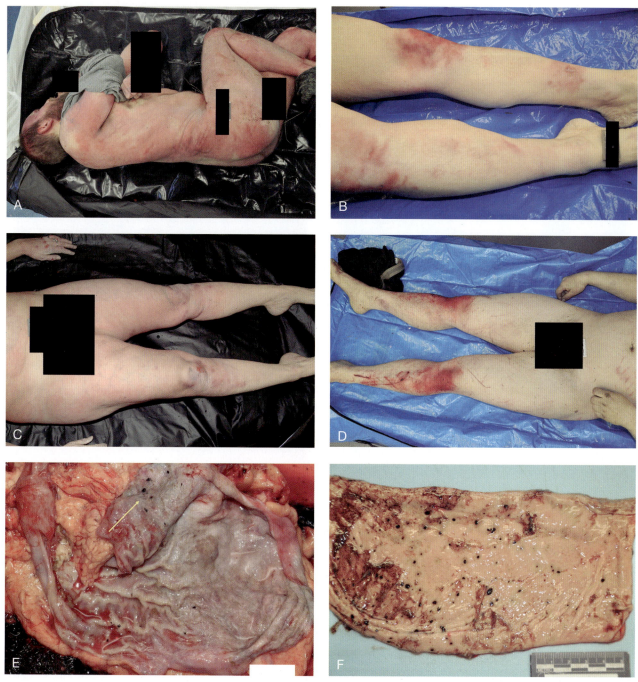

Figure 14.2. Gross and microscopic autopsy and scene findings associated with hypothermia. Autopsy findings of hypothermia include bright red lividity (**A**); frost erythema, which is red discoloration of the knees most commonly and can be combined with abrasions (**B-D**); and Wischnewski spots, which are dark red-black circular discolorations of the gastric mucosa that can be few in number and small (**E** and **F**; arrow indicates Wischnewski spots in **E**), or larger in size and more florid (**G** and **H**), abrasions of the dorsal surface of the hands (**I**), evidence of pathologic undressing at the scene (**J**), and basilar subnuclear vacuolization of the proximal convoluted tubular epithelial cells of the kidney (**K**, high power, H&E).

Figure 14.11g-k (continued)

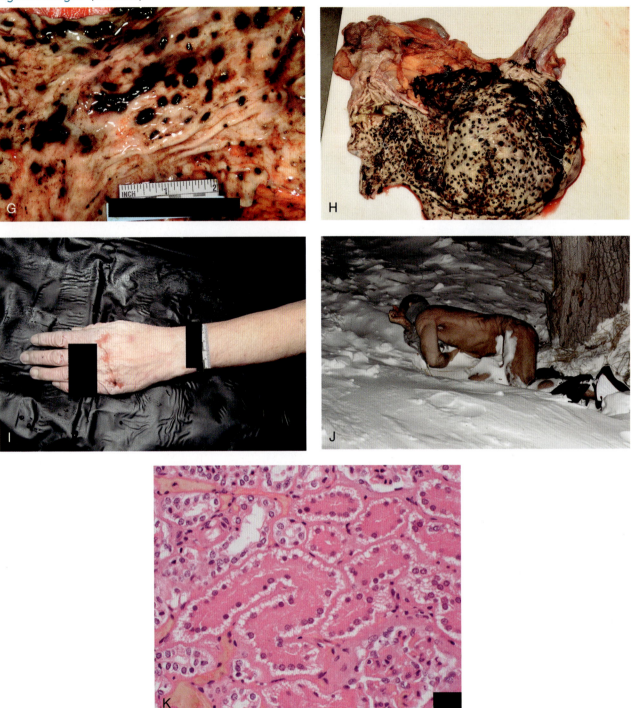

Key scene investigative features in the evaluation of a potential death due to hypothermia[11]

- History regarding the environmental temperatures since decedent was last known alive to when they were found dead
- Recording environmental temperature at the scene
- Documentation of clothing worn by the decedent
- Location of body, especially if found under brush or under an object (hide-and-die syndrome)
- Record temperature of body at scene if appropriate

SAMPLE NOTE: CERTIFICATION OF DEATH FOR INDIVIDUAL WHO POTENTIALLY DIED FROM HYPOTHERMIA AND WHO HAD UNDERLYING NATURAL DISEASE

As the diagnosis of hypothermia is a diagnosis of exclusion, yet its diagnosis designates a non-natural death (eg, an accident vs natural manner of death), without confirmatory information otherwise, the best approach is probably to list hypothermia as the cause of death and the natural disease as contributory, or the natural disease as the cause of death and the hypothermia as contributory, with a manner of accident applied in each situation.

AUTOPSY FINDINGS ASSOCIATED WITH HYPOTHERMIA

WISCHNEWSKI SPOTS

Gross Appearance

Dark red-black or brown-black circular discolorations of the gastric mucosa (Figure 14.2E-H).

Microscopic Appearance

Aggregates of finely stippled yellow-black or brown-black pigment, which represent hematinized hemoglobin (Figure 14.3).[4]

Other Associations

Wischnewski spots are also associated with diabetic ketoacidosis.

Important Points

Wischnewski spots reported in articles are found in 0% to 90% of cases of hypothermia and are more likely to occur in younger decedents than older decedents.[12] While the length of exposure to the cold temperature and the degree of the cold temperature have been suggested to play a role in the development of Wischnewski spots, this fact is debated.[12]

FROST ERYTHEMA

Gross Appearance

Red discoloration of the knees and elbows (the extensor surfaces) but can also affect the scrotum (Figure 14.2B-D).[8]

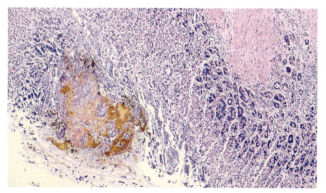

Figure 14.3. Microscopic appearance of Wischnewski spot. Microscopic examination of Wischnewski spots will reveal aggregates of finely stippled yellow to black pigment at the mucosal surface (low power, H&E).

Microscopic Appearance
Hyperemia and dermal edema.[11]

SUBNUCLEAR VACUOLIZATION OF THE PROXIMAL CONVOLUTED TUBULAR EPITHELIAL CELLS
Gross Appearance
Although the condition cannot be diagnosed grossly, it can be suspected when the kidney is paler tan-yellow in color instead of its normal darker red, with the caveat that a significant hemorrhage leading to blood loss could cause a similar appearance.

Microscopic Appearance
At the basal portion of the proximal convoluted tubular epithelial cells are vacuoles. The vacuoles will stain with periodic acid-Schiff (PAS) (Figure 14.2K).[4]

VACUOLATION OF PANCREATIC ADENOID CELLS[9]
Microscopic Appearance
Optically clear vacuoles in the pancreatic adenoid cells.

Other Associations
The vacuoles were also identified in alcoholics but only in those with chronic pancreatitis.

DESCRIPTION OF SNOW IMMERSION
Snow immersion most commonly occurs in the setting of skiing, with a skier falling into a snow well near a tree, or when a snowmobiler triggers an avalanche and is buried in the snow.[13,14] The mechanism of death is asphyxiation. An autopsy is the best way to rule out another cause of death such as blunt force injuries.

BODIES FOUND IN THE WATER
INTRODUCTION
While the autopsy features of drowning have been discussed in the chapter on asphyxia, bodies found in the water is essentially a different topic. To assume that all bodies found in the water have drowned is a major error. Although certain pathologic findings are associated with drowning, drowning is a diagnosis of exclusion and other causes of death must be ruled out through investigation and autopsy.

Key questions to answer when investigating a body found in the water[15]
- Was the victim alive at the time they entered the water?
- Why did the decedent enter the water?
- Why was the decedent unable to survive in the water?

DID THE DECEDENT DROWN?
How to Determine
As described in the chapter on asphyxia, drowning is a diagnosis of exclusion, although certain autopsy findings are associated with drowning, including hyperinflated lungs and an oral foam cone, with fluid in the sphenoid sinus consistent with immersion of the head in water. With an increased length of time spent in the water and subsequent decomposition, or with resuscitative measures performed after the body was recovered from the water, these features can be erased or at least obscured.

WHAT ENVIRONMENTAL AND HUMAN FACTORS WERE INVOLVED?

Importance to Consider

When investigating a drowning death, it is important to consider why the decedent entered the water, and, once they entered the water, why were they not able to survive. Environmental factors such as depth and temperature of the water, speeds of currents, obstacles within the water (eg, tree branches and other objects which could entangle the decedent), and potential hazards in the water (eg, abnormal source of electricity leading to electrocution, potential chemicals in the water) may have played a role in the decedent's inability to survive once they entered the water.[15]

Human factors can affect both the pre-event and the event stage.[15] Pre-event factors (ie, factors that led to the drowning) can include the mental state of the decedent, their physical state, their toxicologic status (eg, whether intoxicated or drug-impaired), and their ability to survive in the water environment (eg, Are they able to swim, and if so, are they able to swim well enough for the conditions?). Event factors, or those that directly contributed to the inability of the decedent to survive in the water environment, would include pre-existing natural disease such as a seizure disorder or cardiovascular disease.

SAMPLE NOTE: CERTIFYING THE DEATH OF AN INDIVIDUAL IN THE WATER WHO HAS UNDERLYING CARDIOVASCULAR DISEASE

If an individual through autopsy and investigation is found to have drowned and was found to have underlying heart disease (or another potential cause of sudden death), the death certificate could be certified in many ways, depending upon the circumstances of the death.

If an older male with significant cardiovascular disease entered a hostile water environment (eg, strong river currents) and was not prepared to handle that environment, the cause of death could be certified as Drowning, with no significant contributory conditions listed as the environmental factors alone are enough to explain the drowning.

If an older male with significant cardiovascular disease entered a safe water environment and sustained a cardiac event and drowned, whether witnessed or not, and was unable to be pulled from the water for a period of time, the cause of death would be certified as Drowning, and the cardiovascular disease listed as a significant contributory condition.

If an older male with significant cardiovascular disease entered a safe water environment and sustained a witnessed cardiac event and collapsed into the water but was immediately removed from the water and resuscitative measures were implemented, but unsuccessfully, the cause of death could be certified entirely upon the cardiovascular disease itself, with no mention of drowning listed.

PEARLS & PITFALLS

When investigating the death of an individual whose body was found in the water, scene investigation is very important in determining both the cause and manner of death and the circumstances of the death. Given the non-specific features of drowning, the variable state that the body can be in when it is finally found in the water (eg, from full preserved to completely skeletonized), the variable types of water in which a person may drown (from salt water to fresh water, from clean water to polluted water), and the presence or absence of resuscitative measures, among others, the best approach to investigating the death of a person found in the water is to not depend upon the autopsy alone to provide all the necessary information but instead to correlate the scene investigation with the autopsy findings to assess for consistency, and, if inconsistencies are found, use those to guide the determination of the cause and manner of death.[15] For example, if a deceased body is found in the water by a passerby, but autopsy identifies a patterned abrasion of the back of the head and underlying skull fracture and subdural hemorrhage, with a lack of hyperinflated lungs and oral foam cone in a non-resuscitated individual, the findings are not consistent with drowning.

> **PEARLS & PITFALLS**
>
> When a body is found in the water, it is not uncommon to identify multiple sharp force injuries of that body. When a body is floating in the water, it can easily be struck by a boat, with the propeller of the boat creating multiple parallel linear injuries of the skin, which can vary from abrasions to deep incised wounds. However, a swimmer can also be struck by a boat in the water, with the contact with the propeller creating injuries that cause death.[16] Distinguishing antemortem trauma from postmortem trauma in bodies found in the water can be difficult depending upon the amount of time the body is in the water, not only will decomposition affect the ability to distinguish the antemortem from postmortem wounds but, when the body is in the water, blood from an antemortem injury can be washed from the soft tissue, giving the wound a postmortem appearance.

POSTMORTEM ARTIFACTS ASSOCIATED WITH BODIES FOUND IN THE WATER

When the body is in the water, a variety of postmortem artifacts can occur. Any skin that is exposed can become dried, with a hard yellow-brown appearance, whereas the skin that is immersed remains wet (Figure 14.4A and B). While in the water, a variety of creatures can chew on the body, from small creatures such as crayfish/crawdads and leeches to fish and snakes to large creatures such as alligators and bears. Another important consideration is that, depending upon the location of the water, snapping turtles feeding on the body can bite off segments of tissue with a sharp angle, which could mimic antemortem sharp force injuries. In addition, depending upon the nature of the water that the body is in, the outer layer of exposed skin can become coated with a mixture of silt and algae (Figure 14.5A and B). This layer can easily be removed with a flexible ruler or other such object with a straight edge by scrapping the surface of the body (Figure 14.5C). This layer of adherent material should be removed so that the skin surface can examined in its entirety for injuries or other findings of significance.

SCUBA DIVING-RELATED DEATHS

CAUSES OF DEATH ASSOCIATED WITH SCUBA DIVING

Deaths that occur during scuba diving are usually due to one of three main mechanisms: drowning or other form of asphyxia, natural disease, or barotrauma, with drowning being the most common cause of death and with ischemic heart disease being the main cause of natural disease-related deaths in scuba divers.[17,18] Pulmonary barotrauma is due to

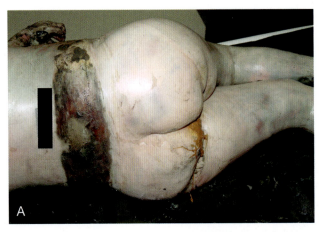 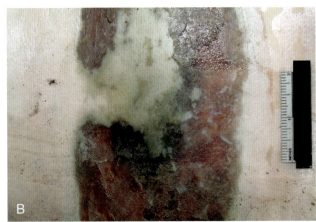

Figure 14.4. Exposed skin in drowned body. This individual in (A and B) was wearing a shirt and pants; however, the shirt was displaced upward, exposing the lower back, with the skin sloughing and the underlying exposed dermis drying producing the band of discoloration across the lower back.

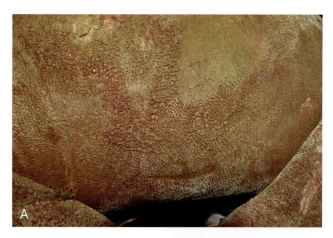
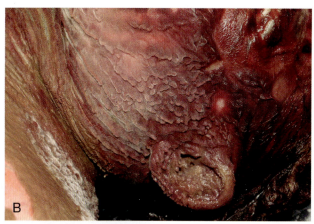
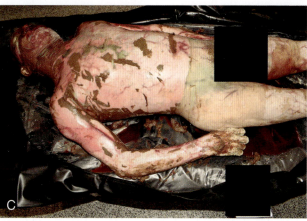

Figure 14.5. Adherent silt and algae on the body. In (**A** and **B**), the decedent has a thin layer of loosely adherent silt and algae on the body. This layer can (and should) be removed from the skin surface prior to final examination. The layer is easily removed with a flexible ruler that is scrapped along the surface (**C**).

pulmonary over-distension and leads to gas emboli, which can obstruct the cerebral vessels or other vessels.[19] Immersion pulmonary edema has also been described in scuba divers, with the scuba diver often, but not always, having underlying cardiac disease.[20,21] In immersion pulmonary edema, the decedent will have no history of aspiration but will have a history of rapid respiratory difficulties despite an appropriate source of oxygen.[22]

HOW TO TEST FOR GAS EMBOLISM AND BAROTRAUMA IN A SCUBA-RELATED DEATH

A radiograph of the chest may reveal a pneumothorax or be able to identify the intravascular gas bubbles.[23,24] Computed tomography or magnetic resonance image can identify the gas bubble in the vessels.[25] Subcutaneous emphysema may also be present.[26] Casadesús et al describe both opening the pericardial sac under water to assess for gas emboli as well as a more thorough dissection in which the vasculature to and from the heart is ligated at various points.[27] The authors provide numerous images to illustrate the procedure.

PEARLS & PITFALLS

Scuba-related deaths can be very complex, involving a scene investigation that may be complicated by being underwater as well as evaluation of the complex equipment used in a sport that many forensic pathologists most likely have little to no familiarity with. The best approach to a scuba diving accident is multi-disciplinary with input from individuals who understand the complexities of such deaths, including how to properly evaluate the decedent's equipment.[28]

ELECTROCUTION

INTRODUCTION

Electrocution can occur in two forms: low voltage and high voltage, with low-voltage electrocution due to exposure to electrical circuits in the household or similar circumstances, and with high-voltage electrocutions being 1000 V or higher and typically due to exposure to lightning, power lines, or similar circumstances.

GROSS APPEARANCE

The burns created in the skin during an electrocution when small can be a circular to oval and dried yellow region.[29] The size of the burn will vary with the nature of the electrocution. With a high-voltage electrocution, a much larger segment of the skin can be involved (Figure 14.6). In a low-voltage electrocution, no burn pattern may be apparent; however, in a high-voltage electrocution, the damage to the skin will most often be quite obvious. Examination of the clothing can also assist in identification of an electrocution (Figure 14.7). One form of high-voltage electrocution is due to lightning, which produces a characteristic skin change, called a Lichtenberg figure, which is a red fernlike or branching temporary discoloration on the skin.[30]

MICROSCOPIC APPEARANCE

Electrocution can lead to intraepidermal blister formation, a basket weave pattern in the keratin, and nuclear streaming, with stretching and narrowing of the shape (Figure 14.8A and B).[4,29] Elastic fibers in the dermis are disrupted.[29] Similar microscopic changes can be found in skin from drying, freezing, and thermal injury.[29]

> **PEARLS & PITFALLS**
>
> Scene investigation can be crucial in the accurate diagnosis of a low-voltage electrocution. Low voltage electrocutions can often leave no marks on the body, or very non-specific marks; however, finding a person down on their kitchen floor with a drill in their hand and evidence that the drill passed into the wall and clipped a power line can easily identify the cause of death.

DOG ATTACKS

INTRODUCTION

Fatal dog attacks are relatively uncommon but when they occur they are often caused by pit bulls, rottweilers, or German shepherds. Also, the fact that a body was attacked by dogs does not necessarily indicate that the dog attack is the cause of death, as postmortem feeding by

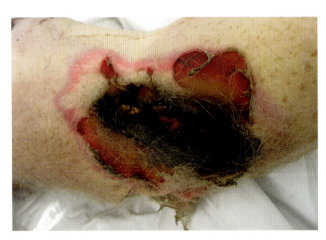

Figure 14.6. High-voltage electrocution. The decedent came into contact with a high-voltage wire, which left a linear charred area of the skin surrounded by a rim of sloughed skin and erythema.

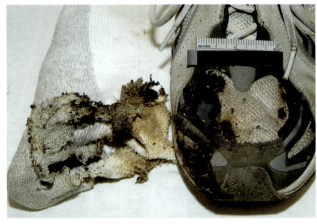

Figure 14.7. High-voltage electrocution. In the case of an electrocution, examination of the clothing may reveal burn marks from passage of the electricity.

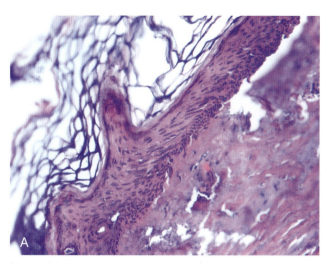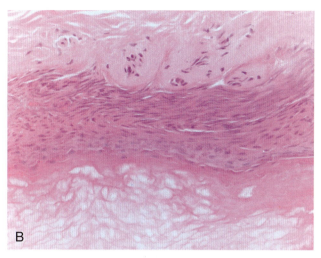

Figure 14.8. Microscopic examination of electrocution. In (A), there is a basket weave pattern to the keratin, streaming of the nuclei, and disruption of the fibers in the dermis (high power, H&E), in (B), are similar changes, albeit the nuclear streaming is the most pronounced.

the animal can also occur. In this situation, identification of an antemortem vital reaction to the dog bites would be important to distinguish the two circumstances (Figure 14.9A and B).

AUTOPSY FINDINGS ASSOCIATED WITH FATAL DOG ATTACK

DeMunnynck describe dog bites as having a puncture site with adjacent tear, with the puncture wound made by the canine and other teeth causing stretch-type lacerations, or hole and tear pattern.[31] Associated with these bite marks will be claw marks, which are parallel superficial abrasions (Figure 14.10). The bite mark pattern is caused by the dog biting and shaking the decedent. Bite mark analysis can be performed with dog bites as well.[31]

PEARLS & PITFALLS

DeMunnynck advocates extensive analysis of the dog(s) involved in the incident to include collection of trace evidence (to link the dog to the decedent), exclusion of infectious disease in the dog(s) such as rabies, toxicology analysis to detect for stimulating substances in the dog, examination of the dog's oral cavity, including making a cast, documentation of any possible identifying features on the dog to assist with identification of the owner if they are unknown, and examination of the intestinal contents of the dog, looking for tissue, blood, and clothing fragments.[31] To make many of these observations would, of course, require the death of the dog and subsequent necropsy of the dog.

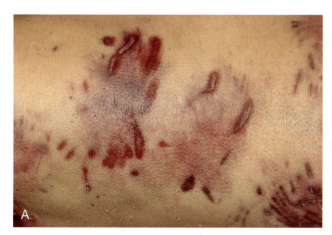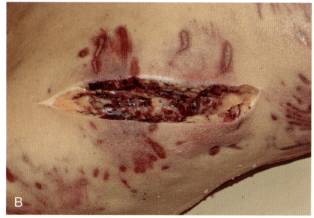

Figure 14.9. Dog mauling. Initially, this individual was believed to have been deceased prior to the dog attack, and the dog attack was believed to be postmortem. However, on the back, two dog bite marks were identified (A) and incision into the skin revealed hemorrhage in the underlying adipose tissue (B), consistent with the individual being alive at the time the wounds were inflicted. If necessary, bite mark analysis of the injuries could be performed.

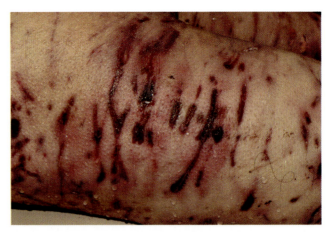

Figure 14.10. Claw marks from dog attack. On the thigh are numerous parallel linear abrasions, which are consistent with scratches from the dogs.

SNAKE BITE

INTRODUCTION

Of around 45,000 snakebites in the United States per year, 8000 are from venomous snakes and cause five to six deaths.[32] Poisonous snakes in the United States include pit vipers such as copperheads, cottonmouths, and rattlesnakes, and coral snakes. Pit viper venom is composed of various types of transaminase, hyaluronidase, phospholipase, phosphodiesterase, and endonuclease (RNase [ribonuclease] and DNase [deoxyribonuclease]); whereas coral snake venom contains phospholipase A2 and an α-neurotoxin.[32] The diagnosis of a snake bite at autopsy requires a consideration of the condition, knowledge of potential exposure (either from the scene or historical description), and interpretation of autopsy findings.

PATHOLOGIC FEATURES OF PIT VIPER INJURY

Autopsy findings associated with death due to a pit viper bite could include puncture sites, edema, possible bullae (which can contain clear watery fluid or hemorrhagic fluid), lymphangitis and ecchymosis (which can take hours to develop), and coagulopathy and shock.[32]

CLINICAL FEATURES OF PIT VIPER INJURY

Individuals who have been bitten by a pit viper will report pain, nausea and vomiting, perioral paresthesia, tingling of extremities, fasciculations, and abnormal taste, including metallic or minty. Shock, altered mental status, tachycardia, hypotension, and respiratory distress can develop.[32] If the individual has a period of survival after the event, this historical information may be determined through witness interviews.

PATHOLOGIC FEATURES OF CORAL SNAKE INJURY

Autopsy findings associated with a coral snake bite as compared to a pit viper bite are minimal, being essentially none.[32]

CLINICAL FEATURES OF CORAL SNAKE INJURY

Individuals who have been bitten by a coral snake will report tremors, increased salivation, altered sensations, and cranial nerve manifestations (including ptosis and dysphagia), with paralysis of respiratory musculature causing death.[32] This historical information may be available through witness statements and assist in the determination of the cause of death.

SPIDER BITE[33]

INTRODUCTION

Two poisonous spiders to which individuals in the United States may be exposed are black widow (genus *Latrodectus*) and recluse (genus *Loxosceles*), both brown recluse and Chilean recluse. Bites due to either the black widow or the recluse spider are rarely lethal.

PATHOLOGIC FEATURES OF BLACK WIDOW BITE

Autopsy findings associated with a black widow bite are often only minimal inflammation at the site of the bite; however, there may be no pathologic findings at all.

CLINICAL FEATURES OF BLACK WIDOW BITE

Patients often have moderate to severe pain, and symptoms begin within 2 hours of the bite to include muscle spasm and rigidity, which begin at site of bite, and spread to the trunk and face. Systemic symptoms can include arthralgia, diaphoresis, fever, nausea and vomiting, and other features.[33] Given that the spider bite may go unrecognized, historical information through witnesses may assist in determining the cause of death.

PATHOLOGIC FEATURES OF RECLUSE BITE

Autopsy findings associated with a recluse spider bite are inflammation at the site of the bite, with the inflammation spreading over time.

CLINICAL FEATURES OF RECLUSE BITE

Patients often have minimal pain at the spider bite site, and symptoms occur 3 to 7 days after the bite, and include arthralgia, fever, chills, and rash. The fever can lead to febrile seizures and both hemoglobinuria and myoglobinuria, which can precipitate acute renal failure.[33]

OTHER FORMS OF ANIMAL ATTACK ENCOUNTERED BY FORENSIC PATHOLOGISTS

In addition to dogs, snakes, and spiders, forensic pathologists in the United States can also encounter injuries due to interactions with bears, crocodiles, alligators, cattle or horses, moose, deer and elk, sharks, animals in the zoo, fire ants, killer bees, scorpions, and others.[34-41] While injuries from animals can be a variety of blunt and sharp force injuries, injuries inflicted by alligators and sharks tend to have some degree of crush-type injury.[37]

HIGH-ALTITUDE PULMONARY EDEMA/ HIGH-ALTITUDE CEREBRAL EDEMA[42]

FEATURES OF HIGH-ALTITUDE CEREBRAL EDEMA

While the mechanism leading to cerebral edema developing in a high-altitude environment is uncertain, the changes are often centered on the splenium of the corpus callosum and the cerebral edema that develops can lead to herniation and death.

FEATURES OF HIGH-ALTITUDE PULMONARY EDEMA

In certain individuals, a rapid ascent or heavy exertion in a high altitude environment can lead to pulmonary edema, especially in individuals with other risk factors including pre-existing risk factors, a previous episode of high-altitude illness, or a normal residence in a low altitude region.

AUTOPSY FINDINGS IN HIGH-ALTITUDE PULMONARY EDEMA

High-altitude pulmonary edema can cause death. Autopsy findings can include edema, hemorrhage in the alveoli, thrombi in the small capillaries, and hyaline membranes.[43]

NEAR MISSES

Near Miss #1: This individual was found outside in the cold weather. Neither scene investigation nor autopsy identified any suspicious findings or evidence of trauma. The cranium was found to have a diastatic fracture of the sagittal suture, which normally occurs with cerebral edema (Figure 14.11). There was some posterior congestion and subgaleal hemorrhage along the line of the diastatic fracture. The diastatic fracture was interpreted as an artifact due to the freeze-thaw cycles the body had gone through, with expansion of the cerebral parenchyma.

Near Miss #2: This elderly woman was found dead in her unheated and unlit garage. She was partially undressed and a patch of blood on the concrete was identified near her (Figure 14.12). The scene image is at least suggestive of a suspicious death; however, no significant injuries other than abrasions of the knees were identified at autopsy. She was believed to have entered the garage, become disoriented, and been unable to find her way out. No pathologic evidence of a recent stroke or other acute intracerebral event was identified.

Near Miss #3: This individual was found floating in the water, with a duffel bag loaded with masonry stone roped to his chest (Figure 14.13). While the finding is at least suspicious for a homicide, with an attempt to dispose of the body in the water, neither scene investigation nor autopsy identified another cause of death other than drowning. The decedent had Huntington chorea. The masonry stone could be matched to stone at his residence. The manner of death was certified as suicide.

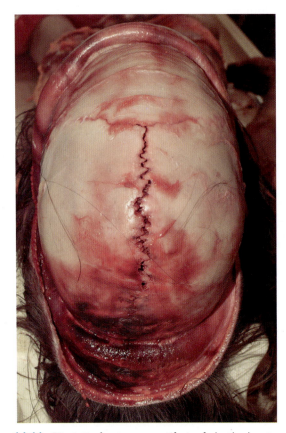

Figure 14.11. Diastatic fracture as artifact of death due to hypothermia.

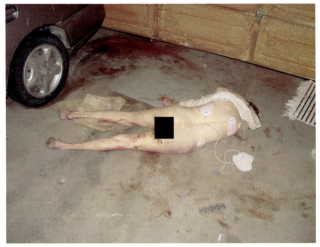

Figure 14.12. Hypothermia-related death, with blood on floor and pathologic undressing, creating a suspicious death scene.

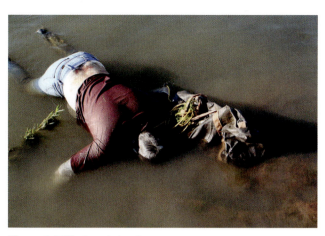

Figure 14.13. Suicide by drowning.

Near Miss #4: This individual was witnessed to jump up and grab a high-voltage wire. The wire came to rest on his neck, and the burn created mimics an incised wound, with even damage to the underlying thyroid cartilage (Figure 14.14).

Near Miss #5: This individual was found dead outdoors and covered with snow (Figure 14.15). The scene investigation suggested hypothermia as the cause of death; however, the individual had a seizure disorder that was due to past head trauma. Autopsy did not reveal features of hypothermia such as frost erythema or Wischnewski spots; however, a death due to hypothermia can occur without those pathologic features being identified at autopsy. In this situation, the decedent essentially has two potential causes of death, both of which are a diagnosis of exclusion (ie, hypothermia and traumatic seizure disorder). The wording of the death certificate could employ both, one as the cause of death and one as contributory, or only one, leaving the other off the death certificate. Although it did not matter in this case, as both causes of death were associated with an accidental manner of death, if there is a discrepancy in manners between two competing causes of death, choosing the non-natural manner is probably the best option.

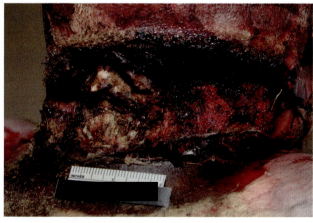

Figure 14.14. Electrocution burn injury mimicking an incised wound. Contact with the high-voltage wire caused the skin at the neck to split and even damaging the underlying thyroid cartilage.

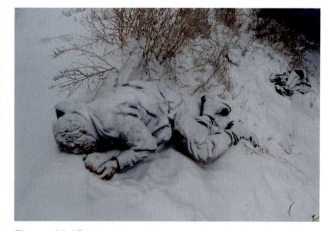

Figure 14.15. Decedent with seizure disorder found outdoors, covered with snow.

References

1. Christiansen LR, Collins KA. Pathologic findings in malignant hyperthermia: a case report and review of literature. *Am J Forensic Med Pathol*. 2004;25(4):327-333.
2. Lugo-Amador NM, Rothenhaus T, Moyer P. Heat-related illness. *Emerg Med Clin North Am*. 2004;22(2):315-327.
3. Quinton RA. Certification of vehicular hyperthermia deaths in the pediatric population. *Acad Forensic Pathol*. 2016;6(4):657-662.
4. Ball CG, Herath JC. Earth, air, water, and fire: histopathology of environmental death. *Acad Forensic Pathol*. 2018;8(3):641-652.
5. Howe JA, Collins KA, King PS, et al. Investigation of elder deaths. *Acad Forensic Pathol*. 2014;4(3):290-304.
6. Palmiere C, Mangin P. Hyperthermia and postmortem biochemical investigations. *Int J Legal Med*. 2013;127(1):93-102.
7. Preuss J, Dettmeyer R, Lignitz E, Madea B. Fatty degeneration of myocardial cells as a sign of death due to hypothermia versus degenerative deposition of lipofuscin. *Forensic Sci Int*. 2006;159:1-5.
8. Turk EE, Sperhake JP, Pueschel K, Tsokos M. An approach to the evaluation of fatal hypothermia. *Forensic Sci Med Pathol*. 2005;1(1):31-35.
9. Preuss J, Lignitz E, Dettmeyer R, Madea B. Pancreatic changes in cases of death due to hypothermia. *Forensic Sci Int*. 2007;166(2-3):194-198.
10. Palmiere C, Teresiński G, Hejna P. Postmortem diagnosis of hypothermia. *Int J Legal Med*. 2014;128(4):607-614.
11. Turk EE. Hypothermia. *Forensic Sci Med Pathol*. 2010;6:106-115.
12. Bright F, Winskog C, Byard RW. Wischnewski spots and hypothermia: sensitive, specific, or serendipitous. *Forensic Sci Med Pathol*. 2013;9:88-90.
13. Van Tilburg C. Non-avalanche-related snow immersion deaths: tree well and deep snow immersion asphyxiation. *Wilderness Environ Med*. 2010;21(3):257-261.
14. Kizer KW, MacQuarrie MB, Kuhn BJ, Scannell PD. Deep snow immersion deaths. *Phys Sportsmed*. 1994;22(12):48-61. doi:10.1080/00913847.1994.11947718
15. Davis JH. Bodies found in the water: an investigative approach. *Am J Forensic Med Pathol*. 1986;7(4):291-297.
16. Ihama Y, Ninomiya K, Noguchi M, Fuke C, Miyazaki T. Fatal propeller injuries: three autopsy case reports. *J Forensic Leg Med*. 2009;16(7):420-423.
17. Lippmann J, Lawrence C, Davis M. Scuba diving-related fatalities in New Zealand, 2007 to 2016. *Diving Hyperb Med*. 2021;20;51(4):345-354.
18. Lippmann J, Taylor DM. Medical conditions in scuba diving fatality victims in Australia, 2001 to 2013. *Diving Hyperb Med*. 2020;50(2):98-104.
19. Aquila I, Pepe F, Manno M, et al. Scuba diving death: always due to drowning? Two forensic cases and a review of the literature. *Med Leg J*. 2018;86(1):49-51.
20. Edmonds C, Lippmann J, Fock A. Immersion pulmonary edema: case reports from Oceania. *Undersea Hyperb Med*. 2019;46(5):581-601.
21. Evain F, Louge P, Pignel R, Fracasso T, Rouyer F. Fatal diving: could it be an immersion pulmonary edema? Case report. *Int J Legal Med*. 2022;136(3):713-717.
22. Vinkel J, Bak P, Juel Thiis Knudsen P, Hyldegaard O. Forensic case reports presenting immersion pulmonary edema as a differential diagnosis in fatal diving accidents. *J Forensic Sci*. 2018;63(1):299-304.
23. Wheen LC, Williams MP. Post-mortems in recreational scuba diver deaths: the utility of radiology. *J Forensic Leg Med*. 2009;16(5):273-276.
24. Williamson JA, King GK, Callanan VI, Lanskey RM, Rich KW. Fatal arterial gas embolism: detection by chest radiography and imaging before autopsy. *Med J Aust*. 1990;153(2):97-100.
25. Ozdoba C, Weis J, Plattner T, Dirnhofer R, Yen K. Fatal scuba diving incident with massive gas embolism in cerebral and spinal arteries. *Neuroradiology*. 2005;47(6):411-416.
26. Türkmen N, Akan O, Cetin S, Eren B, Gürses MS, Gündoğmuş UN. Scuba diver deaths due to air embolism: two case reports. *Soud Lek*. 2013;58(2):26-28.

27. Casadesús JM, Aguirre F, Carrera A, Boadas-Vaello P, Serrando MT, Reina F. Diagnosis of arterial gas embolism in SCUBA diving: modification suggestion of autopsy techniques and experience in eight cases. *Forensic Sci Med Pathol*. 2018;14(1):18-25.
28. Smart DR, Sage M, Davis FM. Two fatal cases of immersion pulmonary oedema—using dive accident investigation to assist the forensic pathologist. *Diving Hyperb Med*. 2014;44(2):97-100.
29. Jin X, Chen D, Li X, et al. Advances in forensic diagnosis of electric shock death in the absence of typical electrical marks. *Int J Legal Med*. 2021;135(6):2469-2478.
30. DiMaio VJM, Molina DK. *DiMaio's Forensic Pathology*. 3rd ed. CRC Press; 2022.
31. DeMunnynck K, Van de Voorde W. Forensic approach of fatal dog attacks: a case report and literature review. *Int J Leg Med*. 2002;116(5):295-300.
32. Gold BS, Barish RA, Dart RC. North American snake envenomation: diagnosis, treatment, and management. *Emerg Med Clin North Am*. 2004;22(2):423-443, ix.
33. Diaz JH, Leblanc KE. Common spider bites. *Am Fam Physician*. 2007;75(6):869-873.
34. De Giorgio F, Rainio J, Pascali V, Lalu K. Bear attack–a unique fatality in Finland. *Forensic Sci Int*. 2007;173(1):64-67.
35. Chattopadhyay S, Shee B, Sukul B. Fatal crocodile attack. *J Forensic Leg Med*. 2013;20(8):1139-1141.
36. Schoeb TR, Heaton-Jones TG, Clemmons RM, et al. Clinical and necropsy findings associated with increased mortality among American alligators of Lake Griffin, Florida. *J Wildl Dis*. 2002;38(2):320-337.
37. Bury D, Langlois N, Byard RW. Animal-related fatalities–Part I: Characteristic autopsy findings and variable causes of death associated with blunt and sharp trauma. *J Forensic Sci*. 2012;57(2):370-374.
38. Byard RW, Gilbert JD, Brown K. Pathologic features of fatal shark attacks. *Am J Forensic Med Pathol*. 2000;21(3):225-229.
39. Prahlow JA, Barnard JJ. Fatal anaphylaxis due to fire ant stings. *Am J Forensic Med Pathol*. 1998;19(2):137-142.
40. França FO, Benvenuti LA, Fan HW, et al. Severe and fatal mass attacks by "killer" bees (Africanized honey bees–Apis mellifera scutellata) in Brazil: clinicopathological studies with measurement of serum venom concentrations. *Q J Med*. 1994;87(5):269-282.
41. Hughes RL. A fatal case of acute renal failure from envenoming syndrome after massive bee attack: a case report and literature review. *Am J Forensic Med Pathol*. 2019;40(1):52-57.
42. Gallagher SA, Hackett PH. High-altitude illness. *Emerg Med Clin North Am*. 2004;22:329-355.
43. Hultgren HN, Wilson R, Kosek JC. Lung pathology in high-altitude pulmonary edema. *Wilderness Environ Med*. 1997;8(4):218-220.

POSTMORTEM TOXICOLOGY 15

CHAPTER OUTLINE

Introduction 444
- Autopsy findings of a drug overdose 444
- Obtaining specimens for toxicologic analysis 447
- Interpretation of toxicologic results 450
- Description of postmortem redistribution and its importance 451
- Specific drugs encountered by forensic pathologists 453

Metabolites of Common Drugs 454

Ethanol 454

INTRODUCTION

Forensic pathologists routinely autopsy individuals whose cause of death is a drug overdose. The potential list of drugs used by decedents can include both prescription medications (eg, opioid medications, psychiatric-type medications) and illicit substances (eg, methamphetamine, cocaine). Prescription medications can also be used illicitly (eg, someone selling their prescribed medication to another person). And medication that is normally considered a prescription medication can also be produced illicitly (eg, fentanyl). While some individuals who die as the result of a drug overdose will have a long history of drug use, others may have no history of drug use. The episode of drug use that led to death is usually for recreational purposes or occasionally suicidal purposes but drugs can also be forcefully or clandestinely given to another person with the intent of harming or killing them.

While the scene investigation can provide evidence in support of a drug overdose as the cause of death (eg, drug paraphernalia found adjacent to the body with evidence of recent drug use such as burned material on tin foil or a suicide note combined with the presence of empty recently prescribed pill containers) and while autopsy findings can be suggestive of a drug overdose (eg, cerebral edema in a young individual with no other cause for the edema identified), toxicologic analysis of body fluids is required to confirm the cause of death as a drug overdose. In addition, even though a scene investigation and autopsy findings may not be suggestive of a drug overdose, subsequent analysis of body fluids obtained at autopsy may in fact reveal that the cause of death is a drug overdose.

> **PEARLS & PITFALLS**
>
> A useful resource for identifying pills found at the scene or with the body at autopsy is www.drugs.com. When the shape of the pill (eg, round or oval), the color of the pill (eg, white, orange), and the imprint(s) on the pill are entered into the database, the identity of the pill will be listed.

Key steps in identifying a drug overdose as the cause of death
- Identify scene and/or autopsy findings that suggest a drug overdose
- Obtain appropriate samples for toxicologic analysis
- Interpret toxicology testing results

Autopsy findings of a drug overdose: While no autopsy findings are diagnostic of a drug overdose, and to identify a drug overdose, toxicologic analysis of the body fluids must be performed, when a person dies as the result of a drug overdose, some external and internal examination findings as well as some microscopic findings are commonly found at autopsy.

On external examination, autopsy findings associated with a drug overdose include conjunctival edema (ie, a mucoidlike conjunctiva) and an oronasal foam cone, which are associated with opioid-type drug overdoses (Figure 15.1A and B). An oronasal foam cone is not specific for a drug overdose and can be found in a variety of other deaths, including drowning and other causes (Figure 15.2A-D). With some survival and with damage to the liver (eg, in an acetaminophen overdose (Figure 15.3A and B)), the conjunctiva may have a yellow discoloration (ie, scleral icterus). Regarding eye findings in a drug overdose, Flaagøy et al. indicate that ethanol may contribute to the development of petechial hemorrhages.[1] In addition to ocular findings, other external evidence of drug use or at least findings consistent with drug use and the associated lifestyle are track marks on the body (Figure 15.4A and B), aggressive dental caries, periodontitis, and poor oral hygiene (Figure 15.5).[2] Track marks can occur in a variety of locations including the upper extremities, the scrotum, and the feet.

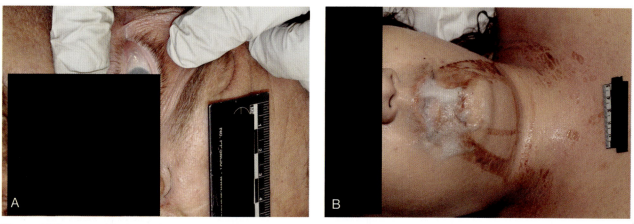

Figure 15.1. External findings of a drug overdose. Both conjunctival edema (**A**) and an oronasal foam cone (**B**) can be found in a drug overdose, most often when the substance used was an opiate or opioid.

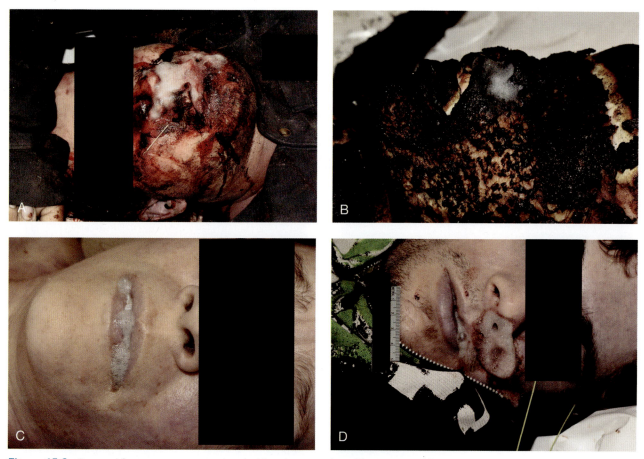

Figure 15.2. Oronasal foam cones not associated with a drug overdose. These oronasal foam cones occurred associated with a motor vehicle accident (**A**), a fire death (**B**), a subarachnoid hemorrhage after a ruptured berry aneurysm (**C**), and an atlanto-occipital dislocation (**D**). In all cases, the toxicologic testing did not disclose a drug overdose.

On internal examination, findings associated with an opioid-type drug overdose include cerebral edema (Figure 15.6), congested lungs (which can exude white frothy fluid upon palpation), a full bladder, and formed feces in the proximal and transverse colon as opioids tend to slow transit through the bowel. Regarding congested lungs and their subsequent increased weight, the ratio of lung to heart weight could serve as a negative marker for a drug overdose.[3] Occasionally a plastic bag will be found in the stomach or remainder of the gastrointestinal tract (Figure 15.7A and B). And, in some areas, especially where drug trafficking occurs across borders, multiple packages containing drugs can be found in the

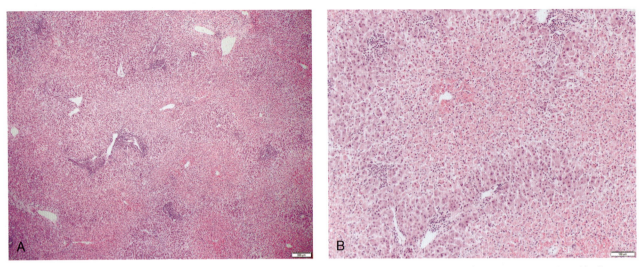

Figure 15.3. Acetaminophen toxicity. The liver is from an individual who overdosed with acetaminophen. Low power (**A**) and high power (**B**) show marked centrilobular necrosis of the hepatocytes, with only a thin rim of periportal hepatocytes being histologically viable.

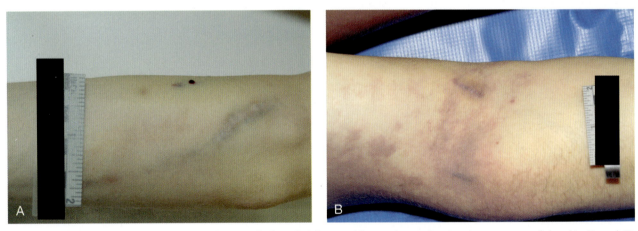

Figure 15.4. Track marks. Track marks are linear and often slightly raised hemorrhagic discolorations or scars of the skin (**A** and **B**). Distinguishing between a track mark and a traumatic scar in any given case can be challenging; however, if necessary, excision of the location and histologic evaluation for foreign material may assist in the differentiation.

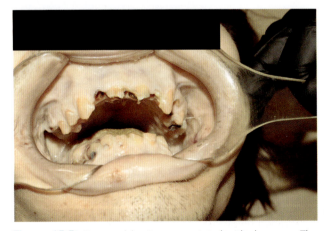

Figure 15.5. Poor oral hygiene associated with drug use. The teeth of drug users are often in poor shape, with prominent dental caries, erosion of teeth, and complete loss of teeth.

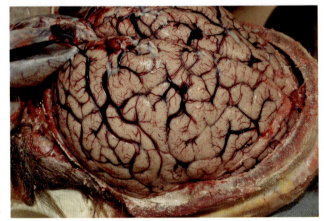

Figure 15.6. Cerebral edema occurring as the result of a methadone overdose. As opioid overdoses can cause death more slowly, the body has time to develop changes including cerebral edema and bronchopneumonia. The gyri are flattened and the sulci are effaced.

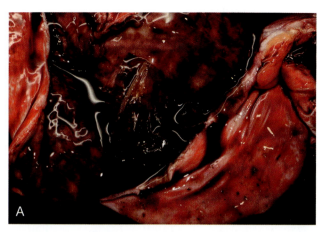 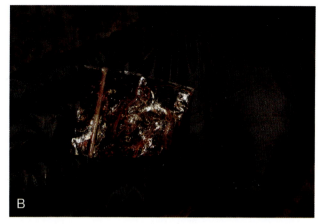

Figure 15.7. Baggie in stomach. When confronted by police, individuals may choose to swallow a baggie of drugs, which can lead to an overdose. At autopsy, the baggie can often be identified in the stomach (**A** and **B**).

gastrointestinal tract. Microscopic examination of the lungs may reveal bronchopneumonia. Pathologic findings that commonly result from intravenous drug use and its complications can also be identified at autopsy including bacterial endocarditis, which can result in septic emboli and abscesses in the heart, the brain, and other organs, and complications of blood borne pathogens can also be found, such as hepatitis or immunosuppression leading to fungal infections. Cocaine and methamphetamine can trigger tears of blood vessels and contribute to various forms of hemorrhage, including intracerebral hemorrhage, aortic dissection, and rupture of aneurysms. In intravenous drug users, microscopic examination of the lung can reveal polarizable foreign material (Figure 15.8A-D).

PEARLS & PITFALLS

While the ingestion of ethylene glycol, a chemical found in antifreeze, is not by itself lethal, alcohol dehydrogenase will convert the ethylene glycol to oxalic acid, which will accumulate in the kidney and can lead to death. Microscopic examination of the kidney will reveal oxalic acid crystals (Figure 15.9A and B). The fungus *Aspergillus niger* can also produce oxalic acid, which will often remain localized around the distribution of the fungus, but can enter the circulation and deposit in the kidney.[4,5] In addition, oxalic acid crystals in kidney can occur due to massive vitamin C administration associated with fluid resuscitation in burn units.[6] Methanol when ingested will be converted by alcohol dehydrogenase to formaldehyde.

PEARLS & PITFALLS

Methamphetamine use is associated with a clinically recognized methamphetamine-associated cardiomyopathy, described as unexplained heart failure that develops in individuals who use methamphetamine.[7] The cardiomyopathy is associated with left ventricular dilation and fibrosis.[8] Methamphetamine is associated with pulmonary hypertension due to the preferential accumulation of the drug in the lung.[8]

Obtaining specimens for toxicologic analysis: Blood for toxicologic analysis can be taken from a variety of locations: femoral, heart, subclavian, inferior vena cava, and, if necessary, body cavity. Based upon the effects of postmortem redistribution in most cases, peripheral blood (eg, femoral blood) is favored over central blood (eg, heart) for analysis of drug concentrations. Blind sticks of the heart should not be performed, as other organs such as the stomach might be hit by the sampling needle, which can result in concentrations of drugs and alcohol that are not representative of the decedent's

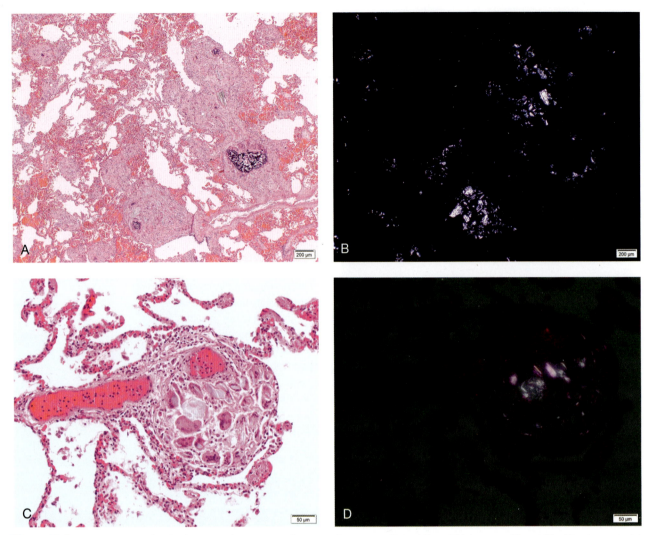

Figure 15.8. Foreign material in the lung in an intravenous drug user. Low power (A and B) and high power (C and D) of foreign material in the lung, seen best with polarized light (B and D). Although the foreign material can often be seen with just regular light microscopy, routinely polarizing the lung tissue can often reveal an unexpected finding. In (C and D), the foreign material is clearly associated with a blood vessel, as would be expected given the route of entry.

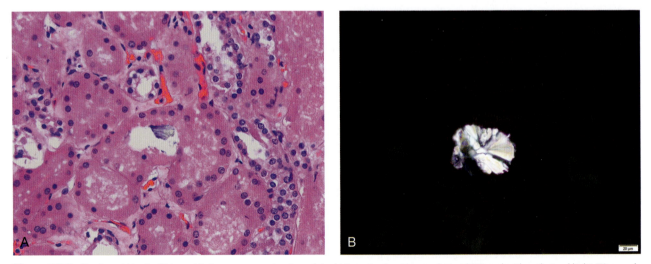

Figure 15.9. Oxalic acid in the kidney. High power examination of the kidney, both with unpolarized (A) and with polarized light (B) reveals the oxalic acid crystals. In addition to ethylene glycol exposure, some species of *Aspergillus* produce oxalic acid, and oxalic acid can be a component of kidney stones.

antemortem state.[9] If subclavian blood is drawn from near the midline, technically, it would seem that the airway can be hit, which could contain vomitus. If the decedent just ingested the drug and vomited, it could result in an artificially elevated concentration of a drug. In addition to blood, other specimens routinely obtained at autopsy include vitreous fluid, urine, and bile. If blood is not available for analysis, such as in a decomposed body, liver and skeletal muscle can be obtained. Brain is also a potential tissue to be used for toxicologic analysis and may assist with evaluation of concentrations of some opioids, including codeine, fentanyl, oxycodone, and tramadol.[10] For fetal autopsies, meconium can serve as a sample for drug analysis. Hair, blood spot cards, and bone may also serve as a source for drug analysis.[11,12]

PEARLS & PITFALLS

A postmortem urine drug screen can assist a forensic pathologist in determining what pathway their autopsy examination will take, and can help guide postmortem toxicologic analysis. If no urine is present, a small amount of sterile saline can be introduced into the bladder (ie, a bladder wash) and then aspirated and used for the urine drug screen.

PEARLS & PITFALLS

While blood can often be obtained simply through direct puncture of the femoral vasculature via a needle inserted through the skin, in some cases such as when the decedent has exsanguinated, this simple procedure does not obtain an adequate amount of blood. Two methods can be employed to increase the yield. First, if one individual draws blood while a second person massages the lower extremity, blood can be forced into the femoral region and aspirated from the vasculature. Second, if blood cannot be obtained by needle puncture of the vasculature in the femoral region even with the assistance of another person, an incision can be made in the skin to directly access the vasculature. In doing so use caution to not transect the femoral artery and vein, as this can impair subsequent embalming procedures.

FAQ: Can cavity blood be used for analysis?

Answer: When an individual is shot, stabbed, or sustains another event causing blood loss into a body cavity (eg, an aortic dissection), obtaining enough blood from the vasculature for toxicologic analysis can be difficult. While the body cavity blood can be collected and submitted for qualitative analysis (ie, to determine what drugs are present), it should not be used for quantitative analysis as the concentrations of drugs in the body cavity blood will not likely accurately represent the concentrations in the peripheral blood.[13]

PEARLS & PITFALLS

If a subdural hemorrhage is the cause of death, analysis of the blood within the clot may be more consistent with the toxicologic concentration of a substance in the decedent's blood at the time of the injury than the concentration in the postmortem autopsy blood obtained via needle from the vasculature.[14] Any drug present in the subdural hemorrhage is outside the normal flow of blood and may not be metabolized as quickly as the drug would be if it were in the normal circulation. As there is some period of survival during the development of a subdural hemorrhage, the drug in the circulated blood will be metabolized to a lower concentration than what was present when the injury occurred.

> **PEARLS & PITFALLS**
>
> When separate toxicologic analyses find discrepant results (eg, between hospital blood and autopsy blood, or between autopsy blood from different regions of the body), one consideration is different testing modalities. Johnson et al. present a case where discrepant ethanol results were found between the hospital laboratory and the forensic laboratory.[15] The two laboratories used different testing modalities, one of which was sensitive to lipemia, but the other modality was not, and the decedent had lipemia.

> **PEARLS & PITFALLS**
>
> If an individual is suspected to have sustained a drug overdose and subsequently died in the hospital, it is important to obtain their admission blood for testing, as the delay between the time of admission and the time of death will allow for continued metabolism of the drug and the postmortem specimen obtained at autopsy will not allow for an accurate determination of the lethal drug concentration. Unfortunately, hospitals will only hold blood for a certain period of time. A pre-existing arrangement with hospitals to hold admission blood on suspected drug overdoses for a longer period of time may help preserve these specimens for future testing if necessary.

Interpretation of toxicologic results: While the toxicology lab will provide both qualitative results (what drug is present) and quantitative results (how much of a drug is present), the forensic pathologist must interpret these results in the context of the scene investigation, medical history, and autopsy findings. To do so, a forensic pathologist should have access to one or more references that list toxic and lethal drug concentrations.[16-23] When interpreting toxicology results, it must be remembered that, with rare exception, the pathologist is only given one drug concentration (ie, the concentration of the drug in the postmortem blood). The pathologist is not usually given previous drug concentrations as they are most often not available, so care must be used in the interpretation of that one concentration as to whether the individual would have died as a result of the drug concentration that was present, whether the individual would have been impaired, or what amount of the drug the individual may have used. Over-interpreting or under-interpreting the results of a single point measurement can easily be done if the forensic pathologist is not careful.

To interpret drug concentrations for prescription medication, the name of the medication, the strength of the medication per pill (ie, milligrams of medication per pill), the date of death, the date the prescription was filled, the number of pills dispensed, and the number of pills remaining must be known. In addition, information regarding the decedent's history of prescription medication or illicit drug use is valuable, especially with opioid medications as the decedent may have tolerance to the drug. For example, the interpretation of the concentration of oxycodone in a deceased individual who was a naive user is different than if the deceased individual had been prescribed and had taken oxycodone for 10 years and has likely developed tolerance. Another consideration is that obese individuals and those with heart or lung disease may have less of a physiologic reserve and may have increased susceptibility to the toxic effects of opioids and other drugs.[24] Diseases of the liver and kidney may also contribute to altered metabolism of the medication.

In addition to considering the amount of drug taken, potential tolerance to the drug or increased sensitivity to the medication's effects, and the effects of postmortem redistribution, which will be discussed below, the forensic pathologist must consider numerous factors that can affect the concentration of drug identified in the postmortem sample and should be considered when interpreting the toxicology results. Kamphuis et al. determined that the degree of decomposition, the position of the body when found, the route of drug administration, and resuscitation efforts can all affect the central blood/peripheral blood ratio for morphine.[25] Zilg et al. also found that the ratio of central to peripheral blood drug concentration increased with increasing postmortem interval.[26] And, activity of cytochrome P450 (CYP) enzymes, including CYP1A2, CYP3A4, CYP2C19, and CYP2D6, may also affect the metabolism of drugs and hence potentially predispose to drug overdose.[27-32]

Key factors to consider when interpreting postmortem drug concentrations
- Scene investigation findings, including pill counts
- Source of the specimen used for analysis
- Postmortem redistribution
- Potential tolerance
- Decomposition
- Underlying medical conditions, including liver or kidney disease
- Activity of CYP enzymes

Description of postmortem redistribution and its importance: Postmortem redistribution is the change in concentration of a drug that occurs between death and the time of autopsy blood sampling.[33] Jones and Pounder determined that the postmortem concentrations of certain drugs (ie, imipramine, desipramine, and codeine) varied depending upon where the blood sample was taken from (eg, femoral vs heart blood) while other drugs (ie, ethanol and acetaminophen) did not have such variance.[34] Additional authors have explored this phenomenon with other drugs. Gerostamoulos et al. obtained blood from deceased bodies twice, once at admission to the morgue and then at autopsy and compared the concentrations.[35] The average time between the initial drawing of specimens and autopsy was 64 hours. Methadone, 2-ethylidene-1,5-dimethyl-3,3-diphenylpyrrolidine (EDDP), fluoxetine, mirtazapine, and sertraline had statistically significant increases in concentrations between the two specimens. 6-acetylmorphine, 9-hydroxy-risperidone, and caffeine each had a statistically significant decrease in the concentration between the two specimens. Mantinieks et al. report postmortem/antemortem ratios for 42 drugs, with all anti-depressants having a ratio of >1 and benzodiazepines having a ratio <1.[36] Based upon previous works by Saitman et al, McIntyre (2014), McIntyre et al (2012), and McIntyre et al (2014), McIntyre (2016) presented a theoretical postmortem redistribution factor for 44 drugs, which indicate the drug's propensity for postmortem redistribution.[37-41] The author discusses numerous confounding factors such as time between death and autopsy and incomplete distribution of drugs in the body; however, the listing of drugs provides a reference as to which drugs are more likely to be susceptible to postmortem redistribution (eg, sertraline, fluoxetine, desipramine) and which drugs are likely to be more resistant (eg, gabapentin, ethanol, acetaminophen, bupropion).

Pounder and Jones offered two potential explanations for postmortem redistribution: (1) postmortem release of drugs from organs such as the lung or liver where they are concentrated in a living person and (2) incomplete distribution of the drug during life (eg, death occurring shortly after the overdose and before an equilibrium level can be achieved in the blood).[34] Pounder and Jones opined that postmortem redistribution comes from postmortem diffusion of drugs along a concentration gradient.[33] In the living person, the lung and the liver can have higher concentrations of a drug than the blood, so, after death, drugs from these organs can diffuse into the heart blood, and then, blood drawn from the heart could have artificially elevated concentrations of certain drugs. Jones and Pounder found an up to eightfold concentration difference between central and peripheral blood for some drugs, with central blood having the higher drug concentrations, which shows that drugs affected by postmortem redistribution are more likely to have falsely elevated concentrations in central blood than peripheral blood.[34]

Numerous authors have commented on the importance of postmortem redistribution. Pounder and Jones stated that "…'postmortem drug redistribution' creates major difficulties in the interpretation of the significance of postmortem drug concentrations in the blood" and "Perhaps most importantly, the phenomenon of 'postmortem drug redistribution' undermines the reference value of databases of drug concentrations in postmortem blood where the site of origin of the sample is unknown."[33] Prouty and Anderson state, "In many more instances than was previously thought, it is desirable or necessary to analyze peripheral blood and tissue specimens to provide a proper foundation to render an opinion as to the role of a drug in the death of an individual."[42] Hilberg et al. stated that "The present study [the authors] confirms that the drug concentration in femoral blood is closer to antemortem levels than cardiac blood."[43] However, as some drugs show a higher concentration in femoral blood than heart blood (such as marijuana) the authors did recommend that several specimens be taken. Andreson et al. succinctly summarized the concept of postmortem redistribution saying, "The phenomenon of PMR [postmortem redistribution] has been known for many years. PMR results in higher concentrations of drugs in blood samples than true concentrations at time of death, possibly leading to misinterpretation by inexperienced persons, and potentially having serious consequences."[44] Unfortunately, Brockbals et al. opined that no accurate methods to predict postmortem redistribution are available.[45]

> **PEARLS & PITFALLS**
>
> Fentanyl is subject to postmortem redistribution, which can render interpretations of postmortem heart blood concentrations and even femoral blood concentrations problematic. Olson and Palamalai indicate that liver is a better source for determination of postmortem fentanyl concentrations.[46,47]

> **PEARLS & PITFALLS**
>
> When trying to determine whether a particular concentration of a drug is lethal, while references can be used for comparison, routine searching in www.PubMed.gov can help identify case reports and other useful articles, which can provide potential information regarding lethal concentrations. For example, Cantrell et al. reported a fatality due to a gabapentin overdose, whereas, if a forensic pathologist is not using the most up-to-date and thoroughly cited reference, some drugs may not have established lethal concentrations.[48] The decedent described by Cantrell et al. had a peripheral blood concentration of 37 mg/L.

SAMPLE NOTES: WORDING OF CAUSE OF DEATH WHEN A DRUG OVERDOSE

The cause of death from a drug overdose can be worded in several ways. If a single drug is responsible for death, the cause of death could be worded "Toxic effects of methamphetamine" or "Methamphetamine toxicity," or "Drug overdose (methamphetamine)," among others. If more than one drug is considered responsible, all drugs that are thought to have played a role should be included on the death certificate. Instead of "Mixed drug toxicity," "Mixed drug toxicity (methamphetamine and fentanyl)" would be preferable.

SAMPLE NOTE: MANNER OF DEATH WITH A DRUG OVERDOSE

The two predominant schools of thought seem to be that, without specific information from the investigation to indicate otherwise, that drug overdoses are an accident, or that drug overdoses are an undetermined manner of death. As drug use is most commonly done for recreational purposes, listing the manner as accident is acceptable; however, as there is a known risk of death associated with drug use and that drug use can be seen as an intentional act with the potential for self-harm, certifying the manner as undetermined is also acceptable. As the interpretation of postmortem drug concentrations can be subjective, certifying the manner of death as a suicide based only upon the drug concentration without supportive scene investigation findings such as a suicide note or clear purposeful ingestion of a lethal number of pills should be done with caution. Office policies and pathologist's training, experience, and preferences will guide manner of death determination for drug overdoses; however, consistency is important.

> **FAQ:** Can the amount of a substance ingested or injected be determined from the postmortem drug concentration (ie, from the postmortem drug concentration can the number of pills taken by the decedent be determined)?
>
> **Answer:** While a formula can be used based upon the volume of distribution of the substance, as my (WLK) statistics professor said (paraphrasing), "It is math. If you put a number into the formula, you will get an answer, but it may not be the right answer." So, while the calculation can be performed, any results should be interpreted with extreme caution. Using an example with amitriptyline, Maskell illustrated the inaccuracy of drug dose calculations based upon postmortem concentrations; however, the amount of ethanol consumed can potentially be estimated with the Widmark equation.[49,50]

Specific drugs encountered by forensic pathologists: While the potential number of drugs that a forensic pathologist might encounter is legion, a relatively small number of drugs are encountered with frequency. Common illicit substances encountered include fentanyl, methamphetamine, heroin, cocaine, and marijuana. Common prescription medications encountered include many psychiatric-type medications (eg, fluoxetine, amitriptyline, bupropion), anti-seizure medications (eg, phenytoin), and opioids (morphine, oxycodone, hydrocodone, fentanyl).

PEARLS & PITFALLS

Not all methamphetamine identified during toxicologic analysis is the illicit substance. Methamphetamine occurs in two forms: d-methamphetamine and l-methamphetamine. d-methamphetamine is the illicit substance. Vicks Vapolnhaler™ contains l-methamphetamine, which can be detectable in the plasma.[51,52] l-methamphetamine may also be detectable in the urine following use of Vicks Vapolnhaler™.[52,53] A metabolite of selegiline is l-methamphetamine.[54] Routine toxicology testing does not distinguish between d- and l-methamphetamine and, if a specific identification is required, a send-out to a major toxicology laboratory would be necessary.

PEARLS & PITFALLS

Heroin has a half-life of 2 to 6 minutes, and its metabolite 6-monoacetylmorphine has a half-life of 6 to 25 minutes.[55] While the presence of 6-monoacetylmorphine (6-MAM) in the urine helps confirm that morphine in the blood is from heroin use, if 6-MAM is not present, a morphine:codeine ratio of >1 in the blood or the urine has also been associated with heroin use.[55,56] Vitreous humor is an excellent source for 6-MAM testing if urine is unavailable.[57]

PEARLS & PITFALLS

When decedents have a fentanyl patch in place, the peripheral blood concentration of fentanyl can increase in the postmortem interval.[58] Also, inter-laboratory and intra-laboratory differences in results on fentanyl testing can reportedly be as much as 25 ng/mL.[58]

PEARLS & PITFALLS

Dust cleaners, which are refrigerant-based propellants, are often abused through huffing. If suspected, toxicologic analysis for 1,1-difluoroethane or tetrafluoroethane should be performed. Huffing can also be done with paint, which contains toluene. Gold and silver paints have the highest concentration of toluene. Chronic use of toluene can lead to solvent vapor abuse leukoencephalopathy, and the brain can have the consistency of formalin-fixed tissue.[59] If toluene huffing is suspected as a cause of death, the blood sample should not be saved in a gel separator tube, as gel separator tubes can be a source of toluene in subsequent testing.[60]

TABLE 15.1: Important Metabolites

Parent Compound	Metabolites
Cocaine	Benzoylecgonine, ecgonine methyl ester, cocaethylene (when combined with ethanol)
Codeine	Morphine
Diazepam	Nordiazepam, oxazepam, temazepam
Fentanyl	Norfentanyl
Heroin	Morphine, 6-monoacetylmorphine
Hydrocodone	Hydromorphone
Methadone	EDDP
Methamphetamine	Amphetamine
Nordiazepam	Oxazepam
Oxycodone	Oxymorphone, noroxycodone
Temazepam	Oxazepam

EDDP, 2-ethylidene-1,5-dimethyl-3,3-diphenylpyrrolidine.

METABOLITES OF COMMON DRUGS

Introduction: An understanding of metabolites can help a forensic pathologist correctly determine which drugs are present because the metabolites of some drugs are also a drug of their own that can be used independently (eg, amphetamine is a prescribed medication and amphetamine is also a metabolite of methamphetamine) (Table 15.1). Also, some metabolites are active and could contribute to the mechanism of death, whereas other metabolites are inactive.

Common important parent-metabolite combinations are fentanyl/norfentanyl, hydrocodone/dihydrocodeine, methadone/EDDP, and oxycodone/oxymorphone. If the metabolite to parent concentration ratio is low, acute consumption is suggested; however, if the parent drug/metabolite concentration ratios is low, longer term use may be the explanation.[61]

PEARLS & PITFALLS

Illicit substances such as cocaine, heroin, and other drugs can have cutting agents such as various sugars or acetaminophen added to increase the bulk amount of the drug product.[62] Adulterants can also be added, which act to modify the effects of the drug. Adulterants can include caffeine, lidocaine, phenacetin, levamisole, and diltiazem.[62]

PEARLS & PITFALLS

While prescription fentanyl will breakdown to norfentanyl, which will be detected on toxicologic analysis, illicit fentanyl can be contaminated with various fentanyl analogs, which can also be detected upon toxicologic analysis. 4-ANPP (4-anilino-N-phenethylpiperidine) and acetyl fentanyl are impurities in the process of fentanyl production, and 4-ANPP is also a metabolite of fentanyl analogs.[63]

ETHANOL

Introduction: Ethanol is commonly encountered during the toxicologic analysis of postmortem blood derived from autopsy. When ethanol is found, several questions can arise: (1) Can it be determined if an individual was drinking at the time of death? (2) Does alcohol form postmortem? (3) How can postmortem production of alcohol be distinguished from antemortem consumption of alcohol? and (4) Is chronic alcoholism a cause of death? Each of these questions will be addressed below.

FAQ: Can it be determined if an individual was drinking at the time of death?

Answer: Two methods to help answer this question are to compare ethanol concentrations in various postmortem fluids (eg, blood, vitreous, and urine), and to measure other substances in the blood, such as ethyl glucuronide and ethyl sulfate. Ito et al. found that with the concentration of alcohol in rats, for 10 minutes after oral administration (the early absorption phase) the highest concentration was in cardiac blood, followed by vitreous fluid, and then urine. For 20 to 50 minutes after oral administration (late absorption phase), the highest concentration was vitreous fluid, followed by cardiac blood and then urine. For 60 to 120 minutes after oral administration (distribution phase) the highest concentration was vitreous humor, followed by urine and then cardiac blood. For 180 minutes after oral administration (excretion), the highest concentration was urine, followed by vitreous humor and then cardiac blood. The authors reported that their results with rats were comparable to studies on nine cadavers.[64] Another method to help determine if an individual was drinking at the time of their death uses the ratio of ethyl glucuronide to ethyl sulfate in blood.[65]

FAQ: Does alcohol form postmortem? How can postmortem production of alcohol be distinguished from antemortem consumption of alcohol?

Answer: Due to bacteria within the body, ethanol will form in the postmortem period.[66] Bacteria can also potentially produce aldehydes, ketones, and aromatics.[66] In their study, Oshaug et al. found that almost 25% of cases with a positive ethanol are likely to have formed that ethanol postmortem, and it was formed entirely postmortem in about 15% of cases.[67] Of course, for any given practice, this number will vary based upon the characteristics of the decedent population and average length of time before bodies are found as well as average length of time between discovery of the body and autopsy. The concentration of ethanol and the fluids in which the ethanol is found may help determine the likelihood of antemortem consumption. Oshaug et al. found that the ethanol concentration when associated with postmortem production was most often less than or equal to 0.2 g/kg, but concentrations of >1.0 g/kg were found in almost 5% of cases.[67] The presence of alcohol in the urine and/or vitreous fluid, which are resistant to postmortem production, most likely indicates that the ethanol in the blood was consumed antemortem.[68] Postmortem diffusion of alcohol from the stomach can also artifactually raise the concentration of ethanol detected by forensic analysis.[69] The storage of the blood sample can also affect postmortem production. Samples stored in EDTA (ethylenediaminetetraacetic acid) tubes compared to sodium fluoride tubes, and samples stored at 37 °C vs those stored at 4 °C both will have a significant production of ethanol.[70]

Measurements of substances other than ethanol may also help distinguish antemortem consumption from postmortem production. Higher alcohols, including 1-propanol, 1-butanol, and isobutanol, are markers of postmortem alcohol production. In addition, Matoba et al. determined that the concentration of n-butyric acid may be used to determine whether the alcohol present in the autopsy sample is due to postmortem production, which has a high concentration of n-butyric acid.[71] Acetaldehyde can also potentially be used as a marker of postmortem production.[72] In contrast, ethylglucuronide and ethylsulfate are markers for antemortem alcohol use.[67,73-75]

FAQ: Is chronic alcoholism a cause of death?

Answer: Chronic alcoholics who die suddenly often have a fatty liver, and no or minimal alcohol in their system.[76] With no or minimal alcohol in the blood, alcohol withdrawal including with seizures can occur. In addition, alcohol withdrawal can induce increased QT variability and thus the risk for sudden death.[77] In support of this risk, Baykara et al. and Sorkin and Sheppard found a higher incidence of arrhythmia and sudden death in individuals with chronic alcoholism than their control group.[78,79] In addition, chronic alcoholics can have other electrolyte abnormalities. Low magnesium can contribute to long QT interval and risk for sudden death.[80] Ketoacidosis may also be a source of some sudden deaths in alcoholics.[81,82]

PEARLS & PITFALLS

As toxicologic testing is important for the determination of cause of death in a large percentage of deaths investigated by a forensic pathologist and is a useful adjunct test in other investigations (eg, motor vehicle accidents), a good relationship between the forensic pathologist and their chosen toxicology laboratory is important. This relationship can allow the forensic pathologist to obtain additional information regarding their testing or consultation regarding how to proceed with testing. In addition, the toxicology laboratory can communicate limits of testing to the forensic pathologist (eg, whether ethyl glucuronide is tested for) and can communicate the role of reference labs.

PEARLS & PITFALLS

As of 2023, forensic pathologists are routinely encountering novel drugs as a cause of death. It is important to understand that some of these new substances are difficult to analyze. When investigating a death that may have resulted from a novel substance, the forensic pathologist must consider several questions. First of all, can the analysis be performed? Testing for some drugs may require significantly more sample, samples in blood tubes that are not routinely used at autopsy, or serum samples instead of blood samples. Second, what is the value of the analysis? For example, cathinones are unstable as is psilocybin. Third, how can the drug concentration be interpreted? Determining a lethal concentration for drugs requires a case series or large sample size, and, with minimal cases of a particular drug available, determining whether a particular drug concentration is lethal is problematic.

Summary: Interpretation of postmortem drug concentrations is often not simple and no single drug concentration should be interpreted in a complete vacuum. A good scene investigation, including pill counts, and, often, evaluation of the medical records, including prescribed drug therapy, is important in the determination of what a particular postmortem drug concentration implies. For example, a femoral blood methadone concentration of 0.42 mg/L in a college student with no medical history and who is on no prescription medication and who was found dead in his bed after a party the night before, is consistent with a cause of death of methadone toxicity. However, a prostitute with the same concentration of methadone in her blood who is prescribed methadone by a clinic and is found naked and in a sexually suggestive position in the back of a van with subtle findings of strangulation, did not die from methadone toxicity as a methadone concentration of 0.42 mg/L would be consistent with therapeutic use. Given the circumstances and autopsy findings, the cause of death is most likely strangulation, or, at the very least, undetermined. But to call this death a methadone overdose is to ignore the circumstances.

> **FAQ:** In suspected drug overdoses, is a full autopsy required?
>
> **Answer:** The NAME Autopsy Standards describe that a forensic pathologist shall perform a forensic autopsy if the death is by apparent intoxication with alcohol, drugs, or poison, unless a significant interval has passed, and the medical findings and absence of trauma are well documented.[83] If a decedent has no known underlying medical history that could cause death and the death is associated with scene findings consistent with a drug overdose, not performing an autopsy could actually potentially result in not identifying a cause of death, as presumed drug overdoses sometimes do not have toxicologic findings to support that presumption; however, if a decedent has known underlying medical history that could lead to a sudden death (eg, hypertension and smoking history in an older male), why cannot toxicology be performed without an autopsy, using the medical history as a cause of death if the toxicology results are not contributory? One argument is that toxicology results should not be interpreted without autopsy findings because, in addition to the lethal drug concentration, the decedent may have undiagnosed lethal natural disease or trauma. However, for the purpose of public health records, it could be argued that the cause of death can be determined based upon the toxicology results in lieu of an autopsy. If the scene investigation is consistent with a drug overdose, and the toxicologic analysis reveals a lethal concentration of a prescription medication or illicit substance, that the cause of death could be determined to be a drug overdose would seem reasonable. However, if criminal charges are to be brought against another person for the death of the individual, an autopsy should always be performed. Without the autopsy findings to confirm the absence of another cause of death, it can easily be argued to the jury that the concentration of drug alone in the body is not enough for the conviction of another person for the death.
>
> Dye et al. determined that without an autopsy forensic pathologists would only classify the cause of death correctly in drug-related deaths in 73% of cases.[84] The authors opined that their findings indicated that a full autopsy is required to classify the COD/MOD in cases of suspected drug toxicity correctly. However, Nashelsky and Lawrence's study indicated that without an autopsy, pathologists would only determine the correct cause of death in around 70% of cases overall and would even miscertify the manner of death in a small percentage of cases, indicating that external examinations are not accurate in cause of death determination.[85] However, for presumed natural deaths, external examinations are accepted as an appropriate method, which argues that in select cases, toxicologic analysis combined with scene investigation, medical record review, and external examination to determine the cause and manner of death in a drug overdose is no less accurate.

References

1. Flaagøy SH, Morild I, Maehle BO, Lilleng PK. Petechial hemorrhages and ethanol in deaths from intoxication. *J Forensic Sci*. 2016;61(5):1266-1269.
2. Teoh L, Moses G, McCullough MJ. Oral manifestations of illicit drug use. *Aust Dent J*. 2019;64(3):213-222.
3. Gustafsson T, Eriksson A, Wingren CJ. The utility of lung weight to heart weight ratio as a means to identify suspected drug intoxication deaths in a medico-legal autopsy population. *J Forensic Sci*. 2021;66(4):1329-1333.
4. Limaiem F, Blibech H, Bouhajja L, Ben Farhat L, Louzir B. Pulmonary aspergilloma with prominent oxalate deposition. *Clin Case Rep*. 2022;10(11):e6667.
5. Roehrl MH, Croft WJ, Liao Q, Wang JY, Kradin RL. Hemorrhagic pulmonary oxalosis secondary to a noninvasive *Aspergillus niger* fungus ball. *Virchows Arch*. 2007;451(6):1067-1073.
6. Buehner M, Pamplin J, Studer L, et al. Oxalate nephropathy after continuous infusion of high-dose vitamin C as an adjunct to burn resuscitation. *J Burn Care Res*. 2016;37(4):e374-e379.
7. Somma V, Osekowski M, Paratz E, Bonomo Y. Methamphetamine-associated cardiomyopathy: an addiction medicine perspective. *Intern Med J*. 2023;53(1):21-26.

8. Kevil CG, Goeders NE, Woolard MD, et al. Methamphetamine use and cardiovascular disease. *Arterioscler Thromb Vasc Biol.* 2019;39(9):1739-1746.
9. Logan BK, Lindholm G. Gastric contamination of postmortem blood samples during blind-stick sample collection. *Am J Forensic Med Pathol.* 1996;17(2):109-111.
10. Nedahl M, Johansen SS, Linnet K. Postmortem brain-blood ratios of codeine, fentanyl, oxycodone and tramadol. *J Anal Toxicol.* 2021;45(1):53-59.
11. Ververi C, Vincenti M, Salomone A. Recent advances in the detection of drugs of abuse by dried blood spots. *Biomed Chromatogr.* 2023;37(7):e5555. doi: 10.1002/bmc.5555. Epub 2022 Dec 4.
12. Vandenbosch M, Pajk S, Van Den Bogaert W, Wuestenbergs J, Van de Voorde W, Cuypers E. Postmortem analysis of opioids and metabolites in skeletal tissue. *J Anal Toxicol.* 2022;46(7):783-790.
13. Hardin GG. Postmortem blood and vitreous humor ethanol concentrations in a victim of a fatal motor vehicle crash. *J Forensic Sci.* 2002;47(2):402-403.
14. Kugelberg FC, Jones AW. Interpreting results of ethanol analysis in postmortem specimens: a review of the literature. *Forensic Sci Int.* 2007;165(1):10-29.
15. Johnson KM, Gunsolus IL, Tlomak W. Critical analysis of laboratory testing methodologies when interpreting conflicting results at autopsy. *Am J Forensic Med Pathol.* 2021;42(1):51-53.
16. Baselt RC. *Disposition of Toxic Drugs and Chemicals in Man.* 8th ed. Biomedical publications; 2008.
17. Molina DK. *Handbook of Forensic Toxicology for Medical Examiners.* CRC Press; 2009.
18. Winek CL, Wahba WW, Winek CLJr, Balzer TW. Drug and chemical blood-level data 2001. *Forensic Sci Int.* 2001;122(2-3):107-123.
19. North Carolina Office of the Medical Examiner. Toxicology; 2017. Accessed January 1, 2022. https://www.ocme.dhhs.nc.gov/toxicology/index.shtml
20. Edvardsen HME, Aamodt C, Bogstrand ST, Krajci P, Vindenes V, Rognli EB. Concentrations of psychoactive substances in blood samples from non-fatal and fatal opioid overdoses. *Br J Clin Pharmacol.* 2022;88(10):4494-4504.
21. Ketola RA, Ojanperä I. Summary statistics for drug concentrations in post-mortem femoral blood representing all causes of death. *Drug Test Anal.* 2019;11(9):1326-1337.
22. Jones AW, Holmgren A, Ahlner J. Post-mortem concentrations of drugs determined in femoral blood in single-drug fatalities compared with multi-drug poisoning deaths. *Forensic Sci Int.* 2016;267:96-103.
23. Spiller HA. Postmortem oxycodone and hydrocodone blood concentrations. *J Forensic Sci.* 2003;48(2):429-431.
24. Dolinak D. Opioid toxicity. *Acad Forensic Pathol.* 2017;7(1):19-35.
25. Kamphuis AEM, Borra LCP, van der Hulst R, et al. Postmortem redistribution of morphine in humans: important variables that might be influencing the central blood/peripheral blood ratio. *Forensic Sci Int.* 2021;329:111094.
26. Zilg B, Thelander G, Giebe B, Druid H. Postmortem blood sampling-Comparison of drug concentrations at different sample sites. *Forensic Sci Int.* 2017;278:296-303.
27. Hansen J, Palmfeldt J, Pedersen KW, et al. Postmortem protein stability investigations of the human hepatic drug-metabolizing cytochrome P450 enzymes CYP1A2 and CYP3A4 using mass spectrometry. *J Proteomics.* 2019;194:125-131.
28. Rahikainen AL, Vauhkonen P, Pett H, et al. Completed suicides of citalopram users-the role of CYP genotypes and adverse drug interactions. *Int J Legal Med.* 2019;133(2):353-363.
29. Jornil J, Nielsen TS, Rosendal I, et al. A poor metabolizer of both CYP2C19 and CYP2D6 identified by mechanistic pharmacokinetic simulation in a fatal drug poisoning case involving venlafaxine. *Forensic Sci Int.* 2013;226(1-3):e26-e31.
30. Jin M, Gock SB, Jannetto PJ, Jentzen JM, Wong SH. Pharmacogenomics as molecular autopsy for forensic toxicology: genotyping cytochrome P450 3A4*1B and 3A5*3 for 25 fentanyl cases. *J Anal Toxicol.* 2005;29(7):590-598.
31. Wong SH, Wagner MA, Jentzen JM, et al. Pharmacogenomics as an aspect of molecular autopsy for forensic pathology/toxicology: does genotyping CYP 2D6 serve as an adjunct for certifying methadone toxicity? *J Forensic Sci.* 2003;48(6):1406-1415.
32. Jannetto PJ, Wong SH, Gock SB, Laleli-Sahin E, Schur BC, Jentzen JM. Pharmacogenomics as molecular autopsy for postmortem forensic toxicology: genotyping cytochrome P450 2D6 for oxycodone cases. *J Anal Toxicol.* 2002;26(7):438-447.

33. Pounder DJ, Jones GR. Postmortem drug redistribution-a toxicological nightmare. *Forensic Sci Int*. 1990;45(3):253-263.
34. Jones GR, Pounder DJ. Site dependence of drug concentrations in postmortem blood-a case study. *J Anal Toxicol*. 1987;11(5):186-190.
35. Gerostamoulos D, Beyer J, Staikos V, Tayler P, Woodford N, Drummer OH. The effect of the postmortem interval on the redistribution of drugs: a comparison of mortuary admission and autopsy blood specimens. *Forensic Sci Med Pathol*. 2012;8(4):373-379.
36. Mantinieks D, Gerostamoulos D, Glowacki L, et al. Postmortem drug redistribution: a compilation of postmortem/antemortem drug concentration ratios. *J Anal Toxicol*. 2021;45(4):368-377. doi:10.1093/jat/bkaa107
37. Saitman A, Fitzgerald RL, McIntyre IM. Evaluation and comparison of postmortem hydrocodone concentrations in peripheral blood, central blood and liver specimens: a minimal potential for redistribution. *Forensic Sci Int*. 2015;247:36-40.
38. McIntyre IM. Liver and peripheral blood concentration ratio (L/P) as a marker of postmortem drug redistribution: a literature review. *Forensic Sci Med Pathol*. 2014;10(1):91-96.
39. McIntyre IM, Sherrard J, Lucas J. Postmortem carisoprodol and meprobamate concentrations in blood and liver: lack of significant redistribution. *J Anal Toxicol*. 2012;36(3):177-181.
40. McIntyre IM, Navarrete A, Mena O. Postmortem distribution of guaifenesin concentrations reveals a lack of potential for redistribution. *Forensic Sci Int*. 2014;245:87-91.
41. McIntyre IM. Analytical data supporting the "theoretical" postmortem redistribution factor (F_t): a new model to evaluate postmortem redistribution. *Forensic Sci Res*. 2016;1(1):33-37.
42. Prouty RW, Anderson WH. The forensic science implications of site and temporal influences on postmortem blood-drug concentrations. *J Forensic Sci*. 1990;35(2):243-270.
43. Hilberg T, Rogde S, Morland J. Postmortem drug redistribution-human cases related to results in experimental animals. *J Forensic Sci*. 1999;44(1):3-9.
44. Andreson H, Gullans A, Veselinovic M, et al. Fentanyl: toxic or therapeutic? Postmortem and antemortem blood concentrations after transdermyl fentanyl application. *J Analytical Toxicol*. 2012;36:182-194.
45. Brockbals L, Wartmann Y, Mantinieks D, et al. Postmortem metabolomics: strategies to assess time-dependent postmortem changes of diazepam, nordiazepam, morphine, codeine, mirtazapine and citalopram. *Metabolites*. 2021;11(9):643.
46. Olson KN, Luckenbill K, Thompson J, et al. Postmortem redistribution of fentanyl in blood. *Am J Clin Pathol*. 2010;133(3):447-453.
47. Palamalai V, Olson KN, Kloss J, et al. Superiority of postmortem liver fentanyl concentrations over peripheral blood influenced by postmortem interval for determination of fentanyl toxicity. *Clin Biochem*. 2013;46(7-8):598-602.
48. Cantrell FL, Mena O, Gary RD, McIntyre IM. An acute gabapentin fatality: a case report with postmortem concentrations. *Int J Legal Med*. 2015;129(4):771-775.
49. Maskell PD. Just say no to postmortem drug dose calculations. *J Forensic Sci*. 2021;66(5):1862-1870.
50. Maskell PD, Cooper GAA. The contribution of body mass and volume of distribution to the estimated uncertainty associated with the Widmark equation. *J Forensic Sci*. 2020;65(5):1676-1684.
51. Newmeyer MN, Concheiro M, da Costa JL, Flegel R, Gorelick DA, Huestis MA. Oral fluid with three modes of collection and plasma methamphetamine and amphetamine enantiomer concentrations after controlled intranasal l-methamphetamine administration. *Drug Test Anal*. 2015;7(10):877-883.
52. Wyman JF, Cody JT. Determination of l-methamphetamine: a case history. *J Anal Toxicol*. 2005;29(7):759-761.
53. Smith ML, Nichols DC, Underwood P, et al. Methamphetamine and amphetamine isomer concentrations in human urine following controlled Vicks VapoInhaler administration. *J Anal Toxicol*. 2014;38(8):524-527.
54. Kupiec TC, Chaturvedi AK. Stereochemical determination of selegiline metabolites in postmortem biological specimens. *J Forensic Sci*. 1999;44(1):222-226.
55. Ellis AD, McGwin G, Davis GG, Dye DW. Identifying cases of heroin toxicity where 6-acetylmorphine (6-AM) is not detected by toxicological analyses. *Forensic Sci Med Pathol*. 2016;12(3):243-247.

56. Konstantinova SV, Normann PT, Arnestad M, Karinen R, Christophersen AS, Mørland J. Morphine to codeine concentration ratio in blood and urine as a marker of illicit heroin use in forensic autopsy samples. *Forensic Sci Int.* 2012;217(1-3):216-221.
57. Maskell PD, Wilson NE, Seetohul LN, et al. Postmortem tissue distribution of morphine and its metabolites in a series of heroin-related deaths. *Drug Test Anal.* 2019;11(2):292-304.
58. Krinsky CS, Lathrop SL, Zumwalt R. An examination of the postmortem redistribution of fentanyl and interlaboratory variability. *J Forensic Sci.* 2014;59(5):1275-1279.
59. Kornfeld M, Moser AB, Moser HW, Kleinschmidt-DeMasters B, Nolte K, Phelps A. Solvent vapor abuse leukoencephalopathy. Comparison to adrenoleukodystrophy. *J Neuropathol Exp Neurol.* 1994;53(4):389-398.
60. Dyne D, Cocker J, Streete PJ, Flanagan RJ. Toluene, 1-butanol, ethylbenzene and xylene from Sarstedt Monovette serum gel blood collection tubes. *Ann Clin Biochem.* 1996;33(pt 4):355-356.
61. Concheiro M, Chesser R, Pardi J, Cooper G. Postmortem toxicology of new synthetic opioids. *Front Pharmacol.* 2018;9:1210.
62. Dolinak D. *Forensic Toxicology: A Physiologic Perspective*. Academic Forensic Pathology Incorporated; 2013.
63. Stanton JD, Whitley P, LaRue L, Bundy WL, Dawson E, Huskey A. Fentanyl analog positivity among near-real-time urine drug test results in patients seeking health care. *Drug Alcohol Depend.* 2020;217:108264.
64. Ito A, Moriya F, Ishizu H. Estimating the time between drinking and death from tissue distribution patterns of ethanol. *Acta Med Okayama.* 1998;52(1):1-8.
65. Wang L, Zhang W, Wang R, et al. Estimating the time of last drinking from blood ethyl glucuronide and ethyl sulphate concentrations. *Sci Rep.* 2022;12(1):14262.
66. Cernosek T, Eckert KE, Carter DO, Perrault KA. Volatile organic compound profiling from postmortem microbes using gas chromatography-mass spectrometry. *J Forensic Sci.* 2020;65(1):134-143.
67. Oshaug K, Kronstrand R, Kugelberg FC, Kristoffersen L, Mørland J, Høiseth G. Frequency of postmortem ethanol formation in blood, urine and vitreous humor—Improving diagnostic accuracy with the use of ethylsulphate and putrefactive alcohols. *Forensic Sci Int.* 2022;331:111152.
68. Levine B, Smith ML, Smialek JE, Caplan YH. Interpretation of low postmortem concentrations of ethanol. *J Forensic Sci.* 1993;38(3):663-667.
69. Marti V, Augsburger M, Widmer C, Lardi C. Significant postmortem diffusion of ethanol: a case report. *Forensic Sci Int.* 2021;328:111046.
70. Ahmad S, Aamir M, Kirmani SI, Haroon ZH, Bibi A, Khalid UB. Effect of temperature and preservative on neo-ethanol formation in postmortem whole blood samples. *J Coll Physicians Surg Pak.* 2021;31(10):1159-1162.
71. Matoba K, Murakami M, Fujita E, et al. The usefulness of measuring n-butyric acid concentration as a new indicator of blood decomposition in forensic autopsy. *Leg Med.* 2022;57:102071.
72. Chen X, Dong X, Zhu R, et al. Abnormally high blood acetaldehyde concentrations suggest potential postmortem ethanol generation. *J Anal Toxicol.* 2021;45(7):748-755.
73. Alsayed SN, Alharbi AG, Alhejaili AS, et al. Ethyl glucuronide and ethyl sulfate: a review of their roles in forensic toxicology analysis of alcohol postmortem. *Forensic Toxicol.* 2022;40(1):19-48.
74. Dip A, Mozayani A. Evaluation of the compatibility of ethyl glucuronide and ethyl sulfate levels to assess alcohol consumption in decomposed and diabetic postmortem cases. *J Anal Toxicol.* 2021;45(8):878-884.
75. Wang H, Li B, Wang F, et al. Determination of ethyl glucuronide and ethyl sulfate in human whole blood and vitreous humor by LC-MS-MS and applications to the interpretation of postmortem ethanol findings. *J Anal Toxicol.* 2021;45(5):484-489.
76. Templeton AH, Carter KL, Sheron N, Gallagher PJ, Verrill C. Sudden unexpected death in alcohol misuse—an unrecognized public health issue? *Int J Environ Res Public Health.* 2009;6(12):3070-3081.
77. Bär KJ, Boettger MK, Koschke M, et al. Increased QT interval variability index in acute alcohol withdrawal. *Drug Alcohol Depend.* 2007;89(2-3):259-266.
78. Baykara S, Ocak D, Berk ŞŞ, Köroğlu S. Analysis of QT dispersion, corrected QT dispersion, and P-wave dispersion values in alcohol use disorder patients with excessive alcohol use. *Prim Care Companion CNS Disord.* 2020;22(1):19m02541.

79. Sorkin T, Sheppard MN. Sudden unexplained death in alcohol misuse (SUDAM) patients have different characteristics to those who died from sudden arrhythmic death syndrome (SADS). *Forensic Sci Med Pathol*. 2017;13(3):278-283.

80. Moulin SR, Mill JG, Rosa WC, Hermisdorf SR, Caldeira LC, Zago-Gomes EMP. QT interval prolongation associated with low magnesium in chronic alcoholics. *Drug Alcohol Depend*. 2015;155:195-201.

81. Komáreková I, Janík M. Ethanol-induced ketoacidosis as a possible neglected cause of sudden death in chronic alcohol consumers. *Soud Lek*. 2014;59(4):48-50.

82. Yanagawa Y, Sakamoto T, Okada Y. Six cases of sudden cardiac arrest in alcoholic ketoacidosis. *Intern Med*. 2008;47(2):113-117.

83. NAME Standards Committee. *Forensic Autopsy Performance Standards*. National Association of Medical Examiners; 2020. (sunset 2025).

84. Dye DW, McGwin G, Atherton DS, McCleskey B, Davis GG. Correctly identifying deaths due to drug toxicity without a forensic autopsy. *Am J Forensic Med Pathol*. 2019;40(2):99-101.

85. Nashelsky MB, Lawrence CH. Accuracy of cause of death determination without forensic autopsy examination. *Am J Forensic Med Pathol*. 2003;24(4):313-319.

SUICIDE 16

CHAPTER OUTLINE

Introduction   464

Basic Considerations When Determining That the Manner of Death Is Suicide   464

Gunshot Wound Homicide vs Gunshot Wound Suicide   465
- Comparison of Features in Homicide vs Suicide Gunshot Wounds   465

Sharp Force Injuries Homicide vs Sharp Force Injuries Suicide   466
- Comparison of Features in Homicide vs Suicide Sharp Force Injury   466

Asphyxial Homicide vs Asphyxial Suicide   468
- Comparison of Features in Homicide vs Suicide Asphyxia   468

Near Misses   473

INTRODUCTION

To certify the manner of death as suicide, the forensic pathologist must determine that an injury was self-inflicted, that the decedent intended to kill or harm themselves, and that the decedent understood the consequences of their actions. Intent can be expressed in an explicit manner or in an implicit manner. A suicide note or a phone call to a family member stating their plan to kill themself would be examples of explicit intent. Having expressed how lonely they were or how much pain they were in the day previous to the suicide can be considered implicit intent.

Suicides are commonly encountered by forensic pathologists and can be one of the more controversial types of deaths that they must handle. Family members can be adamantly opposed to the determination of a manner of death as suicide and can create difficulties for the forensic pathologist who certifies such a manner against the family's wishes, even when the forensic pathologist has accurately identified the suicide. The strongest and most effective argument for certifying a manner of death as suicide is created by careful documentation and analysis of the death scene and the autopsy findings and a thorough collection of medical and social history (including financial history) about the decedent that best supports that the injury was the result of an intentional and self-inflicted action.

KEY FEATURES to Identify Implicit Intent[1]

- Evidence that decedent prepared for death (eg, getting finances in order for their next of kin)
- History that decedent expressed hopelessness, emotional or physical pain, their goodbyes, or that they acknowledged their upcoming death
- Evidence that decedent tried to learn about methods to cause their death
- Evidence that the decedent impaired rescue (eg, a locked door to the room where they committed suicide) (Figure 16.1)
- History of previous suicide attempt, suicidal threat, or suicidal ideation
- History of recent stressful events or a significant loss
- History of depression or other serious mental disorder

> **FAQ:** How common are suicide notes?
>
> **Answer:** Suicide notes are often not identified during a suicide scene investigation. Byard and Austin indicate that in 198 suicides investigated during the course of 1 year only a minority of the decedents left suicide notes.[2] In their 52 confirmed motor vehicle suicides, Milner and DeLeo found that 38.5% of the individuals left suicide notes.[3] Crego (personal communication) in an informal study found four suicide notes associated with 16 deaths in 1 year that were determined to be a suicide. While it is uncommon for a decedent to leave a suicide note at the scene, comments on social media left by the decedent may reveal their intent. Reviewing the decedent's social media accounts may provide evidence to support a suicide manner of death determination.

BASIC CONSIDERATIONS WHEN DETERMINING THAT THE MANNER OF DEATH IS SUICIDE

Numerous reports exist in the medical literature where the authors have evaluated a series of deaths and compared the features of homicide to suicide, often finding significant differences between the two manners of death among their cases.[4-8] While to the inexperienced observer these articles may appear to provide a patterned approach to distinguishing homicides from suicides, the characteristics of groups do not necessarily apply to an individual. In this regard, it must be remembered that in forensic pathology the autopsy represents a case report, a unique situation. Findings that are rare or even non-existent in a collection

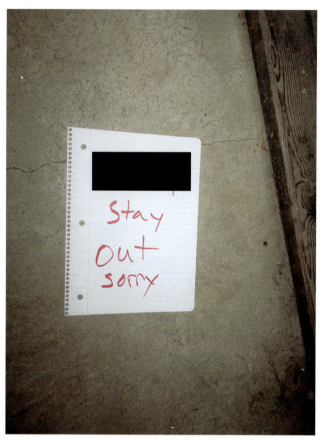

FIGURE 16.1. Note on door associated with suicide. While the note on the door was a simple warning not to come into the room, it would indicate implicit intent, in trying to keep a person from finding the body. The cause of death was a suicidal ligature strangulation with a bungee cord.

of 150 suicide deaths may indeed be present in the suicide death being investigated by the forensic pathologist. As such, the key features listed below are meant to be a guide when investigating deaths and not an absolute marker for one manner of death vs another.

GUNSHOT WOUND HOMICIDE VS GUNSHOT WOUND SUICIDE

COMPARISON OF FEATURES IN HOMICIDE VS SUICIDE GUNSHOT WOUNDS

Karger et al. reviewed 284 suicides and 293 homicides. Of the 284 suicides, 268 had only one gunshot wound, 13 had two, and one each had three, four, and five, with no suicide victims having greater than five wounds.[9] In comparison, of the 293 homicide victims, 135 had one gunshot wound, with a reducing number of victims in each category as the numbers of wounds went from 2 to 23. Of the 306 wounds in suicides, 273 were contact or near contact, with 33 being intermediate and none being distant.[9] In comparison, of the 698 wounds in homicides, 542 were distant, with 52 being contact or near contact. Of the 306 suicide wounds, 252 were of the head and 50 were of the chest. In comparison, with the homicide wounds, one-third were of the head, one-fifth of the back, and one-fifth of the chest.[9] Based upon this study, a suicidal gunshot wound is more likely to be singular, contact in range, and of the head, whereas a homicidal gunshot wound is more likely to be two or more in number, distant in range, and involve a more broad range of the body. While these observations are useful, they do not represent an absolute. For example, Boxho reported an individual who shot themselves in the trunk 14 times with a .22 caliber long rifle, of which Karger et al. had no individual who died as the result of a suicide with that number of gunshot wounds.[9,10]

Karger et al. also looked at location of wounds on the head and pathways of the projectiles.[9] The authors had several conclusions: (1) In suicidal gunshot wounds of the right temple, the pathway is front-to-back and upward or parallel and that a back-to-front and/or downward pathway from this entrance location does not likely indicate a suicide; (2) In a suicidal gunshot wound of the mouth, the typical pathway is upward, with downward a rarity; and (3) In a suicidal gunshot wound of the back of the head or neck, the pathway is usually upward.[9] However, an individual can certainly fire a weapon and achieve a downward or back-to-front pathway in a suicide. Therefore, while a general understanding of the pattern of findings commonly encountered between homicides and suicides such as Karger et al. described is useful, remembering that the specific case being investigated by the forensic pathologist may not follow the general pattern is vital.[9] Each death must be investigated on its own merits.

KEY FEATURES to Consider When Distinguishing Homicidal From Suicidal Gunshot Wounds

- Determine whether the pathway(s) and number of gunshot wounds is consistent with having been self-inflicted
- Careful examination of the scene in a through-and-through gunshot wound can identify where the projectile passed into a surrounding structure and can establish the position of the decedent when the gun was discharged
- Consideration of relative range of fire in that a suicidal wound with stippling or no gunshot residue must be adequately explained
- Determine whether the relationship of the weapon to the body at the scene is consistent with a suicide, appreciating that a weapon can end up some distance from the body after the shot is fired

PEARLS & PITFALLS

When an individual shoots themselves with a shotgun or a rifle, one question can be whether they were able to reach the trigger to discharge the weapon, because, if they were not, the scene may be staged to appear as a suicide, when the manner of death is actually a homicide. One measurement at autopsy that is not routinely obtained but could help prove or disprove such a consideration is a measurement from the axilla to the fingertip, which could show that the individual could or could not reach the trigger. Also, at the scene any device that could be used to reach the trigger (eg, a stick) should be documented.

SHARP FORCE INJURIES HOMICIDE VS SHARP FORCE INJURIES SUICIDE

COMPARISON OF FEATURES IN HOMICIDE VS SUICIDE SHARP FORCE INJURY

Brunel et al. in a study of 118 sharp force injuries fatalities found that wounds of the head, limbs, hands, nape of the neck, and back were more indicative of a homicide, whereas injuries in suicides were on the anterior portion of the trunk, the neck, and the forearms.[11] If cartilage or bone was involved, the wound was more likely to be a homicide. Vertically oriented wounds were more likely to be a homicide, whereas horizontal wounds were more likely to represent a suicide. Defensive wounds were more likely to indicate a homicide and hesitation marks were more likely to indicate a suicide[11] (Figure 16.2A-F). Karger et al. found that in 65 cases of suicide due to sharp force injuries that the number of injuries varied from 1 to 37; however, one-third of cases only had one injury.[12] Incised wounds were most common on the wrist, elbow, or neck and stab wounds were most common on the anterior surface of the chest. About half of their cases involved stabbing through clothing and about half of their cases involved injuries to more than one body site. Importantly, the authors indicated that deviation from the typical pattern in the study group was not infrequent.[12]

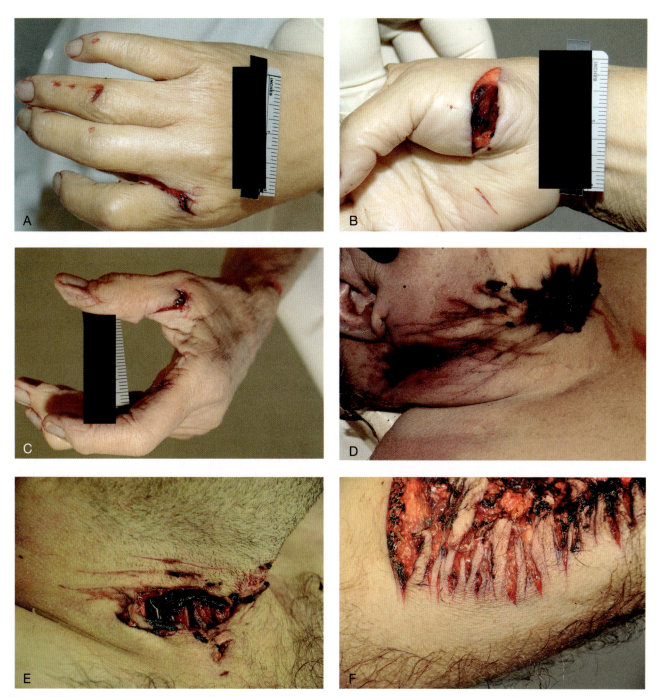

Figure 16.2. Defensive-type injuries and hesitation marks. Defensive-type injuries are incisions, stab wounds, gunshot wounds, or blunt force injuries of the upper or lower extremities that are consistent with the decedent placing their extremity between them and their attacker. (**A-C**) are defensive-type incisions of the hands, from the decedent grabbing the knife or trying to block the knife attacks. With sharp force injuries, the hands are often bloody when first viewed at autopsy. All the blood should be removed and the hands examined for such injuries, which can vary from small to large in size, and can be easy to overlook when found in creases, such as between the digits. Hesitation marks occur when the decedent makes superficial incisions in the skin before cutting deeper. (**D and E**) are hesitation marks associated with suicidal incisions of the neck and (**F**) is hesitation marks associated with suicidal incisions of the forearm. The presence of defensive-type injuries unless not otherwise explained is consistent with a homicide; however, the lack of defensive-type injuries does not mean that the manner of death is not a homicide. Hesitation marks are strongly associated with suicides.

Kernal et al. reviewed 349 homicides and 54 suicides due to sharp force injuries and found that homicides had more injuries; more commonly had stab wounds than incised wounds; involved the head, chest, and back more commonly, with suicides more commonly involving the extremities and abdomen than homicides.[13] In homicides, additional non-sharp force injuries were more likely to be found than in suicides. Hesitation marks were found in 35% of suicides and defensive injuries were found in 31% of homicides.[13]

Lupi Manso et al. found that homicides were more likely stab wounds and involved the neck and trunk, whereas suicides were more likely to be incised wounds involving the neck and upper extremities.[14] Homicidal stab wounds were more likely to be oblique in orientation. Homicides tend to involve damage to clothing, injury to bone or cartilage, and the presence of other non-sharp force injuries.[14]

KEY FEATURES: Characteristic Patterns in Self-Inflicted Sharp Force Injuries[13-15]
- Incised wounds are most commonly found on the ventral surface of the wrists and neck in suicides.
- Stab wounds are most commonly found overlying the heart or the abdomen in suicides.
- Sparing of eyes, lips, nipples, and genitalia (unless the decedent has mental illness) was found in suicides.
- Incised wounds tend to be multiple and predominantly parallel in suicides.
- Wounds consistent with a tentative or hesitant nature are often present in suicides.
- Wounds consistent with defensive-type injuries are more often present in homicides.
- Presence of clothing damage suggests homicide.
- Presence of additional injuries suggest homicide.

ASPHYXIAL HOMICIDE VS ASPHYXIAL SUICIDE

COMPARISON OF FEATURES IN HOMICIDE VS SUICIDE ASPHYXIA

While a textbook example of strangulation has conjunctival petechiae, abrasions and contusions and even fingernail marks of the neck, hemorrhage into the neck musculature, and fractures of the hyoid bone and/or thyroid cartilage and a textbook example of hanging has none of these findings, there is much overlap between the two causes of death in actual practice. The extent of injuries of the neck in a strangulation can vary depending upon the amount of effort put forth by the decedent in preventing the strangulation (ie, fighting against the attacker is more likely to lead to injuries of the skin of the neck and hemorrhage in the neck musculature). However, if a person is quickly overwhelmed by their attacker, they may have minimal to no injuries. A subsequently staged suicide can be very challenging if not impossible to identify. Oshima did indicate that muscular hemorrhages around the scapula may help distinguish a staged hanging after a homicide from a suicidal hanging.[16]

KEY FEATURES in Ligature Strangulation, Homicide vs Suicide[17]
- No or insignificant hemorrhage in neck structures in suicides
- More than one circumference of the noose around the neck in suicides, which could be reflected in the ligature furrow on the skin
- Absence of defensive-type injuries in suicide
- Less significant mechanical injuries in suicides

> **PEARLS & PITFALLS**
>
> Autoerotic asphyxia is a type of accidental death that can easily mimic a suicide. In an autoerotic asphyxial death, the decedent will have prepared a mechanism to induce asphyxia during a sex act. The mechanism may be simple or quite complex. To correctly identify an autoerotic asphyxia, the forensic pathologist must be aware of the condition, and during the scene investigation, it is important to determine if there is an escape mechanism (ie, some way for the individual to terminate the asphyxial mechanism). Pornographic material is often present at the scene (Figure 16.3). If death occurs, there has most often been a failure of the escape mechanism.

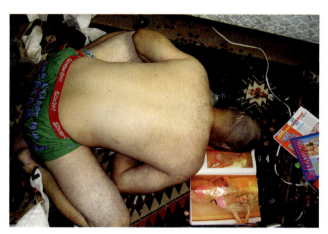

Figure 16.3. Autoerotic asphyxia. This individual was found face down in their room with a plastic bag over their head (comment: the plastic bag had been removed prior to the arrival of the coroner). Also present was a nitrous oxide canister under the left shoulder. The decedent's penis was exposed and pictures of a nude female were on the floor in front of him. While the death could be misinterpreted as a suicidal smothering because of the plastic bag over the head, the cause of death was correctly identified as an autoerotic asphyxia and the manner of death was accident. (Courtesy of Sheriff-Coroner Craig Doolittle.)

PEARLS & PITFALLS

An individual who is experienced with neck holds or chokeholds can easily incapacitate and subsequently kill another person, likely leaving few if any marks on the body, externally or internally. A subsequent staged hanging would be difficult to identify at autopsy. During any scene investigation involving a hanging, determining whether any close contacts of the decedent had this ability may be useful information.

PEARLS & PITFALLS

Suicides can be masked both by the decedent and by their family upon discovery to attempt to make the death appear as an accident or homicide. Good scene investigation is vital to the correct determination of manner of death in a suicide.[18]

PEARLS & PITFALLS

Certain types of deaths can represent a suicide; however, based upon the nature of the death, proving a suicide is difficult or disagreed upon. These types of deaths include Russian roulette (with forensic pathologists disagreeing on whether the manner is accident or suicide), drug and alcohol intoxications, drowning, and single-passenger single-vehicle motor vehicle accidents.[1,2]

FAQ: When deciding between suicide, accident, or undetermined as the cause of death, which factors tend to cause a pathologist to favor undetermined vs suicide?

Answer: Lindqvist and Gustafsson, in their review of 122 cases of suicide and undetermined manner of death, found that poisoning and drowning deaths, an absence of suicidal communication, and a lack of circumstantial evidence that was consistent with a suicidal intent were features in the investigation that caused a pathologist to favor undetermined as the manner of death instead of suicide.[19]

PEARLS & PITFALLS

When a deceased body is found in the water and that body is bound, that the decedent was the victim of a homicide must be considered; however, in individuals who commit suicide by drowning, they may also bind themselves[20] (Figure 16.4).

FAQ: Do the number of injuries help determine the manner of death in homicide vs suicide?

Answer: No. A individual committing suicide can inflict numerous injuries upon themself and can use more than one method when one fails or as a backup in case their primary method does fail (Figs. 16.5A-D; 16.6A-H). Karger and Vennemann reported an individual who committed suicide by inflicting more than 90 stab wounds on themself.[21] Austin et al. reported an individual who died as the result of 24 incised and stab wounds, an individual with three .22 caliber contact gunshot wounds of the head, and an individual with blunt force injuries of the head and a lethal concentration of clozapine.[22] Maghin et al. reported an individual who died as the result of two contact gunshot wounds of the head with a 7 mm handgun.[23]

PEARLS & PITFALLS

When documenting factors to support a suicide manner of death, identification of previous suicide attempts in the medical record, or evidence of past self-harm can provide support (Figure 16.7).

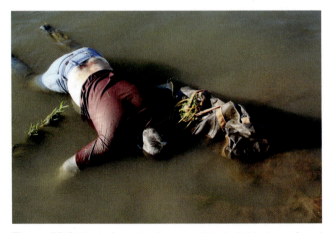

Figure 16.4. Body found in the water. The individual was found tied to a duffle bag weighted with architectural stone. Autopsy identified no injuries and investigation was consistent with a suicide. The stone was matched to the same type of stone at the decedent's house.

FAQ: When the scene investigation is consistent with a suicide, is an autopsy required?

Answer: The answer to this question will depend upon office policies and the preference, training, and experience of the forensic pathologist, with some offices always performing complete autopsies when the manner of death is suicide, and with other offices performing external examinations or partial autopsies (eg, head only to recover a projectile). However, two points are important to consider: (1) suicides can be some of the most contentious deaths that a forensic pathologist will investigate, with families often arguing that suicides are actually homicides or accidents, (2) a complete autopsy will always be a more thorough evaluation of the death than an external examination or partial autopsy. If the office policy is to perform a complete autopsy when the manner of death is suicide and the family objects, the repercussions of not performing an autopsy must be explained to the family and their acceptance documented. If the office policy allows for an external examination or partial autopsy and the scene investigation identifies any unusual circumstances or if the family requests an autopsy or is known to question the manner of death, the best course would be to perform a complete autopsy.

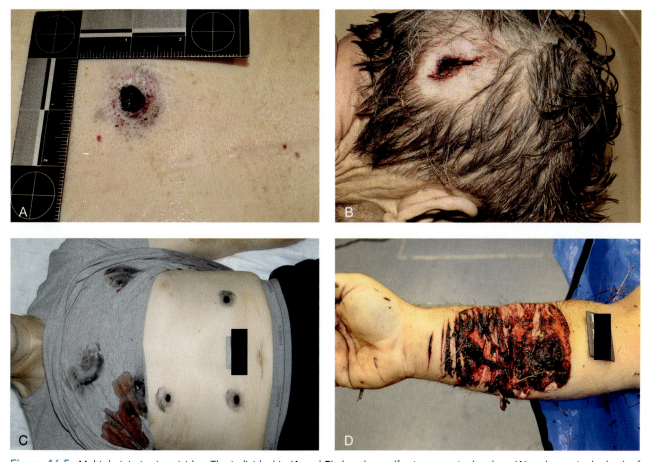

Figure 16.5. Multiple injuries in suicides. The individual in (**A** and **B**) shot themself twice, once in the chest (**A**) and once in the back of the head (**B**). The scene and investigation were consistent with a suicide. The individual in (**C**) shot themself three times in the abdomen. Gunshot wounds of the chest and abdomen will not be instantly lethal, and can actually be associated with a significant delay prior to death, which can allow for several gunshot wounds to be inflicted by the decedent prior to their final demise. The individual in (**D**) cut their forearm numerous times, and also incised their neck.

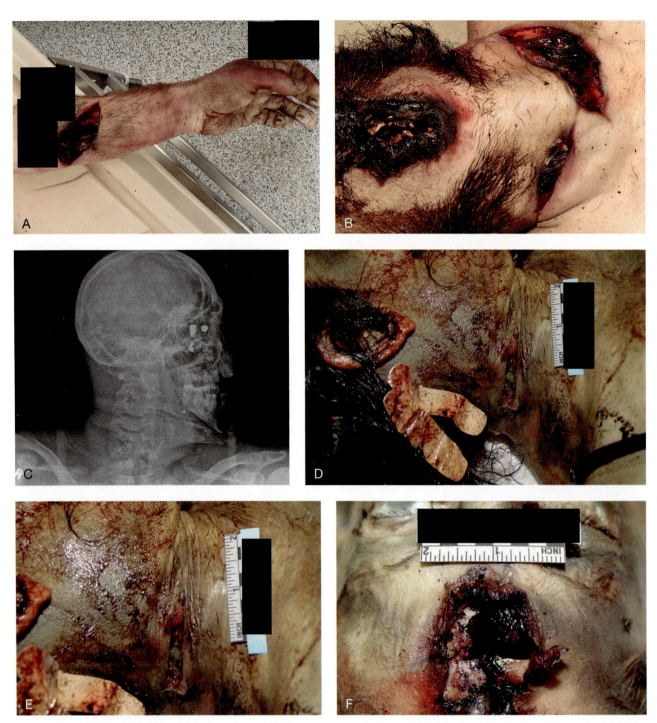

Figure 16.6. Suicides with more than one method used. The decedent in (**A-C**) incised their wrist and neck (**A** and **B**) and shot themself also, with the gunshot entrance in the chin region (**B** and **C**). The decedent in (**D-F**) incised their neck, placed Band-Aids over the injuries (**D** and **E**), and then shot themself (**F**). The purpose of the Band-Aids may have been to limit the bleeding, keeping the area cleaner for their family. The individual in (**G** and **H**) shot themself on the train tracks, apparently under the assumption that if the gunshot wound did not cause their death, that being run over by the train would.

Figure 16.6 (continued)

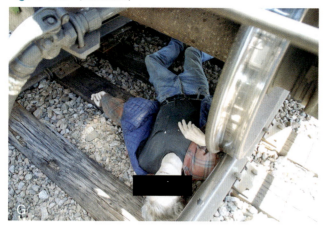
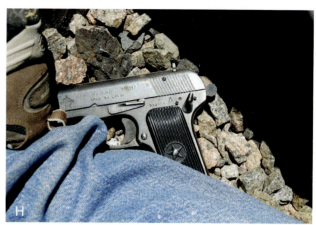

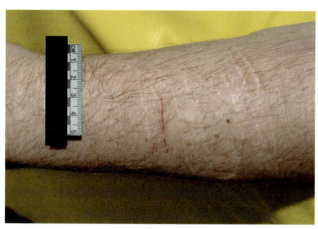

Figure 16.7. Scars on the ventral surface of the forearms. Figure 16.7 illustrates remote incisions of the forearm. In decedents who have committed suicide, searching for such scars, which can be found on the upper and lower extremities and the trunk, provides evidence in support of past episodes of self-harm, which can support a determination that their manner of death is a suicide.

NEAR MISSES

Near Miss #1: While injuries of the upper or lower extremities in addition to similar injuries of the head, neck, or trunk can be consistent with a defensive-type injury, based upon the position of the decedent and the pathway of the projectile, injuries of the extremities can occur in suicide.[24]

Near Miss #2: While intra-oral gunshot wounds are a common location for a suicidal gunshot wound, intra-oral gunshot wounds can occur as the result of a homicide.[25]

References

1. Rosenberg ML, Davidson LE, Smith JC, et al. Operational criteria for the determination of suicide. *J Forensic Sci*. 1988;33(6):1445-1456.
2. Byard RW, Austin A. The role of forensic pathology in suicide. *Forensic Sci Med Pathol*. 2011;7:1-2.
3. Milner A, De Leo D. Suicide by motor vehicle "accident" in Queensland. *Traffic Inj Prev*. 2012;13(4):342-347.
4. Foote CW, Doan XL, Vanier C, Cruz B, Sarani B, Palacio CH. Suicide versus homicide firearm injury patterns on trauma systems in a study of the National Trauma Data Bank (NTDB). *Sci Rep*. 2022;12(1):15672.

5. Kalesan B, Mobily ME, Vasan S, Siegel M, Galea S. The role of interpersonal conflict as a determinant of firearm-related homicide-suicides at different ages. *J Interpers Violence*. 2018;33(15):2335-2351.
6. Druid H. Site of entrance wound and direction of bullet path in firearm fatalities as indicators of homicide versus suicide. *Forensic Sci Int*. 1997;88(2):147-162.
7. Stone IC. Characteristics of firearms and gunshot wounds as markers of suicide. *Am J Forensic Med Pathol*. 1992;13(4):275-280.
8. Karlsson T, Ormstad K, Rajs J. Patterns in sharp force fatalities—a comprehensive forensic medical study: part 2. Suicidal sharp force injury in the Stockholm area 1972-1984. *J Forensic Sci*. 1988;33(2):448-461.
9. Karger B, Billeb E, Koops E, Brinkmann B. Autopsy features relevant for discrimination between suicidal and homicidal gunshot injuries. *Int J Legal Med*. 2002;116(5):273-278.
10. Boxho P. Fourteen shots for a suicide. *Forensic Sci Int*. 1999;101(1):71-77.
11. Brunel C, Fermanian C, Durigon M, de la Grandmaison GL. Homicidal and suicidal sharp force fatalities: autopsy parameters in relation to the manner of death. *Forensic Sci Int*. 2010;198(1-3):150-154.
12. Karger B, Niemeyer J, Brinkmann B. Suicides by sharp force: typical and atypical features. *Int J Legal Med*. 2000;113(5):259-262.
13. Kemal CJ, Patterson T, Molina DK. Deaths due to sharp force injuries in Bexar County, Texas, with respect to manner of death. *Am J Forensic Med Pathol*. 2013;34(3):253-259.
14. Lupi Manso N, Ribeiro IP, Ignacio AR. Sharp force fatalities: differentiating homicide from suicide through a retrospective review (2012-2019) of autopsy findings in Lisbon (Portugal). *Forensic Sci Int*. 2021;327:10959.
15. Mazzolo GM, Desinan L. Sharp force fatalities: suicide, homicide, or accident? A series of 21 cases. *Forensic Sci Int*. 2005;147(suppl l):S33-S35.
16. Oshima T, Ohtani M, Mimasaka S. Muscular hemorrhages around the scapula provide insight on the manner of asphyxia: a preliminary study. *Am J Forensic Med Pathol*. 2021;42(2):130-134.
17. Maxeiner H, Bockholdt B. Homicidal and suicidal ligature strangulation—a comparison of the postmortem findings. *Forensic Sci Int*. 2003;137(1):60-66.
18. Ermenc B, Prijon T. Suicide, accident? The importance of the scene investigation. *Forensic Sci Int*. 2005;147(suppl l):S21-S24.
19. Lindqvist P, Gustafsson L. Suicide classification-clues and their use. A study of 122 cases of suicide and undetermined manner of death. *Forensic Sci Int*. 2002;128(3):136-140.
20. Todt M, Ast F, Wolff-Maras R, Roesler B, Germerott T. Suicide by drowning: a forensic challenge. *Forensic Sci Int*. 2014;240:e22-e24.
21. Karger B, Vennemann B. Suicide by more than 90 stab wounds including perforation of the skull. *Int J Legal Med*. 2001;115(3):167-169.
22. Austin AE, Guddat SS, Tsokos M, Gilbert JD, Byard RW. Multiple injuries in suicide simulating homicide: report of three cases. *J Forensic Leg Med*. 2013;20(6):601-604.
23. Maghin F, Antonietti A, Farina D, Benedetti P, Verzeletti A. A case of suicide by double gunshot wounds to the head: the ability to act after the first shot. *Int J Legal Med*. 2019;133(5):1469-1476.
24. Cecchini MJ, Shkrum MJ. A self-inflicted gunshot wound with an unusual hand injury. *Am J Forensic Med Pathol*. 2019;40(1):47-48.
25. Zietlow C, Hawley DA. Unexpectedly homicide. Three intraoral gunshot wounds. *Am J Forensic Med Pathol*. 1993;14(3):230-233.

HISTOLOGY AT AUTOPSY

CHAPTER OUTLINE

Introduction 476

Frequency of Histologic Examination at Autopsy 476

Histologic Examination of the Brain at Autopsy 478

Near Misses 479

INTRODUCTION

The rate of performance of microscopic examination at forensic autopsy varies from office to office and from pathologist to pathologist, with some offices and some forensic pathologists routinely performing histologic examination on essentially all cases, and with some offices and some forensic pathologists performing histologic examination on few deaths and only when necessary to determine the cause and manner of death. The National Association of Medical Examiners requires a forensic pathologist to perform (ie, "shall perform") a histologic examination if gross examination, toxicologic analysis, and/or scene investigation did not reveal a cause of death.[1]

Key uses of histology in forensic pathology[2]
- Confirm gross diagnoses (eg, if a mass is found in the kidney)
- Identifying pathologic findings as some lesions are only found microscopically
- Determine the cause of death with some conditions (eg, myocarditis, encephalitis)
- Identify cells/tissue requiring further investigation (eg, tissue fragments found on clothing or cytology from a bullet[3]

FREQUENCY OF HISTOLOGIC EXAMINATION AT AUTOPSY

Per de la Grandmaison et al., neither of the agencies accrediting forensic pathology offices (National Association of Medical Examiners and College of American Pathologists) requires histologic examination in all cases, and the medical literature offers conflicting reports regarding the utility of histologic examination, with Langlois indicating it was contributory to the cause of death in 53% of cases and Molina et al indicating the cause of death was altered based upon microscopic examination in only one case, albeit only 25% of the cases were natural deaths.[4-6] One reason for the possible discrepancy may be based upon definitions. Identifying microscopic conditions that contribute to the diagnosis of the cause of death may not be necessary to actually determine the cause of death. For example, in diabetic ketoacidosis, the cause of death will be diagnosed based upon the vitreous electrolyte analysis. While basilar vacuolization in the proximal convoluted tubular epithelial cells is found in diabetic ketoacidosis, the identification of the microscopic finding is not necessary to determine the cause of death in the background of finding elevated glucose and ketones in the vitreous fluid.

> **FAQ:** What causes of death would be missed if histologic examination is not performed?
>
> **Answer:** While not a complete list, de la Grandmaison et al included myocarditis, artery fibromuscular dysplasia, and fat embolism as causes of death that would be missed without microscopic examination as none of these conditions would produce a gross finding (albeit with extensive myocarditis, patchy pallor may be present).[4] To this list, among other conditions, could be added encephalitis, myelitis, leukemia, acute hypophysitis, and hypertrophic cardiomyopathy (if the microscopic changes are distributed evenly throughout the left ventricle), all of which would not be identified based only upon gross examination (Figures 17.1A and 17.1B). de la Grandmaison also included ischemic heart disease, acute myocardial ischemia, cardiomyopathy, acute pneumonia, and acute pancreatitis in the list of causes of death that were determined only by histologic examination; however, while these conditions may not be entirely identifiable at gross examination, there are frequently gross findings to suggest the presence of the disease process, with histologic examination performed for confirmation of the gross impression.[4] For example, acute pneumonia will often produce patchy areas of firm parenchyma in the lung, so, while a color change may not be apparent, palpation of the parenchyma would guide sampling for histologic purposes.

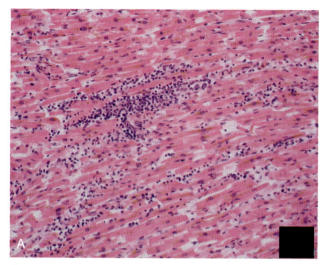

Figure 17.1A. Lymphocytic myocarditis. While myocarditis can cause gross pallor of the myocardium, the change is very nonspecific. Proper confirmation of myocarditis requires microscopic examination of the myocardium.

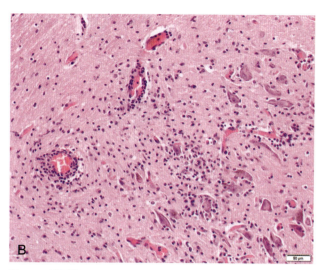

Figure 17.1B. Encephalitis. The three features of viral encephalitis (microglial nodules, inflammatory cells in the Virchow-Robin spaces, and neuronophagia) can be identified upon histologic examination of the cerebral parenchyma but would be missed if only gross examination is done.

> **FAQ:** Can histologic analysis assist with the evaluation of traumatic injuries?
>
> **Answer:** de la Grandmaison et al discuss possible uses of histologic examination in the evaluation of traumatic injuries such as dating injuries, allowing for more precision on gunshot wounds (ie, helping to determine entrance and exit wounds, with histology potentially being able to help identify soot or bullet wipe), and helping to distinguish whether a defect found on gross examination is an injury or not.[4] While the exact dating of an injury cannot be done via histologic examination, the presence of neutrophilic infiltrates or hemosiderin or evidence of organization (eg, granulation tissue or fibrosis) could help provide a relative time frame in which the injury occurred. Depending upon the circumstances of the death, this relative time frame may be enough to contribute substantially to the investigation of the death. In addition, histologic analysis of a lesion can help separate a natural disease process from a traumatic process. For example, histologic examination could allow for the pathologist to distinguish between livor mortis and a bruise, if the distinction was not clear based upon the gross examination.

PEARLS & PITFALLS

In addition to identifying disease processes that are related to the cause of death, de la Grandmaison et al found that numerous disease processes not necessarily related to the cause of death were frequently not identified at gross examination or were misidentified at gross examination.[4] These conditions included hepatic steatosis, cirrhosis, chronic hepatitis, chronic interstitial lung disease, granulomas, neoplasia, nephrosclerosis, and chronic nephritis. To this list could be added acute pyelonephritis and others. Using microscopic examination as a supplement to the gross examination at autopsy can help better delineate many pathologic conditions.

PEARLS & PITFALLS

One common problem faced during forensic autopsy is the identification of early ischemic injury in the myocardium. The earliest histologic changes to help diagnose an acute myocardial infarct take at least several hours to manifest; however, immunohistochemical studies utilizing myoglobin, cardiac troponin I, and C5b-9 complex may be able to be utilized to diagnosis early acute myocardial ischemia and narrow the time frame.[7,8]

HISTOLOGIC EXAMINATION OF THE BRAIN AT AUTOPSY

Common reasons to examine the brain histologically at autopsy are to assess for hypoxic/ischemic injury, diffuse axonal injury, an infectious process such as encephalitis, or neurodegenerative disease. Based upon the forensic pathologist's training and experience, they may wish to consult a neuropathologist for examination of the brain; however, sending a whole brain to a distant location if the neuropathologist is not locally available may be challenging, and retention of the brain is not always favored by the family of the decedent. Knowing which sections of the brain to examine histologically would allow a forensic pathologist to cut the brain and retain the necessary sections for histologic examination while allowing for the remainder of the brain to be released with the body.[9]

> **PEARLS & PITFALLS**
>
> The brain in adults, children, and infants is often examined histologically to assess for the presence of ischemic injury (ie, red neurons). In adults, areas to best check for ischemic injury are the border zone regions (ie, the border zone between vascular distribution of two or more vessels), the posterior hippocampus (Ammon's horn), the dentate nucleus of the cerebellum, and the globus pallidus.[10] In infants, areas to best check for ischemic injury are thalamus, hippocampus, and dorsal brainstem.[11] In neonates, the components of the Papez circuit (entorhinal cortex, amygdala, hippocampus, fornix and thalamus), basal ganglia, and brainstem should be sampled to assess for ischemic injury.[12,13]

> **PEARLS & PITFALLS**
>
> A commonly encountered artifact that mimics ischemic injury is dark neuron change. In dark neuron change, the nucleus looks pyknotic, which can mimic ischemic injury; however, the neuronal cytoplasm is basophilic instead of eosinophilic. In ischemic injury, cytoplasmic eosinophilia precedes nuclear changes (Figure 17.2A-D). Dark neuron change is considered to be an artifact due to brain handling prior to fixation but is commonly misinterpreted, highlighting the importance of being aware of this histologic finding.[14,15] Dark neuron change in the dentate gyrus of the hippocampus has been associated with type I diabetes mellitus.[16]

Key locations in the brain to sample when assessing for diffuse axonal injury[10]
- Corpus callosum, mid to posterior region
- Posterior limb of the internal capsule
- Rostral pons in region of cerebellar peduncle
- Other regions to sample: medulla, genu of the corpus callosum, and cervical spinal cord

Key locations in the brain to sample when assessing for an unspecified neurodegenerative disease[9,10]
- Middle frontal gyrus
- Anterior cingulate gyrus
- Superior and middle temporal gyri
- Hippocampus and entorhinal cortex
- Inferior parietal lobule
- Primary motor cortex
- Caudate nucleus
- Globus pallidus
- Thalamus and subthalamic nucleus

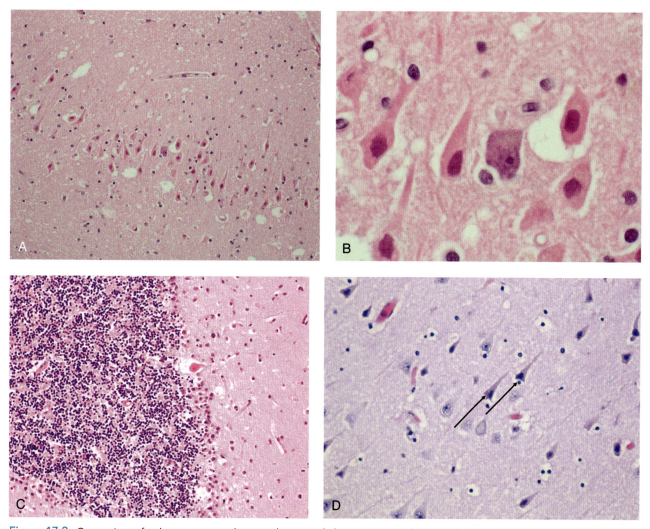

Figure 17.2. Comparison of red neurons secondary to ischemia vs dark neurons secondary to artifact. Red neurons (**A-C**) have eosinophilia of the cytoplasm, pallor of the nucleus, and often rounded external texture with loss of cellular processes, whereas dark neurons (arrows) have a contracted dark nucleus and a contracted and hyperbasophilic cytoplasm (**D**).

- Hypothalamus
- Midbrain including substantia nigra
- Pons with locus coeruleus
- Medulla
- Cerebellum and dentate nucleus

Key high-yield general locations of the brain to examine in infants and children[17]

- Hippocampus (bilateral, if asymmetric)
- Cerebral cortex with leptomeninges
- Basal ganglia
- Brainstem, including medulla

NEAR MISSES

Near Miss #1: Interpretation of histologic changes from autopsy is impaired by decomposition, which causes a loss of basophilia, general pallor of the tissue, and loss of tissue architecture. However, while decomposition can significantly impair interpretation of tissue, it is still possible for significant microscopic findings to be identified (Figure 17.3A).

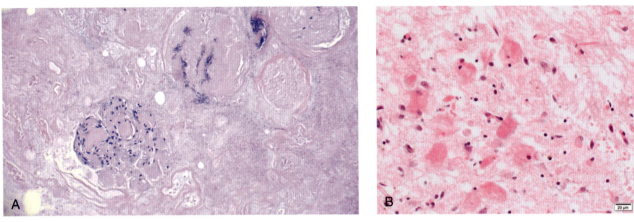

Figure 17.3. Artifacts encountered with microscopic examination. (A) is a decomposed kidney, with essentially complete loss of nuclear and cellular basophilia and pallor of the tissue; however, the characteristic Kimmelstiel-Wilson lesion associated with diabetes mellitus is identifiable in one of the glomeruli. (B) has scattered large red cells, which are anucleate squamous cells, shed from the histotechnologist's fingers.

In addition to decomposition, forensic pathologists must also be aware of artifacts encountered by surgical pathologists, including disruption of tissue (eg, chatter), floaters (ie, tissue displaced from one location to another), and other findings (eg, anucleate squamous cells originating from the histotechnologist's hands (Figure 17.3B)).

References

1. National Association of Medical Examiners. *Forensic Autopsy Performance Standards.* National Association of Medical Examiners; 2020.
2. Dettmeyer RB. The role of histopathology in forensic practice: an overview. *Forensic Sci Med Pathol.* 2014;10(3):401-412.
3. Nichols CA, Sens MA. Recovery and evaluation by cytologic techniques of trace material retained on bullets. *Am J Forensic Med Pathol.* 1990;11(1):17-34.
4. de la Grandmaison GL, Charlier P, Durigon M. Usefulness of systematic histological examination in routine forensic autopsy. *J Forensic Sci.* 2010;55(1):85-88.
5. Langlois NEI. The use of histology in 638 coronial post-mortem examinations of adults: an audit. *Med Sci Law.* 2006;46(4):310-320.
6. Molina DK, Wood LE, Frost RE. Is routine histopathologic examination beneficial in all medicolegal autopsies? *Am J Forensic Med Pathol.* 2007;28:1-3.
7. Kumar V, Abbas AK, Aster JC. *Robbins Basic Pathology.* 10th ed. Elsevier; 2018.
8. Campobasso CP, Dell'Erba AS, Addante A, Zotti F, Marzullo A, Colonna MF. Sudden cardiac death and myocardial ischemia indicators. A comparative study of four immunohistochemical markers. *Am J Forensic Med Pathol.* 2008;29(2):154-161.
9. Love S, *Current Topics in Pathology: Neuropathology, A Guide for Practising Pathologists*: Springer; 2001.
10. Dolinak D, Matshes E. *Medicolegal Neuropathology: A Color Atlas.* CRC Press; 2002.
11. Ellison D, Love S, Chimelli L, et al. *Neuropathology: A Reference Text of CNS Pathology.* 2nd ed. Mosby; 2004.
12. Zheng Q, Viaene AN, Freeman CW, Hwang M. Radiologic-pathologic evidence of brain injury: hypoperfusion in the Papez circuit results in poor neurodevelopmental outcomes in neonatal hypoxic ischemic encephalopathy. *Childs Nerv Syst.* 2021;37(1):63-68.
13. Pasternak JF, Predey TA, Mikhael MA. Neonatal asphyxia: vulnerability of basal ganglia, thalamus, and brainstem. *Pediatr Neurol.* 1991;7(2):147-149.
14. Jortner BS. The return of the dark neuron. A histological artifact complicating contemporary neurotoxicologic evaluation. *Neurotoxicology.* 2006;27(4):628-634.

15. Soontornniyomkij V, Chang RC, Soontornniyomkij B, Schilling JM, Patel HH, Jeste DV. Loss of immunohistochemical reactivity in association with handling-induced dark neurons in mouse brains. *Toxicol Pathol*. 2020;48(3):437-445.
16. Ahmadpour SH, Haghir H. Diabetes mellitus type 1 induces dark neuron formation in the dentate gyrus: a study by Gallyas' method and transmission electron microscopy. *Rom J Morphol Embryol*. 2011;52(2):575-579.
17. Folkerth RD, Nunez J, Georgievskaya Z, McGuone D. Neuropathologic examination in sudden unexpected deaths in infancy and childhood: recommendations for highest diagnostic yield and cost-effectiveness in forensic settings. *Acad Forensic Pathol*. 2017;7(2):182-199.

EMBOLISM 18

CHAPTER OUTLINE

Introduction 484

Pulmonary Thromboemboli 484
- Circumstances Under Which Pulmonary Thromboemboli Occur 484
- How to Identify 484
- Complications of a Pulmonary Thromboembolus 484
- Aging of Pulmonary Thromboemboli 486

Air Embolism 490
- Circumstance Under Which Air Emboli Occur 490
- How to Identify 490

Fat Embolism 490
- Circumstances Under Which Fat Emboli Occur 490
- Clinical Signs of Fatty Emboli 490
- How to Identify 490

Amniotic Fluid Embolism 492
- Circumstance Under Which Amniotic Fluid Emboli Occur 492
- Clinical Signs of Amniotic Fluid Emboli 492
- How to Identify 492

Bullet Embolism 493
- Circumstances Under Which a Bullet Embolism Occurs 493
- How to Identify at Autopsy 493

Septic Embolism 493
- Description of Septic Embolism 493
- Circumstances Under Which Septic Emboli Occur 493
- How to Identify at Autopsy 493
- Location of Emboli 493

Cholesterol Crystal Embolism 494
- Circumstances Under Which Cholesterol Crystal Emboli Occur 494
- How to Identify at Autopsy 494

Other Forms of Embolism 494

Near Misses 496

INTRODUCTION

Various types of emboli are encountered by forensic pathologists, including thromboemboli, air emboli, fat emboli, amniotic fluid emboli, tumor emboli (both gross and microscopic), septic emboli (eg, fragments from vegetations in infective endocarditis), and bullet and other foreign body emboli. Each type of embolus is found under characteristic circumstances; however, if the embolus is not suspected or at least considered during the autopsy procedure, it can easily be missed and not identified, which can impair the determination of the cause and manner of death as well as lead to potentially unanswered questions.

PULMONARY THROMBOEMBOLI

CIRCUMSTANCES UNDER WHICH PULMONARY THROMBOEMBOLI OCCUR

Pulmonary thromboemboli occur due to thrombi that embolize to the lungs. These thrombi most often form in the veins in the lower extremities but can also originate from veins in the upper extremities and from veins in the pelvis. The thrombi break loose from the point where they formed and ultimately enter the pulmonary circulation and can cause sudden death, especially when they lodge at the bifurcation of the pulmonary artery into the right and left main stem pulmonary arteries (ie, a saddle embolus). The main cause of the thrombi in the lower extremities is immobility or relatively decreased mobility, with obesity, trauma, sepsis, chronic illness, and recent surgery being contributors.[1] As immobility or relatively decreased mobility is the main mechanism by which thrombi in veins of the lower extremity occur, for the purpose of death certification, the reason for that diminished ability to ambulate must be determined. If the cause of the decreased mobility is traumatic (eg, a fractured ankle from a fall), the manner of death is non-natural whereas if the cause of the decreased mobility is non-traumatic (eg, obesity), the manner of death is natural. Other factors to consider that increase the risk for the formation of thrombi include inherited coagulopathies (mutations in factor V Leiden or prothrombin or deficiencies of protein C or S, anti-thrombin, or plasminogen), central venous catheters, ventriculoatrial shunts, arteriovenous malformations, inflammatory bowel disease, and cystic fibrosis.[1]

HOW TO IDENTIFY

While the identification of a pulmonary thromboembolus is not difficult in most cases as the lesion forms an obstructing mass within the pulmonary vasculature, it is possible to miss the diagnosis based upon the way in which the organs are removed from the body (eg, if the lungs are removed independently from the heart, and the pulmonary thromboemboli do not extend past the pulmonary artery main stem branch point and into the lungs, the thromboembolus will likely be missed as the dissection will disrupt the location of the thromboembolus). While the organ-by-organ approach can still be used for the autopsy, in cases where a pulmonary thromboembolus is suspected, the pulmonary artery can be opened in-situ to inspect for a thrombus, or the heart and lung block can be removed en bloc. Also, when the lung is transected at the hilum, the presence of a thromboembolus can be noted at that time also. Being able to distinguish a true antemortem thrombus from a postmortem clot is vital. A true antemortem thrombus has some characteristic features: fibrin deposition on the surface (Figure 18.1A and B); distension of the vessel in which the thromboembolus is found (Figure 18.1C and D); a branching pattern that does not fit the vessel in which the thrombus is found (Figure 18.1E); and presence of lines of Zahn, either grossly or microscopically (Figure 18.1F-H).

COMPLICATIONS OF A PULMONARY THROMBOEMBOLUS

When a pulmonary thromboembolus obstructs >60% of the vascular distribution, sudden death can occur.[2] Although the terms saddle pulmonary thromboembolism and massive pulmonary thromboembolism are often used interchangeably to refer to the same entity; it is important to know that not all saddle thromboemboli are massive thromboemboli and the terms should not be used interchangeably.[3] The difference between a massive and a non-massive pulmonary thromboembolus is based upon clinically available criteria, and would not be determinable at autopsy.[4] A massive pulmonary thromboembolus leads to shock and hemodynamic collapse.[3] A saddle vs a non-saddle pulmonary thromboembolus refers to the location of the thrombus (Figure 18.2A and B). Some authors indicate that

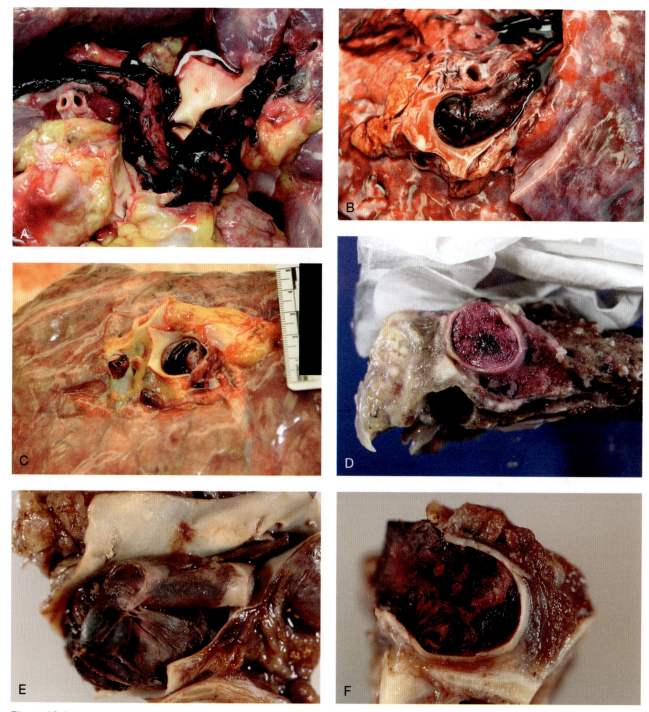

Figure 18.1. Features of a true antemortem thrombus. (**A**) is a saddle thromboembolus and (**B**) is a thromboembolus in the main stem of a left or right pulmonary artery (comment: not determinable from the image as to side). Both have a rough and focally tan-white surface, which would be consistent with fibrin deposition. (**C** and **D**) illustrate how a thromboembolus will distend the lumen of the vessel in which it is impacted. (**E**) illustrates a thromboembolus that has fibrin deposited at the surface and distends the vessel but also has a branching pattern that is inconsistent with the vessel in which it was found. When a deep vein thrombus forms, it has a branching pattern that matches the vessel in which it forms, but, when it embolizes, the branching pattern does not match any longer, whereas a postmortem clot that forms in the pulmonary vessel will branch accordingly to the vessel in which it is found. (**F**), while not ideal, illustrates the layered appearance of an antemortem thrombus, whereas (**G** and **H**) are well-defined examples of such layering of red blood cells alternating with fibrin, and are referred to as lines of Zahn.

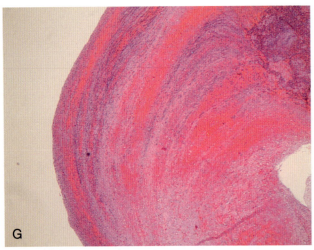
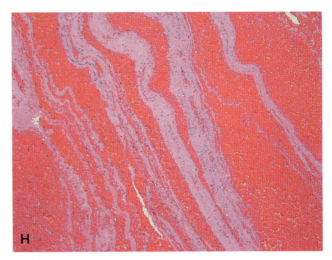

Figure 18.1. Continued

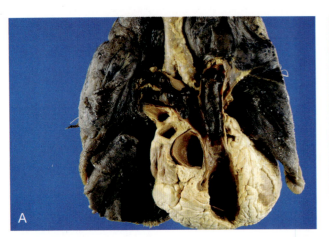
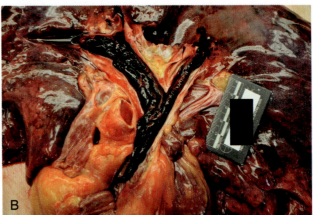

Figure 18.2. Saddle pulmonary thromboembolus. Both (**A** and **B**) illustrate a saddle thromboembolus, with the embolus present in the main stem pulmonary artery, and extending into both the left and right main stem pulmonary artery.

saddle thromboemboli have a higher risk for causing death than non-saddle emboli do, whereas other authors indicate that both saddle and non-saddle emboli are associated with similar mortality rates.[3]

In addition to sudden death, pulmonary thromboemboli, when they reach a peripheral location in the lung, can cause infarcts (Figure 18.3A-G). The presence of a peripheral infarct can provide additional support that a thrombus in the proximal pulmonary arteries is antemortem and not postmortem (ie, if the decedent has a pulmonary infarct due to an older pulmonary thromboembolus, it is more likely that they recently had a larger thromboembolus that obstructed proximally). Finally, recurrent pulmonary thromboemboli could lead to pulmonary hypertension and right ventricular hypertrophy.

AGING OF PULMONARY THROMBOEMBOLI

While an exact age of a pulmonary thromboembolus likely cannot be established, gross and microscopic examination of the thrombus could determine a relative age as to whether the pulmonary thromboembolus is more acute or organizing (Figure 18.4A-J). Recent thromboemboli would be mostly red blood cells and fibrin, at least focally in a layered pattern, whereas when the pulmonary thromboembolus ages, there will be adherence of the thrombus to the pulmonary arterial wall, and ultimately resolution or fibrotic replacement of the thrombus.

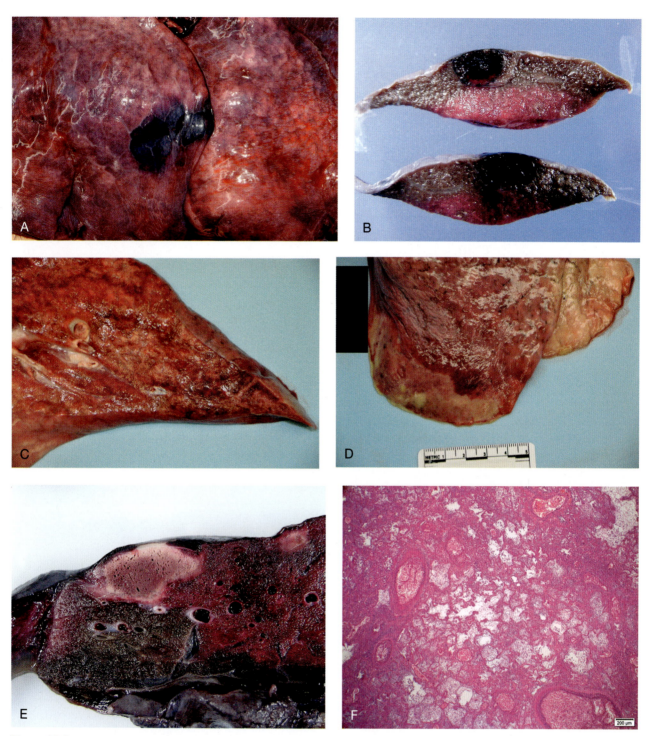

Figure 18.3. Features of pulmonary infarcts secondary to peripheral pulmonary thromboemboli. Infarcts secondary to peripheral pulmonary thromboemboli are located at the pleural surface and form a wedge, with the tip of the wedge often at the location of the thromboembolus. Initially, the infarcts are hemorrhagic and appear red, but with organization can become more firm. (**A** and **B**) are hemorrhagic infarcts and (**C-E**) are two examples of a more organized infarct, having a yellow-tan discoloration. Microscopic examination of the infarct will reveal coagulative necrosis, with preservation of architecture in the early phase of the infarct, but loss of nuclear and cellular basophilia (**F** and **G**). Congestion is also present in the earlier stages of the infarct.

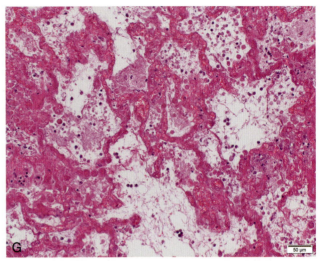

Figure 18.3. Continued

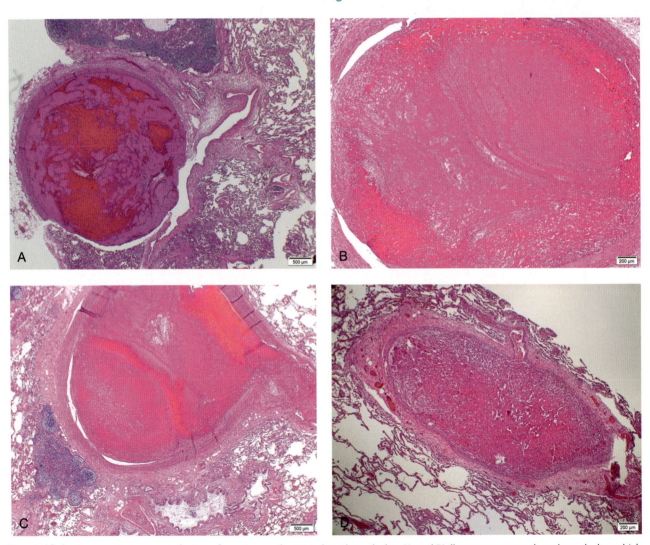

Figure 18.4. Gross and microscopic features for aging a pulmonary thromboembolus. (**A** and **B**) illustrate an acute thromboembolus, which are composed of red blood cells, fibrin, and white blood cells with minimal to no organization identifiable at the periphery. The layered architecture of a thrombus is more apparent in (**B**). (**C-E**) illustrate organization of the thrombus, with some ingrowth of fibroblasts at the periphery of the thrombus in (**C** and **D**), and with (**E**) having extensive peripheral fibrosis and new blood vessel formation. (**F**) illustrates an organized thromboembolus present at a branching point in the pulmonary artery. The thrombus is adherent to the wall of the vessel and light tan-white in coloration, secondary to fibrous replacement. (**G**) is an organized thromboembolus identified in a peripheral vessel, and is composed of mostly just cellular fibrosis with no remnants of red blood cells or fibrin, other than within revascularized channels. (**H**) is of two pulmonary thromboemboli of different ages, with the thrombus to the right being composed of essentially just red blood cells and fibrin, and with the thrombus to the left having extensive organization with fibrosis and neovascularization, but also with some residual fibrin and red blood cells. (**I** and **J**) illustrate examples of an acute thromboembolus on an older thromboembolus (comment: both are from different autopsies).

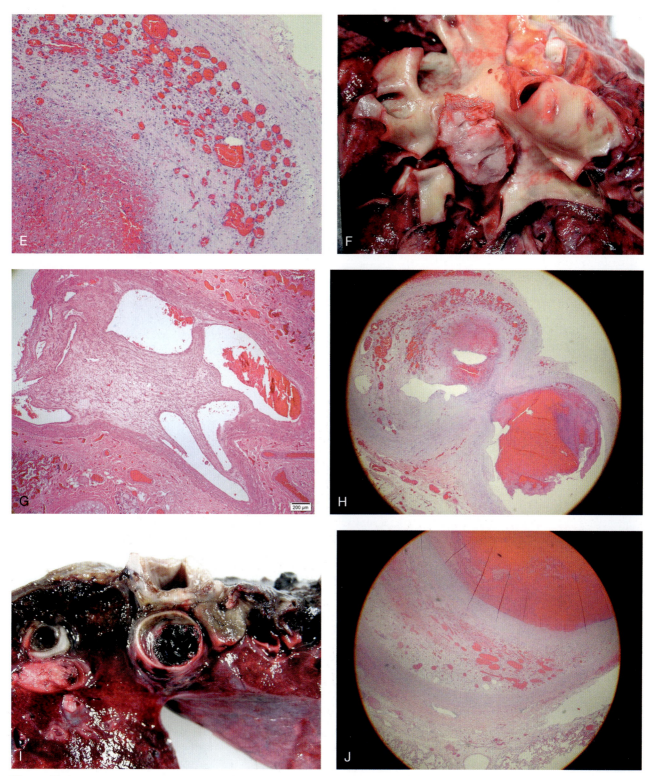

Figure 18.4. Continued

AIR EMBOLISM

CIRCUMSTANCE UNDER WHICH AIR EMBOLI OCCUR

Sharp force injuries or gunshot wounds of the neck that involve a vein, which can allow for air to be pulled into the blood circulation, are common sources of air emboli in forensic autopsies.[5] Other causes of air emboli include intravenous infusion and oral-vaginal sex in which air is forcefully blown into the vaginal cavity or when air enters the circulation through a vaginal laceration.[6,7] When sudden death follows a medical or surgical procedure or when death occurs during the birthing process, an air embolism should also be suspected.[8]

HOW TO IDENTIFY

If an air embolus is suspected, a chest radiograph should be performed.[8] When the chest is opened, the sternum should be sectioned near the level of the second rib so as to avoid injury to the great vessels, following which the pericardium is opened and the space is filled with water, after which the left and right ventricles of the heart are punctured to release air.[8] The amount of air in the heart can be measured.[8] Agarwal et al describe ligating the internal thoracic arteries prior to removal of the chest plate followed by clamping of all major vessels and subsequent removal of the heart en bloc, which was opened in a basin of water.[6] Other possible features at autopsy that could indicate an air embolus include the right side of the heart containing a large amount of red frothy blood and the lungs containing minimal blood.[6]

FAT EMBOLISM

CIRCUMSTANCES UNDER WHICH FAT EMBOLI OCCUR

While the most common situation under which fat emboli occur is the breaking of long bones or the pelvis, fat emboli have also been reported in the setting of trauma to fat, surgical operations, osteomyelitis, injury to fatty liver, alcoholic cirrhosis, and gluteal lipoinjection.[9-12]

CLINICAL SIGNS OF FATTY EMBOLI

While not all individuals with fatty emboli will be symptomatic, those individuals who are symptomatic manifest petechial hemorrhages, changing mental status, and progressive respiratory failure.[13] While the petechial rash would be visible at autopsy, the other features are not but may be identified through witness accounts of the decedent's pre-terminal events.

HOW TO IDENTIFY

Fatty emboli in the lung can be identified via Oil Red O or Sudan Black staining on frozen section tissue from the lungs, or post-fixation of lungs with osmium tetroxide, and subsequent staining[14,15] (Figure 18.5A and B). Determining the relevance of fat emboli can be problematic as fat emboli are a common finding at autopsy; however, if the fatty emboli are visible in all regions of the lung section and have an antlerlike configuration, the decedent most likely has a massive fat embolism.[14]

> **FAQ:** What is the difference between fatty emboli and bone marrow emboli?
>
> **Answer:** Fatty emboli and bone marrow emboli have a different appearance, with bone marrow emboli including hematopoietic cells (Figure 18.6). Fatty emboli and bone marrow emboli occur under similar circumstances; however, the finding of bone marrow emboli is generally considered of academic interest and is rarely of a significant enough level to cause death.[16]

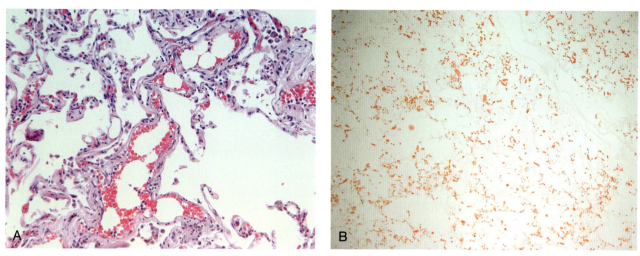

Figure 18.5. Fatty emboli. Fat emboli will appear as clear spaces in the pulmonary vasculature (**A**). An Oil Red O stain on frozen lung tissue will highlight the fatty emboli (**B**).

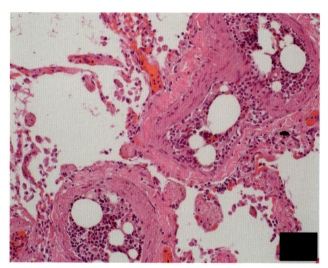

Figure 18.6. Bone marrow emboli. In addition to the clear spaces representing adipose tissue, there are aggregates of hematopoietic cells in the embolus.

PEARLS & PITFALLS

Pulmonary and even cerebral fat emboli occur in a large number of individuals who have terminal resuscitative measures performed. Pulmonary fat emboli can be identified in around 80% of individuals who receive external cardiac massage, and around 25% of these individuals can have cerebral fat emboli.[17] Therefore, the presence of such emboli is often an incidental finding and not directly related to the cause of death.

PEARLS & PITFALLS

Fat emboli can produce clinical symptoms or produce no clinical symptoms. Fatty emboli that cause symptoms, and which can lead to death, often occur after long bone or pelvic fractures (occurring in from 0.5% to 10% of cases, depending upon the number of fractures); whereas fatty emboli that do not produce clinical symptoms and are unassociated with death can occur after all long bone fractures and other conditions, both traumatic and non-traumatic.[18] At autopsy, distinguishing incidental fatty emboli from fatty emboli that caused death can be challenging. Bunai et al indicate that histologic grading of the extent of fatty emboli can be subjective and instead offered a method using image analysis to quantitate the amount of fat, which can be correlated with the probability that the fatty emboli are significant.[18]

AMNIOTIC FLUID EMBOLISM

CIRCUMSTANCE UNDER WHICH AMNIOTIC FLUID EMBOLI OCCUR

Amniotic fluid emboli occur during pregnancy, and should always be considered as a cause of the sudden unexplained death of a pregnant female.

CLINICAL SIGNS OF AMNIOTIC FLUID EMBOLI

While the clinical features of amniotic fluid embolism are variable from case to case, they generally include features associated with hypotension, hypoxia, and coagulopathy[19]

HOW TO IDENTIFY

Amniotic fluid emboli can be identified on histologic examination of the lungs, with anucleate squamous cells in the vessels (Figure 18.7A-C). In addition, mucus may be a large component of an amniotic fluid embolus. An Alcian Blue stain would assist in the identification of the amniotic fluid embolus in this situation (Figure 18.7D).

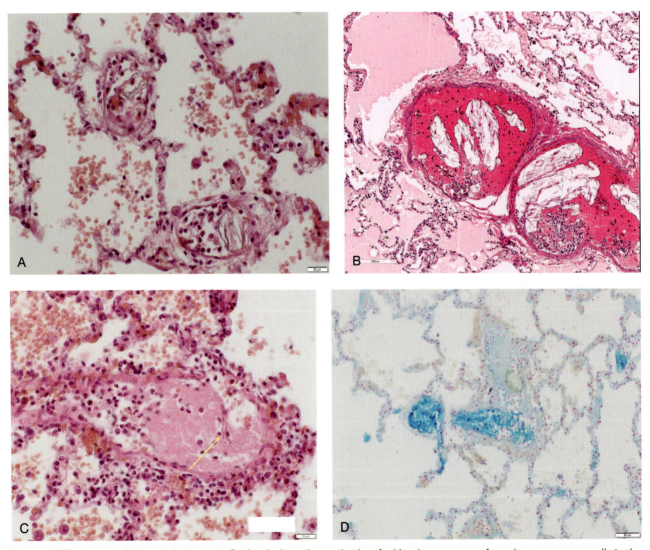

Figure 18.7. Amniotic fluid emboli. Amniotic fluid emboli can be easily identified by the presence of anucleate squamous cells in the pulmonary vasculature (**A** and **B**); however, in some circumstances, the number of anucleate squamous cells is more sparse (arrow) and can be difficult to identify (**C**). As a component of amniotic fluid is mucus, an Alcian Blue stain can assist in the identification of the emboli (**D**).

BULLET EMBOLISM

CIRCUMSTANCES UNDER WHICH A BULLET EMBOLISM OCCURS

In an individual who is shot, if the projectile penetrates but does not perforate a vessel, the projectile can be carried in the flow of blood to a point distant from the pathway of the gunshot wound (Figure 18.8).

HOW TO IDENTIFY AT AUTOPSY

Since the projectile usually lodges in the vasculature at some distance from the pathway of the projectile, unless additional radiographic imaging is performed because a bullet embolus is suspected (eg, after the entrance/exits and projectiles recovered do not add up equally) or a full body imaging study is done, bullet emboli can easily be missed at autopsy and the projectile not recovered.

SEPTIC EMBOLISM

DESCRIPTION OF SEPTIC EMBOLISM

A septic embolism is an embolus composed of an admixture of fibrin and bacterial organisms.

CIRCUMSTANCES UNDER WHICH SEPTIC EMBOLI OCCUR

The most frequent source of septic emboli is infective endocarditis.

HOW TO IDENTIFY AT AUTOPSY

While a septic embolus can be suspected at autopsy by the finding of an embolic source such as infective endocarditis and small white or yellow lesions in organ parenchyma, the microscopic examination will confirm the presence of the embolus, which is often an aggregate of bacterial organisms surrounded by acute inflammatory cells (Figure 18.9).

LOCATION OF EMBOLI

The distribution of septic emboli is going to depend upon the location of the infectious source and the presence or absence of a patent foramen oval. When septic emboli originate from vegetations on the cardiac valves, the most common downstream points of impact are the brain, the spleen, the kidneys, the lungs, the heart, and the liver.

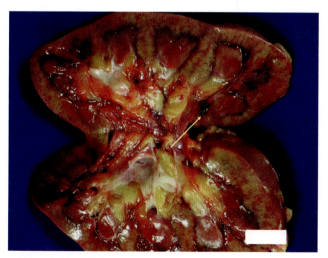

Figure 18.8. Birdshot embolus to the kidney (arrow).

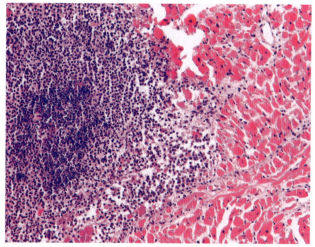

Figure 18.9. Septic embolus. There is a large aggregate of bacterial cocci surrounded by a rim of neutrophils. This septic embolus was secondary to infective endocarditis and the septic embolus was identified in the myocardium.

CHOLESTEROL CRYSTAL EMBOLISM

CIRCUMSTANCES UNDER WHICH CHOLESTEROL CRYSTAL EMBOLI OCCUR

The most frequent source of cholesterol crystals are ruptured atherosclerotic plaques.[20] Cholesterol crystal emboli can be a delayed complication of vascular surgery.[21]

HOW TO IDENTIFY AT AUTOPSY

Microscopic examination will reveal cholesterol clefts in the vessel (Figure 18.10A and B).

OTHER FORMS OF EMBOLISM

Rarely, an embolus from a cardiac myxoma or papillary fibroelastoma or other tumor can present at autopsy.[22-24] While an embolus from a cardiac myxoma or papillary fibroelastoma could be macroscopic, tumor emboli from other tumors are often microscopic. Other potential emboli encountered at autopsy include a mechanical or porcine valve embolizing into the aorta after a ring abscess or catastrophic failure of an aortic valve replacement, polymer material following surgery, bile following certain liver procedures, and barium sulfate.[25-27]

> **PEARLS & PITFALLS**
>
> Postmortem clotting of blood can mimic pulmonary thromboemboli or other thrombi. In a postmortem clot, most frequently there is separation of the red blood cells and the serum, producing a currant jelly (the red blood cells) and a chicken fat (the serum) pattern; however, this clear distinction is not always visible in postmortem clots in the lung (Figure 18.11A and B). To distinguish an antemortem pulmonary thromboembolus from a postmortem clot, examine the cut section of the vessel. A pulmonary thromboembolus will distend the vessel as the thrombus wedges into vessel. Examine the surface of the thrombus. Often a delicate lacy architecture will be present at the surface, which is fibrin related to early organization of the thrombus. Finally, examine the overall shape of the thrombus. A postmortem clot will have a branching pattern that fits the distribution of the vessels around it (ie, the postmortem clot formed in the vessels), whereas the branching pattern of the pulmonary thromboembolus will not fit the branching pattern of the vessel where it was found (ie, it formed in another location and embolized; the branching pattern would fit the distribution of the vessels where the thrombus formed, not where it ultimately lodged).

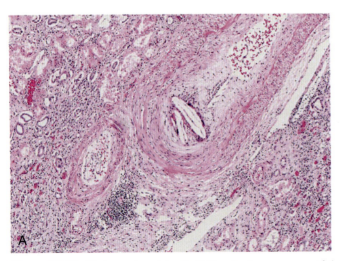
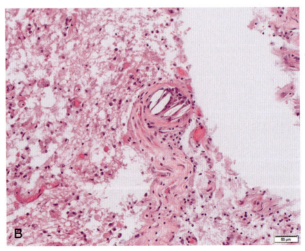

Figure 18.10. Cholesterol crystal emboli. The classic appearance of cholesterol crystals is easily identifiable in the vessel in the kidney (**A**) and in the spinal cord (**B**). Both occurred secondary to vascular procedures that resulted in embolization of cholesterol crystals.

FAQ: Are lower extremity dissections necessary when a pulmonary thromboembolus is identified?

Answer: While dissection of the lower extremities can reveal a source of the pulmonary thromboembolus (ie, the deep vein thrombosis) (Figure 18.12), it is possible for the entire deep vein thrombus to embolize and there to be none to be found upon dissection of the lower extremity. Histologic examination of the deep vein thrombus can identify features which may assist in determining the time frame for the development of the deep vein thrombosis, and finally, dissection of the lower extremities may reveal subtle previously undiagnosed or unidentified trauma, which contributed to the development of the deep vein thrombus and would determine the manner of death. However, dissection of the lower extremities can impair the embalming process and potentially hinder funeral services in that leakage from the dissection especially if done posterior may be a problem. Whether or not to perform a dissection of the lower extremities after identification of a pulmonary thromboembolus will depend upon the training and experience of the forensic pathologist, the nature of the death investigation, and potentially office policies.

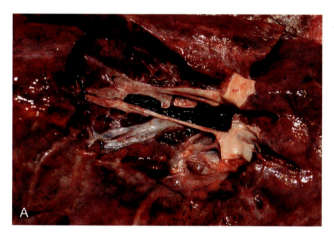 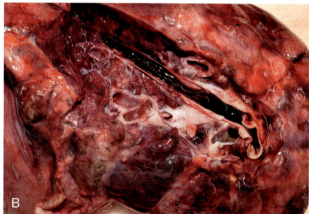

Figure 18.11. Postmortem clots. In (**A**), the clot branches into the adjacent vessels, has no fibrin at the surface, and does not distend the vessel. In (**B**), the clot does not clearly distend the vessel; however, the branching pattern also does not appear to fit the vessel in which the clot was identified. The clot in (**B**) occurred in an individual who died within hours after a traumatic event.

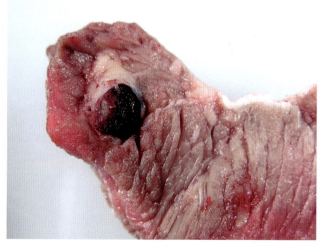

Figure 18.12. Deep vein thrombus. Distending the vein in the musculature is a thrombus.

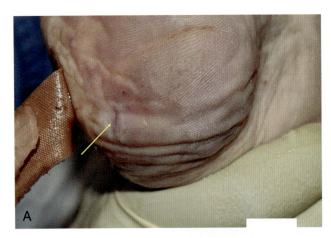
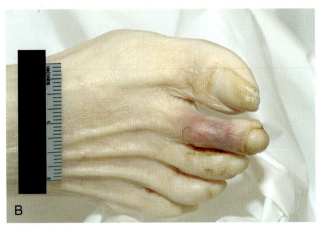
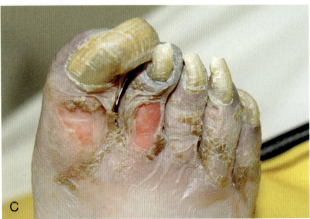

Figure 18.13. Examination of feet revealing probable source for decreased mobility. In (**A**), the decedent had a small bandage on their foot, with an underlying healing laceration of the skin (arrow). The pain of this injury, even though the injury is trivial, could have contributed to decreased mobility, and was therefore listed as the underlying cause of death, and the manner was certified as accident. In (**B**), the decedent has a pulmonary thromboembolus and examination of the feet revealed a fracture of the 2nd digit of the right foot. The manner of death was certified as accident. In (**C**), the decedent had long toenails and growth of the great toenail into the adjacent toe. This condition would potentially cause pain, and lead to decreased mobility.

NEAR MISSES

Near Miss #1: A neoplasm of the pulmonary artery, such as an intimal sarcoma, could be misinterpreted as a pulmonary thromboembolus.[28]

Near Miss #2: When a pulmonary thromboembolus has been identified as the cause of death, it is very important to examine the feet of the decedent very closely. A small lesion of the foot may indicate a reason for recent impaired mobility and thus, risk for deep vein thrombosis and subsequent pulmonary thromboembolus (Figure 18.13A-C). In addition, during the investigation of the death it is important to find out from the friends and family of the decedent if they had any recent injury that impaired their mobility. A strained ankle may impair mobility but would not be identified by a routine autopsy, unless the lower extremities were dissected and some form of hemorrhage was found within the joint capsule or surrounding soft tissue.

Near Miss #3: A heart removed for valvular transplant purposes was interpreted by the cardiovascular pathologist as having an isolated acute myocardial infarct of the right ventricle due to coronary artery atherosclerosis. However, autopsy had identified a pulmonary thromboembolus. Pulmonary thromboemboli can be associated with inflammatory infiltrates and myocyte necrosis in the right ventricle, and be misinterpreted as an acute myocardial infarct (Figure 18.14A and B).[29]

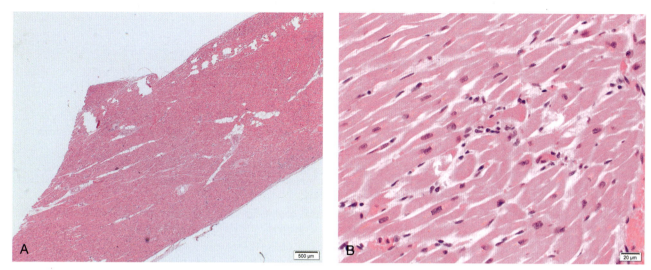

Figure 18.14. Inflammation of right ventricle associated with pulmonary thromboembolus. (**A**) reveals the very patchy nature of the inflammatory infiltrates. (**B**) illustrates a patch of coagulative necrosis associated with an acute inflammatory infiltrate.

References

1. Byard RW. Fatal embolic events in childhood. *J Forensic Leg Med*. 2013;20:1-5.
2. Kumar V, Abbas AK, Aster JC. *Robbins Basic Pathology*. 10th ed. Elsevier; 2018.
3. Alkinj B, Pannu BS, Apala DR, Kotecha A, Kashyap R, Iyer VN. Saddle vs Nonsaddle pulmonary embolism: clinical presentation, hemodynamics, management, and outcomes. *Mayo Clin Proc*. 2017;92(10):1511-1518.
4. Blondon M, Jimenez D, Robert-Ebadi H, et al. Comparative clinical prognosis of massive and non-massive pulmonary embolism: a registry-based cohort study. *J Thromb Haemost*. 2021;19(2):408-416.
5. Adams VI, Hirsch CS. Venous air embolism from head and neck wounds. *Arch Pathol Lab Med*. 1989;113(5):498-502.
6. Agarwal SS, Kumar L, Chavali KH, Mestri SC. Fatal venous air embolism following intravenous infusion. *J Forensic Sci*. 2009;54(3):682-684.
7. Lohner L, Sperhake JP, Puschel K, Burandt EC, Heinemann A, Anders S. Vaginal laceration leading to air embolism during consensual sexual intercourse. *Int J Legal Med*. 2021;135(1):341-346.
8. Bajanowski T, West A, Brinkmann B. Proof of fatal air embolism. *Int J Legal Med*. 1998;111(4):208-211.
9. Peltier LF. Fat embolism: a perspective. *Clin Orthopaedics Res*. 2004;422:148-153.
10. Sakashita M, Sakashita S, Sakata A, et al. An autopsy case of non-traumatic fat embolism syndrome. *Pathol Int*. 2017;67(9):477-482.
11. Cantu CA, Pavlisko EN. Liposuction-induced fat embolism syndrome. *BMJ Case Rep*. 2017;2017:bcr2017219835.
12. Bayter-Marin JE, Cárdenas-Camarena L, Aguirre-Serrano H, Durán H, Ramos-Gallardo G, Robles-Cervantes JA. Understanding fatal fat embolism in gluteal lipoinjection: a review of the medical records and autopsy reports of 16 patients. *Plast Reconstr Surg*. 2018;142(5):1198-1208.
13. Akhtar S. Fat embolism. *Anesthesiol Clin*. 2009;27(3):533-550.
14. Dettmeyer RB. The role of histopathology in forensic practice: an overview. *Forensic Sci Med Pathol*. 2014;10(3):401-412.
15. Milroy CM, Parai JL. Fat embolism, fat embolism syndrome and the autopsy. *Acad Forensic Pathol*. 2019;9(3-4):136-154.
16. Fisher JH. Bone marrow embolism. *Am J Pathol*. 1951;27(4):701-702.
17. Olds K, Byard RW, Langlois NEI. Injuries associated with resuscitation-an overview. *J Forensic Leg Med*. 2015;33:39-43.
18. Bunai Y, Yoshimi N, Komoriya H, Iwasa M, Ohya I. An application of a quantitative analytical system for the grading of pulmonary fat embolisms. *Forensic Sci Int*. 1988;39(3):263-269.

19. Shamshirsaz AA, Clark SL. Amniotic fluid embolism. *Obstet Gynecol Clin North Am.* 2016;43(4):779-790.
20. Sato Y, Okamoto K, Fukuda M, et al. An autopsy case of acute pancreatitis caused by cholesterol crystal embolization. *Intern Med.* 2021;60(6):839-845.
21. Fries C, Roos M, Gaspert A, et al. Atheroembolic disease–a frequently missed diagnosis: results of a 12-year matched-pair autopsy study. *Medicine.* 2010;89(2):126-132.
22. Dell'Aquila M, Carbone A, Pennacchia I, Stigliano E, Oliva A, Arena V. Sudden death by massive systemic embolism from cardiac myxoma. Role of the clinical autopsy and review of literature. *Cardiovasc Pathol.* 2020;49:107244.
23. Uga S, Ikeda S, Matsukage S, et al. An autopsy case of acute cor pulmonale and paradoxical systemic embolism due to tumour cell microemboli in a patient with breast cancer. *BMJ Case Rep.* 2012;2012:bcr2012006682.
24. Okazaki S, Abe T, Takayanagi N, et al. Pulmonary tumor embolism due to squamous cell carcinoma of the uterine cervix: a case report. *In Vivo.* 2018;32(2):337-343.
25. Mehta RI, Perrin RJ, Baldzizhar R, Mehta RI. polymer coating embolism: cause of cerebral vasculopathy and death following congenital heart repair in two infants. *J Neuropathol Exp Neurol.* 2017;76(11):978-980.
26. Brozinsky S, DeSoto-Lapaix F, Jimenez FA, Ostrowitz A. Bile emboli: a complication of PTD. *J Clin Gastroenterol.* 1981;3(2):135-137.
27. Lunetta P, Ojanpera I, Sajantila A. Fatal iatrogenic $BaSO_4$ embolism: morphological and ultrastructural findings confirmed by X-ray microanalysis and ICP-AES. *Forensic Sci Int.* 2007;172(2-3):203-207. doi:10.1016/j.forsciint.2006.11.009
28. Rijal R, Mridha AR, Arava SK, Behera C. Primary intimal sarcoma of the pulmonary artery misdiagnosed as pulmonary thromboembolism: a case confirmed at medicolegal autopsy. *J Forensic Sci.* 2021;66(1):403-406. doi:10.1111/1556-4029.14592
29. Orde MM, Puranik R, Morrow PL, Duflou J. Myocardial pathology in pulmonary thromboembolism. *Heart.* 2011;97(20):1695-1699.

MICROBIOLOGIC ANALYSES

CHAPTER OUTLINE

Introduction   500

INTRODUCTION

Postmortem microbiology can include cultures, polymerase chain reaction testing, and serologic studies. While postmortem microbiology studies can provide a useful adjunct in the determination of which bacterial, viral, or fungal organism is the cause of an infection, whether or not performing routine blood, lung, or cerebrospinal cultures at the time of autopsy is useful when no infectious source is present can be debated.

Description of general mechanisms causing positive postmortem cultures[1-3]: A positive postmortem culture can represent the etiologic agent of an identified infectious source (eg, meningitis or an abscess in the lung); however, a culture can be positive for other reasons. The most common other reason for a positive postmortem culture is contamination, for which the risk can be lessened by using sterile procedure when collecting the specimen. Another potential cause of a positive culture that does not reflect an antemortem process is postmortem spread of the organism. Two mechanisms for postmortem spread of organisms are transmigration, which will occur over time after death, and the possibility of agonal spread. In agonal spread, it is believed that microorganisms enter into the blood through damaged tissue from shock (eg, intestinal necrosis).

KEY FEATURES of postmortem microbiology[2,3]

- Contamination of samples produces the most artifact.
- A pure pathogen is most likely a significant organism.
- Cultures of *Streptococcus pneumoniae*, *Streptococcus pyogenes*, and *Staphylococcus aureus* usually represent a significant infection.
- Polymicrobial cultures and cultures with coagulase-negative *Staphylococcus* and mixed intestinal flora are most likely contaminants.[3]
- Postmortem spread (most likely through transmigration) is not a significant factor for the first 24 to 48 hours after death.[3]

FAQ: Are routine postmortem bacterial cultures useful?

Answer: Riedel describes that other authors both question the utility of postmortem cultures and support the utility of postmortem cultures.[3] Riedel opines that the use of routine postmortem cultures provides little useful information.[3]

PEARLS & PITFALLS

Post-splenectomy patients are at risk for severe infections, including infections associated with encapsulated organisms such as *S. pneumoniae*, which can have a high mortality.[4,5] The decedent may have no underlying infectious focus such as pneumonia, and only a culture of the postmortem blood will identify the cause of death.

References

1. Fernández-Rodríguez A, Burton JL, Andreoletti L, et al. Post-mortem microbiology in sudden death: sampling protocols proposed in different clinical settings. *Clin Microbiol Infect.* 2019;25(5):570-579.
2. Morris JA, Harrison LM, Partridge SM. Postmortem bacteriology: a re-evaluation. *J Clin Pathol.* 2006;59:1-9.
3. Riedel S. The value of postmortem microbiology cultures. *J Clin Microbiol.* 2014;52(4):1028-1033.
4. Tahir F, Ahmed J, Malik F. Post-splenectomy sepsis: a review of the literature. *Cureus.* 2020;12(2):e6898.
5. Rizzo M, Magro G, Castaldo P. OPSI (overwhelming postsplenectomy infection) syndrome: a case report. *Forensic Sci Int.* 2004;146(suppl):S55-S56.

VITREOUS ELECTROLYTE ANALYSIS

CHAPTER OUTLINE

Introduction 502

Vitreous Electrolyte Patterns 502

Hyponatremia 503
- Causes of Fatal Hyponatremia 503
- Clinical Features of Hyponatremia 503
- How to Determine at Autopsy 503

Hyperglycemia 503
- How to Determine at Autopsy 503

Ketoacidosis 504
- How to Determine at Autopsy 504

INTRODUCTION

At the time of autopsy, vitreous fluid is normally obtained, unless it is not available due to the condition of the body (eg, significant trauma with absence of the eye, or secondary to decomposition). While vitreous fluid can be used in toxicologic analyses and is often used for alcohol determinations, the fluid can also be used to evaluate electrolytes. Vitreous fluid electrolyte analysis most often includes measurements of sodium, potassium, chloride, glucose, creatinine, and vitreous urea nitrogen (VUN), which is the postmortem equivalent of blood urea nitrogen (BUN). While electrolyte analysis could be performed on postmortem blood samples, because of the breakdown of red blood cells and other changes that occur after death, the interpretation of electrolyte concentrations based upon results from postmortem blood are unreliable, whereas the vitreous fluid, with a minimal cellular component, offers a much more reliable source for determination of postmortem electrolytes. However, even so, vitreous electrolyte analysis is not without difficulties as postmortem changes can alter the electrolyte concentrations, with increasing concentrations of potassium and decreasing concentrations of glucose.

VITREOUS ELECTROLYTE PATTERNS

Coe described four patterns (Table 20.1) that are commonly identified when postmortem vitreous electrolyte analysis is performed.[1] In the dehydration pattern, the sodium is >155 mEq/L and the chloride is >135 mEq/L. The urea nitrogen will also be elevated, most often between 40 and 100 mg/dL. In the uremic pattern, the urea nitrogen and creatinine concentrations are markedly elevated; however, the sodium and chloride concentrations are not elevated. In the low-salt pattern, the sodium is <130 mEq/L and the chloride is <105 mEq/L and the potassium is <15 mEq/L. In contrast, in the decomposition pattern, the sodium and chloride concentrations are similar to those in the low-salt pattern, but the potassium is >15 mEq/L. The low salt pattern is commonly found in chronic alcoholics. In any given autopsy case, more than one pattern above may be present, and thus, final interpretation of the vitreous electrolyte pattern is best done based upon the totality of the autopsy and scene investigation findings.

> **FAQ:** What are autopsy findings of dehydration?
>
> **Answer:** Autopsy findings consistent with dehydration include sunken eyes, sticky serosal surfaces, decreased skin turgor (which can also occur secondary to loss of skin elasticity), dark urine, and constipation. If historical information is available, it can include reports of dry mucous membranes, decreased sweating, and mental status changes.[2] Vitreous electrolyte analysis is a useful adjunct to the diagnosis of dehydration.[3,4]

TABLE 20.1: Vitreous Electrolyte Patterns

	Sodium	Chloride	Potassium	Urea Nitrogen and Creatinine
Dehydration	>155 mEq/L	>135 mEq/L		Urea nitrogen: 40-100 mg/dL
Uremic	Not elevated	Not elevated		Elevated
Low salt	<130 mEq/L	<105 mEq/L	<15 mEq/L	
Decomposition	<130 mEq/L	<105 mEq/L	>15 mEq/L	

> **PEARLS & PITFALLS**
>
> While a useful adjunct to the autopsy, there are several problems associated with vitreous electrolyte analysis, including variation in values obtained due to different instrumentation used by different labs and low precision with results potentially having high standard deviations, both of which contribute to the difficulty in establishing normal ranges. Also, the decedent may have an unknown disease process that could affect the laboratory value and contribute to difficulties in interpretations.[5,6] However, Thierauf et al analyzed only fifteen sets of eyes to obtain their data, which would also contribute to a high standard deviation, and not necessarily reflect only problems intrinsic to the process of postmortem vitreous electrolyte analysis.[5] Luna concludes that despite challenges in the process, vitreous humor analysis is a useful adjunct in forensic practice.[6]

HYPONATREMIA

CAUSES OF FATAL HYPONATREMIA

Reported causes of fatal hyponatremia identified at autopsy include psychogenic polydipsia, high-endurance exercise, use of amphetamine derivatives (MDMA [3,4-methylenedioxymethamphetamine]), forced water intoxication (in child abuse), and iatrogenic causes.[7] The number of conditions causing hyponatremia itself is much more extensive including vomiting, diarrhea, sweating, burns, salt wasting kidney or cerebral disease, Addison disease, syndrome of inappropriate antidiuretic hormone (SIADH), glucocorticoid deficiency, congestive heart failure, nephrotic syndrome, and cirrhosis, among other conditions.[8,9]

CLINICAL FEATURES OF HYPONATREMIA

The clinical features are non-specific, including malaise and headache.[8]

HOW TO DETERMINE AT AUTOPSY

In their review of the literature, Vanhaebost et al identified six cases in the medical literature where the cause of death was fatal hyponatremia.[7] The reported sodium concentrations varied from 83 mEq/L to 115 mEq/L. However, with time, the sodium and chloride concentrations will also decrease in the postmortem interval due to probable diffusion of those two electrolytes into retinal and choroidal cells.[7] Cerebral edema can be the result of acute hyponatremia.[8] Vanhaebost et al conclude that determining hyponatremia in the postmortem period should not be done solely based upon the concentration of sodium in the vitreous fluid, unless the underlying cause was water intoxication.[7]

HYPERGLYCEMIA

HOW TO DETERMINE AT AUTOPSY

Vitreous glucose concentration is a reliable marker for elevated glucose in the decedent, and, in combination with analysis for ketone bodies, can be used to diagnose diabetic ketoacidosis. Karlovsek reportedly indicates that a postmortem concentration of 234 mg/dL of glucose could indicate hyperglycemia with a fatal outcome; however, the analysis of the vitreous fluid for ketone bodies to supplement the determination is also appropriate.[10,11] If glucose is elevated, but ketones are negative, the forensic pathologist should determine whether D50 was given, because with survival time, this could elevate the vitreous glucose.

> **FAQ:** Should the vitreous fluid from each eye be drawn separately and placed into a separate tube and each analyzed separately?
>
> **Answer:** Mulla et al found that the difference in concentration between electrolytes, including calcium, for each eye was insignificant.[12] However, Pounder et al found no significant differences between sodium and chloride concentrations between the left and right eye but did find a significant difference in the concentration of potassium between the two eyes.[13]
>
> **FAQ:** Can a potassium overdose, whether suicidal or homicidal, be diagnosed through vitreous electrolyte analysis at autopsy?
>
> **Answer:** Following death, the vitreous potassium concentration will rise quickly, so, without historical or scene confirmation of the potassium administration, postmortem diagnosis would not be possible.[14,15]

KETOACIDOSIS

HOW TO DETERMINE AT AUTOPSY

Evaluation of the blood, the urine, and the vitreous fluid can be performed to identify ketones. Ketones include acetoacetate, 3-β-hydroxybutyrate (3HB), and acetone. In ketoacidosis, concentrations of ketones are often >3,000 µmol/L, with normal concentrations of ketones being <500 µmol/L.[11] While diabetic ketoacidosis is one cause of ketoacidosis, there are other causes, including alcoholic or starvation ketoacidosis.[11]

While acetone is a ketone body, there are multiple conditions that can lead to acetone in the vitreous fluid (or blood). Acetone can be derived either endogenously or exogenously. Endogenous production of acetone would occur in ketoacidosis (diabetic, alcoholic, or starvation) and in hypothermia, and exogenous introduction of acetone would occur via ingestion of substances with an acetone base such as glues and solvents, or ingestion of isopropanol or alcohol not-intended for consumption, which contains acetone and/or propanol.[16]

> **PEARLS & PITFALLS**
>
> Coe indicates that the postmortem diagnosis of hypoglycemia is essentially impossible as the glucose concentration in the vitreous fluid declines after death[1]; however, perhaps with confirmatory clinical information and a very brief postmortem interval, the vitreous glucose could potentially be used as a way to detect hypoglycemia. One cause of lethal hypoglycemia could be an insulin overdose. Such a situation can be diagnosed via postmortem analysis of both insulin and C peptide concentrations. If the insulin concentration is elevated and the C peptide concentration is decreased, the most likely cause is exogenous insulin administration.[11] The reported concentrations for lethal level of insulin; however, is debated. Reportedly, authors have proposed from 100 µIU/mL to 800 µIU/mL as the lower range of a lethal concentration.[11]

> **PEARLS & PITFALLS**
>
> The presence of isopropyl alcohol in the body fluids can provide a diagnostic challenge as it can indicate ingestion or inhalation of the alcohol; however, acetone can also be converted to isopropyl alcohol and thus can be present in decedents with ketoacidosis and in patients who die as the result of hypothermia or who are chronic alcoholics.[11] To distinguish those situations (ie, intake of isopropyl alcohol vs ketoacidosis) testing for 3HB can be performed, with 3HB present in individuals who are in ketoacidosis, but not due to ingestion or inhalation.[11]

> **PEARLS & PITFALLS**
>
> In addition to testing for sodium, chloride, potassium, urea nitrogen, creatinine, and glucose, the vitreous fluid may be used for testing for other substances, such as ethanol and various drugs, and can also play a role in the investigation of drowning deaths, such as elevation of sodium and chloride concentrations in salt water drowning.[17-19]

References

1. Coe JI. Postmortem chemistry of blood, cerebrospinal fluid and vitreous humor. In: Tedeschi CG, Eckert WC, Tedeschi LG, eds. *Forensic Medicine*. Vol. 2. WB Saunders; 1977.
2. Howe JA, Collins KA, King PS, et al. *Investigation of elder deaths*. 2014;4(3):290-304.
3. Whitehead FJ, Couper RT, Moore L, Bourne AJ, Byard RW. Dehydration deaths in infants and young children. *Am J Forensic Med Pathol*. 1996;17(1):73-78.
4. Huser CJ, Smialek JE. Diagnosis of sudden death in infants due to acute dehydration. *Am J Forensic Med Pathol*. 1986;7(4):278-282.
5. Thierauf A, Musshoff F, Madea B. Postmortem biochemical investigations of vitreous humor. *Forensic Sci Int*. 2009;192(1-3):78-82.
6. Luna A. Is postmortem biochemistry really useful? Why is it not widely used in forensic pathology. *Leg Med*. 2009;11:527-530.
7. Vanhaebost J, Palmiere C, Scarpelli MP, Bou Abdallah F, Capron A, Schmit G. Postmortem diagnosis of hyponatremia: case report and literature review. *Int J Leg Med*. 2018;132(1):173-179.
8. Byramji A, Cains G, Gilbert JD, Byard RW. Hyponatremia at autopsy: an analysis of etiologic mechanisms and their possible significance. *Forensic Sci Med Pathol*. 2008;4(3):149-152.
9. Kemp WL, Koponen MA, Meyers SE. Addison disease: the first presentation of the condition may be at autopsy. *Acad Forensic Pathol*. 2016;6(2):249-257.
10. Karlovsek MZ. Postmortem diagnosis of diabetes mellitus and diabetic coma: a comparison of HbA1, glucose, lactate and combined glucose and lactate values in vitreous humor and in cerebrospinal fluid. In: Jacob B, Bonte W, eds. *Advances in Forensic Sciences: Forensic Criminalistic 2*. Vol. 4. Verlag Dr Köstner; 1995.
11. Palmiere C, Mangin P. Postmortem chemistry update Part I. *Int J Legal Med*. 2012;126(2):187-198.
12. Mulla A, Massey KL, Kalra J. Vitreous humor biochemical constituents: evaluation of between-eye differences. *Am J Forensic Med Pathol*. 2005;26(2):146-149.
13. Pounder DJ, Carson DO, Johnston K, Orihara Y. Electrolyte concentration differences between left and right vitreous humor samples. *J Forensic Sci*. 1998;43(3):604-607.
14. Chaturvedi AK, Rao NG, Moon MD. Poisoning associated with potassium. *Hum Toxicol*. 1986;5(6):377-380.
15. Palmiere C, Scarpelli MP, Varlet V, Baumann P, Michaud K, Augsburger M. Fatal intravenous injection of potassium: is postmortem biochemistry useful for the diagnosis? *Forensic Sci Int*. 2017;274:27-32.
16. Teresiński G, Buszewicz G, Madro R. Acetonaemia as an initial criterion of evaluation of a probable cause of sudden death. *Leg Med*. 2009;11(1):18-24.
17. Garland J, Tse R, Oldmeadow C, Attia J, Anne S, Cala AD. Elevation of post mortem vitreous humour sodium and chloride levels can be used as a reliable test in cases of suspected salt water drowning when the immersion times are less than one hour. *Forensic Sci Int*. 2016;266:338-342.
18. Cala AD, Vilain R, Tse R. Elevated postmortem vitreous sodium and chloride levels distinguish saltwater drowning (SWD) deaths from immersion deaths not related to drowning but recovered from saltwater (DNRD). *Am J Forensic Med Pathol*. 2013;34(2):133-138.
19. Byard RW, Summersides G. Vitreous humor sodium levels in immersion deaths. *J Forensic Sci*. 2011;56(3):643-644.

SUDDEN UNEXPECTED INFANT DEATH

21

CHAPTER OUTLINE

Introduction 508

Checklist for Investigation of a Sudden Unexpected Infant Death 508

Description of SUID (sudden unexplained infant death) and SIDS (sudden infant death syndrome) 510

Identifying an overlay or other asphyxial death at autopsy 510

Microbiology Studies 512

Near Miss 513

INTRODUCTION

Sudden unexpected infant deaths will frequently be encountered by forensic pathologists. While child abuse must always be considered when an infant dies suddenly, this chapter will focus on non-traumatic deaths. Common scenarios include infants who die while sleeping in a crib or who are bed-sharing with adults or who are in another unsafe sleeping environment. Definitive natural disease causes of death (eg, myocarditis, encephalitis, ruptured berry aneurysm) are not frequently identified at autopsy as the cause of a sudden unexpected infant death; instead, the most common differential diagnosis is a sudden unexplained natural death (ie, one with no gross or microscopic abnormalities) or an asphyxial-type death, which can include death while bed-sharing or death under another unsafe sleeping condition. Unfortunately, distinguishing between a sudden unexplained natural death and an asphyxial-type death is problematic.

CHECKLIST for Investigation of a Sudden Unexpected Infant Death

- [ ] Performance of a scene investigation including completion of the Centers for Disease Control and Prevention's sudden unexpected infant death investigation (SUIDI) form and photos of a doll re-enactment (Figure 21.1) (the scene investigation should include investigation of the location where the infant was found unresponsive and not just the hospital bed where death was pronounced)
- [ ] Documentation of important risk factors for SUID: bed-sharing, prone sleep position, and maternal tobacco use[1]
- [ ] Documentation of sleeping conditions for infant, including type of bedding present
- [ ] If witnesses/caregivers report injury prior to death, documentation of the specifics of the injury
- [ ] Review of medical records to obtain birth history, neonatal screen results, and information about subsequent doctor's visits
- [ ] Obtain full body radiographs and/or computed tomography scan
- [ ] Perform complete autopsy, which can include middle ears, optic nerves and eyes, and back dissection, depending upon the preference of the pathologist and office policies
- [ ] Obtain fluids for toxicologic analysis, including vitreous electrolyte analysis
- [ ] If applicable, obtain heart blood and cerebrospinal fluid for bacterial cultures, and nasal swabs for viral polymerase chain reaction analysis
- [ ] Obtain specimen for metabolic testing
- [ ] Obtain specimen for genetic testing
- [ ] Perform histologic examination of the organs

PEARLS & PITFALLS

With full-body radiographs, the bones of the forearms and the legs tend to overlap, which can obscure findings. Two methods to counteract this tendency are to place the infant face down for the radiographs, which tends to straighten out the legs, or to loosely bind the thighs together, which can also straighten out the legs.

FAQ: When evaluating an infant death, how many histologic sections are necessary?

Answer: In their evaluation of 510 sudden unexpected deaths of infants, Weber et al found that 166 deaths were ultimately explained, and of those deaths, a little over 50% were explained by histologic examination of the lungs, the heart, the liver or the kidneys, with sections of the spleen, thymus, pancreas, and adrenal glands not identifying a cause of death in any case.[2] While histologic examination of the thymus may not identify a cause of death, it will allow for identification of thymic involution (Figure 21.2A-C), which can be a significant marker for stress, such as could occur with abuse or neglect, or as a marker for an immune system deficiency.[3,4] Although the histologic examination of organs in an infant forensic autopsy is often unrevealing, broad sampling of the organs is the best option to ensure a thorough evaluation of the unexpected death.

PEARLS & PITFALLS

When selecting sections for histologic analysis in the case of a sudden unexpected infant death, microscopic examination of the diaphragm may yield significant findings as to a cause of death, including inflammation.[5] In addition, even in infants, the atrioventricular node can be identified by microscopic examination.

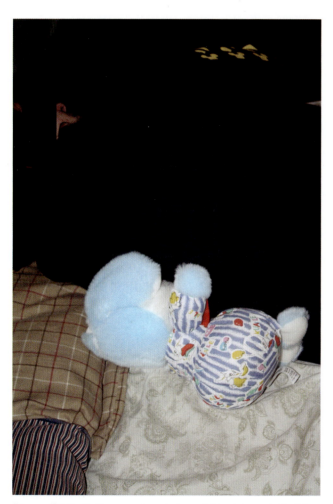

Figure 21.1. Doll re-enactment. A useful tool to assist in infant death investigations is a doll re-enactment, in which the caregiver is asked to position a doll in the position in which the infant was placed down to sleep, in the position in which the infant was last known alive, and the position in which the infant was found dead. Figure 21.1 illustrates how the infant was found by the caregiver. Although the doll re-enactment is best performed with a realistic doll, to help reduce potential emotional response from the caregiver, a stuffed animal or other doll can be used.

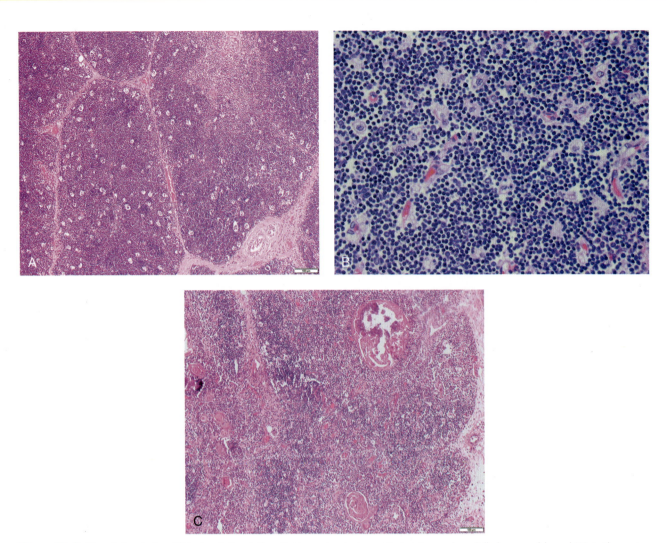

Figure 21.2. Thymic involution. With thymic involution, the boundary between the cortex and medulla become blurred (**A**). In the cortex will be numerous macrophages (**B**). In the medulla will be a prominent number of large Hassall corpuscles (**C**).

Description of SUID (sudden unexplained infant death) and SIDS (sudden infant death syndrome): Both SUID and SIDS are or have been used when a scene investigation, toxicologic analysis, and autopsy fail to determine a cause of death. The term "sudden infant death syndrome" (SIDS) was developed by Beckwith et al and came to be used as the cause of death when an infant between 1 month and 1 year of age, usually between the ages of 2 and 4 months, died unexpectedly, with a subsequent negative scene investigation, autopsy, and toxicologic analysis.[6] The manner of death was natural. However, among forensic pathologists, a switch from SIDS/natural to SUID/undetermined for cause and manner of death has occurred for several reasons including that the diagnosis of SIDS has been used too liberally and traumatic deaths have been mistakenly diagnosed as SIDS, but also because distinguishing between a sudden natural death with no autopsy findings and an asphyxial-type death cannot be done adequately.[7-14] However, in the medical literature, the term SIDS is still routinely used in the year 2023. Although clinicians tend to use SIDS, they recognize the importance of the sleeping environment, with prone or side sleeping and bed sharing as risk factors for SIDS and also that a firm crib mattress and no soft bedding are important considerations to prevent SIDS.[15] The main distinction between the forensic pathology and clinical physician approach to sudden unexpected infant deaths would therefore apparently not be whether SIDS or SUID is more appropriate but whether an infant dying in an asphyxial environment is a non-natural death.

Identifying an overlay or other asphyxial death at autopsy: Case reports describe autopsy findings associated with asphyxial deaths. For example, Nya et al report an infant who was overlaid by the mother's breast during breastfeeding.[16] Autopsy identified congestion in the right frontal region of the face, bilateral conjunctival petechiae, congestion with petechiae of the right frontal scalp, and few petechiae of the lungs. However, the autopsy findings of asphyxia including overlay are non-specific and the pertinent findings are either debated or considered minuscule or non-existent.[17,18] Brown et al best describe the difficulty as "There is no set of autopsy criteria that is pathognomonic for asphyxial deaths," and "…determination of the cause and manner of death in most newborn, infant, and young childhood asphyxial deaths is not possible based on the autopsy findings alone. Rather, the diagnosis is often based on scene investigation, witness statements, and even confessions."[19]

FAQ: What is the importance of intra-thoracic petechiae?

Answer: Intra-thoracic petechiae (ie, petechiae of the thymus, pleura, and epicardium) are frequent findings during an infant autopsy (Figure 21.3A-D). Potential causes that have been considered are SIDS, overlay with thoracic compression, cardiopulmonary resuscitation, and body position. Kleemann et al found that intra-thoracic petechiae were significantly more common in SIDS cases than the control group, which comprised natural deaths and traumatic deaths.[20] Beckwith indicates that vigorous respiratory efforts associated with upper airway obstruction may be the mechanism of formation of the intra-thoracic petechiae in SIDS.[21] Richardson and Adams, through stimulation of the laryngeal chemoreflex in piglets leading to death through prolonged apnea, induced intra-thoracic petechiae, with the number of intra-thoracic petechiae increased in piglets pretreated with hypoxic gases.[22] Based upon their study of 473 cases of SIDS, Krous et al found that the incidence of intra-thoracic petechiae did not vary between infants found face up and those found face down, and the authors concluded that their study did not support external upper airway obstruction due to a face down position as contributory to the causation of intra-thoracic petechiae, but instead that the intra-thoracic petechiae were from internal upper airway obstruction, which would be in agreement with Beckwith.[21,23] The work of Krous would seem to indicate that situations such as smothering, which could occur during bed-sharing, would not lead to intra-thoracic petechiae. With regard to distinguishing whether or not an infant was overlaid based upon the presence of intra-thoracic petechiae, Weber et al found no significant difference in the incidence of intra-thoracic petechiae between co-sleeping and non-co-sleeping deaths, but did find a significant difference in the incidence of fresh intra-alveolar hemorrhage between co-sleeping and non-co-sleeping, with fresh intra-alveolar hemorrhage more common in infants who died while co-sleeping.[24] Becroft et al identified that nasal and intra-pulmonary hemorrhages were statistically associated with bed-sharing, but intra-thoracic petechiae were not.[25] However, in a review of 14 cases of hanging and wedging deaths in infants and children, Moore and Byard identified intra-thoracic petechiae in four of six wedging deaths and intra-thoracic petechiae in two of eight partial hanging cases.[26] In their review of 484 infant autopsies, Fracasso et al found pleural, pericardial, epicardial, thymic, and/or peritoneal petechiae in deaths due to sudden infant death syndrome, sepsis, airway infections, asphyxia, and trauma.[27] While some pathologists use intra-thoracic petechiae, specifically pleural and epicardial petechiae, as a sign of compression of the trunk and a feature of overlay, the literature would not seem to support this interpretation, and caution in their interpretation is most likely appropriate.

PEARLS & PITFALLS

The finding of facial, conjunctival, or cutaneous petechiae of the chest should not be equated with intra-thoracic petechiae. Petechiae in these three locations are concerning for other conditions, including sepsis, forceful coughing or vomiting, inflicted trauma, or asphyxia due to chest compression.[28]

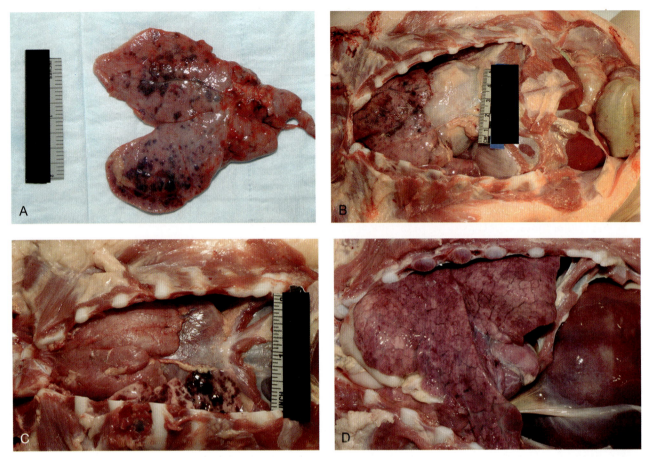

Figure 21.3. Intra-thoracic petechiae Intra-thoracic petechiae can involve the thymus (**A** and **B**), the pleural surface (**C** and **D**), and the epicardium. The petechiae can vary from coarse (**C**) to fine (**D**).

> **FAQ:** How much of a risk for sudden death is bed-sharing?
>
> **Answer:** Bed-sharing is viewed as a significant risk factor for sudden unexpected infant death; however, bed-sharing is a common practice. Gilmour et al indicate that in their survey of women in Canada who gave birth in the last 5 years, about 33% indicated that their infant had slept on a surface with another person every day or nearly every day.[29] Only 40% had never bed-shared. Breastfeeding and facilitation of sleep for mother and infant were listed as reasons for bed-sharing. In comparing SIDS deaths and explained infant deaths, which were often due to an infectious cause, Möllborg et al identified that bed-sharing was significantly more common in the SIDS group (albeit breastfeeding was also more common in this group).[30] Baddock et al indicate that physiologic and behavioral factors play a role in an infant's risk for death during bed-sharing.[31] Also, the risk for sudden death with bed-sharing is increased when the mother smokes.[32,33] Given the relatively common practice of bed-sharing, if the practice represented a significant risk to all infants it seems that infant deaths in such a situation would be more common; however, that the practice represents a risk to some infants is clear.

MICROBIOLOGY STUDIES

Introduction: In the evaluation of sudden unexpected infant deaths, a variety of microbiological studies can be performed, including bacterial cultures of the blood, the cerebrospinal fluid, the lung, and the spleen. In addition to bacterial cultures, virology studies (either culture or molecular studies) can also be performed. According to their survey of 154 offices, with 54 responding, Brooks and Gill indicate that routine virologic and bacteriologic cultures are not performed by all offices, with routine cerebrospinal fluid cultures the least likely to be performed (with only about 50% of offices doing so), and routine viral studies the most likely to be performed, with around 90% of offices doing routine virology studies as part of the workup of sudden unexpected infant deaths.[34]

> **FAQ:** Are routine virological studies required for sudden unexpected infant death investigation?
>
> **Answer:** Weber et al reviewed 546 SUID autopsies and a virus was identified in only 18 cases (4%).[35] The viruses identified included enterovirus, respiratory syncytial virus, herpes simplex virus, cytomegalovirus, adenovirus, influenza virus, and human immunodeficiency virus. In only seven of the 18 cases was the virus identified determined to be the cause of death.
>
> **FAQ:** What is the difference between a sudden unexpected infant death and a sudden unexplained infant death?
>
> **Answer:** Although the terms can be used relatively interchangeably, when an infant dies who is not expected to die, the death could be considered a sudden unexpected infant death; however, if that infant undergoes an autopsy, as is appropriate, and that autopsy does not identify a cause of death, then the death could be considered a sudden unexplained infant death.

> **PEARLS & PITFALLS**
> Cow's milk allergy can cause apnea in infants.

Summary: Infant deaths are challenging to investigate and, unfortunately, are the cases in which the cause of death, despite an extensive evaluation, is most likely to remain unidentified. Whether the cause of death is certified as Sudden unexplained infant death (SUID), with a manner of undetermined, or whether the cause of death is certified as Sudden infant death syndrome (SIDS), or a similar such wording, with a manner of natural, is dependent upon the training, experience, and preference of the forensic pathologist, and office policies, although among forensic pathologists, SUID/Undetermined appears to be favored.

NEAR MISS

Near Miss #1: Repeat deaths in the same family do not indicate homicide. If the family has a genetic disorder associated with sudden death, that family can easily have several infant deaths. Eminoglu et al reported the death of an infant with very long-chain acyl CoA dehydrogenase deficiency, which was initially considered a homicide.[36]

References

1. Knight LD, Hunsaker DM, Corey TS. Cosleeping and sudden unexpected infant deaths in Kentucky: a 10-year retrospective case review. *Am J Forensic Med Pathol.* 2005;26(1):28-32.
2. Weber MA, Pryce JW, Ashworth MT, Malone M, Sebire NJ. Histological examination in sudden unexpected death in infancy: evidence base for histological sampling. *J Clin Pathol.* 2012;65(1):58-63.
3. Fukunaga T, Mizoi Y, Yamashita A, et al. Thymus of abused/neglected children. *Forensic Sci Int.* 1992;53(1):69-79.
4. Varga I, Bódi I, Mešťanová V, Kováč M, Klein M. Association between histological alterations in the thymus and sudden infant death syndrome. *J Forensic Leg Med.* 2018;55:8-13.

5. Sundararajan S, Ostojic NS, Rushton DI, Cox PM, Acland P. Diaphragmatic pathology: a cause of clinically unexplained death in the perinatal/paediatric age group. *Med Sci Law*. 2005;45(2):110-114.
6. Beckwith JB, Bergman AB, Ray CG, eds. *Sudden Infant Death Syndrome: Proceedings of the Second International Conference on the Causes of Sudden Death in Infants*. University of Washington Press; 1970.
7. Perrot LJ, Nawojczyk S. Nonnatural death masquerading as SIDS (sudden infant death syndrome). *Am J Forensic Med Pathol*. 1988;9(2):105-111.
8. Emery JL. Child abuse, sudden infant death syndrome, and unexpected infant death. *Am J Dis Child*. 1993;147(10):1097-1100.
9. Meadow R. Unnatural sudden infant death. *Arch Dis Child*. 1999;80(1):7-14.
10. Stanton J, Simpson A. Murder misdiagnosed as SIDS: a perpetrator's perspective. *Arch Dis Child*. 2001;85(6):454-459.
11. Sawaguchi T, Nishida H. SIDS doesn't exist. *Am J Forensic Med Pathol*. 2001;22(2):211-212.
12. Mitchell E, Krous HF, Donald T, Byard RW. Changing trends in the diagnosis of sudden infant death. *Am J Forensic Med Pathol*. 2000;21(4):311-314.
13. Bajanowski T, Vennemann M, Bohnert M, et al. Unnatural causes of sudden unexpected deaths initially thought to be sudden infant death syndrome. *Int J Leg Med*. 2005;119(4):213-216.
14. Nashelsky M, Pinckard KJ. The death of SIDS. *Acad Forensic Pathol*. 2011;1(1):92-98.
15. Adams SM, Ward CE, Garcia KL. Sudden infant death syndrome. *Am Fam Physician*. 2015;91(11):778-783.
16. Nya S, Abouzahir H, Belhouss A, Benyaich H. Unexpected death of an infant suffocated in the course of breastfeeding when the mother fell asleep. *Med Leg J*. 2021;89(2):139-142.
17. Behera C, Chauhan M, Bijarnia M. Infant death resulting from sharing a cot with a 10-year-old boy. *Med Leg J*. 2020;23:25817220930550.
18. Collins KA. Death by overlaying and wedging: a 15-year retrospective study. *Am J Forensic Med Pathol*. 2001;22(2):155-159.
19. Brown TT, Batalis NI, McClain JL, et al. A retrospective study of the investigation of homicidal childhood asphyxial deaths. *J Forensic Sci*. 2018;63(4):1160-1167.
20. Kleemann WJ, Wiechern V, Schuck M, Tröger HD. Intrathoracic and subconjunctival petechiae in sudden infant death syndrome (SIDS). *Forensic Sci Int*. 1995;72(1):49-54.
21. Beckwith JB. Intrathoracic petechial hemorrhages: a clue to the mechanism of death in sudden infant death syndrome? *Ann N Y Acad Sci*. 1988;533:37-47.
22. Richardson MA, Adams J. Fatal apnea in piglets by way of laryngeal chemoreflex: postmortem findings as anatomic correlates of sudden infant death syndrome in the human infant. *Laryngoscope*. 2005;115(7):1163-1169.
23. Krous HF, Haas EA, Chadwick AE, Masoumi H, Stanley C. Intrathoracic petechiae in SIDS: a retrospective population-based 15-year study. *Forensic Sci Med Pathol*. 2008;4(4):234-239.
24. Weber MA, Risdon RA, Ashworth MT, Malone M, Sebire NJ. Autopsy findings of co-sleeping-associated sudden unexpected deaths in infancy: relationship between pathological features and asphyxial mode of death. *J Paediatr Child Health*. 2012;48(4):335-341.
25. Becroft DM, Thompson JM, Mitchell EA. Nasal and intrapulmonary haemorrhage in sudden infant death syndrome. *Arch Dis Child*. 2001;85(2):116-120.
26. Moore L, Byard RW. Pathological findings in hanging and wedging deaths in infants and young children. *Am J Forensic Med Pathol*. 1993;14(4):296-302.
27. Fracasso T, Vennemann M, Klöcker M, et al. Petechial bleedings in sudden infant death. *Int J Legal Med*. 2011;125(2):205-210.
28. Byard RW, Krous HF. Petechial hemorrhages and unexpected infant death. *Leg Med*. 1999;1(4):193-197.
29. Gilmour H, Ramage-Morin PL, Wong SL. Infant bed sharing in Canada. *Health Rep*. 2019;30(7):13-19.
30. Möllborg P, Wennergren G, Almqvist P, Alm B. Bed sharing is more common in sudden infant death syndrome than in explained sudden unexpected deaths in infancy. *Acta Paediatr*. 2015;104(8):777-783.

31. Baddock SA, Purnell MT, Blair PS, Pease AS, Elder DE, Galland BC. The influence of bed-sharing on infant physiology, breastfeeding and behaviour: a systematic review. *Sleep Med Rev*. 2019;43:106-117.
32. Scragg R, Mitchell EA, Taylor BJ, et al. Bed sharing, smoking, and alcohol in the sudden infant death syndrome. New Zealand Cot Death Study Group. *BMJ*. 1993;307(6915):1312-1318.
33. MacFarlane ME, Thompson JMD, Wilson J, et al. Infant sleep hazards and the risk of sudden unexpected death in infancy. *J Pediatr*. 2022;245:56-64.
34. Brooks EG, Gill JR, National Association of Medical Examiners NAME Ad Hoc Committee for Bioterrorism and Infectious Disease. Testing for infectious diseases in sudden unexpected infant death: a survey of medical examiner and coroner offices in the United States. *J Pediatr*. 2015;167(1):178-182.e1.
35. Weber MA, Hartley JC, Ashworth MT, Malone M, Sebire NJ. Virological investigations in sudden unexpected deaths in infancy (SUDI). *Forensic Sci Med Pathol*. 2010;6(4):261-267.
36. Eminoglu TF, Tumer L, Okur I, Ezgu FS, Biberoglu G, Hasanoglu A. Very long-chain acyl CoA dehydrogenase deficiency which was accepted as infanticide. *Forensic Sci Int*. 2011;210(1-3):e1-e3.

IN-CUSTODY DEATHS 22

CHAPTER OUTLINE

Introduction 518

Excited Delirium Syndrome 519

Restraint Asphyxia 520

Prone Restraint Cardiac Arrest 520

Conducted Electrical Weapons/Electronic Control Devices 520

INTRODUCTION

In-custody deaths can vary from the expected death of a prison inmate due to a terminal disease process to suicide in a jail cell to a police shooting to a sudden death during restraint with few if any autopsy findings. While each jurisdiction may define in-custody deaths differently as to what constitutes an in-custody death, it is important to consider that many deaths might be best to be treated as such, including deaths where police officers are present, such as in a high-speed chase, or when a person commits suicide during a stand-off with police. Also, deaths that occur in state mental institutions and similar such places, where law enforcement is not directly involved but where the individual is still under the control of a city, county, or state entity, are good to be considered as in-custody deaths. Common types of in-custody deaths involve police shootings and jail hangings. While the details of gunshot wounds and asphyxia are covered in other chapters, this chapter will cover some basic concepts that apply to most if not all in-custody investigations, and will cover the concepts of excited delirium syndrome, restraint asphyxia, and conducted electrical weapons, which are intertwined.

CHECKLIST for In-Custody Deaths

- ☐ Remember that in-custody autopsies are often performed to document what is not present (ie, inflicted injury) as much as to document what is present.
- ☐ Obtain pertinent negative external photos: conjunctivae, oral cavity, hands, wrists and forearms, genitalia, anus, and bottom of feet.
- ☐ Obtain fluids for toxicology, and have a complete toxicologic analysis performed, not just for drugs of abuse.
- ☐ Perform external and internal examination as with other death scenarios.
- ☐ Depending upon the nature of the in-custody death, consider layer-by-layer dissection of the neck, cut-downs to the wrists (to assess for presence of hemorrhage), dissection of the back and extremities, a posterior neck dissection, and cut-downs on the soles of the feet.
- ☐ Remember that in the evaluation of in-custody deaths, more dissection rather than less is usually most appropriate.
- ☐ Obtain pertinent negative internal photos: reflected scalp, cranial cavity with brain in-situ, layer-by-layer anterior neck dissection, reflected skin of anterior and posterior surfaces of the trunk, and dissections of the posterior surface of the extremities.
- ☐ Obtain police statements regarding the death, and, if available, audio and/or video recordings of the event.

PEARLS & PITFALLS

The specifics of the in-custody scenario and availability of video documentation can help guide the subsequent autopsy examination. For example, if the decedent is found in their jail cell dead and was alone and video reveals that no one went into or out of the cell, only the autopsy is required. However, if the decedent was in the jail cell with other prisoners, then, in addition to the autopsy, interviews with the prisoners present are also necessary. If the decedent was arrested and restrained and died during the restraint, review of all videos available and all body cams available is necessary, as different cameras can provide different angles for viewing the death.

EXCITED DELIRIUM SYNDROME

Introduction: The use of the term "excited delirium" appears to have been first used by Wetli and Fishbain (1985) to describe a fatal complication of cocaine intoxication characterized by paranoia followed by violent and bizarre behavior.[1] Five of the seven decedents in their report died while in custody. Previous authors have described patients with both delirium and motor excitation and the term "delirious mania" was first used almost 100 years before Wetli and Fishbain's article to describe a patient who was restless, agitated, and violent.[2,3] Bell mania is another term for delirious mania and is characterized by the acute onset of symptoms, which include mania and delirium.[4] The patients often have a history of mania and/or a family history of bipolar disorder, and the condition is responsive to treatment for mania. Fink and Taylor indicate that catatonia, malignant catatonia, neuroleptic malignant syndrome, toxic serotonin syndrome, delirious mania, catatonic excitement, benign stupor, and oneirophrenia are probably best considered as slight variations of one disease process.[5] In addition, Mash indicates that the terms delirious mania, Bell mania, acute maniacal delirium, and lethal catatonia are previous terms for excited delirium.[6]

Features of excited delirium syndrome: While death from excited delirium has been associated with restraint, both in police custody and in psychiatric patients, excited delirium has also been described in individuals not in police custody, with evidence for bizarre or violent behavior being shown by apparent self-inflicted injuries of the body.[7-10] Excited delirium syndrome, when associated with drug use, is most commonly associated with cocaine, methamphetamine, or designer cathinone abuse, but other drugs have been implicated including mephedrone, synthetic cannabinoids, and 25C-NBOMe.[6,11-15] The mechanism of death in excited delirium syndrome may be multi-factorial and include hyperthermia, catecholamine-induced fatal arrhythmias, which may be secondary to drug use, and a component of positional asphyxia.[16] Long QT syndrome exacerbated by the circumstances may also be a mechanism for sudden death.[17] In support for the suggested mechanism of action, simulated law enforcement encounters were shown to cause acidosis and increased catecholamine concentrations.[18]

Autopsy findings in excited delirium syndrome: Some authors have reported that elevated concentrations of heat shock proteins in combination with decreased concentrations of dopamine transporter concentrations when interpreted in the context of the autopsy findings and reported history may assist with the diagnosis of excited delirium.[19] However, the use of biomarkers to identify excited delirium is not supported by all authors.[20] Gill indicates that in the evaluation of potential deaths due to excited delirium, the forensic pathologist must identify all other conditions which may have played a role in the death and determine their contribution as there are no characteristic autopsy findings for excited delirium.[21]

CHECKLIST of Features of Excited Delirium Syndrome[22]
- ☐ Severe agitation combined with violent and bizarre behavior
- ☐ Extreme paranoia, panic, and fear
- ☐ Tireless despite constant physical exertion
- ☐ Unusual strength
- ☐ High level of pain tolerance
- ☐ Stupor
- ☐ Hot to touch
- ☐ Tachycardia and tachypnea
- ☐ Sweating and mydriasis
- ☐ Seizure

> **FAQ:** Is excited delirium syndrome a condition accepted by all?
>
> **Answer:** Numerous articles discuss the diagnosis of excited delirium syndrome; however, Truscott and Ranson describe the lack of support for excited delirium as a legitimate condition.[22-24] Strömmer et al indicate that, based upon their review of the literature, there is a lack of evidence to support excited delirium as a cause of death in the absence of restraint, and that in these cases, restraint-related asphyxia is the likely cause of death.[25] If death occurs in the prone position, Weedn et al opine that cardiac arrest (ie, prone restraint cardiac arrest) and not restraint asphyxia or excited delirium is the cause of death.[26] Slocum et al indicate that excited delirium should not be used as a diagnosis.[27] Therefore, the acceptance of excited delirium as a medical condition is not universal.

RESTRAINT ASPHYXIA

Introduction: Originally described as positional asphyxia occurring in suspects being transported, asphyxia associated with restraint leading to death during police encounters occurs in other scenarios.[25,28-30] However, while the concept of restraint asphyxia has proponents, there are also opponents. Chan et al disagreed with Reay et al and did not feel that the prone position that suspects were placed into would cause asphyxia.[28,31] In support of this disagreement, some studies indicate that the physiologic changes induced by the restraint may not cause significant asphyxia. In their review of the literature, Vilke indicated that restraint did not significantly affect cardiac function nor would it be enough to cause asphyxia or ventilatory arrest, and that other factors such as drugs and alcohol play a role, but also indicating that the experiments used to make such determinations would not necessarily be able to replicate real life situations.[32] In a study of healthy males stressed after exertion, Childers et al found that a head down, hip flexed position produced no significant change in maximal voluntary ventilation after 5 minutes.[33] Karch provides a review of the concept of restraint asphyxia, and theories regarding the cause of death.[34] Regardless of the debate regarding restraint asphyxia, deaths occurring under such circumstances are rare. In their review of 4,828 consecutive use of force police encounters, Hall et al determined that following police use of force 99.8% of subjects would survive whether in the prone or non-prone position.[35]

PRONE RESTRAINT CARDIAC ARREST

Introduction: Using the term "prone restraint cardiac arrest," two citations were identified in PubMed (Feb 2023). Based upon his review, Steinberg, in contrast to Vilke, apparently concluded that with prone restraint people will have decreased ventilation and/or cardiac output and, that in addition, metabolic acidosis, which occurs with increased physical activity, will be worsened by the decrease in ventilation and cardiac output, leading to cardiac arrest.[32,36] As such, Steinberg proposed the term "prone restraint cardiac arrest." Weedn et al opined that deaths with police restraint were due to prone restraint cardiac arrest and not asphyxiation or excited delirium syndrome.[26] However, Lamperti et al discuss how prone positioning in spontaneously breathing patients with respiratory distress can improve oxygenation, which would seem to question whether or not the prone position alone in restraint situations can lead to death.[37]

CONDUCTED ELECTRICAL WEAPONS/ ELECTRONIC CONTROL DEVICES

Introduction: Conducted electrical weapons are a non-lethal technique that can be used by law enforcement to subdue an aggressive or agitated individual. Whether or not conducted electrical weapons cause death has been debated. Swerdlow et al indicate that if a conducted electrical weapon causes death, the individual should collapse within 10 seconds after use of the device and will have ventricular fibrillation, and if collapse is not immediate or is cardiac asystole or pulseless electrical activity, then the conducted electrical weapon did not cause death.[38] Zipes based upon their review of 8 cases, determined that ventricular fibrillation/tachycardia was the initial rhythm when a conducted electrical weapon caused death; however, if the individual was not resuscitated, asystole would develop.[39] Deaths can occur indirectly as the result of the use of a conducted electrical weapon (ie, not due to the weapon itself, but the effects of rendering the suspect incapacitated). For example, fatal traumatic brain injury can rarely occur after use of the conducted electrical weapon due to the uncontrolled fall that results.[40] Aspiration with resultant pneumonia is also a possible complication.[41]

> **PEARLS & PITFALLS**
>
> A reenactment of the situation leading up to the death may assist in understanding the mechanism of death in a situation that involves police restraint.[42]

> **PEARLS & PITFALLS**
>
> When an in-custody death involves restraint of an aggressive or agitated individual with or without the use of a conducted electrical weapon, the cause of death is not often apparent at autopsy. The investigation of these deaths is very complicated and often the subject of much family and media critique. Each death should be handled very carefully with collection of as much data as possible including not just a thorough autopsy and toxicologic analysis but review of videos, officer statements, and witness statements regarding the death.

SAMPLE NOTE: MANNER OF DEATH DETERMINATION FOR IN-CUSTODY DEATHS

While in many in-custody deaths, the cause and manner of death is fairly straightforward (eg, a suicidal hanging in a jail cell, or a police-involved shooting determined to be a homicide), in a small subset, the cause and manner of death is much more complex and often the wording is unique to the particular features of the death being investigated. However, if the death occurs during active restraint, certifying the manner of death as homicide is most likely the best approach. However, if the death occurs following restraint, at what point to consider the death a homicide is not always clear, although, if the arrest occurs in the ambulance or otherwise during transport, certifying the manner of death not as a homicide is most likely the best approach. Unfortunately, there is otherwise no clear answer as to when the effect of restraint is still pertinent in determining the manner of death.

References

1. Wetli CV, Fishbain DA. Cocaine-induced psychosis and sudden death in recreational cocaine users. *J Forensic Sci.* 1985;30(3):873-880.
2. Vasquez E, Chitwood WR Jr. Postcardiotomy delirium: an overview. *Int J Psychiatry Med.* 1975;6(3):373-383.
3. Carswell J. Case of acute delirious mania: with remarks on diagnosis and treatment. *Glasgow Med J.* 1879;12(11):350-356.
4. Cordeiro CR, Saraiva R, Côrte-Real B, et al. When the Bell rings: clinical features of Bell's mania. *Prim Care Companion CNS Disord.* 2020;22(2):19l02511.
5. Fink M, Taylor MA. The many varieties of catatonia. *Eur Arch Psychiatry Clin Neurosci.* 2001;251:I8-I13.
6. Mash DC. Excited delirium and sudden death: a syndromal disorder at the extreme end of the neuropsychiatric continuum. *Front Physiol.* 2016;7:435.

7. Pollanen MS, Chiasson DA, Cairns JT, Young JG. Unexpected death related to restraint for excited delirium: a retrospective study of deaths in police custody and in the community. *Can Med Assoc J*. 1998;158(12):1603-1607.
8. Morrison A, Sadler D. Death of a psychiatric patient during physical restraint. Excited delirium–a case report. *Med Sci Law*. 2001;41(1):46-50.
9. Stratton SJ, Rogers C, Brickett K, Gruzinski G. Factors associated with sudden death of individuals requiring restraint for excited delirium. *Am J Emerg Med*. 2001;19(3):187-191.
10. Shields LB, Rolf CM, Hunsaker JCIII. Sudden death due to acute cocaine toxicity-excited delirium in a body packer. *J Forensic Sci*. 2015;60(6):1647-1651.
11. Murray BL, Murphy CM, Beuhler MC. Death following recreational use of designer drug "bath salts" containing 3,4-Methylenedioxypyrovalerone (MDPV). *J Med Toxicol*. 2012;8(1):69-75.
12. Penders TM, Gestring RE, Vilensky DA. Excited delirium following use of synthetic cathinones (bath salts). *Gen Hosp Psychiatry*. 2012;34(6):647-650.
13. Lusthof KJ, Oosting R, Maes A, Verschraagen M, Dijkhuizen A, Sprong AGA. A case of extreme agitation and death after the use of mephedrone in The Netherlands. *Forensic Sci Int*. 2011;206(1-3):e93-e95.
14. Labay LM, Caruso JL, Gilson TP, et al. Synthetic cannabinoid drug use as a cause or contributory cause of death. *Forensic Sci Int*. 2016;260:31-39.
15. Kristofic JJ, Chmiel JD, Jackson GF, et al. Detection of 25C-NBOMe in three related cases. *J Anal Toxicol*. 2016;40(6):466-472.
16. Otahbachi M, Cevik C, Bagdure S, Nugent K. Excited delirium, restraints, and unexpected death: a review of pathogenesis. *Am J Forensic Med Pathol*. 2010;31(2):107-112.
17. Bozeman WP, Ali K, Winslow JE. Long QT syndrome unmasked in an adult subject presenting with excited delirium. *J Emerg Med*. 2013;44(2):e207-e210.
18. Ho JD, Dawes DM, Nelson RS, et al. Acidosis and catecholamine evaluation following simulated law enforcement "use of force" encounters. *Acad Emerg Med*. 2010;17(7):e60-e68.
19. Mash DC, Duque L, Pablo J, et al. Brain biomarkers for identifying excited delirium as a cause of sudden death. *Forensic Sci Int*. 2009;190(1-3):e13-e19.
20. Johnson MM, David JA, Michelhaugh SK, Schmidt CJ, Bannon MJ. Increased heat shock protein 70 gene expression in the brains of cocaine-related fatalities may be reflective of postdrug survival and intervention rather than excited delirium. *J Forensic Sci*. 2012;57(6):1519-1523.
21. Gill JR. The syndrome of excited delirium. *Forensic Sci Med Pathol*. 2014;10(2):223-228.
22. Gonin P, Beysard N, Yersin B, Carron PN. Excited delirium: a systematic review. *Acad Emerg Med*. 2018;25(5):552-565.
23. Truscott A. A knee in the neck of excited delirium. *Can Med Assoc J*. 2008;178(6):669-670.
24. Ranson D. Excited delirium syndrome: a political diagnosis? *J Law Med*. 2012;19(4):667-672.
25. Strömmer EMF, Leith W, Zeegers MP, Freeman MD. The role of restraint in fatal excited delirium: a research synthesis and pooled analysis. *Forensic Sci Med Pathol*. 2020;16(4):680-692.
26. Weedn V, Steinberg A, Speth P. Prone restraint cardiac arrest in in-custody and arrest-related deaths. *J Forensic Sci*. 2022;67(5):1899-1914.
27. Slocum S, Fiorillo M, Harding E, et al. In pursuit of inter-specialty consensus on excited delirium syndrome: a scoping literature review. *Forensic Sci Med Pathol*. 2022. doi:10.1007/s12024-022-00548-4.
28. Reay DT, Fligner CL, Stilwell AD, Arnold J. Positional asphyxia during law enforcement transport. *Am J Forensic Med Pathol*. 1992;13(2):90-97.
29. O'Halloran RL, Frank JG. Asphyxial death during prone restraint revisited: a report of 21 cases. *Am J Forensic Med Pathol*. 2000;21(1):39-52.
30. Sathyavagiswaran L, Rogers C, Noguchi TT. Restraint asphyxia in in-custody deaths Medical examiner's role in prevention of deaths. *Leg Med*. 2007;9(2):88-93.
31. Chan TC, Vilke GM, Neuman T. Reexamination of custody restraint position and positional asphyxia. *Am J Forensic Med Pathol*. 1998;19(3):201-205.
32. Vilke GM. Restraint physiology: a review of the literature. *J Forensic Leg Med*. 2020;75:102056. doi:10.1016/j.jflm.2020.102056.
33. Childers R, Cronin AO, Castillo EM, et al. Evaluation of the ventilatory effects on human subjects in prolonged hip-flexed/head-down restraint position. *Am J Emerg Med*. 2021;50:1-4.

34. Karch SB. The problem of police-related cardiac arrest. *J Forensic Leg Med.* 2016;41:36-41.
35. Hall C, Votova K, Heyd C, et al. Restraint in police use of force events: examining sudden in custody death for prone and not-prone positions. *J Forensic Leg Med.* 2015;31:29-35.
36. Steinberg A. Prone restraint cardiac arrest: a comprehensive review of the scientific literature and an explanation of the physiology. *Med Sci Law.* 2021;61(3):215-226.
37. Lamperti M, Gattinoni L. Breathing face down. *Br J Anaesth.* 2022;128(5):745-747.
38. Swerdlow CD, Fishbein MC, Chaman L, Lakkireddy DR, Tchou P. Presenting rhythm in sudden deaths temporally proximate to discharge of TASER conducted electrical weapons. *Acad Emerg Med.* 2009;16(8):726-739.
39. Zipes DP. Sudden cardiac arrest and death following application of shocks from a TASER electronic control device. *Circulation.* 2012;125(20):2417-2422.
40. Kroll MW, Adamec J, Wetli CV, Williams HE. Fatal traumatic brain injury with electrical weapon falls. *J Forensic Leg Med.* 2016;43:12-19.
41. Plenzig S, Verhoff MA, Gruber H, Kunz SN. Aspiration-related pneumonia after Taser exposure—a multiple causations mechanism. *Forensic Sci Int.* 2021;326:110906.
42. O'Halloran RL. Reenactment of circumstances in deaths related to restraint. *Am J Forensic Med Pathol.* 2004;25(3):190-193.

ELDER ABUSE 23

CHAPTER OUTLINE

Introduction 526

Risk Factors for Elder Abuse 526

Senile Ecchymoses 528
- Description 528
- Causes 528

Decubitus Ulcers 528
- Description 528
- Causes 528
- Risk Factors for Decubitus Ulcers 528
- Classification of Decubitus Ulcers 529
- Complications of Decubitus Ulcers 530
- Important Point 530

Near Misses 530

INTRODUCTION

Elder abuse is not so much a completely separate topic from other basic forensic pathology concepts, but more just an acknowledgment of a need for careful analysis in specific situations. As with child abuse, elder abuse can include inflicted injury (blunt and sharp force and gunshot wounds) but also neglect, which can manifest as weight loss due to inadequate caloric intake or as dehydration due to inadequate fluid intake but also as untreated medical conditions or untreated minor injuries, which subsequently become a significant problem. If the cause of death is elder abuse, the manner of death should be certified as homicide; however, the pathologist must also be aware of age-related changes that can mimic abuse and not overcall neglect.[1] In addition, unfortunately, distinguishing willful neglect from poverty and ignorance can be challenging.

> **FAQ:** What are the most common forms of elder abuse?
>
> **Answer:** The most common form of elder abuse is neglect, with around 50% of elder abuse cases involving some form of neglect. Physical abuse occurs in about 25% of cases. Sexual abuse is relatively rare, with <1% of elder abuse cases involving sexual abuse.[2]

RISK FACTORS FOR ELDER ABUSE[2]

Age of >75 years
History of dementia, depression, or other mental illness
Inability of decedent to care for themselves
Caregiver who is a substance abuser

Key autopsy features of elder abuse[1-3]

- Dehydration
- Bruises, especially when over bony prominences and when of varying ages
- Patterned injuries, including bite marks
- Burns (eg, cigarette burns (Figure 23.1A) or scalds)
- Malnutrition/starvation (unless explainable by a natural disease process) (Figure 23.1B)
- Poor hygiene (including long and dirty hair and nails; excoriations of perianal skin; excessive dental plaque) (Figure 23.1C-G)
- Untreated decubitus ulcers
- Contractures
- Over medication or under medication
- Inadequate treatment/no treatment of medical conditions (Figure 23.1H)
- Fractures
- With sexual assault occurring: genital, anal, or breast lesions
- Trauma of the back, palms or soles, nose, intraoral, and chin
- Presence of lice

> **PEARLS & PITFALLS**
>
> In the case of possible elder abuse, knowledge about the caregivers may help in the determination. Ortmann et al indicate that caregivers who are more likely to perpetuate abuse will be unemployed, in social isolation, and dependent upon the victim, both financially and mentally.[4] The level of education of the caregiver is not a risk factor, as individuals with high levels of education can contribute to elderly abuse.[4]

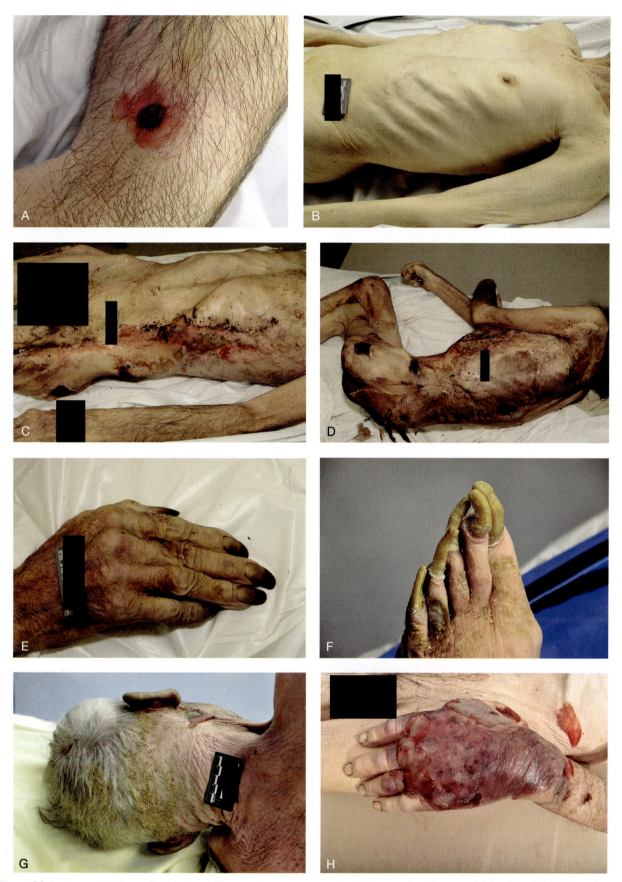

Figure 23.1. Autopsy findings of elder abuse. Cigarette burns, among other injuries, can be a feature of elder abuse (**A**). Malnourishment can lead to significant weight loss; however, cachexia associated with a neoplasm can present as a similar picture (**B**). Poor hygiene, which can be a feature of elder abuse, can include poor skin care (**C** and **D**), long untrimmed and dirty fingernails and toenails (**E-F**), and extensive dandruff (**G**), all of which can indicate the basic needs of the decedent were not being met. Another autopsy finding can be untreated medical conditions. In (**H**), the decedent has cellulitis of the left hand.

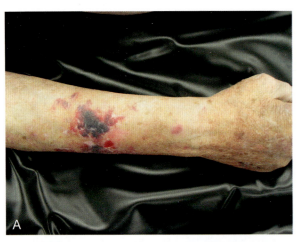
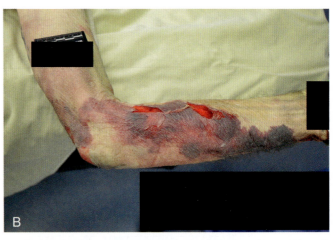

Figure 23.2. Senile ecchymoses. Senile ecchymoses are a common finding on the upper extremities of elderly decedents. Although trauma leads to the bruising, the degree of trauma necessary to cause the bruising is minor and not necessarily indicative of inflicted injury. Senile ecchymoses can vary from extensive hemorrhage (**A**) to one or a few small bruises (**B**).

SENILE ECCHYMOSES

DESCRIPTION

Bruises of the upper extremities, which can vary from a few scattered lesions to essentially diffuse bruising from the wrists to the shoulders (Figure 23.2A and B).

CAUSES

Atrophy of the skin, weakened support of blood vessels, and solar damage cause decreased elasticity that can lead to large ecchymoses with just minimal trauma.[1]

> **PEARLS & PITFALLS**
>
> In the setting of anticoagulant medications, drug-induced thrombocytopenia, various disease processes (eg, liver disease, Cushing syndrome), and age-related changes such as acquired factor V or VIII deficiency or dysfunctional platelets, elderly individuals can potentially have a higher propensity to bleed with more minimal trauma.[1] Because of these factors, apparent extensive bruising should not automatically be attributed to severe inflicted trauma.

DECUBITUS ULCERS

DESCRIPTION

Ulcers associated with reduced mobility that occur on the skin overlying bony prominences, such as the sacrum, but which can also occur on the lower extremities at the ankles (Figure 23.3A-E).

CAUSES

Decubitus ulcers are caused by some combination of pressure over a body prominence, which contribute to shearing forces on the skin leading to destruction of the skin, and compromise of the blood flow.[5] Other terms for decubitus ulcers are pressure ulcer and bed sore.

RISK FACTORS FOR DECUBITUS ULCERS

Bed-bound/non-ambulatory decedents and decedents with diabetes mellitus, incontinence, peripheral vascular disease, and anemia are at risk for decubitus ulcers.[3] With good conscientious nursing care, the risk for decubitus ulcers can be greatly reduced.[6]

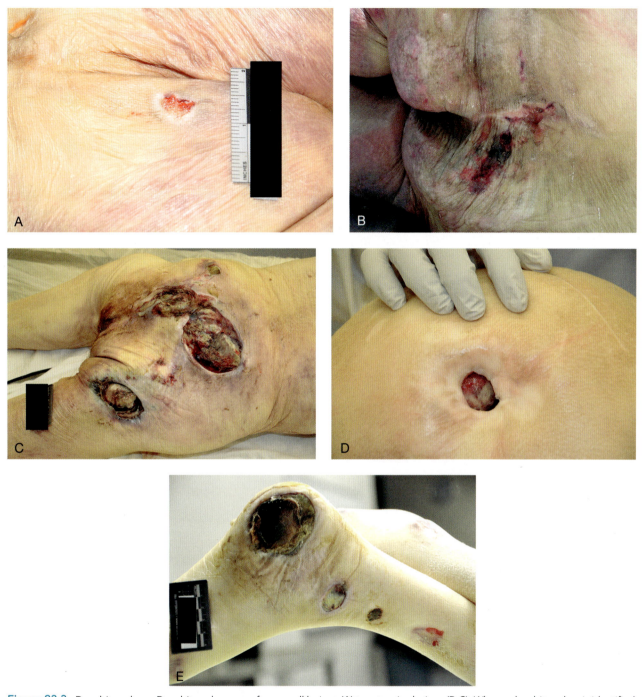

Figure 23.3. Decubitus ulcers. Decubitus ulcers vary from small lesions (**A**) to extensive lesions (**B-C**). When a decubitus ulcer is identified, its extent, as far as involvement of the dermis, underlying musculature, or bone should be documented (**D**). A section of the underlying bone can help rule out or identify osteomyelitis associated with the decubitus ulcer. Decubitus ulcers can also involve the lower extremities (**E**).

CLASSIFICATION OF DECUBITUS ULCERS

There are four stages by which a decubitus ulcer can be classified[5]:
Stage I: No tissue loss and non-blanchable erythema of the skin.
Stage II: Partial-thickness ulcer with minimal tissue necrosis.
Stage III: Full-thickness ulcer that extends to the dermis.
Stage IV: Full-thickness ulcer that extends through the dermis and into the muscle and/or bone.

COMPLICATIONS OF DECUBITUS ULCERS

Decubitus ulcers can lead to osteomyelitis, pneumonia, and sepsis, which can result in death.[3]

IMPORTANT POINT

While decubitus ulcers could be seen as a failure of care, the patient's underlying disease processes and condition of their skin may be as much of a factor in the development of decubitus ulcers as the care of the decedent is. In support of this idea, nursing homes with similar methods of care have been reported to have significant differences in the rate of decubitus ulcer formation.[5]

> **PEARLS & PITFALLS**
>
> If an elderly decedent has pneumonia or suspected sepsis due to decubitus ulcers, it is helpful to culture the decubitus ulcer itself as well as the lung and/or blood. The confirmation of the same organism in all areas can indicate that the decubitus ulcer was the source of the systemic infection.[3]

> **PEARLS & PITFALLS**
>
> In addition to the autopsy findings, scene investigation is very important in the determination of elder abuse. The scene investigation can reveal the specifics of living conditions, such as presence or absence of heating and cooling, presence or absence of food, access to running water and sewer, and whether the individual has the medical aids they require such as medication, hearing aids, and dentures.[1]

NEAR MISSES

Near Miss #1: The decedent with these senile ecchymoses (Figure 23.4) was sent to the medical examiner's office for autopsy, with the bruises believed to have been indicative of a homicide. Autopsy did not reveal any other findings of concern for elder abuse. The manner of death was natural.

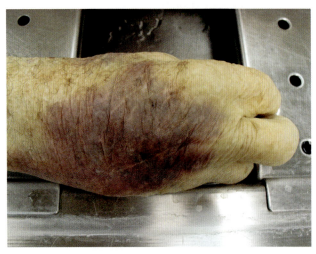

Figure 23.4. Senile ecchymosis misinterpreted as inflicted trauma by investigators.

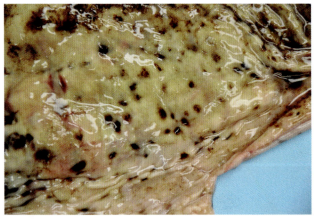

Figure 23.5. Wischnewski spots identified in decedent with signs of elder abuse.

Near Miss #2: A decedent with features of elder abuse, including decubitus ulcers and untreated minor injuries, also had Wischnewski spots, which are most frequently associated with diabetic ketoacidosis and hypothermia (Figure 23.5).

References

1. Collins KA, Presnell SE. Elder neglect and the pathophysiology of aging. *Am J Forensic Med Pathol.* 2007;28(2):157-162.
2. Geroff AJ, Olshaker JS. Elder abuse. *Emerg Med Clin N Am.* 2006;24(2):491-505.
3. Howe JA, Collins KA, King PS, et al. *Investigation of elder deaths.* 2014;4(3):290-304.
4. Ortmann C, Fechner G, Bajanowski T, Brinkmann B. Fatal neglect of the elderly. *Int J Legal Med.* 2001;114(3):191-193.
5. Campbell C, Parish LC. The decubitus ulcer: facts and controversies. *Clin Dermal.* 2010;28(5):527-532.
6. Holmes JHIV, Guileyardo JM, Barnard JJ, DiMaio VJ. Pressure sores in a Christian Science sanatorium. *Am J Forensic Med Pathol.* 1993;14(1):10-11.

ANTHROPOLOGY 24

CHAPTER OUTLINE

Introduction 534

Non-Human Versus Human 534
- Introduction 534
- Identification of Non-Human Bones 534

Biological Profile 536
- Introduction 536

Sex 536
- How Determined 536
- Pelvic Features of Sex 538
- Cranial Features of Sex 539

Age 539
- How Determined 539
- Pubic Symphysis 540
- Auricular Surface 540
- Rib Ends 540
- Cranial Suture Closure 540

Ancestry 543
- How Determined 543
- Morphologic Analysis for Ancestry 543

Stature 543
- How Performed 543

Variants and Natural Disease 546
- Introduction 546

Near Misses 549

INTRODUCTION

When skeletal remains are found, the first question that must be answered is whether the remains are human or non-human. Once the remains are determined to be human, whether the remains are of historical or forensic interest should be determined, as remains of historical interest do not need to be removed from the ground for examination, if that step can be avoided. When the skeletal remains are examined, the number of individuals present is determined, and, as best as possible, for each individual the skeletal inventory (ie, which bones are present) and the biological profile (the ancestry, the sex, the age, and the stature) will be determined. Accurate identification of the four components of the biological profile will depend upon the skeletal remains present (eg, with a complete skeleton, a much more accurate biological profile can be determined than if the skeletal remains present are only the femur). In examining the skeletal remains, anatomic variants, trauma (antemortem, perimortem, or postmortem), natural disease, and postmortem alterations can be identified.

NON-HUMAN VERSUS HUMAN

INTRODUCTION

While a wide range of animal skeletal remains can be identified by the public and brought to law enforcement or the coroner or medical examiner, commonly found bones include those of deer, pigs, and domestic animals. Common bones found include the scapula (Figure 24.1A), ribs (Figure 24.1B), the femur and tibia (Figure 24.1C-G), metacarpals and metatarsals (Figure 24.1H), and vertebrae (Figure 24.1I). Distinguishing human from non-human ribs can be difficult for an inexperienced observer, but one feature that can help is that non-human ribs are straighter than human ribs, an apparent result of the orientation of the chest of an animal downward and toward the ground instead of straight ahead. While non-human metacarpals and metatarsals can be distinguished from each other, the term "metapodial" can be used as a general term to refer to both types of bones. Most non-human bones have the name of their human counterpart; however, the human talus is the equivalent of the non-human astragalus.

IDENTIFICATION OF NON-HUMAN BONES

Non-human bones are not infrequently submitted to a coroner or medical examiner's office for identification; however, many medical examiners may feel uncertain about determining human from non-human especially with bones such as the ribs, the vertebrae, the phalanges, and even the long bones, as many non-human bones are similar to their human counterpart (Figure 24.2A-D). While medical students study the skeletal system in detail, recalling all the landmarks and familiarity with those landmarks is often not something all forensic pathologists feel comfortable with. The availability of a human skeleton in the morgue and reference texts on human and non-human osteology can allow for easy identification of most non-human bones.[1]

> **PEARLS & PITFALLS**
>
> After skinning, the forepaws and hind paws of bears that have been shot by a hunter are often discarded. When the soft tissue decomposes and mummifies, the remains can easily mimic a human hand or foot and are subsequently identified by the public and brought to the coroner or medical examiner for review (Figure 24.3A). The overall morphology of the bear paw is different in that the shortest digit is on the opposite side from the human hand or foot; however, a radiograph of a bear paw will reveal numerous sesamoid bones, which helps confirm the origin (Figure 24.3B). If necessary, the soft tissue can be removed. The difference in morphology comparing the individual bear bones to a human hand or foot is apparent to the experienced observer.

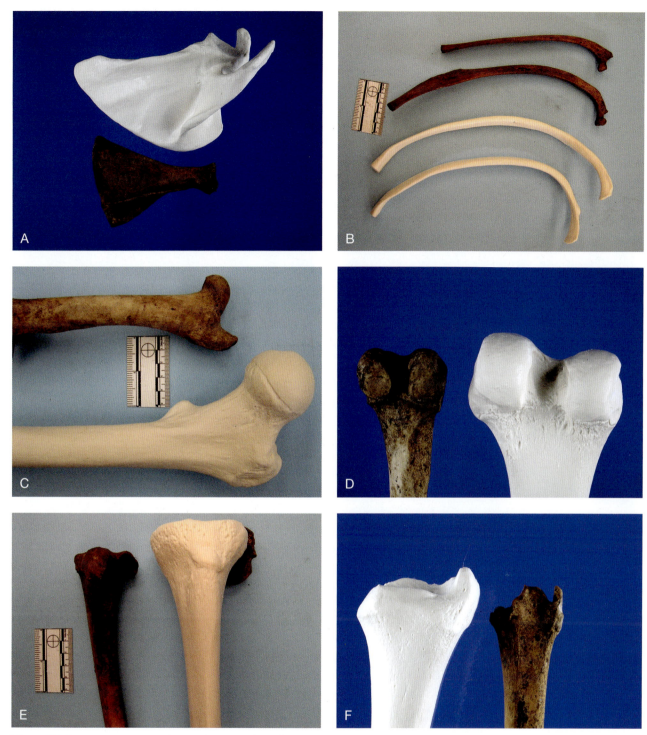

Figure 24.1. Human versus non-human bones. In these figures, all except (H) are a non-human bone compared to a plastic replica of a human skeletal element. (A) (scapula), (B) (ribs), (C) (proximal femur), (D) (distal femur), (E) (proximal tibia), (F) (distal tibia), (G) (proximal tibia), and (I) (vertebra) illustrate differences between human bones and deer bones, which are commonly identified by the public and brought in for inspection. (H) is a metapodial. The distal end of the metapodial appears as a pulley, and has no similar comparative structure in the human skeletal system. Metapodials are commonly identified and brought for inspection.

Figure 24.1g-i (continued)

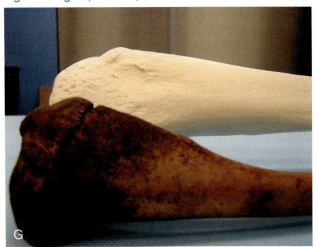
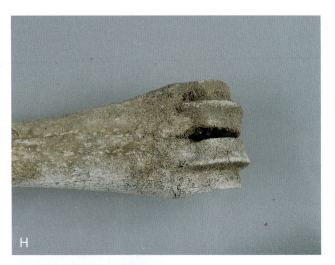
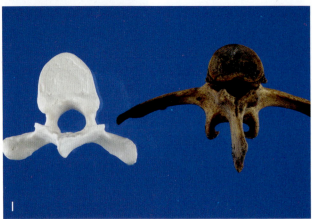

> **PEARLS & PITFALLS**
> The finding of skeletal remains together with human objects (eg, clothing, tools, or weapons) at the same site is not an infrequent occurrence; however, the association of the two does not necessarily indicate that the skeletal remains are of human origin. While this finding can be concerning to individuals who are unfamiliar with the appearance of non-human bones, quick identification of the origin of the skeletal remains can alleviate concerns (Figure 24.4A and B). Also, as with human skeletal remains, animal bones can have natural disease (eg, healed fracture or osteoarthritis) and traumatic injuries (eg, saw marks) (Figure 24.5).

BIOLOGICAL PROFILE

INTRODUCTION

The biological profile as determined by examination of skeletal remains would include their age at death, their ancestry, their sex, and their stature. The biological profile is an estimate based upon the skeletal features available to the person examining the remains. The more complete the skeletal remains, the more accurate the biological profile may be.

SEX

HOW DETERMINED

The three best methods for the determination of the sex of the individual from the skeletal remains are through examination of the pelvis, the cranium, and the long bones, specifically measurement of the diameter of the humeral and femoral heads.

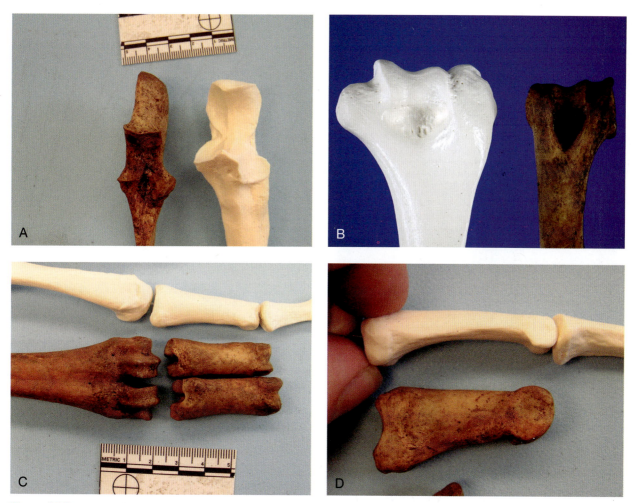

Figure 24.2. Human versus non-human bones. In all four of these figures, a non-human bone has been compared to a plastic replica of a human skeletal element. The proximal ulna (**A**), the distal humerus (**B**), and the phalanges (**C** and **D**) of animals can appear very similar to those of a human to inexperienced forensic pathologists; however, the use of basic references and some practice can easily allow for a distinction to be made, albeit, as the bones become fragmented, the distinction can become more challenging.

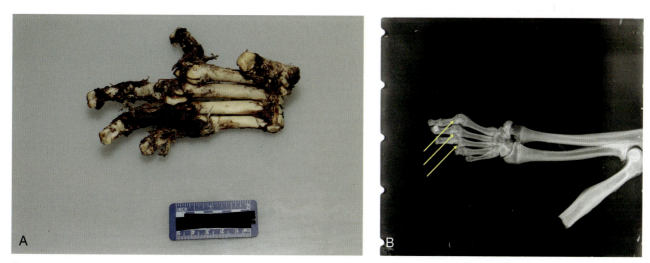

Figure 24.3. Bear paw. The skeletal remains of a bear paw, especially with attached mummified or decomposed soft tissue, can easily mimic a human hand or foot (**A**). A radiograph of the specimen will reveal numerous sesamoid bones (arrows) and can be used to distinguish bear from human (**B**).

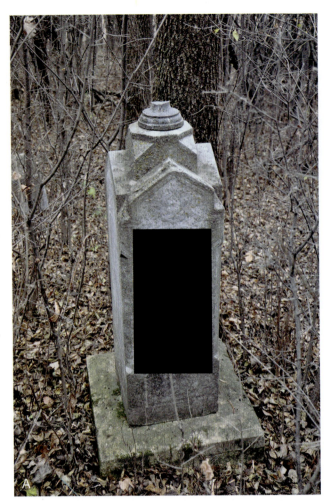
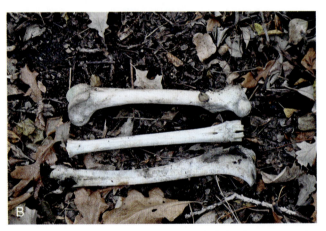

Figure 24.4. Non-human remains identified in a human location. An abandoned cemetery (**A**) was found to have skeletal remains on the surface of the ground. The skeletal remains were examined at the scene and found to be all non-human. Representatives of the collection are in (**B**), a non-human femur, a metapodial, and a non-human tibia.

PELVIC FEATURES OF SEX

The Phenice criteria involve the presence or absence of the ventral arc, the morphology of the subpubic region, and the shape of the medial surface of the ischiopubic ramus (Figure 24.6A-D).[2,3] In a female, a ventral arc will be present (absent in a male), the subpubic region will be concave, and the medial surface of the ischiopubic ramus will be narrow.

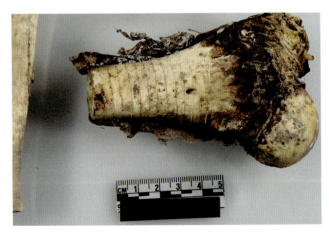

Figure 24.5. Non-human femur with saw marks. Commonly, non-human remains discovered will have been butchered and can easily have traumatic injuries.

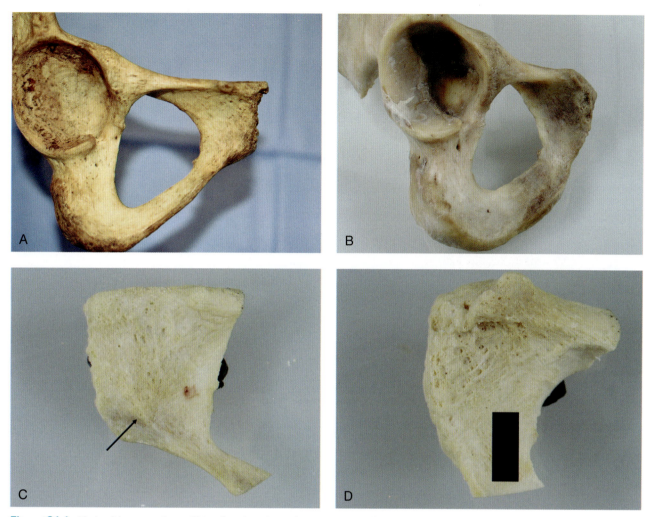

Figure 24.6. Skeletal features of sex. (**A**) is a female pelvis, whereas (**B**) is a male pelvis. One very useful feature of the pelvis to distinguish male and female is the presence (female) or absence (male) of the ventral arc. (**C**) illustrates a ventral arc in the pubic bone of a female (arrow), whereas (**D**) illustrates the absence of a ventral arc in the pubic bone of a male.

Other features of the pelvis that vary between the sexes are the overall shape of the pelvis, which is broader in females, with the sacrum not impinging as much as in males, and the greater sciatic notch is larger in males.

CRANIAL FEATURES OF SEX

To determine the sex, the nuchal crest, mastoid process, supra-orbital margin, supra-orbital ridge, and mental eminence are examined (Figure 24.7A).[4] In females, each will be less well-developed or smaller, whereas in males, each will be more prominently developed or larger. Males have a more depressed nasal root, whereas in females this region is more flat (Figure 24.7B). Many features of sex based upon examination of the cranium can blur with older age. The action of muscles over time on the markings can make an older female appear as a male.

AGE

HOW DETERMINED

In subadults, growth plate closure and tooth development are the best methods to determine the age of the individual (Figure 24.8A-D), whereas in adults, the appearance of the pubic symphysis, the auricular surface, the fourth rib ends, and the status of the cranial sutures are the most commonly used methods.

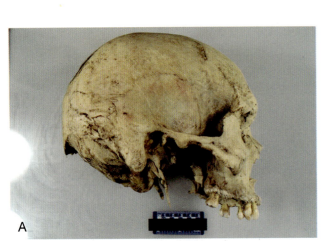
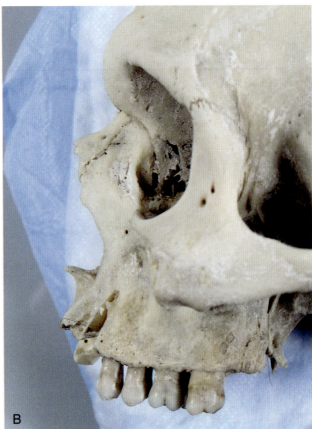

Figure 24.7. Cranial features of sex. (**A**) is a male; note the prominent external occipital protuberance and large mastoid process. (**B**) is also a male, illustrating a prominently depressed nasal root.

PUBIC SYMPHYSIS

The articular surface of the pubic bone undergoes changes with age.[5-10] While the surface of the pubic bone initially is composed of ridges and furrows, with age, these flatten and at the superior and inferior end of the bone, extremities develop. A ventral bevel and rampart and dorsal margin also develop. These combined changes ultimately given the pubic symphysis a rounded appearance with a well-defined rim. With continued age, the surface can begin to break down with pockets in the bone forming. Based upon the changes in the pubic symphysis, an estimated age can be derived from the changes. The Suchey-Brooks system is most commonly used (Figure 24.9A-C).

AURICULAR SURFACE

Like the pubic symphysis, the auricular surface of the pelvis will undergo changes, with the bone becoming denser and developing porosity with age.[11-13]

RIB ENDS

The rib ends, best with the fourth rib, can be examined for changes that occur with age.[14-17] The rib end begins relatively flat, but will develop a central pit. The edges of the rib can become thin extensions, which appear similar to claws. The changes can be used to estimate the age of the individual (Figure 24.10A and B).

CRANIAL SUTURE CLOSURE

While initially open, as an individual ages, the cranial sutures tend to close, filling in with bone and even becoming obliterated with minimal to no residual features in the bone as to their presence. Using these suture closure stages, the age of the individual can be estimated (Figure 24.11).[18]

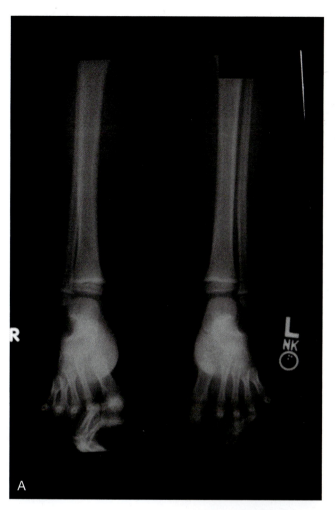
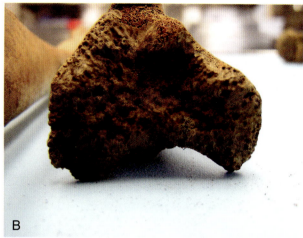
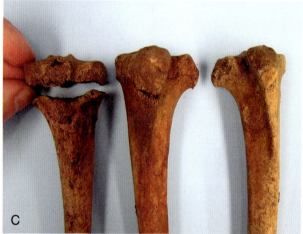
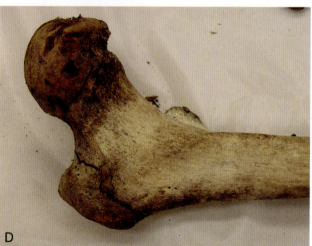

Figure 24.8. Subadult age estimation. (**A**) is a radiograph of a 6-year-old individual. The state of the closure of the growth plates can be used to establish an age at death for the individual. While (**B** and **C**) are non-human, they illustrate features of a subadult, which are similar in humans. When the epiphysis is not fused, the proximal and/or distal ends of the bone will have an appearance similar to wind-blown sand (**B**). With time, the epiphysis will go from unclosed to partially fused to completely fused, as exhibited by the three non-human tibia in (**C**). (**D**) is a juvenile human femur, with fusion of the growth plates at the femoral head and the greater trochanter but with the line of closure still visible.

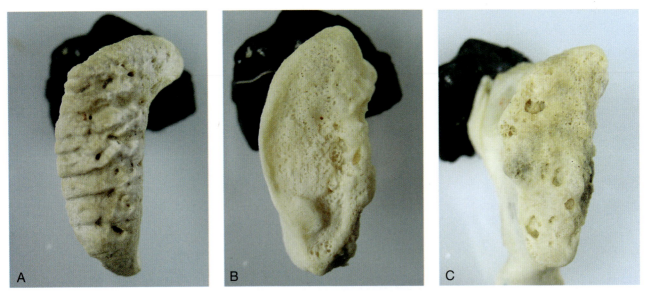

Figure 24.9. Pubic symphysis age estimation. Younger individuals will have prominent ridges and furrows (**A**). With time, the ridges and furrows will flatten and fill in and a ventral rampart and dorsal plateau and upper and lower extremities will develop, giving the pubic symphysis surface a flat and oval appearance, with a rim completely or nearly completely encircling the surface (**B**). With continued aging, the surface will begin to break down, with pores forming and a loss of the rim (**C**).

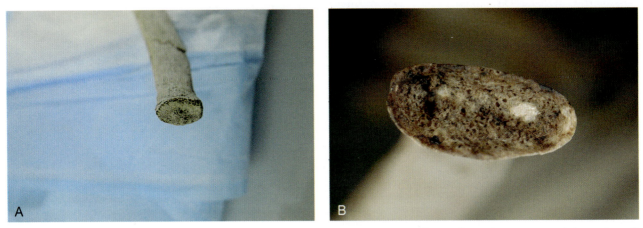

Figure 24.10. Rib end age estimation. In younger individuals, the rib end will be more flat (**A**), but with age, a central depression will develop, among other changes (**B**).

Figure 24.11. Cranial suture age estimation. The sagittal suture to the left side of the figure is completely closed (ie, obliterated) whereas the coronal suture and more proximal portion of the sagittal suture is only partially fused.

ANCESTRY

HOW DETERMINED

The ancestry of the skeletal remains can be estimated via either morphologic features or morphometric features. Using both sliding and spreading calipers, various measurements of the cranium are obtained and the measurements are entered into Fordisc™, which is an available computer program to use to help determine ancestry.[19-22] The ancestral groups most commonly used as divisions are White, Black, Asian, and Native American.

MORPHOLOGIC ANALYSIS FOR ANCESTRY

Based upon Hefner, morphology of the anterior nasal spine, the inferior nasal aperture (Figure 24.12A and B), the inter orbital breadth, the malar tubercle, the nasal aperture width and shape, the nasal bone contour and shape (Figure 24.12C and D), nasal bone overgrowth, the nasofrontal suture, the orbital shape, the palate shape (Figure 24.12E and F), the presence or absence of a postbregmatic depression (Figure 24.12G and H), the posterior zygomatic tubercle, the supranasal suture, the transverse palatine suture, and the zygomaxillary suture (Figure 24.12I and J) can each be examined and used for the determination of ancestry.[23-27] The breadth of variability in each of these morphologic features is the subject of an entire book, the examples provided in this chapter are merely to show some of the range to allow for the reader to appreciate the utility of examination of the human cranium for determination of ancestry.[28] Other features of the cranium and post-cranial elements can also assist in the determination of ancestry including projection of the zygomatic bone (Figure 24.12K and L), alveolar prognathism, appearance of the teeth (including shovel incisors and presence of a Carabelli cusp), the presence of palatine and/or mandibular tori, and the shape of the femoral shaft (Figure 24.12M). Unfortunately, while some morphologic features may be found with greater frequency in one particular group (eg, postbregmatic depression in individuals of African descent), no morphologic feature is absolutely specific to any one ancestral group.

> **PEARLS & PITFALLS**
>
> With Native American remains, the preference is most often, when an option, to leave found historical remains in place. For medical examiners who work in regions where Native American remains are found, it is good to have working knowledge of the regulations in place for the handling of such remains.

STATURE

HOW PERFORMED

Stature estimates are based upon the length of bones in the collection of skeletal remains, using formulas based upon linear regression to determine a height based upon the length of the single bone, or a mixture of bones. Long bones such as the femur or tibia are preferred. The Fordisc™ program is, in addition to ancestry estimates, also able to calculate stature.

> **FAQ:** How accurate is the biologic profile?
>
> **Answer:** All features of the biological profile (ancestry, sex, age, stature) are always best considered estimates. The individual to whom the remains belong may fit the biologic profile or may vary quite a bit from the determination. However, the remains are being examined to assist with the investigation into an unknown individual, and as long as it is understood that the determinations are estimates, the information hopefully will help with the investigation. Some aspects of the profile are fairly accurate (eg, determination of sex from the pelvis) and estimation of age based upon growth plate closure; however, other aspects of the profile are fairly broad (eg, determination of age from cranium).

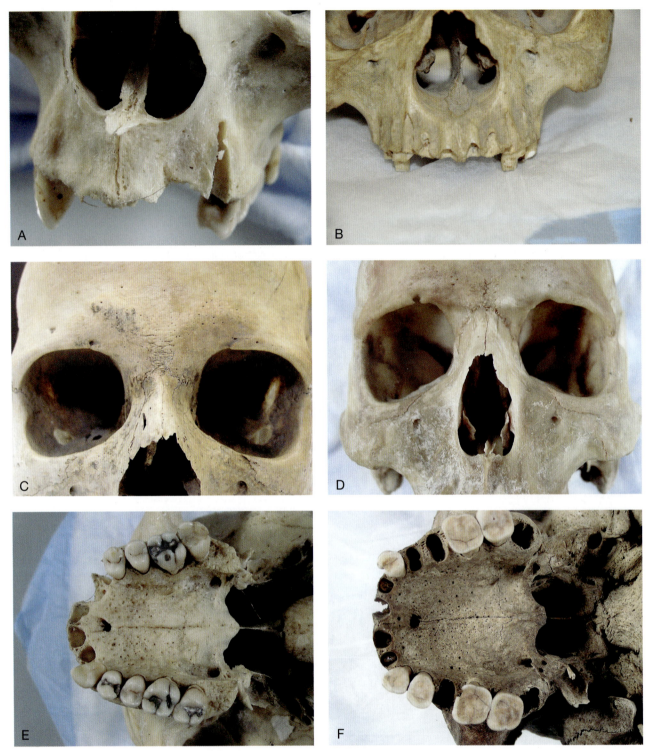

Figure 24.12. Cranial morphologic features for ancestry estimation. The inferior border of the nasal orifice can be more like a wall (ie, a prominent nasal sill) as in (**A**), or more sloped (ie, guttered), with no boundary between the floor of the nasal cavity and the maxilla (**B**). The size of the anterior nasal spine is also useful. The nasal region is of vital importance in the estimation of ancestry, with the shape of the nasal bones, the interorbital breadth, and the width of the nasal orifice all useful observations. In (**C**), the nasal bone contour is more rounded, whereas in (**D**), the nasal bone contour is more tented and steep. Palate shape and appearance of the transverse palatine suture assist in the identification of ancestry (**E** and **F**). A postbregmatic depression is very commonly associated with Black individuals. Figure (**G**) was a White male, with no postbregmatic depression, whereas (**H**) was a Black male, with postbregmatic depression. The zygomaxillary suture has a variable appearance and has been used to help distinguish Native American remains from Whites (**I** and **J**). Projection of the zygomatic bone has been used to help identify Native Americans. (**K**) is a White male, and (**L**) is from a Native American male. Although the cranium is the best marker available to distinguish ancestry, some post-cranial morphologic differences have also been identified. Native Americans (the lower femur in **M**) tend to have flattening of the shaft inferior to the inferior trochanter, whereas whites tend to have a more rounded subtrochanteric femoral shaft.

Figure 24.12g-l (continued)

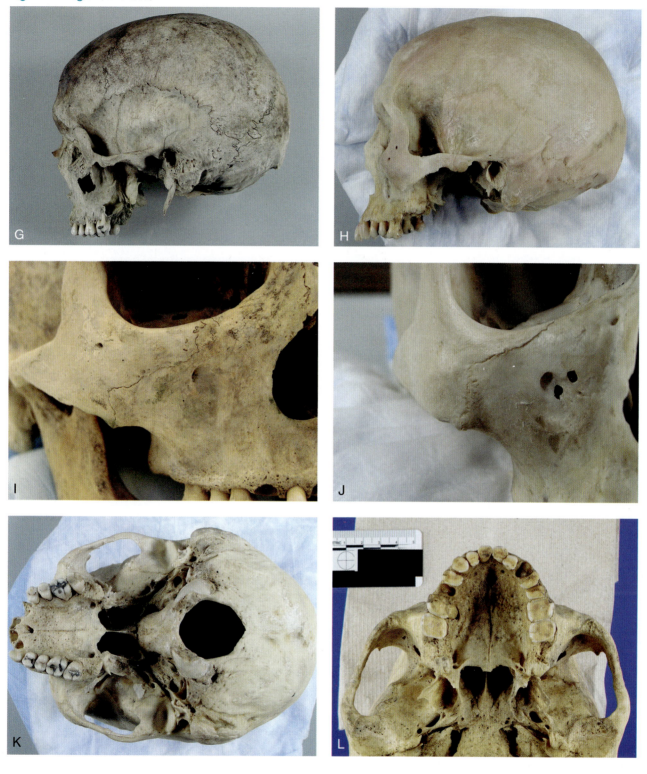

Figure 24.12m (continued)

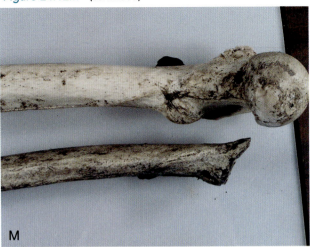

> **PEARLS & PITFALLS**
>
> When bones are identified, having a forensic anthropologist assist with their recovery may yield additional information about the death rather than just from the examination of the bones themselves. How the bones are positioned at the scene, if properly interpreted, may provide information about the position of the body or other information regarding the death and may provide very useful information in the investigation. If the bones are simply picked up at the scene and placed into a box and transported to the forensic anthropologist for examination, this context is lost, and the information that would have been available is also lost.

VARIANTS AND NATURAL DISEASE

INTRODUCTION

The number of osteologic variants and the types of natural disease that can be encountered are the subject of entire books. One natural disease commonly encountered as an incidental finding at autopsy is hyperostosis frontalis, which is an undulating growth on the inner surface of the frontal bone, most commonly encountered in older females (Figure 24.13A). Two commonly encountered cranial anatomic variants at autopsy are a metopic suture (Figure 24.13B) and Wormian bones (Figure 24.13C).

> **PEARLS & PITFALLS**
>
> Anatomic variants can mimic natural disease and trauma. For example, a wide parietal foramen, if enlarged enough, could mimic a gunshot wound or other traumatic defect (Figure 24.14).

> **PEARLS & PITFALLS**
>
> While there are only 206 bones in the human body, ossification of cartilage can lead to additional bones being found with skeletal remains. Commonly, the thyroid and cricoid cartilage can partially or completely ossify and can be found with the skeletal remains (Figure 24.15).

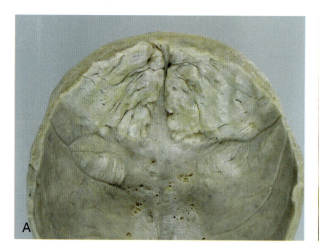
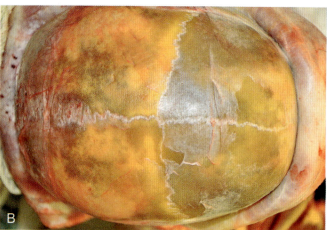
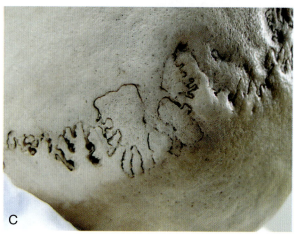

Figure 24.13. Common variants and natural disease. (**A**) is hyperostosis frontalis. (**B**) is a metopic suture, which is a commonly identified cranial variant. A metopic suture is the visible suture between the two frontal bones. This individual also had very prominent golden yellow discoloration of the bone, which has been associated with tetracycline use. (**C**) is a Wormian bone.

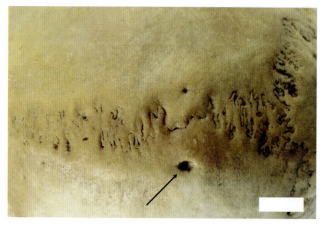

Figure 24.14. Prominent parietal foramen. To each side of the posterior portion of the sagittal suture is a small foramen, the parietal foramen (arrow). However, the parietal foramen can be enlarged. Although the example in the image is not likely to be misinterpreted as a gunshot wound or other traumatic injury, in certain cases, depending upon the size of the foramen, this anatomic variant could be misinterpreted as trauma.

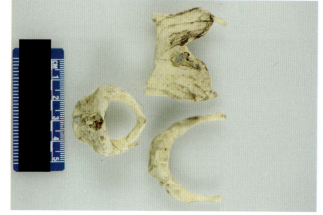

Figure 24.15. Ossified thyroid and cricoid cartilage. In the figure are the hyoid bone, which is fused, and a completely ossified thyroid and cricoid cartilage.

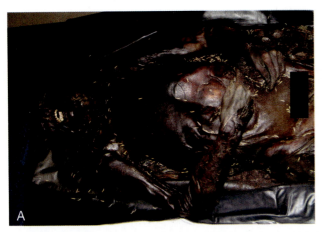 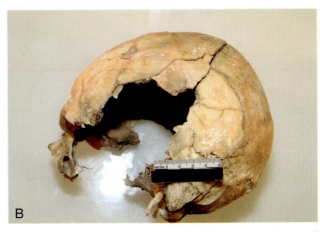

Figure 24.16. Removal and defleshing of skeletal remains to better examine the bone. Although the defleshing of all decomposed remains to better assess the skeletal system is not possible in all cases, in certain situations, such a procedure should be considered, as it is the best way to assess the skeletal system, unless full body radiography or computed tomography scanner is available. In certain situations, removal of the skeletal element of most concern and defleshing can speed the process and provide very useful information (**A** and **B**).

FAQ: What is the utility of analysis of the skeletal remains in a decomposed body?

Answer: The difference in the ability to identify fractures in the decomposed body versus the defleshed skeletal remains is significant.[29] However, retention of the body for the time period required to deflesh and examine all such decedents, which is a labor-intensive process, is not always feasible. When a decomposed body is found to have traumatic injuries, selective defleshing of the skeletal elements of most interest can be performed to speed the process (Figure 24.16A and B).

PEARLS & PITFALLS

In situations where the cranium has sustained significant trauma (eg, shotgun or rifle wound, or multiple blunt force injuries) and is in numerous fragments, the skeletal remains can be cleaned of soft tissue and reassembled using a water-based glue to allow for better documentation of the trauma (Figure 24.17A and B).

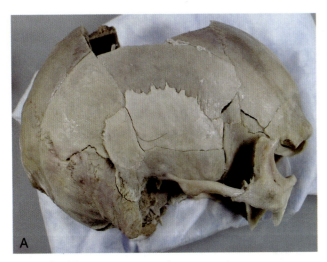 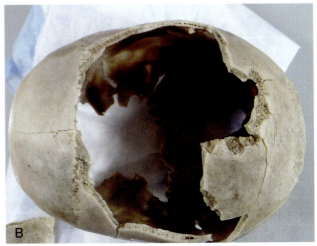

Figure 24.17. Reconstruction of cranium to better assess trauma. This individual was found decomposed with an apparent shotgun wound of the head. The cranial fragments were retained, defleshed, and reassembled (**A** and **B**). Doing so allowed for the pathway of the shot charge to be determined and the wound was consistent with an intraoral shotgun wound or a wound inflicted underneath the chin. As received, determining the pathway of the projectile and ruling out an improbable suicidal shot (eg, the side of the head with a shotgun) and subsequent staging of the scene would not have been possible.

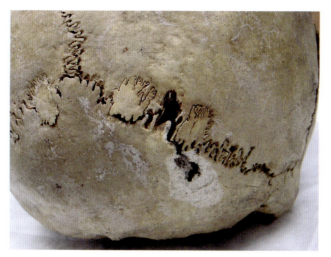

Figure 24.18. Loss of Wormian bone. The loss of a Wormian bone can result in a roughly circular defect in the cranium that could potentially mimic a gunshot wound.

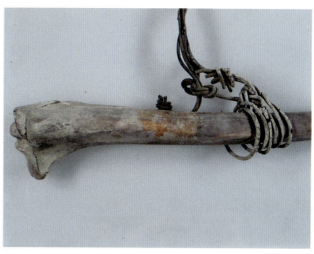

Figure 24.19. Non-human tibia with wire wrapped around the shaft. The bone was found in a river and because of the wire was considered a suspicious finding.

NEAR MISSES

Near Miss #1: When an accessory ossicle falls from its location and is not present with the body to be reassembled, the resultant defect in the cranium can potentially mimic a gunshot wound (Figure 24.18).

Near Miss #2: This tibia was found in the river, with a length of wire wrapped around the shaft (Figure 24.19). Such a finding can be concerning for a concealed homicide; however, the tibia is non-human. The large tibial tuberosity and other morphologic features are not consistent with human origin.

References

1. France D. *Human and Non-human Bone Identification: A Color Atlas*. 1st ed. CRC Press; 2009.
2. Phenice TW. A newly developed visual method of sexing the os pubis. *Am J Phys Anthropol*. 1969;30(2):297-301.
3. McFadden C, Oxenham MF. Revisiting the Phenice technique sex classification results reported by MacLaughlin and Bruce (1990). *Am J Phys Anthropol*. 2016;159(1):182-183.
4. Walker PL. Sexing skulls using discriminant function analysis of visually assessed traits. *Am J Phys Anthropol*. 2008;136(1):39-50.
5. Schanandore JV, Wolden M, Smart N. The accuracy and reliability of the Suchey-Brooks pubic symphysis age estimation method: systematic review and meta-analysis. *J Forensic Sci*. 2022;67(1):56-67.
6. Miranker MA. A comparison of different age estimation methods of the adult pelvis. *J Forensic Sci*. 2016;61(5):1173-1179.
7. Shirley NR, Ramirez Montes PA. Age estimation in forensic anthropology: quantification of observer error in phase versus component-based methods. *J Forensic Sci*. 2015;60(1):107-111.
8. Garvin HM, Passalacqua NV. Current practices by forensic anthropologists in adult skeletal age estimation. *J Forensic Sci*. 2012;57(2):427-433.
9. Kimmerle EH, Konigsberg LW, Jantz RL, Baraybar JP. Analysis of age-at-death estimation through the use of pubic symphyseal data. *J Forensic Sci*. 2008;53(3):558-568.
10. Kimmerle EH, Prince DA, Berg GE. Inter-observer variation in methodologies involving the pubic symphysis, sternal ribs, and teeth. *J Forensic Sci*. 2008;53(3):594-600.
11. Buckberry JL, Chamberlain AT. Age estimation from the auricular surface of the ilium: a revised method. *Am J Phys Anthropol*. 2002;119(3):231-239.
12. Ost AM. Age-at-death estimation from the auricular surface of the ilium: a test of a sex-specific component method. *J Forensic Sci*. 2022;67(3):868-876.

13. Igarashi Y, Uesu K, Wakebe T, Kanazawa E. New method for estimation of adult skeletal age at death from the morphology of the auricular surface of the ilium. *Am J Phys Anthropol.* 2005;128(2):324-339.
14. Hartnett KM. Analysis of age-at-death estimation using data from a new, modern autopsy sample—part II: sternal end of the fourth rib. *J Forensic Sci.* 2010;55(5):1152-1156.
15. Işcan MY, Loth SR, Wright RK. Age estimation from the rib by phase analysis: white males. *J Forensic Sci.* 1984;29(4):1094-1104.
16. Işcan MY. The aging process in the rib: an analysis of sex- and race-related morphological variation. *Am J Hum Biol.* 1991;3(6):617-623.
17. Oettlé AC, Steyn M. Age estimation from sternal ends of ribs by phase analysis in South African Blacks. *J Forensic Sci.* 2000;45(5):1071-1079.
18. Ruengdit S, Troy Case D, Mahakkanukrauh P. Cranial suture closure as an age indicator: a review. *Forensic Sci Int.* 2020;307:110111.
19. Elliott M, Collard M. FORDISC and the determination of ancestry from cranial measurements. *Biol Lett.* 2009;5(6):849-852.
20. Dudzik B, Jantz RL. Misclassifications of hispanics using Fordisc 3.1: comparing cranial morphology in Asian and hispanic populations. *J Forensic Sci.* 2016;61(5):1311-1318.
21. Ramsthaler F, Kreutz K, Verhoff MA. Accuracy of metric sex analysis of skeletal remains using Fordisc based on a recent skull collection. *Int J Legal Med.* 2007;121(6):477-482.
22. Guyomarc'h P, Bruzek J. Accuracy and reliability in sex determination from skulls: a comparison of Fordisc® 3.0 and the discriminant function analysis. *Forensic Sci Int.* 2011;208(1-3):180.e1-6.
23. Klales AR, Kenyhercz MW. Morphological assessment of ancestry using cranial macromorphoscopics. *J Forensic Sci.* 2015;60(1):13-20.
24. Plemons A, Hefner JT. Ancestry estimation using macromorphoscopic traits. *Acad Forensic Pathol.* 2016;6(3):400-412.
25. Hefner JT. The macromorphoscopic databank. *Am J Phys Anthropol.* 2018;166(4):994-1004.
26. Spiros MC, Hefner JT. Ancestry estimation using cranial and postcranial macromorphoscopic traits. *J Forensic Sci.* 2020;65(3):921-929.
27. Hefner JT. Cranial nonmetric variation and estimating ancestry. *J Forensic Sci.* 2009;54(5):985-995.
28. Hefner JT, Linda KC. *Atlas of Human Cranial Macromorphoscopic Traits.* Elsevier Academic Press; 2018.
29. Kemp W, McKeown A, Symes S, Skelton R. Identification of skeletal fractures before and after removal of soft tissue: a case report. *Am J Forensic Med Pathol.* 2013;34(1):18-22.

ODONTOLOGY 25

CHAPTER OUTLINE

Introduction   552

INTRODUCTION

Examination of human teeth at the time of autopsy is most often for the purpose of identification, although the condition of the teeth themselves can also provide a forensic pathologist some information about the individual in whether they have good dental hygiene and/or apparent access to a dentist for maintenance and treatment. For the purpose of identification, antemortem dental records such as radiographs and clinic notes are necessary to compare to postmortem radiographs. When an odontologist examines the teeth for the purpose of identification, the number of features they can assess is extensive, and includes characteristics of the teeth themselves such as root morphology as well as features of the surrounding regions of the mouth. Even if a forensic pathologist routinely enlists the aid of a forensic odontologist, they should possess a basic level of knowledge of odontology so as to be able to chart the dentition when required. Postmortem odontology also includes the evaluation of bite marks.

Basic terminology for human dentition: Human dentition is numbered from the right upper third molar, which is #1, to the left upper third molar, which is #16, to the left lower third molar, which is #17, to the right lower third molar, which is #32. The teeth have five surfaces. For molars, the mesial surface is anterior-medial (ie, adjacent to the tooth in front), the distal surface is posterior-lateral, the buccal surface is anterior-lateral (ie, toward the inner surface of the cheek), the lingual surface is posterior-medial (ie, toward the tongue), and the occlusal surface is the upper surface of the tooth.[1] For incisors, the mesial surface is the medial surface, the distal surface is the lateral surface, the labial surface is the surface that faces the lips, the lingual surface is the surface that faces the tongue, and the incisal surface is the upper surface of the tooth.

CHECKLIST for Potential Roles of a Forensic Odontologist[2]
- ☐ Identification of decedents, including in mass disaster situations
- ☐ Assistance with sex determination
- ☐ Age estimation, especially for sub-adults
- ☐ Assistance with ancestry determination
- ☐ Bite mark analysis

CHECKLIST for Evaluation of Bite Mark[2,3]
- ☐ Obtain case demographics
- ☐ Visual examination (preferably by the odontologist who will do the analysis)
- ☐ Photography (using an ABFO ruler)
- ☐ Swabs of the lesion for DNA
- ☐ Impressions of the lesion
- ☐ Following swabs, fingerprint powder can be used to make a bite mark print
- ☐ If necessary, the skin with the bite mark can be excised and retained in formalin

PEARL & PITFALLS

When comparing the antemortem and postmortem dental radiographs and notes, two types of discrepancies can occur: explainable or unexplainable.[4] An explainable discrepancy is one that would be potentially expected given the time course between when the antemortem dental records were created and when the individual died. The loss of a tooth or placement or enlargement of an amalgam is an explainable circumstance as both could have occurred during the time course.[4] An unexplainable circumstance is one that cannot be explained by the time course alone. The presence of a native tooth in the postmortem radiograph which is absent from the antemortem radiograph is unexplainable.[4]

> **PEARLS & PITFALLS**
>
> A postitive dental identification can be made based upon the features of a single amalgam or restoration as long as the features are an exact match between the antemortem and postmortem radiographs.[5-7] One important factor to consider is the angle at which the radiograph is taken because even a slight variance in the angle between the two radiographs can distort the appearance of the amalgam and preclude identification.[5-7]

> **FAQ:** Can a forensic pathologist make a positive dental identification without the aid of a forensic odontologist?
>
> **Answer:** In most cases, the forensic pathologist has access to not just the dental records but also the circumstantial information regarding the decedent and can make a positive identification using circumstances in combination with dental examination. However, if the identification may undergo the scrutiny of courtroom proceedings, confirmation of the identification by a forensic odontologist may be preferred. And, if the comparison is based only upon natural features of the teeth (eg, the root morphology), unless the forensic pathologist has specific training in such an identification, consultation with a forensic odontologist is a better option. Whether or not the forensic pathologist makes an identification based upon circumstances in combination with comparison of restorations in antemortem and postmortem radiographs is dependent upon the forensic pathologist's training, experience, preference, and office policies.

> **PEARLS & PITFALLS**
>
> Even when antemortem dental records are not available, a forensic odontologist may still be able to assist with the identification. Through a process of postmortem dental profiling, the forensic odontologist can potentially provide information about the decedent's age, ancestry, sex, and socio-economic status as well as possibly information about the decedent's diet, habits, and dental or systemic diseases.[4]

> **PEARLS & PITFALLS**
>
> Features on antemortem photographs can be used to identify individuals in the postmortem period.[8]

> **PEARLS & PITFALLS**
>
> While removal of the upper and lower teeth for the purpose of identification is destructive and should be reserved only for those decedents that would not be able to be viewed (eg, decomposed bodies and bodies with extensive thermal injuries), an approach from the intracranial cavity can be used to assist in identification of viewable bodies, without damage to the external features of the head.[9]

References

1. Clemente CD. *Anatomy: A Regional Atlas of the Human Body*. 3rd ed. Urban and Schwarzenberg; 1987.
2. Gupta S, Agnihotri A, Chandra A, Gupta OP. Contemporary practice in forensic odontology. *J Oral Maxillofac Pathol*. 2014;18(2):244-250.
3. Dolinak D, Matshes E, Lew E. *Forensic Pathology: Principles and Practice*. Elsevier Academic Press; 2005.
4. Pretty IA, Sweet D. A look at forensic dentistry—Part 1: The role of teeth in the determination of human identity. *Br Dent J*. 2001;190(7):359-366.
5. Phillips VM, Stuhlinger M. The discrimination potential of amalgam restorations for identification: part 1. *J Forensic Odontostomatol*. 2009;27(1):17-22.
6. Phillips VM, Stuhlinger M. The discrimination potential of amalgam restorations for identification: part 2. *J Forensic Odontostomatol*. 2009;27(1):23-26.
7. Zondag H, Phillips VM. The discrimination potential of radio-opaque composite restorations for identification: part 3. *J Forensic Odontostomatol*. 2009;27(1):27-32.
8. Silva RF, Franco A, Souza JB, Picoli FF, Mendes SDSC, Nunes FG. Human identification through the analysis of smile photographs. *Am J Forensic Med Pathol*. 2015;36(2):71-74.
9. Byrd RC, Berman GM. A surgical method for solving the problem of accessing the oral structures during autopsy for the identification of viewable remains—[An] intracranial technique involving the removal of a small area of the temporal bone to access the TMJ area. *Proceedings of the 48th Annual Meeting of the American Academy of Forensic Sciences, February 19-24, 1996*. Nashville, TN.

MASS DISASTERS

26

CHAPTER OUTLINE

Introduction 556

INTRODUCTION

Mass disasters can occur secondary to a range of events, including terrorist attacks, mass shootings or other types of mass homicidal events, large scale accidents (eg, car wrecks on the freeway involving hundreds of vehicles), and natural disasters (eg, tornados or hurricanes). Mass disasters are, of course, not predictable and because of their extent, tax local resources, including the medical examiner's office or coroner's office responsible for deaths in the jurisdiction. Mass disasters will involve the medical examiner or coroner's office working with numerous other agencies, including the Federal Bureau of Investigation, FAA (*Federal Aviation Administration*), National Transportation Safety Board, and DMORT (Disaster Mortuary Operational Response Team), depending upon the size and nature of the mass disaster. What is a mass disaster for one location will not be a mass disaster for another location. For example, 2,996 people died in the terrorist attacks of 9/11 and the population of New York City at the time was 8,044,000. The 9/11 event was definitely a mass disaster. A car accident with two fatalities in the town of Plentywood, MT (population of 1,668 in 2021) would involve a larger percentage of the local population, but would not be considered a mass disaster. To handle a mass disaster, each medical examiner's office or coroner's office should have a plan in place for dealing with a number of decedents that far exceeds their normal capacity. Frequently, medical examiner offices publish their plan in some form online, and this plan can be obtained and modified by the medical examiner's or coroner's office that requires their own plan.

PEARLS & PITFALLS

Airports are required to have mass disaster preparations, which include mock disasters. The coroner's office or medical examiner's office may be able to participate in these drills to help prepare for a mass disaster.

FAQ: Do the decedents in a mass disaster require the same level of examination as those seen in the routine course of daily events?

Answer: To be certain, each examination must be performed to ensure that a positive identification and correct determination of cause and manner of death is made as well as that evidence necessary to evaluate the mass disaster is collected; however, depending upon office policies and the nature of the mass disaster, more liberal use of external examinations and/or limited autopsies may allow for the office responsible for the investigation to both handle the mass disaster effectively and at the same time perform their vital functions in an acceptable fashion.

PEARLS & PITFALLS

Depending upon the geographic location of the medical examiner's office, airplane crashes with small airplanes may be a fairly common occurrence. While these types of accidents are not often mass disasters, depending upon the medical examiner's office size, the crash of a ten person aircraft could easily tax their resources. In any airplane crash, collection of toxicology specimens for the FAA is required. Having a "Tox Box" on hand in the event of such a need is important, and even though the amount and breadth of fluid and tissue required for submission are extensive, the process is fairly streamlined and should not be a burden.

STILLBIRTHS 27

CHAPTER OUTLINE

Introduction 558

Basic Information Regarding Handling of a Stillborn Infant 558

Basic Features of a Stillborn Fetus 558

Examination of the Placenta 559

Chorioamnionitis 559
- Autopsy Findings 559
- Potential Mimics 560

Placental Abruption 560
- Autopsy Findings 560

Meconium Aspiration 561
- Autopsy Findings 561

Near Miss 561

INTRODUCTION

While stillborn fetuses are not commonly autopsied by forensic pathologists, when trauma or drug use was determined to be a likely cause for a stillbirth, an autopsy is often more likely to be performed. Of importance in the discussion of stillbirths is the distinction between a stillborn fetus and a live-born infant, which, at autopsy, can be a challenging if not often impossible distinction.

BASIC INFORMATION REGARDING HANDLING OF A STILLBORN INFANT

A "fetus" is the term given to a product of conception from the eighth week of gestation to birth. If an infant is born alive and subsequently dies, a death certificate will be issued. For stillborns, depending upon state statutes, a fetal death certificate will usually be issued if the weight of the fetus is at least 350 g, or if the fetus has reached 20 weeks of gestation. Therefore, not all fetal deaths require a death certificate. Perinatal refers to the period from the 28th week of gestation through the first 7 days after delivery. Therefore a perinatal death may refer to a stillborn fetus or a live-born neonate.

If the body is 350 g or greater in weight or 20 weeks of gestation or older, the remains are treated as a fetus and a funeral home should be involved with the removal of the fetus from the hospital. If the conceptus is less than 20 weeks, technically, the remains are referred to as "products of conception" and not a fetus. Therefore, the remains can be treated as a surgical pathology specimen. However, if an intact and identifiable fetus is present, even below the age of 20 weeks and the parents wish for a burial, they should be allowed to do such.

BASIC FEATURES OF A STILLBORN FETUS

Depending upon the time frame from death to delivery, the fetus's body will undergo various changes associated with maceration including red discoloration, skin slippage, overlapping of cranial bones, and autolysis of the internal organs (Figure 27.1).

> **FAQ:** How do you distinguish a live birth from a stillbirth?
>
> **Answer:** Unfortunately this question arises not infrequently and despite its very important connotations, can be very difficult to answer. While floatation of lungs in water has been used as a marker for a live birth (based upon the concept that following a live birth the lungs will fill with oxygen and float in water), the test is hardly absolute, as decomposition with postmortem gas formation could also cause lungs to float, yet would not be indicative of a live birth. If food material is found in the infant's stomach at the time of autopsy, the infant was certainly live born. In addition, a vital reaction in the umbilical cord stump is consistent with a live birth. Another method to determine if a fetus is live-born or stillborn is scene investigation. If the infant is born into water, for example, a toilet or a bathtub, scene investigation or historical information may be able to distinguish a live birth from a stillbirth as a live-born infant would breathe and potentially cause gas bubbles to form in the water. While histologic examination of the lungs revealing expansion of the alveoli may be consistent with the infant having taken breaths, this determination should be done with caution. To be described below, if available with the remains, examination of the placenta may assist in the determination of a live-born versus a stillborn infant.

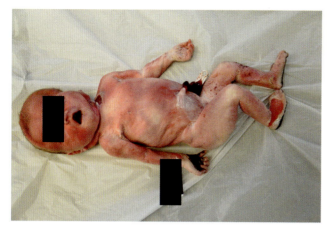

Figure 27.1. Stillborn fetus. While an early stillborn fetus, note the skin slippage on the neck and extremities. The black discoloration on the palm is from hand prints obtained at the hospital for the parents.

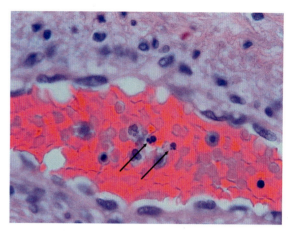

Figure 27.2. Stillborn placental pathology. The earliest change in a stillborn placenta, occurring within hours after the death of the fetus, is intravascular karyorrhexis (arrows) in the chorionic villi (high power).

EXAMINATION OF THE PLACENTA

With stillborn fetuses, examination of the placenta is a vital component of the autopsy. In their review of 946 intrauterine deaths with subsequent submission of the placenta for histologic analysis, Man et al found that in 32% of cases the cause of death resided within the placenta.[1] In addition to the cause of death, histologic changes in the placenta can be used for determining the time since death of the fetus. Genest found that intravascular karyorrhexis in the villi occurred at 6 or more hours from the time of death (Figure 27.2).[2] Stem villi vascular lumen abnormalities including fibroblast septation or total obliteration of the lumen, if multifocal in distribution, are consistent with 2 or more days since death, and if extensive in distribution, are consistent with 2 or more weeks since death.[2] The presence of extensive fibrosis of terminal villi indicates a time frame of 2 or more weeks since death.[2] Thus, if the placenta is present with the fetus, examination of the placenta may therefore be able to help distinguish a live-born infant from a stillborn fetus.

> **FAQ:** How useful is examination of the organs in a stillbirth to determine the cause of death if the organs appear normal upon gross examination?
>
> **Answer:** Man et al found that in 1,046 intrauterine deaths, if the liver, kidneys, adrenal glands, spleen, thymus gland, intestines, pancreas, brain, or thyroid gland appeared grossly normal that microscopic examination did not reveal a cause of death.[3] Only examination of grossly normal lungs provided a cause of death that would not have been determined else wise, which was a case of congenital cytomegalovirus.[3] However, microscopic examination of a normal brain could allow for the identification of red neurons, indicative of hypoxic-ischemic injury.

CHORIOAMNIONITIS

AUTOPSY FINDINGS

Gross examination will reveal a yellow-green discoloration of the fetal surface of the placenta and dull appearance of the membranes. Microscopic examination will reveal a neutrophilic infiltrate in the fetal membranes (Figure 27.3A). Also present can be inflammation of the umbilical cord, which is termed "funisitis" (Figure 27.3B).

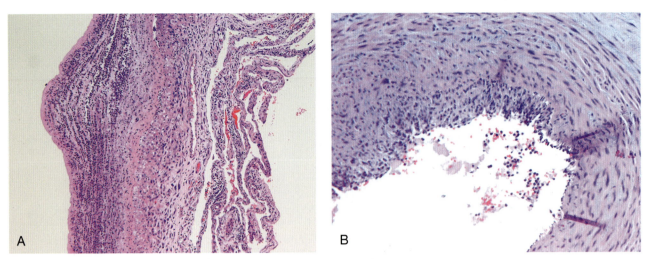

Figure 27.3. Chorioamnionitis and funisitis. In acute chorioamnionitis, a common cause of fetal death, a neutrophilic infiltrate in the chorion will be present (**A**, medium power). Examination of the umbilical cord may reveal inflammation of one or more vessels, which is funisitis (**B**, high power).

POTENTIAL MIMICS

Meconium staining of the fetal membranes can mimic chorioamnionitis because of the yellow-green discoloration; however, microscopic examination will not reveal a neutrophilic infiltrate. It is common to see neutrophils in the decidua attached to the fetal membranes, and this also does not indicate chorioamnionitis.

PLACENTAL ABRUPTION

AUTOPSY FINDINGS

In an acute abruption, no gross morphologic features may be present and the diagnosis depends upon the clinical history. For an abruption that has been present for a longer period of time, compression of maternal cotyledons by adherent hematoma will occur (Figure 27.4A). Microscopic examination of the placenta in the case of abruption can reveal extravasated red blood cells in the chorionic villi (Figure 27.4B).[4]

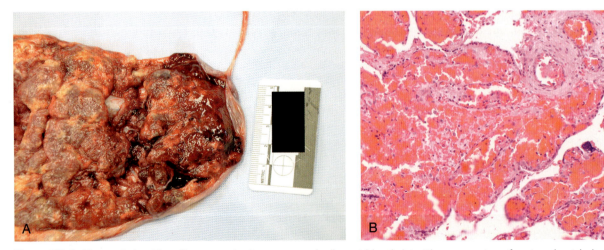

Figure 27.4. Placental abruption. Gross examination may reveal adherent blood clot with compression of maternal cotyledons (**A**). As the distinction between an acute placental abruption and just adherent residual blood from the delivery without the clinical history can be impossible, examination of the placenta can assist. With placental abruption, extravasated red blood cells in the chorionic villi can be present (**B**, high power).

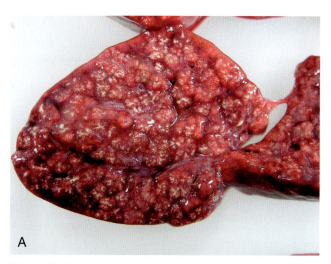
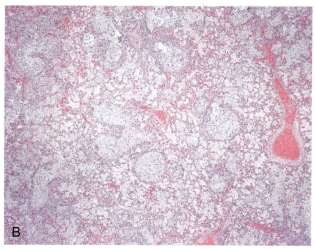

Figure 27.5. Meconium aspiration. While meconium aspiration of some degree is fairly common, extensive meconium aspiration can cause death. In this case, the lungs were gritty upon sectioning and airways packed with anucleate squamous cells are visible grossly (**A**), and confirmed microscopically (**B**, low power).

MECONIUM ASPIRATION

AUTOPSY FINDINGS

With massive meconium aspiration, the lungs can have a gritty texture (Figure 27.5A). Microscopic examination will reveal anucleate squamous cells in the airways and alveoli (Figure 27.5B).

NEAR MISS

Near Miss #1: While fetuses can have a wide range of malformations, including absence of the neurocranium and brain, one eye, or fusion of the lower extremities, occasionally, an apparent malformed fetus is not actually a fetus. A donation at a charitable store (Figure 27.6) scared two workers who called the coroner. Chemical analysis of the fetus revealed plastic.

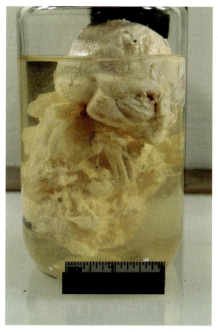

Figure 27.6. Plastic alien fetus.

References

1. Man J, Hutchinson JC, Heazell AE, Ashworth M, Jeffrey I, Sebire NJ. Stillbirth and intrauterine fetal death: role of routine histopathological placental findings to determine cause of death. *Ultrasound Obstet Gynecol.* 2016;48(5):579-584.
2. Genest DR. Estimating the time of death in stillborn fetuses: II. Histologic evaluation of the placenta; a study of 71 stillborns. *Obstet Gynecol.* 1992;80(4):585-592.
3. Man J, Hutchinson JC, Ashworth M, Judge-Kronis L, Levine S, Sebire NJ. Stillbirth and intrauterine fetal death: role of routine histological organ sampling to determine cause of death. *Ultrasound Obstet Gynecol.* 2016;48(5):596-601.
4. Mooney EE, al Shunnar A, O'Regan M, Gillan JE. Chorionic villous haemorrhage is associated with retroplacental haemorrhage. *Br J Obstet Gynaecol.* 1994;101(11):965-969.

COMMON MECHANISMS AT AUTOPSY 28

CHAPTER OUTLINE

Introduction 564

Hypovolemic Shock 564
- Mechanism 564
- Causes of Hypovolemic Shock 564
- Estimation of Effect of Blood Loss 564
- Autopsy Findings of Blood Loss 564

Cardiogenic Shock 564
- Mechanism 564
- Causes of Cardiogenic Shock 565

Septic Shock 565
- Mechanism 565
- Causes of Septic Shock 565

Anaphylactic Shock 565
- Mechanism 565

Neurogenic Shock 565
- Mechanism 565

Autopsy Findings Associated With Shock 565

Autopsy Findings of Cerebral Edema 567
- Complications of Cerebral Edema 568
- Autopsy Findings of Global Hypoxic Ischemic Encephalopathy 568

Near Misses 570

INTRODUCTION

Many conditions that cause a delayed death produce common pathologic end points, which will be identified at autopsy. Delayed death situations can vary from individuals dying at home as a result of an opioid drug overdose to those dying in the hospital after a gunshot wound. However, the common pathologic end points of a delayed death (ie, features of shock including cerebral edema and its complications) must be recognized and interpreted for what they are, which are secondary changes, and not the etiology of the individual's death. Forensic pathologists will encounter individuals who have died of conditions that led to hypovolemic shock, cardiogenic shock, septic shock, anaphylactic shock, and neurogenic shock. The three most common types of shock are cardiogenic, hypovolemic, and septic.[1] The underlying basic mechanism for shock which produces the effects on the organs, is hypoperfusion of the tissue, leading to cell death.

HYPOVOLEMIC SHOCK

MECHANISM

Hypovolemic shock is due to low cardiac output which is the result of low blood volume, which can result from blood or fluid loss.

CAUSES OF HYPOVOLEMIC SHOCK

In the forensic pathology context, hypovolemic shock is most commonly due to a traumatic injury with resultant blood loss, but can also frequently result from a natural disease process. For example, gastrointestinal bleeding due to a bleeding peptic ulcer or due to ruptured esophageal varices occurring in patients with cirrhosis is a relatively common autopsy finding.[2]

ESTIMATION OF EFFECT OF BLOOD LOSS

When an individual is found dead or dies prior to significant resuscitative efforts, whether the amount of blood lost in a traumatic or non-traumatic event is enough to have caused their death is a frequent question. In general, the total blood volume is estimated at 7% of the body weight, and a class IV hemorrhage, which is loss of >40% of the blood volume, is considered a pre-terminal event, with patients potentially dying within minutes.[3] However, this calculation does not consider other factors such as underlying co-morbidities, which might make a person more susceptible to lethal effects from comparatively less blood loss than a healthier individual might be.

AUTOPSY FINDINGS OF BLOOD LOSS

Decreased lividity, pallor of the internal organs, including the kidneys, which can appear much more tan, wrinkling of the splenic capsule, and sub-endocardial hemorrhages in the left ventricular outflow tract are found in individuals who have exsanguinated.[3] Plattner et al found sub-endocardial hemorrhages in 9% of their cases, with half of all exsanguination cases and one-third of cases with isolated brain injury having sub-endocardial hemorrhages.[4]

> **PEARLS & PITFALLS**
> Assessing blood loss at autopsy can be challenging. External blood loss most often cannot be quantitated. Internal blood loss in the body cavities can be measured; however, with the presence of ascites or pleural effusions, the blood loss will be diluted. Blood loss into tissue cannot be accurately quantitated.[3]

CARDIOGENIC SHOCK

MECHANISM

Cardiogenic shock is due to a condition causing heart failure, which leads to insufficient cardiac output that causes end-organ dysfunction, with individuals often being hypotensive.[5]

CAUSES OF CARDIOGENIC SHOCK

Acute myocardial infarct, valvular dysfunction, aortic dissection, myocardial contusion, and myocarditis are causes of cardiogenic shock.[5]

SEPTIC SHOCK

MECHANISM

A systemic inflammatory response syndrome (SIRS) initiated by the causative pathologic condition leads to a release of inflammatory mediators that promote vascular dilation (and subsequent venous blood pooling) and vascular leakage, which result in hypoperfusion of the tissue.[2]

CAUSES OF SEPTIC SHOCK

The systemic inflammatory response syndrome is often triggered by a bacterial infection, severe burns, severe trauma, or pancreatitis.[2]

ANAPHYLACTIC SHOCK

MECHANISM

An immunoglobulin E–mediated response to a substance triggers systemic vasodilation and leakage from the vessels, which leads to hypoperfusion of organs.[2]

NEUROGENIC SHOCK

MECHANISM

Anesthesia or an injury to the spinal cord can trigger loss of vascular tone, which would essentially act as systemic vasodilation, and lead to hypoperfusion of organs.[2]

AUTOPSY FINDINGS ASSOCIATED WITH SHOCK

Gross and/or microscopic findings associated with shock include cerebral edema, border-zone (ie, watershed) infarcts in the brain, sub-endocardial infarction of the heart, sub-endocardial hemorrhage in the left ventricular outflow tract, diffuse alveolar damage, centrilobular changes in the liver including congestion and necrosis, acute tubular necrosis of the kidneys, petechial and larger hemorrhage of the gastric mucosa with resultant bloody fluid in the stomach lumen, and hemorrhagic infarction of the border-zone regions of the gastrointestinal tract, including the region of the cecum, the splenic flexure, and the recto-sigmoid region, resulting in hemorrhagic discoloration of the wall of the gastrointestinal tract and hemorrhage into the mucosa (Figure 28.1A-J).

> **FAQ:** Can acute tubular necrosis/acute tubular injury of the kidneys be accurately diagnosed at autopsy?
>
> **Answer:** Unfortunately, postmortem autolysis can mimic and/or impair the histologic identification of acute tubular necrosis (ATN); therefore, the diagnosis of acute tubular necrosis at autopsy should be done with caution. Kocovski and Duflou studied ten histologic features of renal tubular epithelial cells and their association with necrosis and postmortem change: epithelial proliferation (Ki-67 immunoperoxidase positivity), fibrin thrombi, tubular epithelial whorls, mitoses, casts, autolysis, tubulorrhexis, epithelial flattening, interstitial inflammation, and interstitial expansion.[6] The authors identified that tubular epithelial whorls were found in sixteen ATN cases and were not present in controls. The circumstances of the death and available clinical history may assist in the postmortem diagnosis of acute tubular necrosis. With survival, features of regeneration of the tubular cells may be present such as mitotic figures.

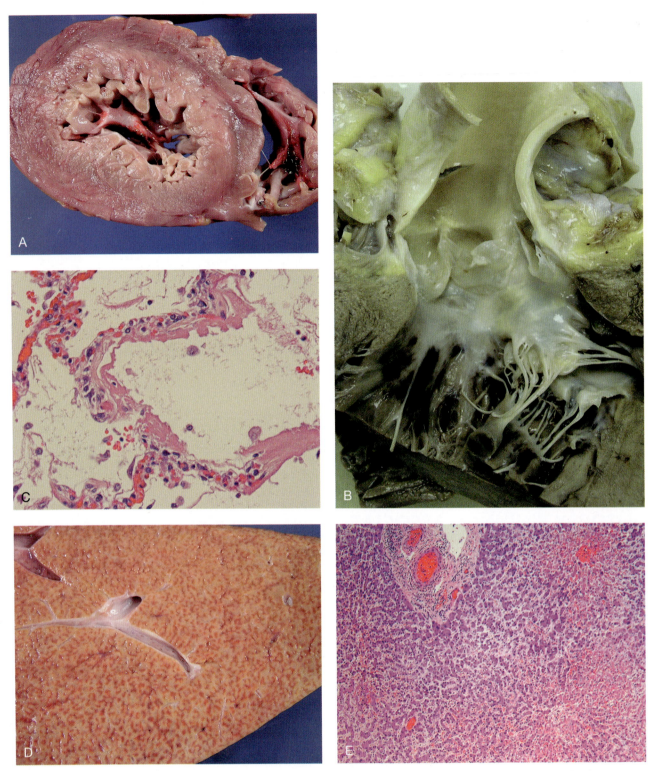

Figure 28.1. Pathologic features of shock. Circumferential sub-endocardial pallor (**A**) can be indicative of sub-endocardial ischemic injury; however, histologic confirmation is required. The change is the result of generalized low blood flow, with the sub-endocardial region the most sensitive region of the heart to ischemic injury. Sub-endocardial hemorrhage in the aortic outflow tract (**B**) is associated with stress, as could occur with shock. Hyaline membranes are a feature of diffuse alveolar damage, which is associated with shock (**C**). Reduced blood flow to the liver leads to injury to the centrilobular hepatocytes, which are the last region of the liver to receive blood and thus the most prone to ischemic injury in states of reduced perfusion. Grossly, the liver will have a nutmeg appearance (**D**) and microscopically, ischemic injury of the centrilobular hepatocytes with preservation of the periportal hepatocytes will be present, which can vary from outright coagulative necrosis to subtle increased eosinophilia of the cytoplasm and pallor of nuclei associated with sinusoidal dilation (**E**, medium power). Acute tubular necrosis is challenging to diagnose in the postmortem period; however, features of acute tubular necrosis would include coagulative necrosis of epithelial cells, flattening and loss of epithelial cells, and dilation of the tubular lumen. The section is from an individual who died in the hospital with clinically diagnosed acute tubular necrosis (**F**, high power). The presence of nucleated cells in the vasa recta may also assist with the diagnosis of acute tubular necrosis (**G**). Intestinal ischemia can vary from a focal distribution, which is most often concentrated at the arterial border-zone regions (**H**), to a more diffuse distribution (**I**). Microscopic examination will reveal extravasated red blood cells in the mucosa (**J**, high power).

Figure 28.1f-j (continued)

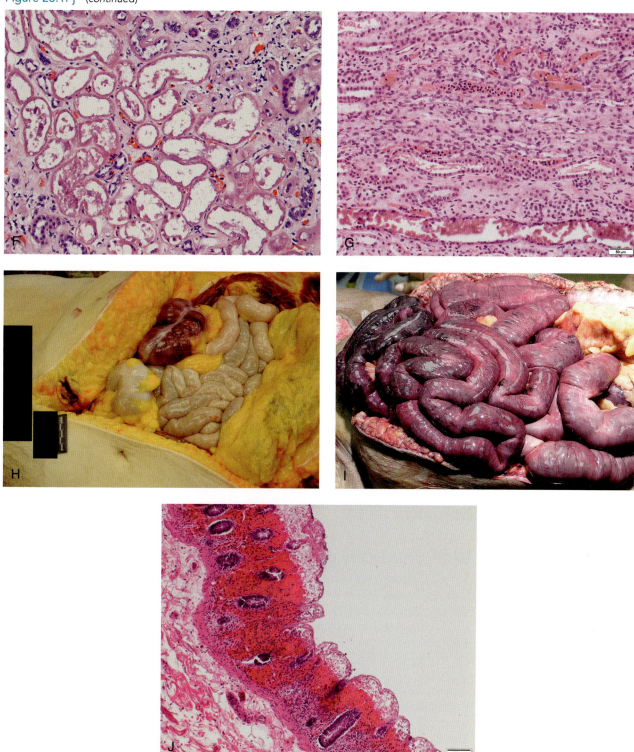

AUTOPSY FINDINGS OF CEREBRAL EDEMA

The gross features of cerebral edema include flattened gyri, effaced sulci, compressed (ie, slitlike) cerebral ventricles, and prominent cerebellar tonsils; however, the interpretation of the findings can be subjective and dependent upon the pathologist, especially when the cerebral edema is not well-developed.[7] Microscopic features of cerebral edema include pale and spongy parenchyma and perivascular distension[7] (Figure 28.2A-D).

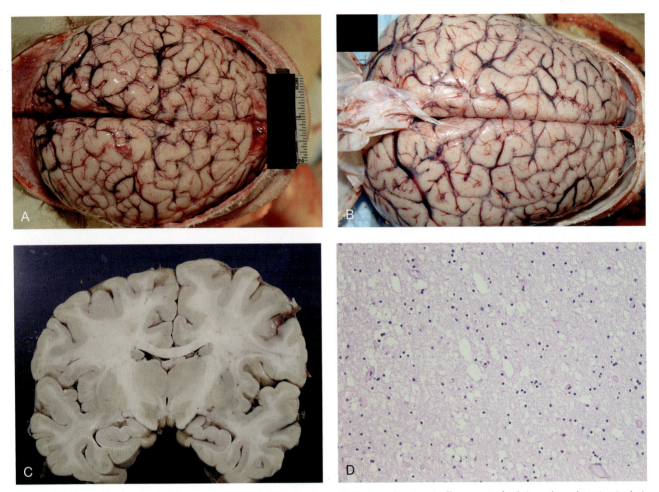

Figure 28.2. Cerebral edema. The gross features of cerebral edema (flattening of gyri and effacement of sulci) can be subjective in their interpretation, varying from more borderline examples (**A**) to more definitive examples (**B**). Cross section of the brain will reveal slitlike ventricles (**C**). Microscopic examination can reveal vacuolation of the white matter (**D**, high power), with caution advised in diagnosing cerebral edema based only upon the microscopic appearance.

COMPLICATIONS OF CEREBRAL EDEMA

Cerebral edema leads to herniation, which can include herniation of the cingulate gyri, unci, and cerebellar tonsils (Figure 28.3A-F). Herniation through a surgical or other type of defect in the cranium can also occur. Herniation of a cingulate gyrus (ie, sub-falcine herniation) can lead to compression of the ipsilateral anterior cerebral artery, which can lead to infarction of the corresponding cerebral hemisphere distribution. Herniation of an uncus (ie, transtentorial herniation) can lead to compression of the ipsilateral posterior cerebral artery and oculomotor nerve. Transtentorial herniation can also lead to compression of the contralateral cerebral peduncle, producing Kernohan notch, and linear hemorrhages in the midbrain/pons (ie, Duret hemorrhage) (Figure 28.4A and B). The compression of the posterior cerebral artery can lead to infarction of the corresponding occipital lobe distribution. Herniation of the cerebellar tonsils can impinge upon the brainstem, leading to respiratory and circulatory failure and death.[1]

AUTOPSY FINDINGS OF GLOBAL HYPOXIC ISCHEMIC ENCEPHALOPATHY

When the brain sustains a diffuse (ie, global) hypoxic-ischemic event, such as can occur with shock, the brain will die. In global hypoxic ischemic encephalopathy, the presence of red neurons, which are indicative of cerebral hypoxia/ischemia, are best searched for in adults in the hippocampus, specifically the CA1 sector, the cerebellum (Figure 28.5), including the dentate nucleus, and the border-zone/watershed regions in the depths of the sulci. Border-zone/watershed regions are any location where the distribution of two major cerebral arteries overlaps. In infants, the thalamus should be included in the regions searched.

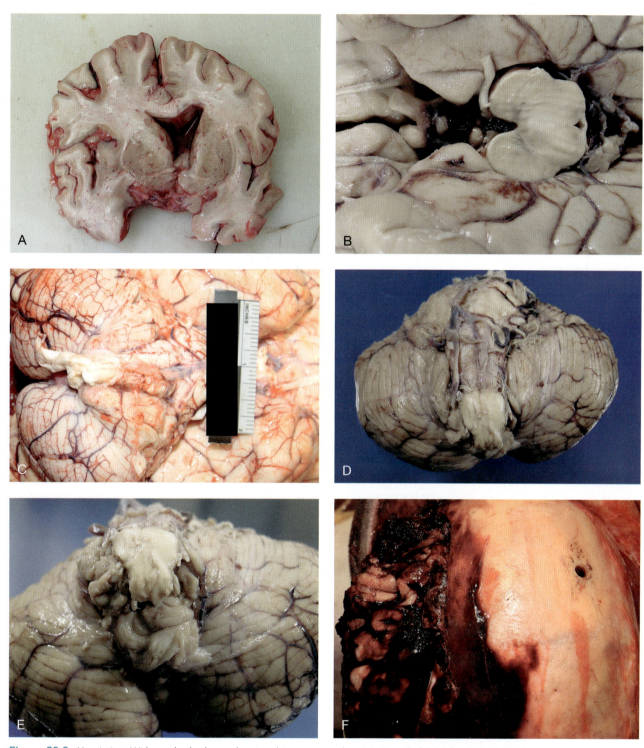

Figure 28.3. Herniation. With cerebral edema, the cingulate gyrus can herniate (ie, sub-falcine herniation) (**A**), the uncus can herniate (ie, transtentorial herniation) (**B**), and the cerebellar tonsils can herniate. Uncal notching is a common postmortem finding and must be interpreted carefully. Hemorrhage or necrosis, such as in **B**, helps confirm the diagnosis but is not commonly present. With tonsillar herniation, the tonsils will be molded against the brainstem (**C-E**). Hemorrhage or necrosis of the cerebellar tonsils helps confirm the diagnosis but is not commonly present. When the decedent has undergone a craniotomy prior to death, the cerebral parenchyma can herniate through the defect in the bone (**F**).

PEARLS & PITFALLS

Arnold-Chiari malformations are associated with elongated cerebellar tonsils, which could mimic cerebellar tonsillar herniation. In an Arnold-Chiari type I malformation, the cerebellum is present 5 mm below the level of the foramen magnum.[8]

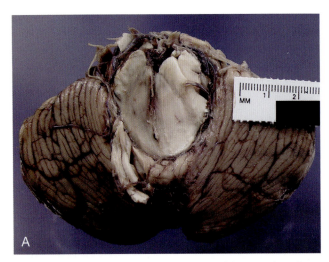
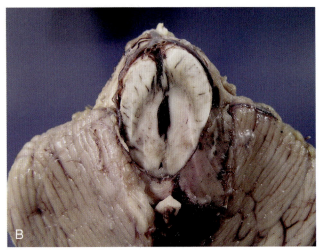

Figure 28.4. Complications of herniation. While a notch in the cerebral peduncle is not visible in (**A**), the image at least illustrates how changes in the brainstem due to cerebral edema can be unilateral, and that one side could affect the other side. (**B**) is an example of a classic linear midline Duret hemorrhage; however, in practice, the morphologic features of a Duret hemorrhage are broader and caution must be used to not confuse a Duret hemorrhage with a primary intracerebral hemorrhage involving the brainstem.

NEAR MISSES

Near Miss #1: A young male riding a motorcycle was involved in a collision. A partial autopsy was performed, which identified 1,600 mL of blood in the right pleural cavity. No fractures of the sternum or ribs were present. The source of the blood was a tear in the right azygos vein. Prior to release of the body, communication with the coroner indicated that the decedent was essentially dead on impact, as emergency medical providers who happened to be in the vehicle behind the decedent stopped and immediately started rendering aid and found him pulseless. As the autopsy findings were not consistent with being immediately lethal, the cranial cavity was opened, revealing a complete atlanto-occipital dislocation. The blood in the right chest cavity is presumed to have been circulated by resuscitative measures.

Near Miss #2: With stress, bare megakaryocyte nuclei can be found in the pulmonary vasculature (Figure 28.6). The nuclei can be quite prominent in number and could potentially be confused for an infectious process or emboli.

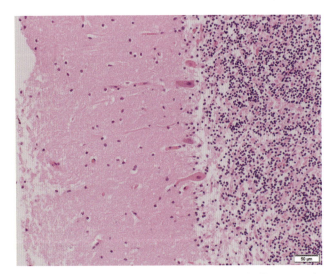

Figure 28.5. Red neurons in cerebellum. With global hypoxic ischemic encephalopathy, more than one area of the brain should be involved (ie, the global aspect). In the image, red neurons in the Purkinje cell layer of the cerebellum are present (high power).

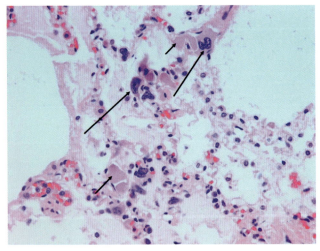

Figure 28.6. Bare megakaryocyte nuclei in individual with disseminated intravascular coagulation (DIC). The alveolar septal capillaries have both microthrombi (short arrows) associated with the DIC as well as bare megakaryocyte nuclei (long arrows) (high power).

References

1. Kumar V, Abbas AK, Aster JC, et al. *Robbins and Kumar Basic Pathology*. 11th ed. Elsevier; 2023.
2. Kumar V, Abbas AK, Aster JC. *Robbins Basic Pathology*. 10th ed. Elsevier; 2018.
3. Potente S, Ramsthaler F, Kettner M, Sauer P, Schmidt P. Relative blood loss in forensic medicine-do we need a change in doctrine? *Int J Legal Med*. 2020;134(3):1123-1131.
4. Plattner T, Yen K, Zollinger U. The value of subendocardial haemorrhages as an indicator of exsanguination and brain injury-a retrospective forensic autopsy study. *J Forensic Leg Med*. 2008;15(5):325-328.
5. Moskovitz JB, Levy ZD, Slesinger TL. Cardiogenic shock. *Emerg Med Clin N Am*. 2015;33(3):645-652.
6. Kocovski L, Duflou J. Can renal acute tubular necrosis be differentiated from autolysis at autopsy? *J Forensic Sci*. 2009;54(2):439-442.
7. Bauer M, Gerlach K, Scheurer E, Lenz C. Analysis of different post mortem assessment methods for cerebral edema. *Forensic Sci Int*. 2020;308:110164.
8. Rosenblum JS, Pomeraniec IJ, Heiss JD. Chiari malformation (update on diagnosis and treatment). *Neurol Clin*. 2022;40(2):297-307.

TREATMENT-RELATED AUTOPSY FINDINGS 29

CHAPTER OUTLINE

Introduction   574

Types of Medical Devices Used   574

External Injuries Caused by Resuscitation Attempts   575

Internal Injuries Caused by Resuscitation Attempts   576

Near Misses   579

INTRODUCTION

Quite frequently, when a forensic pathologist conducts an autopsy, the body has undergone resuscitation attempts. These resuscitation attempts will leave medical devices in place and marks on and within the body that the forensic pathologist must identify and interpret.

> **PEARLS & PITFALLS**
>
> In individuals who are shot or stabbed and subsequently treated in the emergency room and operating room, it is not uncommon for treating physicians to place chest tubes in traumatic defects, or cut through traumatic defects when they do a thoracotomy or exploratory laparotomy. Such artifacts create a challenge for the forensic pathologist; however, careful observation at autopsy combined with a review of the medical records often can sort out the changes.

TYPES OF MEDICAL DEVICES USED

With resuscitation, commonly encountered medical devices include oral endotracheal tubes; nasal and oral gastric tubes; oral or nasal airways; blood pressure cuffs; catheters in the chest; electrocardiography (ECG) patches; defibrillator-pacer patches; various forms of intravascular lines, which can be present in the neck, subclavian regions, antecubital fossae, and femoral regions, among other sites; Foley urinary catheters; and intra-osseous catheters, which are commonly placed in the leg but can also be placed in the shoulder region.

> **FAQ:** Should the placement of medical devices be confirmed in situ before the medical device is removed?
>
> **Answer:** Whether the placement of a medical device is confirmed in situ before its removal is based upon office policies and pathologist preference. The placement of the medical device was done to treat the patient and should not be the cause of death. Whether it was correctly placed could potentially be a civil concern or possibly an issue in criminal proceedings; however, that the device was not partially pulled and replaced prior to examination by the forensic pathologist would be difficult to determine solely based upon the autopsy itself (Figure 29.1).

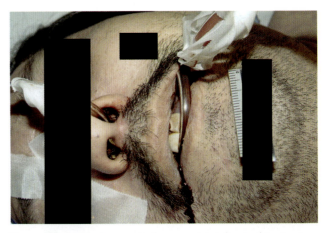

Figure 29.1. Misplacement of nasogastric tube. In this situation, the nasogastric tube curled in the mouth instead of entering the esophagus. However, that the tube was properly placed, pulled after death, and subsequently replaced cannot be ruled out.

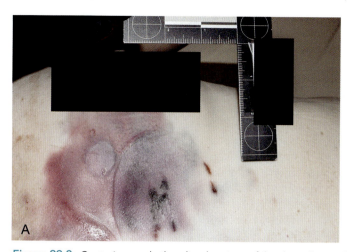
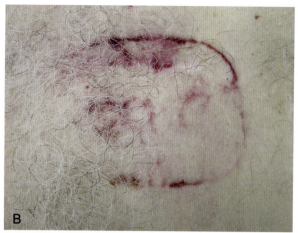

Figure 29.2. Contusions and other discolorations of the chest. Depending upon survival period following resuscitation, contusions of the chest can be quite prominent and can be misinterpreted as inflicted injury (**A**). Defibrillator-pacer patches will produce a rectangular red discoloration of the skin (**B**).

EXTERNAL INJURIES CAUSED BY RESUSCITATION ATTEMPTS

Common external injuries caused by resuscitation attempts include defined rectangular discolorations or irregular dried yellow-orange patches of skin on the chest, sometimes associated with contusions (Figure 29.2A and B), and puncture wounds, which can be on the hands, wrists, antecubital fossae, neck, and, in infants, the feet.

> **PEARLS & PITFALLS**
>
> If the identification of puncture sites is especially important to a particular autopsy case, having the medical team that performed the resuscitation identify any punctures they created is useful. This identification can easily be done with a magic marker, circling the resuscitation-induced puncture sites. Some organizations will have pre-made stickers that they can place to identify therapeutic or postmortem punctures (eg, those associated with organ or tissue recovery) (Figure 29.3).

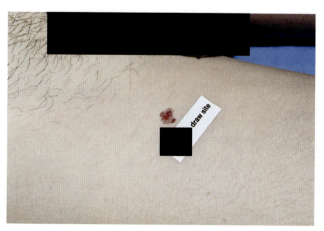

Figure 29.3. Tissue recovery draw site. If tissue recovery occurs prior to examination of the body, stickers placed by the recovery technician can identify postmortem blood draw sites.

INTERNAL INJURIES CAUSED BY RESUSCITATION ATTEMPTS[1-8]

Intubation attempts can cause oral injuries as well as injuries of the neck organs, including even potentially fractures of the hyoid bone or thyroid cartilage, although such fractures would be rare and must be adequately explained (Figure 29.4A-D). If the intubation remains in place for a period of time with survival, contusions, ulcers, and polypoid collections of granulation tissue can all develop at the lateral edge of the vocal cords (Figure 29.5). Compression of the chest can lead to sternum and rib fractures, which are usually anterior or anterior-lateral in location. Compression of the chest can also lead to hemorrhage into the mediastinum, rupture of the pericardial sac and cardiac chambers, and laceration of the liver or spleen (Figure 29.6A-H). Potente et al described rupture of the pericardial sac, left atrium, and right ventricle due to cardiopulmonary resuscitation (CPR) in a 73-year-old woman who died secondary to intra-abdominal hemorrhage that occurred during surgery.[9] The left thoracic cavity contained 1,500 mL of blood. Finally, any device inserted into the body can cause hemorrhage (eg, hemorrhage in the bladder mucosa associated with Foley catheter placement) (Figure 29.7A and B).

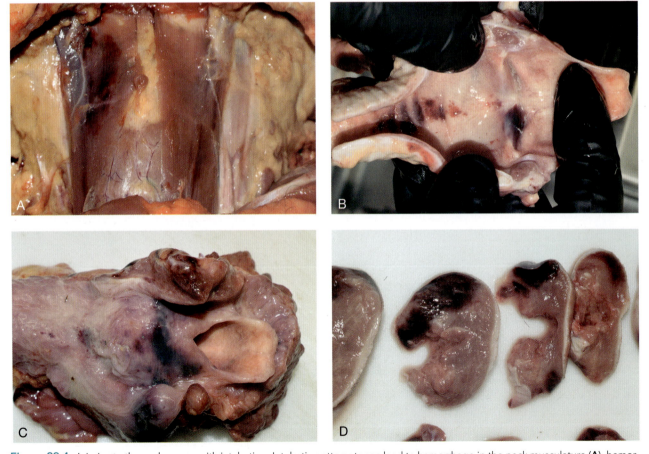

Figure 29 4. Injuries to the neck organs with intubation. Intubation attempts can lead to hemorrhage in the neck musculature (**A**), hemorrhage of the larynx and surrounding soft tissue (**B** and **C**), and hemorrhage in the tongue (**D**). With survival following resuscitation attempts, these hemorrhages can become quite prominent as in (**D**).

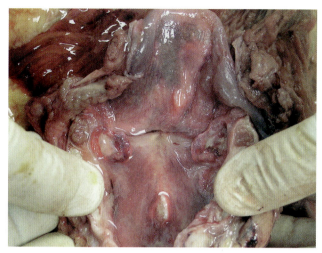

Figure 29.5. Intubation ulcers. With prolonged intubation, ulcers of the lateral aspect of the true vocal cords can develop.

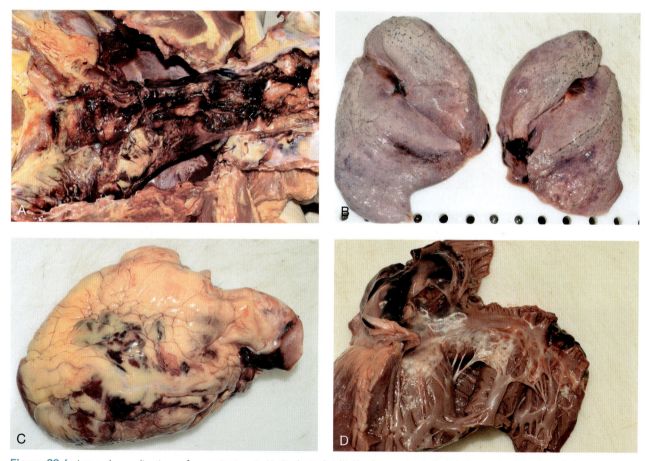

Figure 29.6. Internal complications of resuscitation. In (A-C), the individual had extensive in-hospital resuscitation, which led to prominent mediastinal hemorrhage (A), contusions of the lung (B), and contusions and a small epicardial tear of the heart (C). In (D), this individual who hanged themself in their jail cell sustained a laceration of the right atrium as a result of CPR attempts. In (E and F), the individual also hanged themself in their jail cell, and at autopsy was found to have blood in the pericardial sac (E) and a tear at the right atrium (F). Liver lacerations due to CPR (G and H) will usually be associated with a relatively insignificant amount of hemorrhage (eg, 100-300 mL) in the peritoneal cavity. CPR, cardiopulmonary resuscitation.

Figure 29.6 (continued)

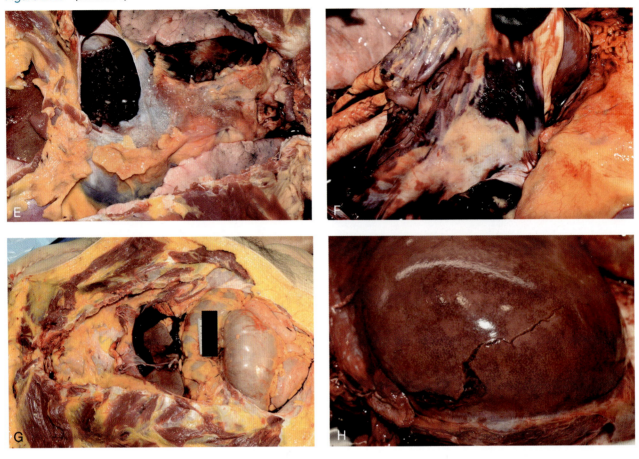

> **PEARLS & PITFALLS**
>
> When an emergent thoracotomy is performed, not infrequently a laceration of the adjacent axilla will be produced (Figure 29.8). Depending upon the cause of death, this iatrogenic injury could be confused with a gunshot wound or stab wound.

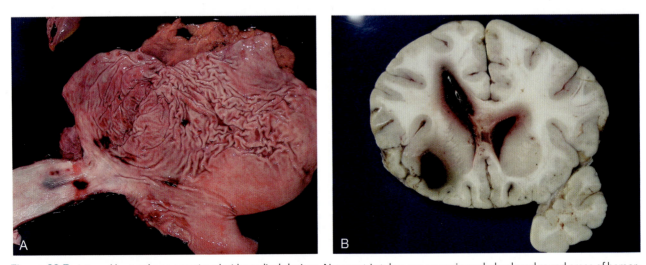

Figure 29.7. Internal hemorrhage associated with medical devices. Nasogastric tubes can cause irregularly placed round areas of hemorrhage in the gastric mucosa (**A**). Ventriculostomy tubes can have hemorrhage along the track (**B**). This hemorrhage must be distinguished from natural disease or trauma.

> **FAQ:** Does resuscitation cause conjunctival petechiae? Does resuscitation cause retinal hemorrhages?
>
> **Answer:** Binenbaum et al, Longmuir et al, and Odom et al found that CPR can cause a few intraretinal hemorrhages in the posterior pole of the eye[10-12]; however, Levinson et al identified diffuse bilateral retinal hemorrhages in an infant with a coagulopathy and prolonged CPR who was found to have died from an anomalous coronary artery.[13] While Hood et al indicate that CPR can cause conjunctival petechiae, based upon their review of 196 cases, Maxeiner and Jekat determined the CPR does not cause conjunctival petechiae.[14,15] The differences among authors would indicate that the answer to the two questions is not absolute and can depend upon the circumstances of the death, and that it is not agreed upon in the literature.

> **PEARLS & PITFALLS**
>
> Blood clot at a source of bleeding is consistent with an antemortem hemorrhage; whereas pooled blood is more consistent with a resuscitation related hemorrhage.[16] While coagulated blood is most commonly evidence of antemortem bleeding, Watanabe et al indicated that coagulated blood in the pericardial sac can occur secondary to resuscitation or postmortem manipulation.[17]

NEAR MISSES

Near Miss #1: Just because medical devices were placed, do not assume that the time of death was close to the time of medical intervention. Depending upon policy and procedures of given ambulance or hospital services, a certain level of attempted resuscitation must be performed, or at least a certain level of confirmation of death must be performed, hence the presence of ECG patches on a decomposed body (Figure 29.9).

Near Miss #2: This individual was stabbed; however, in the left axilla was a lesion related to the thoracotomy site, which could easily be misinterpreted as a stab wound (Figure 29.10A and B).

Near Miss #3: CPR can introduce a significant amount of air into the stomach, which can distend the stomach and be misinterpreted as bleeding into the peritoneal cavity (Figure 29.11).

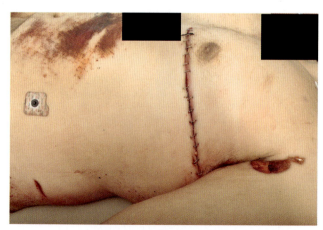

Figure 29.8. Thoracotomy artifact. When thoracotomies are performed, especially in an emergent situation, it is not uncommon to have small lacerations of the adjacent axillary skin. This injury could be misinterpreted as a stab wound or gunshot wound, depending upon the circumstances of the death; however, exploration of the wound will reveal its superficial nature.

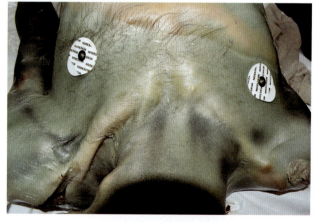

Figure 29.9. ECG patches on a decomposed body. Even bodies that are obviously deceased may have some forms of resuscitation measures applied.

Near Miss #4: Subcapsular hemorrhage in liver from CPR could mimic a subcapsular hemorrhage in HELLP (hemolysis, elevated liver enzymes, low platelet count) syndrome (Figure 29.12A and B).

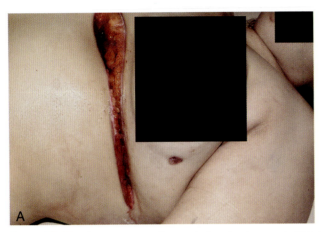
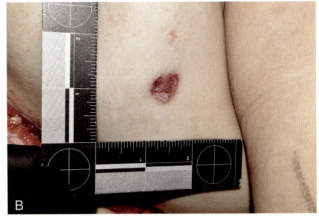

Figure 29.10. Thoracotomy artifact in victim of stab wounds. This individual had an emergent thoracotomy performed as part of resuscitative attempts after she was stabbed. In the left axilla is a lesion that could mimic a stab wound (**A**); however, the dried yellow edges, superficial nature of the wound (**B**), and context are consistent with a treatment artifact related to the thoracotomy.

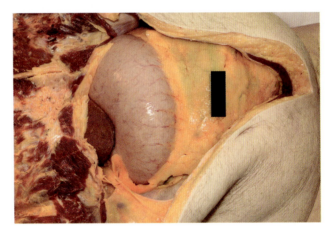

Figure 29.11. Air in the stomach. During CPR, air can enter and distend the stomach. This change will cause the abdomen to be more swollen and can be misinterpreted externally as air or blood in the peritoneal cavity.

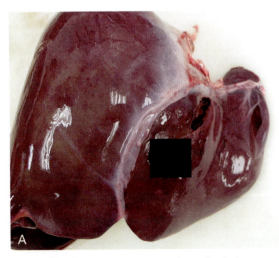
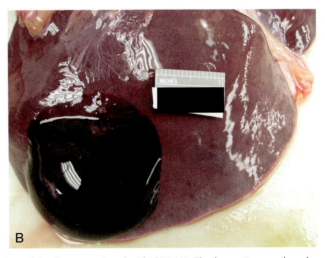

Figure 29.12. Laceration of liver. This individual sustained a laceration of the liver associated with CPR (**A**). The laceration produced a subcapsular hemorrhage (**B**). Subcapsular hemorrhages in the liver are associated with HELLP syndrome for which the artifact could be mistaken.

References

1. Olds K, Byard RW, Langlois NEI. Injuries associated with resuscitation-An overview. *J Forensic Leg Med.* 2015;33:39-43.
2. Hashimoto Y, Moriya F, Furumiya J. Forensic aspects of complications resulting from cardiopulmonary resuscitation. *Leg Med.* 2007;9(2):94-99.
3. Righi FA, Jenkins S, Lin PT. Nonskeletal injuries related to cardiopulmonary resuscitation: an autopsy study. *J Forensic Sci.* 2021;66(6):2299-2306.
4. Ram P, Menezes RG, Sirinvaravong N, et al. Breaking your heart-A review on CPR-related injuries. *Am J Emerg Med.* 2018;36(5):838-842.
5. Milling L, Leth PM, Astrup BS. Life-threatening and suspicious lesions caused by mechanical cardiopulmonary resuscitation. *Am J Forensic Med Pathol.* 2017;38(3):219-221.
6. Hickey TB, Gill GG, Seidman MA, Webber DL. CPR-associated right ventricular rupture in the setting of pulmonary embolism. *CJEM.* 2016;18(6):484-487.
7. Buschmann CT, Tsokos M. Frequent and rare complications of resuscitation attempts. *Intensive Care Med.* 2009;35(3):397-404.
8. Raven KP, Reay DT, Harruff RC. Artifactual injuries of the larynx produced by resuscitative intubation. *Am J Forensic Med Pathol.* 1999;20(1):31-36.
9. Potente S, Ramsthaler F, Kettner M, Sauer P, Schmidt P. Relative blood loss in forensic medicine—do we need a change in doctrine? *Int J Legal Med.* 2020;134(3):1123-1131.
10. Binenbaum G, Forbes BJ, Topjian AA, Twelves C, Christian CW. Patterns of retinal hemorrhage associated with cardiac arrest and cardiopulmonary resuscitation. *J AAPOS.* 2021;25(6):324.e1-324.e4.
11. Longmuir SQ, McConnell L, Oral R, Dumitrescu A, Kamath S, Erkonen G. Retinal hemorrhages in intubated pediatric intensive care patients. *J AAPOS.* 2014;18(2):129-133.
12. Odom A, Christ E, Kerr N, et al. Prevalence of retinal hemorrhages in pediatric patients after in-hospital cardiopulmonary resuscitation: a prospective study. *Pediatrics.* 1997;99(6):E3.
13. Levinson JD, Pasquale MA, Lambert SR. Diffuse bilateral retinal hemorrhages in an infant with a coagulopathy and prolonged cardiopulmonary resuscitation. *J AAPOS.* 2016;20(2):166-168.
14. Hood I, Ryan D, Spitz WU. Resuscitation and petechiae. *Am J Forensic Med Pathol.* 1988;9(1):35-37.
15. Maxeiner H, Jekat R. Resuscitation and conjunctival petechial hemorrhages. *J Forensic Leg Med.* 2010;17(2):87-91.
16. Chatzaraki V, Thali MJ, Ampanozi G. Diagnostic accuracy of postmortem computed tomography for bleeding source determination in cases with hemoperitoneum. *Int J Legal Med.* 2021;135(2):593-603.
17. Watanabe S, Hyodoh H, Shimizu J, Okazaki S, Mizuo K, Rokukawa M. Classification of hemopericardium on postmortem CT. *Leg Med.* 2015;17(5):376-380.

AUTOMOBILE ACCIDENTS 30

CHAPTER OUTLINE

Introduction 584

Characteristic Injuries in a Motor Vehicle Accident 586
- Transection of the Aorta 586
  - Gross Features 586
  - Important Points 586
- Basilar Skull Fracture 586
  - Gross Features 586
- Flail Chest 586
  - Gross Features 586
- Atlanto-Occipital Fracture/Dislocation (See Blunt Force Injuries Chapter) 587
- Dicing 587
  - Gross Description 587
  - Importance 587
- Stretch Abrasions/Lacerations 587

Near Misses 592

INTRODUCTION

In motor vehicle accidents, two main scenarios for the decedent are possible: the decedent was inside the vehicle at the time of the accident or the decedent was outside the vehicle at the time of the accident (ie, a pedestrian struck by a motor vehicle). When a pedestrian is struck by a motor vehicle, either the driver will stop and render aid, or the driver will leave the scene, either knowingly having struck a pedestrian or unknowingly having struck a pedestrian. In the case of a driver leaving the scene, examination of the decedent may provide evidence to better understand the nature of the collision and to identify evidence that may help link the vehicle, if and when it is found, to the decedent. Evidence found on the body, such as paint chips, when analyzed can also potentially provide investigators with information as to the type of vehicle involved. In addition, analysis of fragments of the vehicle found at the scene may also narrow the search for possible vehicles involved in the collision. The main reasons for autopsying individuals who are inside of a vehicle at the time of an accident are to (1) determine the cause of death, (2) distinguish the driver from the passenger(s), (3) collect fluids for toxicologic analysis, and (4) determine if any natural event may have contributed to the accident. In some situations, when a body is found alongside the road, it may not be possible to determine if the individual was a pedestrian struck by a motor vehicle, or an individual who fell or was pushed/thrown from a motor vehicle.

CHECKLIST for a Motor Vehicle Accident (in addition to those for a general forensic autopsy)

- ☐ Obtain report from highway patrol or other agency involved with the investigation of the crash itself.
- ☐ Depending upon the circumstances, consider examination of the vehicle.
- ☐ Consider carboxyhemoglobin testing in individuals who were inside a vehicle.
- ☐ Examine the shoes for evidence of brake pad contact.
- ☐ As neck injuries can be subtle, consider a posterior neck dissection to best examine for injuries at this location.

PEARLS & PITFALLS

Relying on autopsy to determine why an accident occurred is an error.[1] While the autopsy can identify lethal injuries and determine whether the impact caused the death of the individual, it is very unlikely to reveal the cause of the accident. In an older individual with 75% stenosis of a coronary artery due to atherosclerosis, attributing the motor vehicle accident to a cardiac event, while possible, would be inappropriate without further confirmatory evidence, such as a witness seeing the driver grab their chest just before the accident occurred. Scene investigation may provide useful information for understanding why the accident occurred (Figure 30.1).

PEARLS & PITFALLS

Not all individuals who are involved in a vehicular accident die as the result of injuries from the accident, and not all individuals found with a vehicle have sustained injuries. Scene investigation can be very important to interpret these deaths (Figure 30.2).

CHAPTER 30 AUTOMOBILE ACCIDENTS

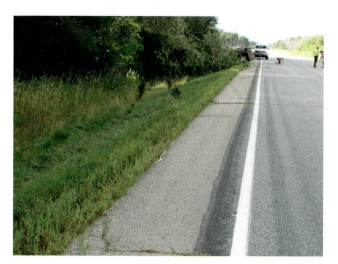

Figure 30.1. Scene investigation of motor vehicle accident revealing cause of accident. The decedent's tire marks just slowly angled off the road until the vehicle impacted vegetation at the side of the road. Investigation revealed the decedent was texting on his phone at the time of the accident.

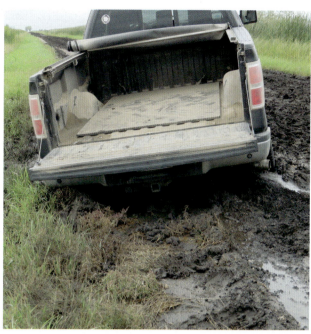

Figure 30.2. Scene investigation to assist in determination of cause of death when motor vehicle is involved. The decedent was found dead in the cab of his truck, which was stuck in deep mud, with the decedent apparently having tried to drive the vehicle out of the mud. Autopsy revealed no injuries and only significant heart disease.

CHECKLIST for a Hit and Run

- ☐ Retain clothing as evidence.
- ☐ Collect a head hair standard and blood standard (to compare to evidence found on the suspected vehicle if/when found).
- ☐ Examine lacerations and other injuries on the body for paint fragments or other fragments of the vehicle (Figure 30.3A and B).
- ☐ Dissect the lower extremities to check for impact site (Figure 30.4).
- ☐ Measure the distance from the bottom of the sole of the foot to the impact site.
- ☐ Consider removing any fractured bone in the lower extremity for better examination.

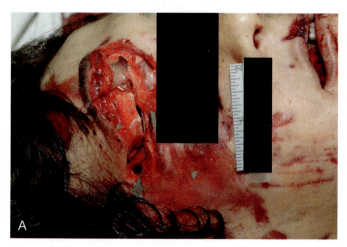
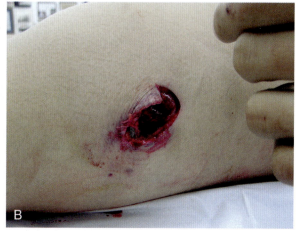

Figure 30.3. Evidence collection from a hit-and-run. In a pedestrian who is struck by a vehicle, sometimes paint chips or other items of evidentiary value can be found in the injuries. In (**A** and **B**), the paint fragments are quite obvious; however, in some circumstances, it requires diligent searching of a large gaping wound to find a tiny fragment of paint from the vehicle.

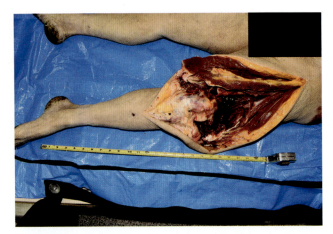

Figure 30.4. Dissection of lower extremities in a pedestrian-related death. When a pedestrian is struck by a motor vehicle, especially if that motor vehicle fled the scene, it is good to dissect the lower extremities to identify the impact site, which will be an area of torn muscle, hemorrhage, and partially to completely liquefied fat. A tape measure can be used to document the location of the impact site and its distance from the sole of the foot, which can help identify the height of the vehicle.

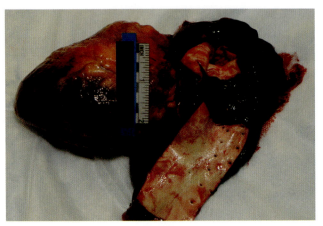

Figure 30.5. Transection of the aorta. A common cause of death in motor vehicle accidents is transection of the aorta, which will most often quickly lead to death through hemorrhage into the left pleural cavity.

CHARACTERISTIC INJURIES IN A MOTOR VEHICLE ACCIDENT

While many different types of injuries can be identified during the examination of a decedent who was involved in a motor vehicle collision, including various types of blunt force injuries, some injuries are frequently identified in this category of deaths and have some characteristic findings.

TRANSECTION OF THE AORTA

Gross Features

A transection of the aorta due to blunt force injuries of the chest most commonly occurs around the region of the ligamentum arteriosum (Figure 30.5). Associated with the tear will be blood in the left pleural cavity.

Important Points

While a transection of the aorta is a common cause of death, with death often occurring shortly after the accident, depending upon the nature of the injury, a delay following the injury and prior to death occurring can happen. Trauma can also contribute to the development of a thoracic aortic aneurysm, with death occurring potentially years after the injury itself.[2]

BASILAR SKULL FRACTURE

Gross Features

In regards to motor vehicle accidents, a basilar skill fracture is often used to describe a fracture of the base of the cranium that involves the middle cranial fossae, the region of the sella turcica, and one or both petrous ridges (Figure 30.6). Associated with the fractures on external examination will be blood draining from one or both external auditory canals.

FLAIL CHEST

Gross Features

The clinical diagnosis of a flail chest, which can cause acute respiratory failure and death, requires that three or more continuous ribs are fractured in two or more locations

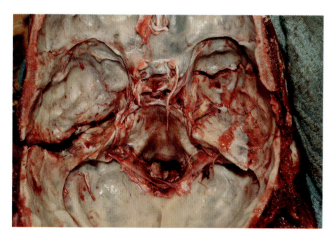

Figure 30.6. Basilar skull fracture. A common cause of death in motor vehicle accidents is a basilar skull fracture. While the base of the cranium includes the orbital plates, the types of basilar skull fractures encountered at autopsy that are responsible for death involve the left and right petrous ridge and/or adjacent floor of middle cranial fossa, and the sella turcica region, but could also potentially involve the floor of the posterior cranial fossa, especially the area immediately adjacent to the foramen magnum.

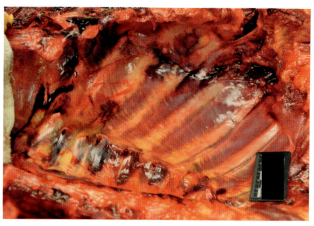

Figure 30.7. Flail chest. An easy diagnosis to forget as a potential cause of death in a motor vehicle accident is a flail chest. To document a flail chest at autopsy, the forensic pathologist needs to show three or more ribs fractured in two or more locations. In the image, more than three of the left sided ribs are fractured anterior and paraspinal. Of course, to document a flail chest adequately, the possibility that cardiopulmonary resuscitation caused the second set of fractures, especially if they are anterior, must be considered.

(Figure 30.7), which causes this segment of ribs to collapse inward toward the lung with respiration and can have a mortality rate of around 35%.[3] Although flail chest is a clinical diagnosis, the pathologic findings consistent with the disease process can easily be identified at autopsy.

ATLANTO-OCCIPITAL FRACTURE/DISLOCATION (SEE BLUNT FORCE INJURIES CHAPTER)[4-7]
DICING
Gross Description

The edges of cubed broken glass from the side windows will produce characteristic "L," "T," and "I" shaped superficial incisions in the skin (Figure 30.8A-C).

Importance

While dicing is not a lethal injury, the finding on the decedent may be able to assist in determining the position of the decedent in the vehicle at the time of the accident. While not absolute, the side of the face with the dicing injuries is often the side that was facing the window (ie, if the dicing injuries are on the right side of the face and right shoulder, the decedent was most likely sitting on the right side of the vehicle; however, this is not absolute as unrestrained bodies can move around quite a bit in a vehicle, especially if the vehicle rolls).

STRETCH ABRASIONS/LACERATIONS
Gross Description

In pedestrians who are struck by a motor vehicle, stretch-type abrasions and lacerations can develop in the femoral region (Figure 30.9A and B). The finding is consistent with an impact to the buttocks.[8]

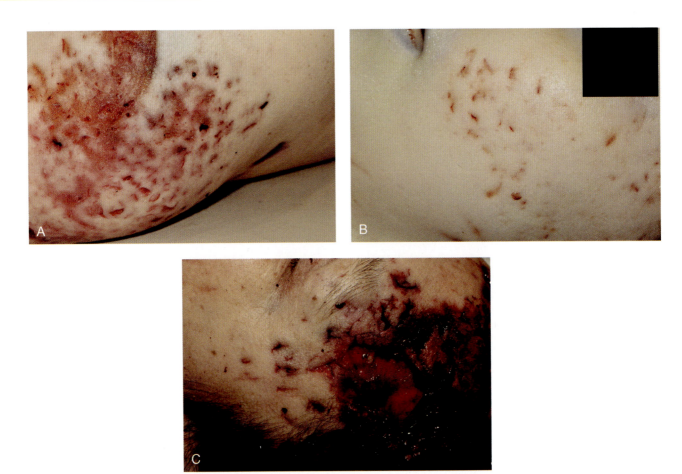

Figure 30.8. (**A-C**) Dicing. While not lethal injuries, dicing injuries caused by contact with cubed glass produced when side windows break may be able to help identify the position of the decedent in the vehicle when the crash occurred. For example, unless there is evidence otherwise, dicing injuries of the right side of the face would be consistent with an individual who was on the passenger side of the car when the crash occurred.

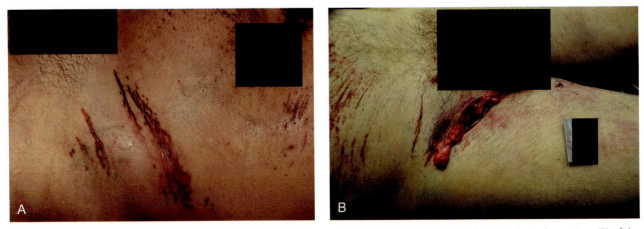

Figure 30.9. Stretch-type injuries of the femoral region. In an impact to a pedestrian, stretch-type abrasions (**A**) or lacerations (**B**) of the femoral region, either unilateral or bilateral, can occur.

FAQ: Can the driver and passenger(s) in a motor vehicle accident be distinguished at autopsy (ie, at autopsy can it be determined whether the decedent was the driver or a passenger in the vehicle)?

Answer: This question is oftentimes asked of forensic pathologists, as in a motor vehicle accident with more than one occupant, the death of all individuals is not certain, and, if the driver survives and the passenger(s) die, criminal charges may be brought against the driver for the death of the passenger, especially if the driver is intoxicated or otherwise impaired. Unfortunately, unrestrained individuals in a motor vehicle can move around quite a bit. While it is sometimes possible to determine whether the decedent was the driver or passenger, especially if seat belt type abrasions are present, or if the scene investigation and evaluation of the car assists (eg, if the car left the roadway and slammed straight into a fence and did not roll, and the decedent is found in the passenger side of the vehicle), in most motor vehicle accidents, the injury patterns are not specific enough to allow for a reliable determination of driver vs passenger based upon the autopsy findings alone. When a seat belt is worn, the patterned injury made by the seatbelt will allow for the determination of whether the decedent was on the right or left side of the vehicle, unless the front seats have a shoulder harness type of seatbelt and the rear seats only a lap belt, in which case, the side and position of the decedent most often cannot be determined (Figure 30.10A-F). In motor vehicle fatalities, the decedent is often not wearing a seat belt, and, in this situation, the pattern from a seat belt is not available as a marker of the decedent's position in the vehicle. Also, in many motor vehicle accidents, the vehicle rolls and/or the occupants are ejected. In these cases, the position of the decedent can change markedly from before the impact to after the impact. Blood, hair, and fingerprints, depending upon their location and the nature of the accident, may allow for determination of driver vs passenger. Also, specific patterned injuries that only the driver or a passenger could have had (eg, impact with an adjacent object) could help distinguish the two. In many motor vehicle accidents with multiple occupants, when one or more persons survives, distinguishing the driver from the passenger would be important for potential legal action against the driver, assuming they survived; however, distinguishing between the driver and passenger often cannot be done.

PEARLS & PITFALLS

Before confirming that a decedent was wearing a seat belt through the identification of an injury on the chest consistent with that scenario, it is prudent to confirm with investigators if there was or was not evidence of seat belt use at the scene. Confirming a seat belt was worn by findings at autopsy when the scene investigation clearly shows that seat belts were not worn can be embarrassing.

FAQ: Can cause of death be determined in a motor vehicle accident without performing an autopsy?

Answer: While some forensic pathologists prefer to perform a complete autopsy on individuals who have died in a motor vehicle accident, other forensic pathologists are comfortable with performing an external examination and identifying evidence of injuries. If brain is found at the external ear or fluid blood can be made to drain from the external ear canal, the findings are consistent with a basilar skull fracture (Figure 30.11A-C). Palpation and/or radiography can reveal a neck fracture or dislocation. A needle inserted into the chest posterior to the level of the heart can identify blood in the chest cavity, and, combined with a radiograph, could confirm a hemothorax, with the radiograph also allowing for the identification of rib fractures or a vertebral column fracture (Figure 30.11D). Whether to perform an external examination vs a complete autopsy can also depend upon whether a legal action will be brought against another person as a result of the death. If someone is to be charged for the death, many attorneys prefer that an autopsy is performed.

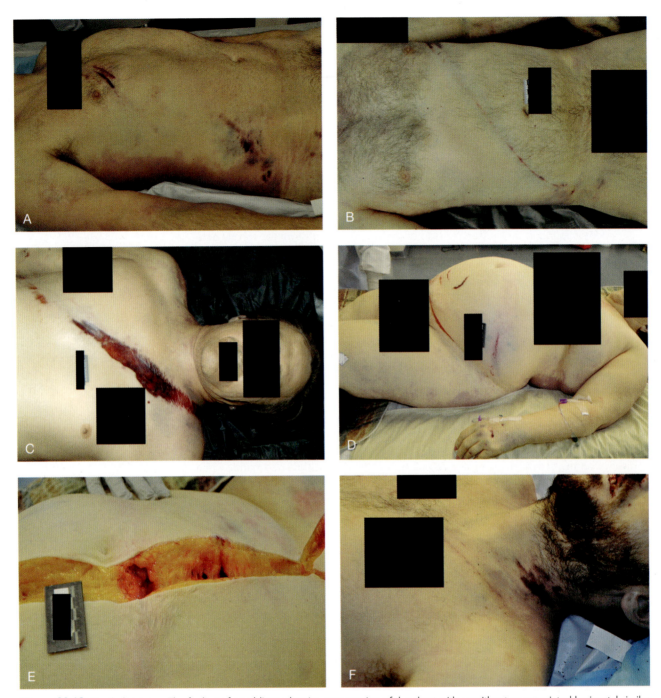

Figure 30.10. Seatbelt injuries. The finding of an oblique abrasion or contusion of the chest with or without an associated horizontal similar injury of the lower abdomen is consistent with a seatbelt. In some cases, the seat belt injury will be faint and/or discontinuous (**A** and **B**), whereas in other cases, the seat belt injury is very well defined (**C**). Associated with the seat belt injury can be laceration of the underlying adipose tissue (**D** and **E**). While seatbelt injuries are commonly on the chest, the neck can also be involved, and, in some cases, may be the only indication that a seat belt was worn (**F**).

> **FAQ:** If there is minimal damage to a vehicle from a low-speed impact and the driver has no external injuries, assuming that the cause of death is natural disease, is an autopsy required?
>
> **Answer:** This determination is best made with all interested parties (eg, forensic pathologist, law enforcement, coroner, attorney, family members) able to voice their preference. With a low-speed or no-speed impact (eg, a driver drove off the road and into a field, or a driver drove off a road and into a house, with minimal damage to the vehicle or the house) and in a driver who has a significant past medical history indicating a strong likelihood that they sustained a sudden cardiac death behind the wheel, unless specifically requested, an autopsy is not necessarily needed.

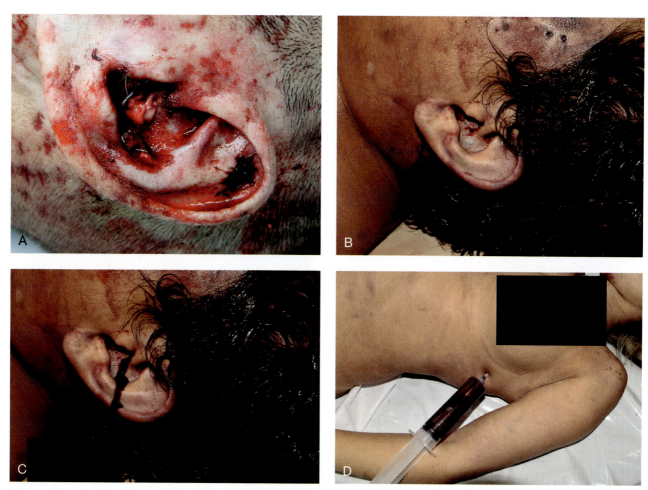

Figure 30.11. Confirmation of internal injuries by external examination. In some cases, fragments of brain will be found in the external auditory canal (**A**), which indicates significant internal trauma. While the brain may be palpably intact, if fluid blood can be drained from the external auditory canal, it is consistent with a basilar skull fracture, with tearing of the vessels at the base of the brain, and blood entering the ear canal through a fracture of the petrous ridge. First, the ear should be cleaned of extraneous blood (**B**), then the head rotated to see if fluid blood will drain from the ear canal (**C**). A needle in the chest can confirm blood in the left pleural cavity (**D**), which can be consistent with an aortic transection. However, rib fractures can also produce bleeding into a pleural cavity. A radiograph of the chest may help further define this injury pattern.

PEARLS & PITFALLS

For motor vehicle accidents, consider carboxyhemoglobin testing to ensure that the accident was not caused by a carbon monoxide leak into the compartment of the car. Also, although individuals found in a vehicle outdoors are often not considered to have died from carbon monoxide toxicity due to the fact that the vehicle is not in an enclosed space such as a garage with the door closed and the carbon monoxide can instead dissipate, if the vehicle is running and there is a defect in the floor of the trunk or elsewhere where exhaust can then enter the vehicle, carbon monoxide toxicity can occur in a vehicle that is outside and not enclosed by a building.

PEARLS & PITFALLS

When a pedestrian is struck by a motor vehicle, one necessary distinction is whether the pedestrian was standing or walking at the time of the impact, or whether they were already on the ground. In their review of 371 pedestrian victims, Teresinski and Madro determined that the finding of bilateral injuries of the sacroiliac joints and external dislocations of hip joints were consistent with the decedent having been run over while they were lying on the ground, whereas unilateral injuries of the sacroiliac joints and central dislocations of the hip joints can indicate the side of impact in an individual who is standing.[9] The authors indicate that these findings can be identified on radiograph.

> **PEARLS & PITFALLS**
>
> For motor vehicle accidents, it is important to have scene photographs available for review, or at the least, a detailed description of how the body was found. In situations where another agency does the scene investigation, good communication is important. Traumatic asphyxia is not an uncommon cause of death in motor vehicle accidents, but, without scene photographs or a good description of the position of the body after the accident, this diagnosis will likely be missed by the forensic pathologist conducting the autopsy.

Key conditions to consider if there is a delayed death following a motor vehicle accident

- Fat embolism
- Splenic laceration with hemorrhage (Figure 30.12)
- Liver laceration with hemorrhage

> **PEARLS & PITFALLS**
>
> While fat embolism syndrome is most commonly associated with fractures of long bones and occurs within 48 hours after the incident,[10] fat embolism can occur in motor vehicle accidents with no osseous injury and can occur within minutes after the injury occurred.[11]

NEAR MISSES

Near Miss #1: In a single-occupant motor vehicle accident with no surviving witness as to the driver's behavior prior to the accident, assuming that just because there was an accident that the driver sustained lethal injuries is an error. Lethal injuries must always be documented before the death is ascribed to the accident.

Near Miss #2: Although individuals can be found with injuries that appear to have a particular origin, one must always be careful in interpreting them in the context of all the autopsy findings and history that is available. While the decedent in Figure 30.13 has an oblique linear abrasion on the trunk, which could easily mimic a seat belt abrasion, the decedent was a pedestrian struck by a vehicle.

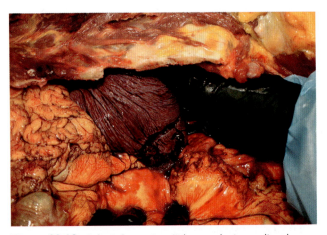

Figure 30.12. Splenic laceration. Either a splenic or a liver laceration can cause bleeding and a delayed death, such as in the case where an individual is responsive when emergency medical services arrives but subsequently becomes unresponsive.

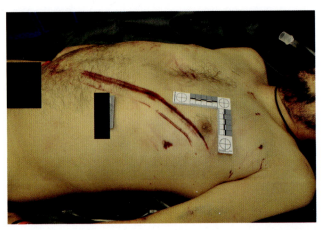

Figure 30.13. Mimic of seatbelt abrasion. While this individual has an oblique abrasion on the trunk that could easily mimic a seatbelt abrasion, this individual was a pedestrian struck by a motor vehicle.

References

1. Fisher RS, Petty CS. *Forensic Pathology: A Handbook for Pathologists*. National Institute of Law Enforcement and Criminal Justice, Law Enforcement Assistance Administration, US Department of Justice; 1977.
2. Keramati AR, Sadeghpour A, Farahani MM, Chandok G, Mani A. The non-syndromic familial thoracic aortic aneurysms and dissections maps to 15q21 locus. *BMC Med Genet*. 2010;11:143.
3. Davignon K, Kwo J, Bigatello LM. Pathophysiology and management of the flail chest. *Minerva Anestesiol*. 2004;70(4):193-199.
4. Adams VI. Neck injuries: I. Occipitoatlantal dislocation—a pathologic study of twelve traffic fatalities. *J Forensic Sci*. 1992;37(2):556-564.
5. Kondo T, Saito K, Nishigami J, Ohshima T. Fatal injuries of the brain stem and/or upper cervical spinal cord in traffic accidents: nine autopsy cases. *Sci Justice*. 1995;35(3):197-201.
6. Tepper SL, Fligner CL, Reay DT. Atlanto-occipital disarticulation. Accident characteristics. *Am J Forensic Med Pathol*. 1990;11(3):193-197.
7. Živković V, Nikolić S, Strajina V, Babić D, Djonić D, Djurić M. Pontomedullary lacerations in unhelmeted motorcyclists and bicyclists: a retrospective autopsy study. *Am J Forensic Med Pathol*. 2012;33(4):349-353.
8. DiMaio VJM, Molina DK. *DiMaio's Forensic Pathology*. 3rd ed. CRC Press; 2022.
9. Teresiński G, Madro R. Pelvis and hip joint injuries as a reconstructive factors in car-to-pedestrian accidents. *Forensic Sci Int*. 2001;124(1):68-73.
10. Weiss W, Bardana D, Yen D. Delayed presentation of fat embolism syndrome after intramedullary nailing of a fractured femur: a case report. *J Trauma*. 2009;66(3):E42-E45.
11. Bolliger SA, Muehlematter K, Thali MJ, Ampanozi G. Correlation of fat embolism severity and subcutaneous fatty tissue crushing and bone fractures. *Int J Legal Med*. 2011;125(3):453-458.

SPECIAL DISSECTIONS   31

CHAPTER OUTLINE

Introduction 596

Dissection of Middle Ears 596
- When Performed 596
- How Performed 596

Dissection of Optic Nerves and Eyes 596
- When Performed 596
- How Performed 596

Dissection of Vertebral Arteries 597
- When Performed 597
- How Performed 597

Dissection of the Anterior and Posterior Neck 597
- When Performed 597
- How Performed 598

Dissection of the Cervical Vertebral Column 598
- When Performed 598
- How Performed 598

Examination for Pneumothorax 598
- When Performed 598
- How Performed 599

Examination for Air Embolus 599
- When Performed 599
- How Performed 599

Dissection of the Back 599
- When Performed 599
- How Performed 600

Dissection of the Lower Extremities 600
- When Performed 600
- How Performed 600

Dissection of the Sinoatrial and Atrioventricular Nodes 600
- When Performed 600
- How Performed 600

Dissection of the Parathyroid Glands 601
- When Performed 601
- How Performed 601

Examination of Esophagus for Varices 602
- When Performed 602
- How Performed 602

Quick Removal of the Entire Spinal Cord 603
- When Performed 603
- How Performed 603

Underwater Removal of Macerated Infant Brain 603
- When Performed 603
- How Performed 603

Maceration of the Thyroid Cartilage 604
- When Performed 604
- How Performed 604

En Bloc Removal of Female Genitalia and/or Anus (Including the Male Anus) 604
- When Performed 604
- How Performed 604

INTRODUCTION

Depending upon the circumstances of the death, additional procedures that are not routinely conducted during the course of a standard autopsy may be useful in certain situations. These special dissections include examination of the middle ears and optic nerves and eyes (both examinations are most frequently performed in infants as part of the evaluation of deaths suspicious for inflicted trauma), dissection of the vertebral arteries, dissection of the anterior or posterior neck musculature, removal of the cervical vertebral column (in infants), demonstration of a pneumothorax, dissection of the back or lower extremities, dissection of the sinoatrial and atrioventricular nodes, and eversion of the esophagus for varices.

DISSECTION OF MIDDLE EARS

WHEN PERFORMED

During the autopsy of infants the middle ear is most commonly opened to assess for the presence or absence of inflammation. While pus can be identified upon gross examination, if necessary, microscopic examination of the region could be performed to confirm the presence of a neutrophilic infiltrate. In an adult with meningitis, the middle ear can also be opened as one method to identify the source of the infection.

HOW PERFORMED

Using the bone saw, a wedge of the petrous ridge is removed to expose the middle ear (Figure 31.1).

DISSECTION OF OPTIC NERVES AND EYES

WHEN PERFORMED

When the optic nerves and eyes are examined, it is almost always in the context of a suspicious infant death. In addition, office policies and forensic pathologist preference may determine when the optic nerves and eyes are examined.

HOW PERFORMED

To examine the optic nerves alone all that must be done is to remove the orbital plate above the eye, which is done with a bone saw in a triangular cut with the apex distal. The optic nerve is then dissected from the surrounding adipose tissue and skeletal muscle (Figure 31.2). This procedure can be performed routinely in all infant autopsies, as it would

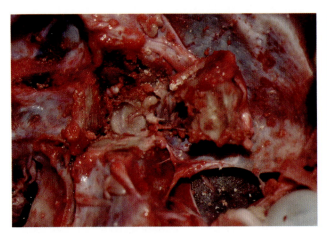

Figure 31.1. Dissection of middle ear. To expose the middle ear, a small wedge of the petrous ridge can be removed.

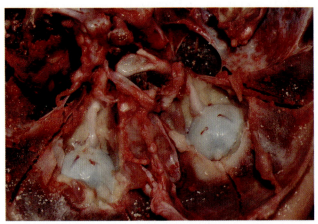

Figure 31.2. Dissection of the optic nerves. A small triangle of bone from the orbital roof is removed. The optic nerves are exposed by dissecting away the surrounding adipose tissue and muscles.

not involve removal of the eye. If the eye itself is removed, this is done by identifying the eye globe invested in the orbital fat, and with gentle traction on the globe with forceps, pulling backwards and cutting the investing tissue, being cautious to not cut the upper or lower eyelids. After removal, the eye is fixed in formalin and then bisected for examination. Challenging to adequately photograph, the retina can be best illuminated either by directly shining a light source into the optic cup or by backlighting the eye with a light source, or both methods can be used.

DISSECTION OF VERTEBRAL ARTERIES

WHEN PERFORMED

If a subarachnoid hemorrhage is identified and the source is not apparent (eg, trauma, a berry aneurysm, or arteriovenous malformation), that the source is a vertebral artery dissection or other anomaly should be considered. While the source for the vertebral artery lesion may reside intracranial, if an intracranial source for the hemorrhage is not identified, an extracranial source within the vertebral artery should be considered.

HOW PERFORMED

The vertebral artery can be examined through contrast injection and subsequent radiography (Figure 31.3), or through direct dissection.[1] Exposure of the vertebral artery via dissection can be done through a posterior approach with removal of the bony canal surrounding each artery.

DISSECTION OF THE ANTERIOR AND POSTERIOR NECK

WHEN PERFORMED

A layer-by-layer dissection of the anterior neck is most often performed to evaluate asphyxial-type deaths (eg, hanging, strangulation), or to assess for occult trauma in situations where the nature of the death is concerning for a strangulation or other form of inflicted injury (Figure 31.4). Given the ease with which an anterior neck dissection can be performed, some forensic pathologists may choose to do the dissection as a routine part of each autopsy. A posterior neck dissection can be performed in similar situations, but is often performed when there

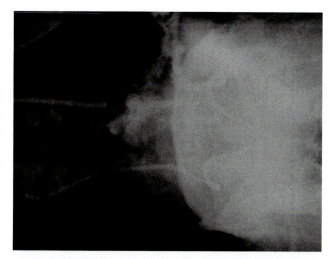

Figure 31.3. Radiography of the vertebral arteries. Although dissection of the vertebral arteries will allow for a gross visual inspection, injection of the vertebral arteries with contrast and subsequent radiography can also allow for examination of the vessels for potential pathology such as a dissection or ruptured aneurysm.

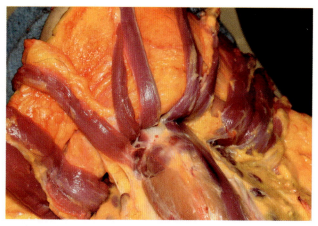

Figure 31.4. Anterior neck dissection. The muscles of the neck are sequentially reflected to examine for hemorrhage. After removal of the neck organs, the pre-vertebral fascia and musculature should also be inspected for hemorrhage. If the neck organs are forced backward against the vertebral column, such as in a strangulation, hemorrhage in this location may result.

is a concern for occult trauma of the neck (eg, a decedent found after a motor vehicle accident with the remainder of the autopsy revealing no lethal traumatic injuries) (Figure 31.5).

HOW PERFORMED

With a layer-by-layer dissection of the anterior neck, each of the anterior neck muscles is sequentially reflected. One way to proceed is the sternocleidomastoid muscles, followed by the omohyoid muscles, followed by the sternohyoid muscles, followed by the sternothyroid muscles. After removal of the neck organs, the pre-vertebral fascia and pre-vertebral musculature should be inspected for hemorrhage. With a posterior neck dissection, the muscle layers are not as clearly defined; however, the muscles are reflected to assess for hemorrhage and to expose the spinous processes of the cervical vertebrae. The laminae are cut and the posterior portion of the cervical vertebrae is removed, revealing the spinal cord. Following removal of the spinal cord, the integrity of the atlanto-axial joint and alar ligaments can be directly inspected. Dolinak and Matshes neuropathology atlas has a good description of the procedure and demonstrative images.[2]

DISSECTION OF THE CERVICAL VERTEBRAL COLUMN

WHEN PERFORMED

The cervical segment of the vertebral column is examined in the investigation of suspicious infant deaths to allow for examination of the spinal nerves and dorsal root ganglia.

HOW PERFORMED

The cervical segment of the vertebral column can either be entirely removed or the dorsal root ganglia and spinal nerves can be examined in situ by removing the surrounding bone.[3,4] If the cervical segment of the vertebral column is removed in its entirety, it is a good idea to fix the entire segment prior to examination. Following the fixation, the segment of cervical vertebral column should be decalcified and can then be serially sectioned to inspect the spinal nerves and dorsal root ganglia.

EXAMINATION FOR PNEUMOTHORAX

WHEN PERFORMED

A pneumothorax commonly occurs secondary to trauma; however, a spontaneous pneumothorax can also occur secondary to a natural disease process such as the rupture of an emphysematous bleb.

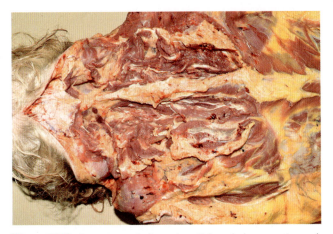

Figure 31.5. Posterior neck dissection. Although the posterior neck muscles are not as easily dissected in a layer-by-layer approach like the muscles in the anterior neck, they can be examined for hemorrhage, and the spinal cord can be exposed via a posterior approach.

HOW PERFORMED

A pneumothorax can easily be detected with a radiograph of the chest; however, a pneumothorax can also be identified through simple dissection procedures. As a routine part of the autopsy dissection, a small segment of intercostal muscle can be scraped from between the ribs (Figure 31.6A and B). With care, the parietal pleura can be left intact, and a pneumothorax can be identified as the lung will not be present at the pleura. A pneumothorax can also be identified by creating a pocket with the reflected chest skin, filling the pocket with water, and incising into the pleural cavity below the level of the water, with air bubbling into the water as a sign of the pneumothorax.

EXAMINATION FOR AIR EMBOLUS

WHEN PERFORMED

An air embolus commonly occurs with penetrating injuries of the neck, such as incised wounds or gunshot wounds, but can occur in a range of other situations.

HOW PERFORMED

A radiograph can reveal an air embolus. In addition, the heart can be opened in situ after filling the pericardial sac with water. Another method is to half fill a syringe with water and draw blood from the right ventricle of the heart and if air is present, it will bubble into the water in the syringe.

DISSECTION OF THE BACK

WHEN PERFORMED

Dissections of the back are performed whenever there is a need to carefully document the presence or absence of trauma to the back. As blunt force injuries may not manifest at the skin surface but may be easily identifiable in the subcutaneous tissue, a back dissection is useful in those situations. Back dissections are commonly performed in the investigation of infant deaths and in-custody deaths but could also be useful in the investigation of elder abuse deaths and other homicides, including strangulation. Dissections of the back can and often do include reflection of the skin of the upper and lower extremities as well. In addition, for in-custody deaths, dissection of the soles of the feet in individuals with darkly pigmented skin, and incisions of the wrists to evaluate for hemorrhage associated with cuff marks can also be performed.

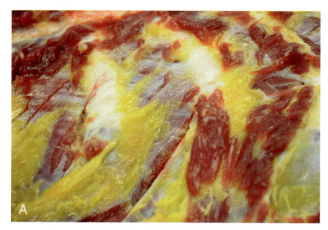
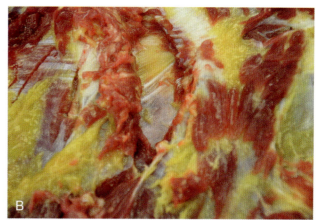

Figure 31.6. Dissection for a pneumothorax. While a chest radiograph can reveal a pneumothorax, the finding can also be identified via dissection. The intercostal musculature between two ribs (**A**) is gently scraped away, leaving the parietal pleura intact. The underlying lung should be identified up against the parietal pleura (**B**).

HOW PERFORMED

Incisions are made into the back often from the shoulder to the midline, and extended to the lower extremities, and the skin is subsequently reflected from the musculature of the back (Figure 31.7). The incisions can, depending upon the nature of the case, be extended to the wrists and ankles. Examination of the arms in cases of child abuse may reveal injuries (ie, where the child was grabbed).

DISSECTION OF THE LOWER EXTREMITIES

WHEN PERFORMED

The lower extremities are most often dissected after a pulmonary thromboembolus is identified in the lungs to confirm the presence of deep venous thrombi in the lower extremities as the source of the embolus in the lung. Identifying and sampling the thrombus in the lower extremities may allow for potential dating of the time frame since the development of the thrombus, which may provide useful information in the investigation. Dissection of the lower extremities is also performed in the evaluation of hit-and-run scenarios to help identify the impact site from the vehicle.

HOW PERFORMED

The skin of the lower extremity is incised, often from a posterior approach, but potentially also from a medial approach or anterior approach. The underlying musculature is sectioned to examine for a thrombus.

DISSECTION OF THE SINOATRIAL AND ATRIOVENTRICULAR NODES

WHEN PERFORMED

In evaluation of a sudden death, when no cause of death is identified at autopsy, examination of the cardiac conduction system can be performed.

HOW PERFORMED

The sinoatrial node is immediately adjacent to the crista terminalis on the side of the superior vena cava and at the junction with the right atrium. By removing the crista

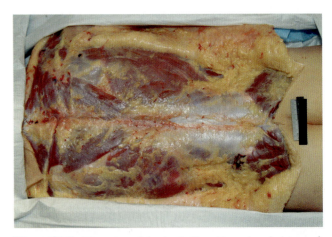

Figure 31.7. Dissection of the back. The skin and underlying soft tissue is reflected, revealing the underlying musculature. The reflection of the skin can be extended to the wrists and ankles, depending upon the circumstances of the autopsy and the need to identify injuries of the back and extremities.

terminalis and sectioning parallel to the muscle bundle, the sinoatrial node can be identified. Often, the sinoatrial nodal artery is visible grossly (Figure 31.8A-D). The atrioventricular node can be isolated using two approaches: from the right ventricular surface, utilizing Koch triangle, or from the left ventricular side. On the left ventricular side, the atrioventricular node is immediately subjacent to the non-coronary cusp of the aortic valve (Figure 31.9A and B). If the non-coronary cusp and underlying myocardium is excised and serially sectioned perpendicular to the cusp, the atrioventricular node can be obtained. In the examination of the sinoatrial or atrioventricular node, fixation of the excised block of tissue in formalin prior to sectioning will facilitate the process.

DISSECTION OF THE PARATHYROID GLANDS

WHEN PERFORMED

As long as the neck organs are removed, the parathyroid glands should be examined in any given autopsy; however, if there is a history of renal failure or of hypercalcemia then the examination is more likely to yield findings.

HOW PERFORMED

The superior parathyroid glands can be easily identified. With reflection of the fascia at the transition from the larynx to the trachea between the thyroid gland and the trachea on the posterior surface, the glands can be identified (Figure 31.10A and B).

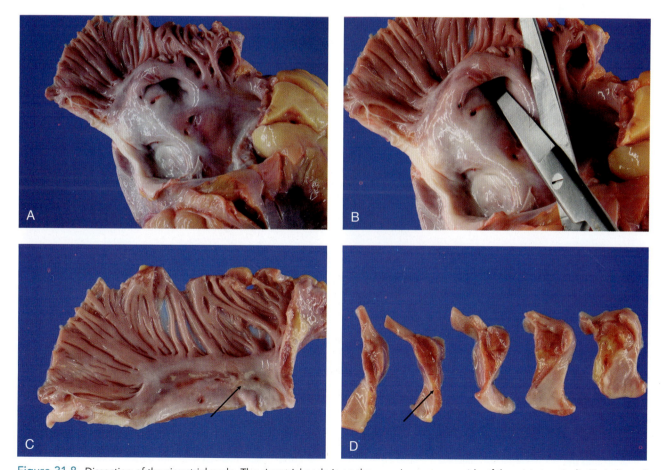

Figure 31.8. Dissection of the sinoatrial node. The sinoatrial node is on the superior vena cava side of the crista terminalis (**A**; indicated by arrow in **C**). The crista terminalis is removed (**B** and **C**) and serially sectioned (**D**). The sinoatrial nodal artery can often be visualized (arrow) (**D**). The sinoatrial node is around this vessel.

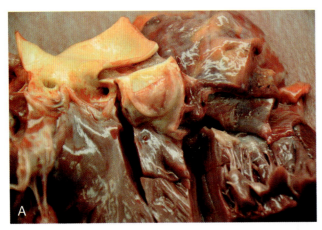 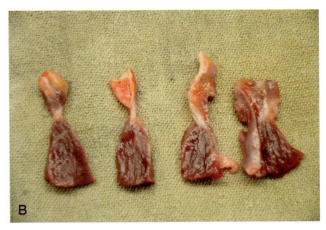

Figure 31.9. Dissection of the atrioventricular node. One approach is to remove the non-coronary cusp of the aortic valve with the subjacent myocardium (where the atrioventricular node is located) (**A**) and serially section this segment of tissue (**B**).

EXAMINATION OF ESOPHAGUS FOR VARICES

WHEN PERFORMED

When the autopsy identifies cirrhosis associated with a gastrointestinal hemorrhage, one likely source is bleeding esophageal varices.

HOW PERFORMED

A nick is made in the stomach close to the gastroesophageal junction. A clamp is passed through the nick to the proximal end of the esophagus (assuming that the esophagus, stomach, and pancreas are in their own separate block and not still attached to the remainder of the organs). The proximal end of the esophagus is secured (ie, pinched) in the clamp, and then the proximal esophagus is pulled through the nick in the stomach (Figure 31.11A and B). This process everts the esophagus and reveals the varices. The process potentially keeps pressure on the esophageal veins, allowing them to stand out, but also prevents their blind cutting if the esophagus into the stomach were to be opened as usual.

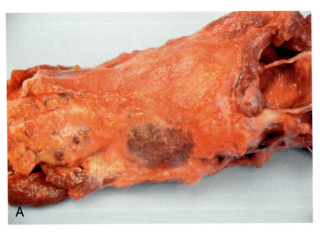 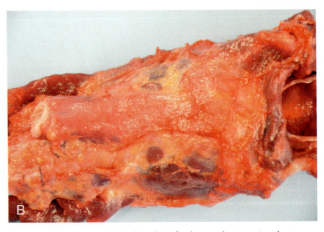

Figure 31.10. Dissection of the parathyroid glands. The superior parathyroid glands can easily be identified near the junction between the larynx and trachea posterior by reflecting the most superficial layer of fascial tissue after removal of the neck organs from the body (**A** and **B**).

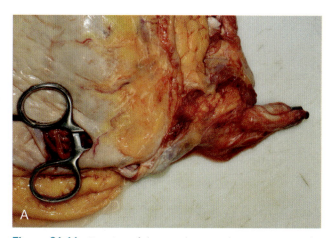 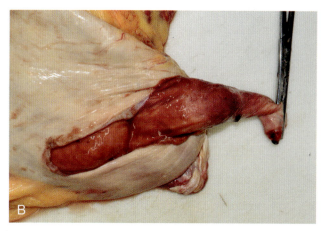

Figure 31.11. Eversion of the esophagus. After creating a nick in the stomach near the gastroesophageal junction (**A**) through which forceps or a clamp is placed, pulling the proximal tip of the esophagus through the nick in the stomach, everting the esophagus (**B**).

QUICK REMOVAL OF THE ENTIRE SPINAL CORD

WHEN PERFORMED

While the spinal cord can be examined for a variety of reasons, including trauma and natural disease, obtaining the entire spinal cord is often only done with infant homicides. And, for trauma, the known or suspected region of the trauma can be directly inspected by opening up that segment of the vertebral column. While the entire spinal cord is best removed from a posterior approach, which, after excising the lamina allows for removal of the dura, the dorsal root ganglia, and the entire spinal cord, a more simple procedure can allow for examination of the spinal cord itself (eg, to assess for the presence of multiple sclerosis or a myelitis).

HOW PERFORMED

A small window to the spinal canal is made in the lower lumbar region of the vertebral column from an anterior approach. After the dura is cut and the spinal cord is exposed, the spinal cord is wrapped with a wet paper towel and with gentle traction, the entire spinal cord can be pulled from the vertebral column. Dolinak and Matshes neuropathology atlas has a good description of the procedure and demonstrative images.[2]

UNDERWATER REMOVAL OF MACERATED INFANT BRAIN

WHEN PERFORMED

For the autopsy of a stillborn infant or an infant who has been in the hospital brain-dead for a period of time, the brain is often macerated and, during normal removal can be easily damaged.

HOW PERFORMED

The head or entire body of the infant is immersed in water.[5] The brain is removed while the head is immersed in water. Essentially, the water will allow the brain to float and maintain its shape. The brain can then be careful transferred from the water to formalin. To assist with the process, the scalp can be reflected prior to immersion in the water, and the area extensively flushed with water so that, when the cranium is opened, the water will stay relatively clear, best allowing for visualization of the brain for removal.

MACERATION OF THE THYROID CARTILAGE[6]

WHEN PERFORMED

Maceration of the thyroid cartilage can be performed in strangulation cases, or in cases that are suspicious for strangulation, to allow for better examination of the neck structures and assess for subtle fractures.

HOW PERFORMED

The soft tissue can be macerated with bleach or a powdered laundry detergent.[6]

EN BLOC REMOVAL OF FEMALE GENITALIA AND/OR ANUS (INCLUDING THE MALE ANUS)

WHEN PERFORMED

To fully evaluate deaths in which sexual trauma may have occurred, the female genitalia and/or anus can be removed en bloc.

HOW PERFORMED

Deep incisions dorsal, ventral, and lateral of the vaginal and/or anal orifice followed by transection of the deep tissue allows the female genitalia and/or anus to be removed in one large block and subsequently opened for examination (Figure 31.12A-C).

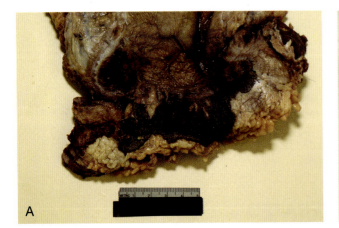
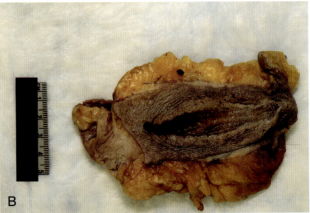
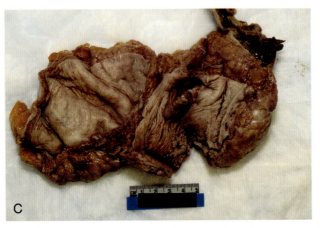

Figure 31.12. Removal of the anus and/or female genital tract. (**A**) is the opened anus block removed from a male to better document injuries. Figures 31.12b-c illustrate removal of the female genital tract, both before (**B**) and after (**C**) opening the specimen.

References

1. Galtés I, Rodríguez-Baeza A, Subirana M, Barbería E, Castellà J, Medallo J. A proposed dissection procedure for vertebral arteries in forensic pathology. *J Forensic Sci*. 2012;57(1):212-214.
2. Dolinak D, Matshes E. *Medicolegal Neuropathology: A Color Atlas*: CRC Press; 2002.
3. Matshes EW, Evans RM, Pinckard JK, et al. Shaken infants die of neck trauma, not of brain trauma. *Acad For Path*. 2011;1(1):82-91.
4. Peterson JE, Love JC, Pinto DC, Wolf DA, Sandberg G. A novel method for removing a spinal cord with attached cervical ganglia from a pediatric decedent. *J Forensic Sci*. 2016;61(1):241-244.
5. Prahlow JA, Ross KF, Salzberger L, Lott EG, Guileyardo JM, Barnard JJ. Immersion technique for brain removal in perinatal autopsies. *J Forensic Sci*. 1998;43(5):1056-1060.
6. LaGoy A, Evangelou EA, Somogyi T, DiGangi EA. Recommended practices for macerating human thyroid cartilage. *J Forensic Sci*. 2020;65(4):1266-1273.

APPENDIX A: SELF-ASSESSMENT QUESTIONS

QUESTIONS

When reviewing the questions, remember that more than one answer is possible; however, based only upon the photograph provided and the four answer choices, one answer is the best choice. In addition, while the complete set of autopsy findings associated with each photo was known to the forensic pathologist when the diagnosis was made, only one photograph is available to answer each question.

Question 1: **The image is from an infant autopsy. Based upon the location and pathologic findings, of the following, what general scenario was the forensic pathologist most likely investigating?**

    A. Drowning
    B. Death while bed-sharing with parents
    C. Suspected inflicted head injury
    D. A motor vehicle accident

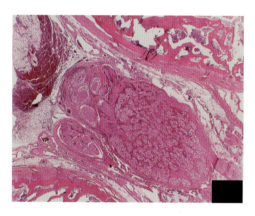

Question 2: **A 23-year-old female was found dead at her residence. Microscopic examination of the lungs revealed the finding in the photo. Of the following, which is most likely to have been found upon gross examination?**

    A. Hyperinflated lungs
    B. A pulmonary thromboembolus
    C. Metastatic tumor
    D. Hypersensitivity myocarditis

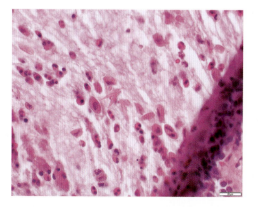

Question 3: A 54-year-old male was found dead in his residence. At autopsy, the following finding was identified. What is the diagnosis?

    A. Anomalous origin of the right coronary artery from the left sinus of Valsalva
    B. Anomalous origin of the left coronary artery from the right sinus of Valsalva
    C. Origin of the circumflex coronary artery from the left sinus of Valsalva
    D. Origin of the conal artery from the right sinus of Valsalva

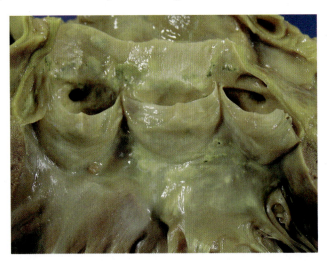

Question 4: The left and right lungs are from a male found dead on the floor in his house. Of the following, which best explains the difference in coloration between the two lungs?

    A. Lobar pneumonia of the right lung
    B. Gunshot wound of the heart, with left hemothorax
    C. Body position
    D. Pulmonary thromboembolus

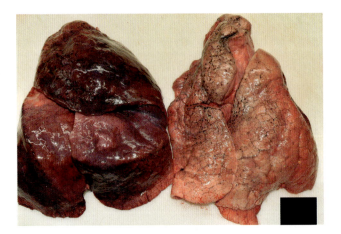

Question 5: A 24-year-old male is found unresponsive in his house. His family last saw him 1 day ago, and he voiced no complaints. At autopsy, lividity was blanching and rigor was well-developed. The finding in the image was found at autopsy. Of the following, what is the most likely cause?

    A. Decomposition

    B. Acute appendicitis

    C. Crohn disease

    D. Dye in food or medication that was ingested

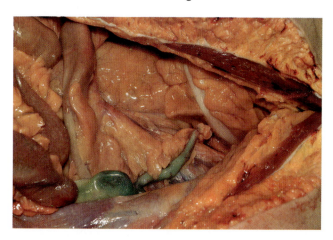

Question 6: A 53-year-old male who has been sick for 3 days, complaining of cough, congestion, and occasional chest pain, is found dead during a welfare check by family. At autopsy, the following finding is identified. Of the following, what is the most likely diagnosis?

    A. Atrial myxoma

    B. Bacterial endocarditis

    C. Pulmonary thromboembolus

    D. Postmortem clot

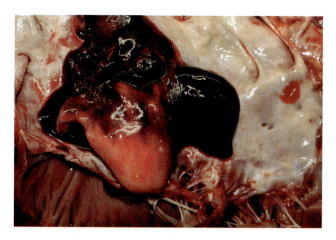

Question 7: A 56-year-old man is found unresponsive outdoors in an alleyway behind a restaurant. At autopsy, the forensic pathologist observes the finding in the image. Of the following, what is the identity of the substance below the left eye?

    A. Rice
    B. Powdered illicit substance
    C. Fly eggs
    D. Benign skin growth

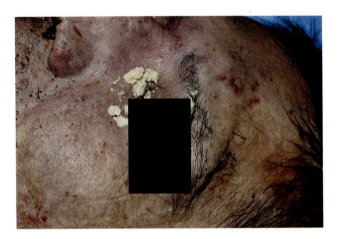

Question 8: A 33-year-old male is found unresponsive in an alleyway in a pool of blood. A weapon is found adjacent to the body. Based upon the cluster of wounds in the image, what was the most likely type of weapon used?

    A. A single-edged knife
    B. A double-edged knife
    C. Closed scissors
    D. Open scissors

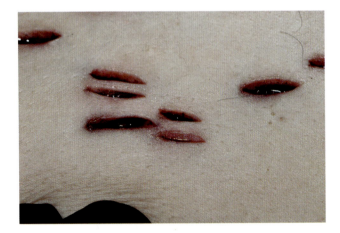

Question 9: A 10-year-old male is involved in a motor vehicle accident. Based upon the pattern of injuries on the neck and trunk, which of the following positions did the boy most likely occupy in the vehicle?

    A. Driver's seat
    B. Front right passenger
    C. Left rear passenger
    D. Unrestrained, sitting on parent's lap

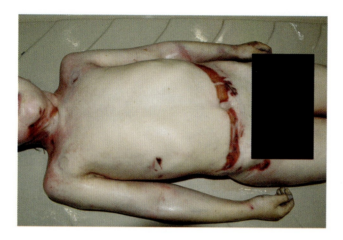

Question 10: The finding illustrated in the photo is identified at autopsy. Of the following, what was the most likely scenario of the decedent's death?

    A. Gunshot wound of the head
    B. Standing height fall
    C. Motor vehicle accident
    D. Sharp force injuries of the neck

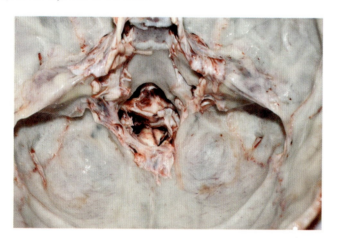

Question 11: The finding illustrated in the photo is identified at autopsy. Of the following, which is the best description for the wound?

    A. Stab wound of the cranium, consistent with ice pick
    B. Entrance gunshot wound
    C. Exit gunshot wound
    D. Keyhole-type entrance gunshot wound

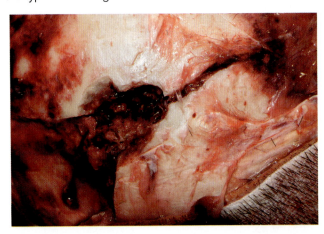

Question 12: A 24-year-old female is found dead at her residence during a welfare check by her parents. Given that the finding in the image is related to her cause of death, of the following, what is scene investigation most likely to reveal?

    A. A bloody knife
    B. Notice of recent doctor's visit for treatment of psoriasis
    C. Tin foil with charred area
    D. Obvious infestation

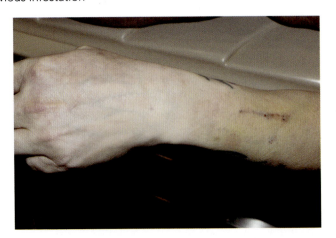

Question 13: A 32-year-old female has complained of a headache for 2 days. She is subsequently found unresponsive in her bed when a co-worker, who has a key to her house, checked on her after she failed to show up for work. The house was locked and the scene investigation revealed no evidence of a disturbance. At autopsy, the finding in the image is identified. Of the following, what was the most likely cause of the finding in the image?

    A. A ruptured berry aneurysm
    B. A vertebral artery dissection
    C. A ruptured arteriovenous malformation
    D. Inflicted blunt force injuries of the head

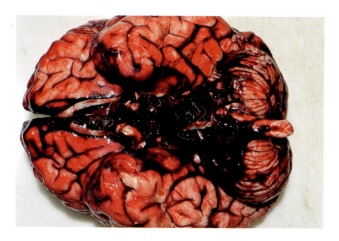

Question 14: During the examination of an individual involved in a motor vehicle accident, the following abrasion was identified. Given the appearance of the wound, which of the following was the pathway in which the wound was formed (ie, in which the object that caused the injury moved in relation to the body)?

    A. Left to right (in the photo)
    B. Right to left (in the photo)
    C. Superior to inferior (in the photo)
    D. Inferior to superior (in the photo)

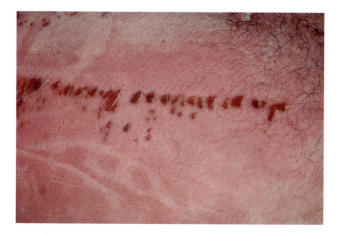

Question 15: **Microscopic examination of the lungs reveals the finding illustrated in the image. Of the following, which condition would best fit the scenario in which the finding in the image might occur?**

    A. Centrilobular necrosis of the liver
    B. Transections of the upper cervical segment of the spinal cord due to a gunshot wound
    C. Central pontine myelinolysis
    D. Ruptured esophageal varices

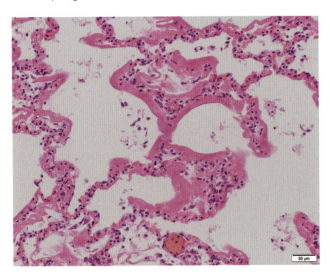

Question 16: **At the vertex of the head, the injury identified in the image was observed at autopsy. Of the following, which choice best describes the finding?**

    A. Entrance gunshot wound
    B. Exit gunshot wound
    C. Laceration from blunt force trauma
    D. Stab wound

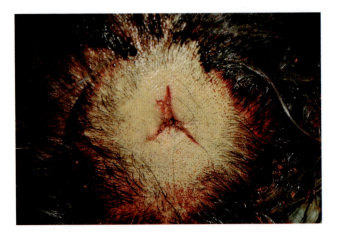

Question 17: At autopsy, the finding illustrated in the lung is identified at autopsy. Of the following, which best explains the pathologic change in the image?

    A. Gunshot wound of the chest with aspiration of blood
    B. Multiple stab wounds of the chest, injuring the lung
    C. Contusion of the lung due to blunt force injuries of the chest
    D. Metastatic angiosarcoma

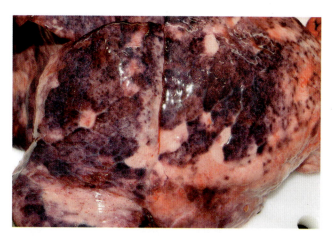

Question 18: An older male was witnessed by his family to fall and strike his head. They wanted to take him to the hospital, but he refused. Three days later, he was found dead. At autopsy, a subdural hemorrhage was found at the right cerebral hemisphere of the brain and was very loosely adherent to the surface. The cerebral hemisphere underlying the hemorrhage had an undulating texture (ie, from the gyri and sulci). Of the following, which would sectioning of the brain be most likely to find?

    A. Herniated and hemorrhagic right uncus
    B. Herniated and hemorrhagic left uncus
    C. Neoplasm of the right cerebral hemisphere
    D. Neoplasm of the left cerebral hemisphere

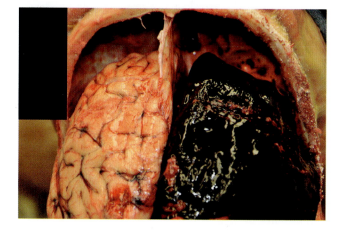

Question 19: **The blood tubes in the image are from two separate autopsies. The individual on the left side of the photo died from a drug overdose. Of the following, what was the most likely cause of death for the individual whose blood is on the right side of the image?**

    A. Bacterial sepsis
    B. Carbon monoxide poisoning
    C. Carbon dioxide poisoning
    D. 1,1-difluoroethane toxicity

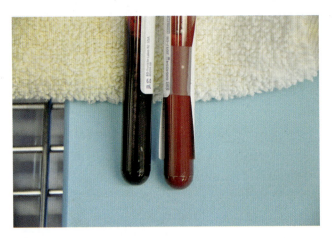

Question 20: **A forensic pathologist is performing an autopsy on a 33-year-old male who was found dead on the sidewalk, several blocks from his house. Examination of the brain reveals the pathologic finding illustrated in the image. Of the following, the autopsy is most likely to reveal which of the following?**

    A. A gunshot wound of the head
    B. A laceration of the occipital region of the scalp
    C. A laceration of the right temple region of the scalp
    D. A ruptured berry aneurysm

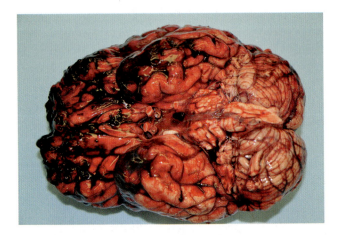

Question 21: The fracture in the image was sustained due to an accidental fall onto the back of the head. Of the following, which is most likely to be observed at autopsy?

    A. Avulsion of a tooth
    B. Hemorrhagic discoloration of the upper eyelids
    C. Unsuspected gunshot wound of the head
    D. Hyperostosis frontalis

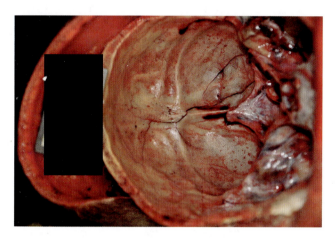

Question 22: Microscopic examination of the kidney in a 27-year-old male reveals the finding illustrated in the image. Of the following, what is the most likely cause of death?

    A. Lead poisoning
    B. Disseminated intravascular coagulation
    C. Diabetic ketoacidosis
    D. Acute pyelonephritis

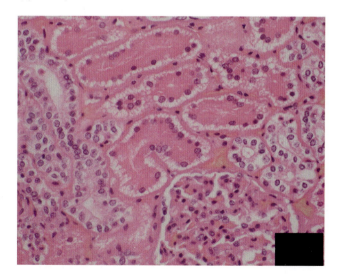

Question 23: A 29-year-old female became unresponsive after a traffic stop by law enforcement. If the finding illustrated in the image is representative of her cause of death, of the following, what is the most likely cause of death?

    A. Metastatic squamous cell carcinoma of the cervix
    B. Sepsis due to necrosis and secondary infection of infarcted uterine polyp
    C. Methamphetamine toxicity
    D. Avulsion of fetus papyraceous

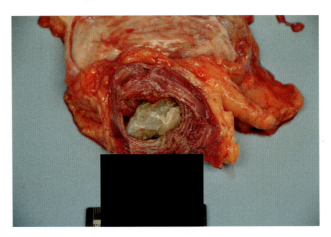

Question 24: A 34-year-old female collapses at work after a short period of difficulty breathing. Autopsy identifies the finding in the image. Of the following, what is the most likely diagnosis?

    A. Postmortem clot
    B. Pulmonary thromboembolus
    C. Pulmonary intimal sarcoma
    D. Intravascular extension of hepatocellular carcinoma

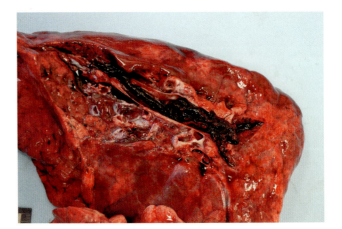

Question 25: **A young child was shot by a parent. Resuscitative efforts were ineffective. At autopsy, the forensic pathologist identifies the following gunshot wound. Of the following, what is the most likely explanation for the peripheral punctate red areas?**

    A. Abrasions from unburned gunpowder
    B. Abrasions from fragments of an intermediary target
    C. Fragments of dried blood
    D. Treatment artifact

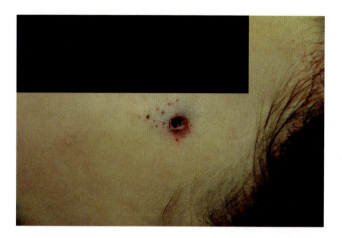

Question 26: **At autopsy, the forensic pathologist identifies the finding illustrated in the image. Of the following, what was the most likely cause of this change?**

    A. Lighting strike
    B. Bacterial sepsis
    C. Decomposition
    D. Self-inflicted injury

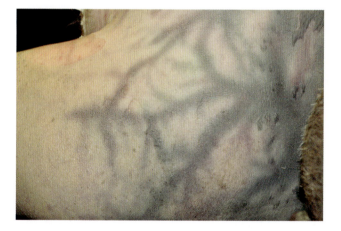

Question 27: The autopsy of a 41-year-old female identifies the pathologic change in the image, in which an aberrant fibrous cord embolized into and became adherent within the right coronary artery. In the determination of whether the subsequent tethering of the cusp led to aortic insufficiency, which of the following findings would best suggest that functional abnormality?

A. Measurement of the aortic valve circumference
B. Dilation of the left ventricle
C. Patch of endocardial fibrosis subjacent to the cusp
D. Microscopic examination of the cord

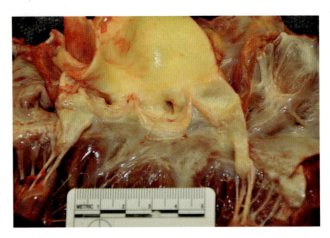

Question 28: Upon removal of the brain and stripping of the dura from the endocardial surface, the forensic pathologist identified the pathologic change illustrated in the image. Of the following, what is the most likely explanation?

A. Contact entrance gunshot wound
B. Distance range gunshot wound with bullet wipe
C. Exit gunshot wound
D. Thermal injury

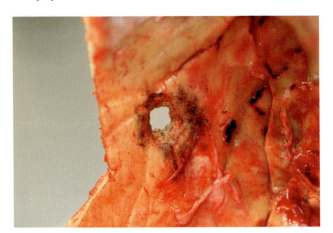

Question 29: **This individual hanged himself. Assuming that the lividity is fixed, of the following, which combination of position of the body when found and time after death that the individual was cut down is most likely?**

    A. Lying, 2 hours
    B. Lying, 12 hours
    C. Standing, 2 hours
    D. Standing, 12 hours

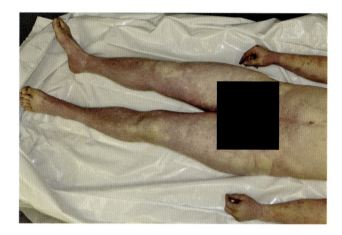

Question 30: **During the autopsy of an infant, the forensic pathologist identifies the finding in the image. Of the following, what is the most likely cause of the abnormality?**

    A. Inflicted trauma
    B. Resuscitation
    C. Neoplasm
    D. Infectious process

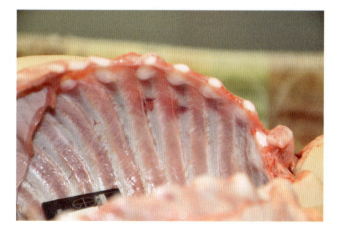

Question 31: At autopsy, a forensic pathologist identifies the following pathologic change in the brain. Of the following, what is the most likely etiology for the pathologic change?

    A. Neurodegenerative changes
    B. Elevated blood pressure
    C. Trauma
    D. Elevated intracranial pressure

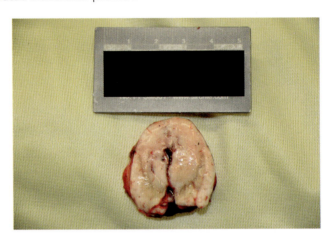

Question 32: A forensic pathologist is examining an individual who shot himself. Which of the following findings is present associated with the gunshot wound?

    A. Pseudostippling
    B. Muzzle abrasion
    C. Shoring of an exit wound
    D. Independent blunt force injuries and a gunshot wound

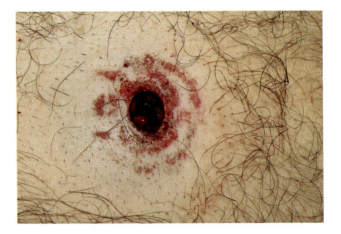

Question 33: A forensic pathologist identifies a pathologic lesion upon sectioning of the brain. Based upon the finding in the image, presuming the diagnosis was made antemortem, what condition would be listed in the decedent's medical records?

    A. Recent intracerebral hemorrhage
    B. Remote cerebral infarct
    C. Metastatic tumor
    D. Multiple sclerosis

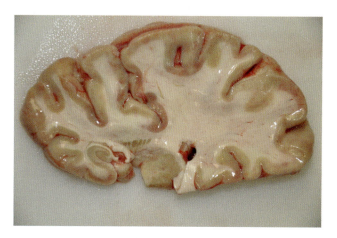

Question 34: A forensic pathologist is examining a decedent who was shot and identifies the wound in the image. Of the following, which best explains the features of this wound?

    A. Contact range
    B. Close range gunshot wound with soot deposition
    C. Gunshot wound with intervening object
    D. Atypical stab wound

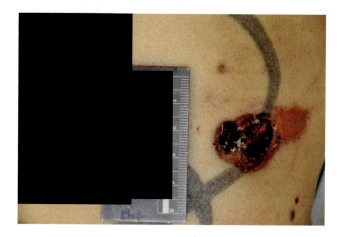

Question 35: A 37-year-old alcoholic homeless female was found unresponsive in an alleyway. The cause of death was ultimately determined to be complications of chronic alcoholism; however, autopsy also revealed the finding in the image. Based upon this pathologic finding, sectioning of the brain could reveal which of the following associated features?

    A. Communicating hydrocephalus
    B. Non-communicating hydrocephalus
    C. Clusters of bacterial cocci in the meninges
    D. Healing contusions of the superior surface of the cerebral hemispheres

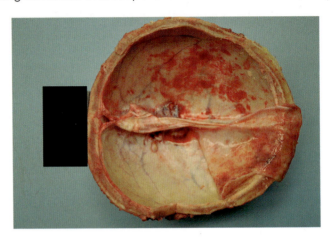

Question 36: A forensic pathologist performs an autopsy on an individual who died in a motor vehicle accident and who was the sole occupant of the vehicle. At autopsy, around 1 liter of blood is identified in the left pleural cavity. Of the following, which feature would be consistent with a flail chest?

    A. The line of anterior rib fractures
    B. The line of posterior rib fractures
    C. Three or more contiguous ribs fractured in two or more locations
    D. Six or more contiguous ribs fractured in two or more locations

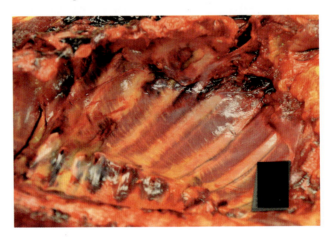

Question 37: An autopsy is being performed on a decedent who was struck by another individual in a bar fight, staggered several steps, and fell unresponsive. Of the following, which pathologic finding is most likely to be identified by internal examination?

A. Atlanto-occipital dislocation
B. Intracerebral hemorrhage
C. Vertebral artery laceration
D. Subdural hemorrhage

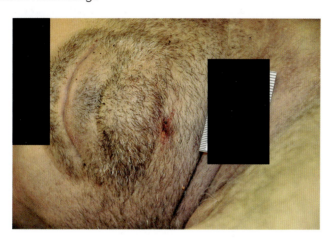

Question 38: The decedent in the image died from a contact gunshot wound of the head, and the following finding was identified at autopsy. Of the following, which best explains the pathologic change?

A. Direct contact with the projectile
B. Subsequent fall on the back of the head after the gunshot
C. Previous injury
D. Kinetic energy transfer and damage from gases

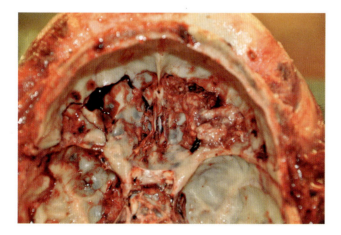

Question 39: Upon opening the gastrointestinal tract, a forensic pathologist identifies the pathologic finding in the image. If the image is associated with the cause of death, which of the following other features may be present at autopsy?

    A. Red discoloration of the knees
    B. Nodular black pigmented skin lesion
    C. Erosion of the esophageal mucosa
    D. Myocarditis

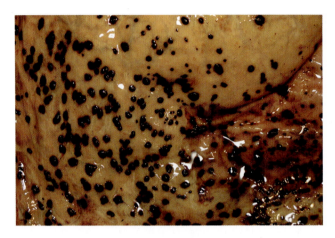

Question 40: A 52-year-old male is found unresponsive at his workplace. An autopsy is performed that identifies no traumatic injuries and the lesion identified in the image. Of the following, what is the most likely etiology for the pathologic change?

    A. Hypertension
    B. Cerebral amyloid angiopathy
    C. Ruptured berry aneurysm
    D. Hemorrhage into a cerebral neoplasm

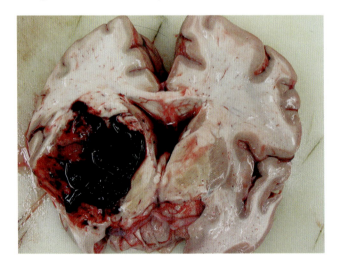

Question 41: A forensic pathologist performs an autopsy on an individual who was in a car accident and had 30 minutes of cardiopulmonary resuscitation performed. Microscopic examination of the lungs reveals the finding in the image. Of the following, what is the diagnosis?

   A. Bone marrow embolus
   B. Fat embolus
   C. Leukemia
   D. Embolization of myelolipoma

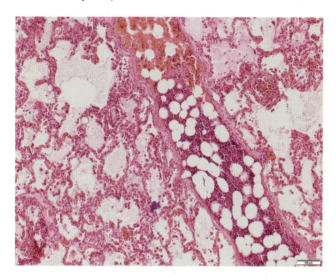

Question 42: A forensic pathologist performs an autopsy on a 49-year-old male who was found unresponsive in his house during a welfare check by friends. Polarization of the lungs reveals the following finding in the image, which is perivascular. The material is found in several foci in each of several sections of the lung. Of the following, what is the most likely cause?

   A. Ethylene glycol ingestion
   B. *Aspergillus niger* infection
   C. Intravenous drug use
   D. Hypercalcemia

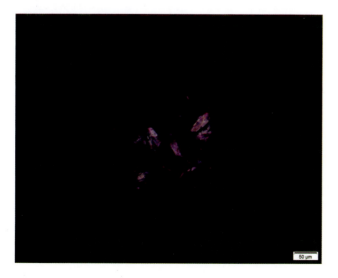

Question 43: **A hiker found the bones in the image and took them to the local coroner's office. The coroner sent them to the anthropologist at the university for examination. Of the following, what best describes the skeletal elements?**

    A. Human cervical vertebrae
    B. Human thoracic vertebrae
    C. Non-human cervical vertebrae
    D. Non-human thoracic vertebrae

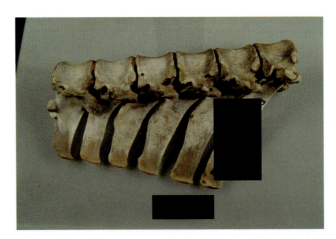

Question 44: **A forensic pathologist autopsied a 45-year-old male who was found dead in their vehicle at a campground. Autopsy identified no cause of death during gross examination; however, the microscopic examination revealed the finding in the image. Of the following, what substance was most likely in the vehicle with the decedent?**

    A. Acetaminophen
    B. Anti-freeze
    C. Mercury
    D. Ethanol

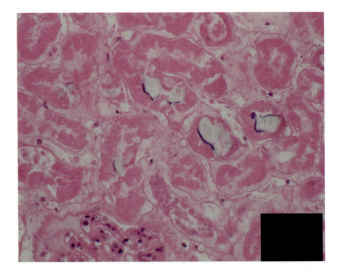

Question 45: **A forensic pathologist performed an autopsy on an individual who died suddenly during the night and was found unresponsive by his wife. Autopsy identified no definitive cause of death by gross examination; however, microscopic examination revealed the finding in the image. Of the following, which condition is most likely to be listed in the decedent's medical records?**

    A. Alzheimer disease
    B. Diffuse Lewy body dementia
    C. Seizure disorder
    D. Hippocampal asymmetry

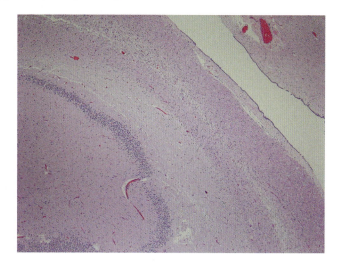

Question 46: **A 31-year-old female was found unresponsive by her husband the morning after she complained of a severe headache but did not want to seek medical care. At autopsy, the forensic pathologist performing the autopsy identified the lesion in the image. Of the following, what is the most likely diagnosis?**

    A. Intraventricular berry aneurysm
    B. Choroid plexus papilloma
    C. Colloid cyst
    D. Foreign body

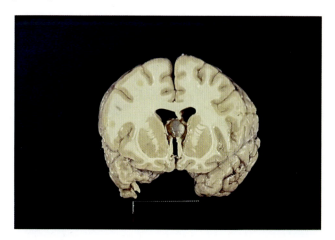

Question 47: **A forensic pathologist is examining microscopic sections of a brain from an individual who had a delayed death in the hospital. Examination of the hippocampus reveals the change illustrated in the image. Of the following regions of Ammon's horn, which is most sensitive to the change in the image?**

    A. CA1
    B. CA2
    C. CA3
    D. CA4

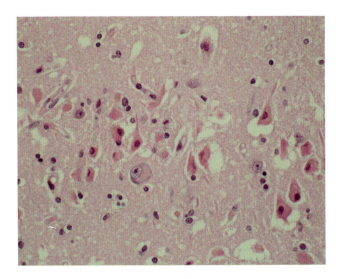

Question 48: **A forensic pathologist is examining a heart from an autopsied body, and identifies two findings in addition to an anomalous cord. Of the following, which most likely are the two findings?**

    A. Anomalous origin of right coronary artery from left sinus of Valsalva and subendocardial hemorrhage
    B. Anomalous origin of left coronary artery from right sinus of Valsalva and subendocardial hemorrhage
    C. Anomalous origin of right coronary artery from left sinus of Valsalva and reperfused infarct
    D. Anomalous origin of left coronary artery from right sinus of Valsalva and reperfused infarct

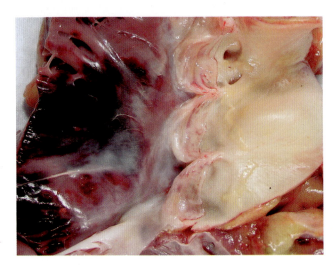

Question 49: **A forensic pathologist is reviewing their microscopic sections from a recent autopsy and identifies the pathologic finding illustrated in the image. Review of the medical records would most likely reveal which of the following diagnoses?**

    A. Multiple myeloma
    B. Hepatitis C
    C. Long-term corticosteroid use
    D. Diabetes mellitus type 2

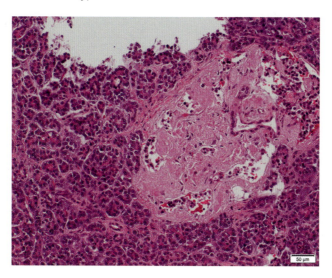

Question 50: **During the autopsy of a driver of a motor vehicle involved in a collision with a fixed object, the forensic pathologist photographs the cranium. Of the following, which term is best used to describe the finding in the image?**

    A. Normal anatomy
    B. Anatomic variant
    C. Trauma
    D. Natural disease process

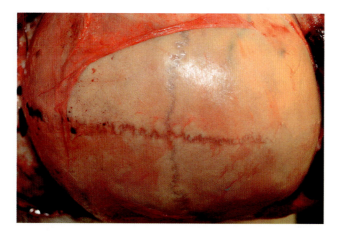

Question 51: A forensic pathologist receives medical records including copies of a CT scan performed on an individual. Of the following, what is the diagnosis?

A. Normal brain
B. Epidural hemorrhage
C. Subdural hemorrhage
D. Subarachnoid hemorrhage

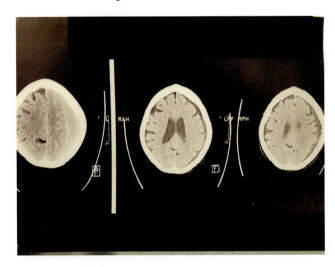

APPENDIX B: SELF-ASSESSMENT ANSWERS

ANSWERS

Answer 1: C (suspected inflicted head injury)

The image is a low-power view of a dorsal root ganglion with extensive extravasated red blood cells. Removal of the cervical segment of the vertebral column or in situ examination of the dorsal root ganglia is most often performed in the evaluation of suspected inflicted head injuries, and the presence of hemorrhage in the dorsal root ganglia would support inflicted head injury. Of course, such an examination could be performed in any circumstance; however, of the choices, C is the most likely under which the exam would be performed, and the hemorrhage would correlate with this scenario.

Answer 2: A (hyperinflated lungs)

The image is a high-power view revealing eosinophils and Charcot-Leyden crystals, which are microscopic features of asthma, which can be a cause of sudden death in a young adult. At autopsy, assuming no resuscitation has occurred, the characteristic gross finding in a sudden death due to asthma is hyperinflated lungs (answer A). While a pulmonary thromboembolus can cause sudden death, the eosinophils and Charcot-Leyden crystals are not a usual feature of such a pathologic change. There is no neoplastic process in the image, and while hypersensitivity myocarditis is associated with eosinophils, it would involve the heart.

Answer 3: C (origin of the circumflex coronary artery from the left sinus of Valsalva)

The non-coronary cusp is in the center of the image, with the right coronary cusp to the left side of the photo and the left coronary cusp to the right side of the photo. The left coronary artery sinus has two ostia. As the right coronary artery arises as normal from the right sinus, A is incorrect. The circumflex coronary artery can arise independently from the left sinus, such as in the image (answer C). The right sinus can have one or two accessory ostia, for the conal artery and the sino-atrial nodal artery; however, these ostia are often quite small.

Answer 4: C (body position)

The body was found on its right side, which caused the right lung to be markedly congested with blood, and the left lung, essentially free of blood. A lobar pneumonia would involve one lobe, and the entire right lung appears equally involved. A hemothorax would result in atelectasis and the left lung is fairly well inflated. A pulmonary thromboembolus could lead to collapse of one or both lungs to some degree.

Answer 5: D (dye in food or medication that was ingested)

There is a bright green discoloration of the colon and appendix, which is most likely due to dye in an ingested food or medication that was ingested (answer D). Given the time frame and other postmortem changes, decomposition is not likely, and the green of decomposition is usually a darker hue. The appendix is not dilated and the surface is smooth and shiny, which are not consistent with appendicitis. Crohn disease can involve the colon but is not often associated with color changes such as in the image.

Answer 6: D (postmortem clot)

The finding has the appearance of postmortem clot (answer D), with the currant jelly and chicken fat textures. Given the symptomatology, the decedent could be septic associated with a pneumonia, which can lead to postmortem clotting. While the left atrium is the usual location for an atrial myxoma, the finding would be much rarer than a postmortem clot, and the neoplasm would likely have a more consistent texture. The smooth texture of the surface would seem inconsistent with the texture of a vegetation, and given that the abnormality is on the mitral valve, a pulmonary thromboembolus without the presence of a patent foramen ovale, would not be possible. In addition, the smooth gelatinous texture and the two separate appearing components of the finding are not consistent with an antemortem thrombus.

Answer 7: C (fly eggs)

The finding on the cheek is fly eggs (answer C), which, especially in an outdoor location, can be deposited very quickly on the body.

Answer 8: A (a single-edged knife)

The patch of skin has multiple stab wounds. Some of the stab wounds have a blunt angle (left side of the wound) and a sharp angle (right side of the wound). This finding is consistent with a single-edged knife (answer A). A double-edged knife would not produce a blunt angle. A closed pair of scissors would produce a wound with two blunt angles. While one angle could tear and become sharp, that that process would repeat itself several times and in the same orientation is much less likely than when the weapon used is a single-edged knife. Open scissors could produce injuries with both a blunt angle and a sharp angle, but the wounds would be paired.

Answer 9: B (front right passenger)

The wide linear abrasion on the right side of the neck and across the lower abdomen is consistent with being restrained. The injury to the right side of the neck could occur from the seatbelt being anchored to the door at the right side of the body; therefore, of the choices, the injury pattern fits best with a front right passenger (answer B).

Answer 10: C (motor vehicle accident)

The autopsy identified an atlanto-occipital dislocation. The bone of the vertebral column is visible in the foramen magnum anterior. Of the choices, the most likely to produce an atlanto-occipital dislocation would be a motor vehicle accident (answer C).

Answer 11: D (keyhole-type entrance gunshot wound)

The cranium has a keyhole-type entrance gunshot wound (answer D). From 12 to 6 o'clock, the defect has a well-defined punched-out appearance, and from 6 to 12 o'clock, there is outward beveling. Therefore, both inward beveling (at 12-6 o'clock) and outward beveling are present, which is the appearance of a keyhole-type gunshot wound.

Answer 12: C (tin foil with charred area)

The finding in the image is consistent with a track mark (answer C), which can be linear scars or discolorations on the upper extremities. Track marks are found in intravenous drug users, and the tin foil with a charred area would be evidence of drug use. Psoriasis is most commonly on the extensor surfaces and involves a more patchy area, and scratching from lice or fleas or other infestation would often be more numerous and parallel (eg, from adjacent fingertips). A scratch from a knife is possible, but the wound has some scabbed appearance. Although answers A and D are possible, of the choices, C is the best.

Answer 13: A (a ruptured berry aneurysm)

The brain has a prominent subarachnoid hemorrhage at the base. While answer choices A to D can all cause a basilar subarachnoid hemorrhage, the most common of the three is a ruptured berry aneurysm (answer A). Given such a finding at autopsy, the hemorrhage should be flushed with running water and the aneurysm identified prior to fixation of the brain (if the brain is going to be retained in formalin). A vertebral artery dissection and ruptured arteriovenous malformation should be considered and searched for if no aneurysm is identified. Subarachnoid hemorrhage concentrated at the base of the brain can occur with inflicted injury, especially if the vertebral artery is injured; however, of the choices, and given the scenario, it is not the most likely choice.

Answer 14: A (left to right (in the photo))

The linear band of discontinuous abrasions has epidermal piling at the right edge (in the photo) of each, which would indicate that the direction of contact with the body was left to right (answer A). While such a finding is uncommon to rare to find, the piling of the epidermis can assist a forensic pathologist in determining the direct of contact, with the epidermis piling at the end of the contact (eg, similar to a snow plow).

Answer 15: A (centrilobular necrosis of the liver)

The finding in the image is hyaline membranes, consistent with diffuse alveolar damage, which occurs in the context most often of sepsis, pneumonia, pancreatitis, and head trauma but is a component of the general morphologic findings associated with shock, as is centrilobular necrosis (answer A). Both B (transections of the upper cervical segment of the spinal cord due to a gunshot wound) and D (ruptured esophageal varices) would cause death quite quickly and would not be as expected to lead to shock. While central pontine myelinolysis is a cause of death, it would not as clearly be associated with diffuse alveolar damage as centrilobular necrosis.

Answer 16: B (exit gunshot wound)

Given the choices, the injury is most consistent with an exit gunshot wound (answer B), having a stellate appearance with no marginal abrasion. With an entrance gunshot wound a central circular defect with a marginal abrasion would be most likely. While a laceration from blunt force trauma cannot be entirely excluded as the depths of the wound cannot be seen in the image, there is no marginal abrasion or contusion, and, given the choices, the exit gunshot wound is most consistent. While a stab wound could be stellate, all three corners are sharp, and there is no evidence of a blunt angle. Like choice C (laceration from blunt force trauma), a stab wound cannot be entirely excluded based only upon the image; however, of the choices, it is less likely than an exit gunshot wound.

Answer 17: A (gunshot wound of the chest with aspiration of blood)

With aspiration of blood, the blood will be bound by the interlobular septa and produce well-defined polygonal areas of hemorrhage, which can be seen at the pleural surface (answer A). There are no injuries of the pleural surface or masses, and contusions of the lung will cross over the interlobular septa, and not usually have such well-defined edges.

Answer 18: A (herniated and hemorrhagic right uncus)

As there was some survival period from the subdural hemorrhage, compression of the right cerebral hemisphere would produce a midline, right to left shift, which could cause herniation of the right uncus (answer A), and with survival, hemorrhage and necrosis due to ischemia of the herniated region. While the left cerebral hemisphere is flattened in the image, this is from compression against the cranium as a result of the right to left shift. While an underlying neoplasm can be the source for a subdural hemorrhage, this would be rare compared to the incidence in a fall.

Answer 19: B (carbon monoxide poisoning)

The blood on the right side of the image is brighter red than the blood on the left side of the image. Of the choices, carbon monoxide poisoning is the best choice (answer B), as the carbon monoxide irreversibly binds to hemoglobin, giving the blood an arterial appearance in the postmortem period.

Answer 20: B (a laceration of the occipital region of the scalp)

The image illustrates subarachnoid hemorrhage and contusions of the inferior surface of the frontal lobes of the brain and the tips of the temporal lobes, which is consistent with contre-coup contusions due to a fall on the back of the head, which could also produce a laceration of the occipital region of the scalp (answer B). With a fall onto the right side of the head (ie, the laceration of the right temple region of the scalp), the subarachnoid hemorrhage and contusions would be on the lateral surface of the left side of the brain. A ruptured berry aneurysm causing death would produce a basilar subarachnoid hemorrhage and would not cause contusions. A gunshot wound of the head that fractured the floor of the anterior cranial fossae could produce this change, but, without injury to the brain such as tears of the parenchyma, that would be much less likely than a fall.

Answer 21: B (hemorrhagic discoloration of the upper eyelids)

With a fall on the back of the head, contre-coup injuries can occur, which can include contusions of the frontal and temporal lobes of the brain, anterior subarachnoid hemorrhage, and fractures of the orbital plates. With fractures of the orbital plates, hemorrhage into the upper eyelids can occur (answer B). The impact would not be more likely to cause avulsion of a tooth, and hyperostosis frontalis would be an unrelated incidental finding, not a cause of the fall, nor a result of the fall. While a witnessed fall has the potential to be from an unsuspected gunshot wound, nothing in the image supports that as the best choice.

Answer 22: C (diabetic ketoacidosis)

The pathologic change is well-developed subnuclear vacuolation of the proximal convoluted tubules, which is associated with ketoacidosis (answer C). Lead poisoning can cause inclusions; disseminated intravascular coagulation could result in microthrombi in the glomeruli; acute pyelonephritis would be associated with neutrophils in the tubules and interstitium.

Answer 23: C (methamphetamine toxicity)

In the vagina is a plastic baggie, which was found to contain methamphetamine (answer C). When individuals are going to be in custody, or in an attempt to smuggle drugs into jail, they may place drugs in a baggie or other container into a bodily orifice (eg, the rectum or vagina), or may attempt to dispose of the drug by swallowing it. Depending upon the composition and integrity of the packaging material, the drug may be secondarily absorbed into the blood and cause death. When an individual dies suddenly in such circumstances, swallowing or otherwise hiding of drug material must be considered and the packaging searched for, which may necessitate opening of the small and large intestine.

Answer 24: B (pulmonary thromboembolus)

The thrombus distends the vessel, has a rough and focally tan external surface, and has a branching pattern that is inconsistent with the vessel in which it is found, which would be consistent with a pulmonary thromboembolus (answer B) instead of a postmortem clot. While answers C and D are possible, each would be very rare.

Answer 25: A (abrasions from unburned gunpowder)

The gunshot was fired at close range, and the entrance wound exhibits stippling, which is from unburned gunpowder particles striking the skin (answer A). Fragments of an intermediary target could create pseudostippling; however, with stippling from gunpowder the punctate defects are all about the same size, whereas with an intermediary target, fragments of different size are most often produced, so the pseudostippling will vary in size and shape. Fragments of dried blood can mimic stippling in a photograph, so, for any photograph to be used in court or for examination by another forensic pathologist, care should be taken to ensure the surrounding skin is cleaned of debris. Stitching could potentially mimic stippling.

Answer 26: C (decomposition)

The change is marbling, which is a common postmortem finding due to changes induced by bacterial proliferation following death (answer C). A lightning strike can produce a Lichtenberg figure (or ferning), which has a somewhat similar appearance in that both are branching; however, the image also has skin slippage, and decomposition is much more common than a fatal lightning strike. While bacterial sepsis can quicken decomposition, it is not by itself a necessary cause of marbling, which can easily occur in individuals who die from a non-infectious cause.

Answer 27: C (patch of endocardial fibrosis subjacent to the cusp)

With valvular insufficiency, a regurgitant jet lesion is created that can strike the endocardial surface of the outflow tract and create a patch of fibrosis (answer C). While aortic insufficiency would result in dilation of the left ventricle (due to volume increase), dilation of the ventricle can be a difficult determination at autopsy. Dilation of the aortic valve root can lead to insufficiency, but the mechanism created by this lesion would not necessarily be dilation of the aortic root, and there is overlap in the measurements. Microscopic examination of the cord, which was performed, could identify the tethered nature of the cord to the right coronary artery intima but not whether insufficiency was produced.

Answer 28: A (contact entrance gunshot wound)

The defect has circumferential inward beveling, which is consistent with an entrance gunshot wound. There is soot on the bone, which would indicate the weapon was discharged while in contact with the body (answer A). While bullet wipe, or deposition of soot and other grime from the bullet, on the tissue that the projectile passes through can mimic soot, the bullet wipe should be on tissue contacted by the projectile, whereas in the image, there is soot some distance from the defect in the bone.

Answer 29: D (standing, 12 hours)

The fixed lividity is present in the lower half of the body; therefore, the distribution of the lividity is consistent with a standing position, instead of a lying position. If the body was cut down within 2 hours after being found, the lividity would have re-distributed; therefore, a time frame of 12 hours of the two choices is most consistent.

Answer 30: B (resuscitation)

Several right sided ribs have anterior rib fractures, which are marked by the thin red lines. While both inflicted trauma and resuscitation could cause rib fractures, given the essential lack of hemorrhage, the rib fractures most likely occurred at or around the time of death, and resuscitation-related rib fractures (answer B) are fairly common findings, whereas inflicted trauma is much less common.

Answer 31: D (elevated intracranial pressure)

The section of the midbrain has a midline hemorrhage. While both hypertension and cerebral edema can lead to hemorrhages in the brainstem, the hemorrhages due to cerebral edema with resultant herniation are classically midline (answer D), whereas the hemorrhages due to hypertension are more globular, and, in the section, there is no other feature to otherwise separate the two conditions or to indicate trauma, which can produce hemorrhage, however, to produce a single midline hemorrhage would be unlikely.

Answer 32: B (muzzle abrasion)

Surrounding the wounds are curvilinear abrasions, which are consistent with a muzzle abrasion (answer B).

Answer 33: D (multiple sclerosis)

At the depth of the lateral fissure is a gray-pink discoloration of the white matter, which is consistent with a multiple sclerosis plaque (answer D). A remote cerebral infarct would be cystic. A metastatic tumor would likely be more well-defined but could be found at the gray-white junction. A recent intracerebral hemorrhage could be slitlike but should have a yellow-brown discoloration from the hemosiderin deposition.

Answer 34: C (gunshot wound with intervening object)

The entrance wound has an atypical shape, instead of being circular, and has an irregular marginal abrasion. When the projectile deforms prior to striking the skin, the entrance wound produced is often atypical with features such as in the image. This deformation is produced by the projectile striking an intervening object prior to hitting the skin (answer C).

Answer 35: A (communicating hydrocephalus)

The underlying surface of the dura mater has a resolving subdural hemorrhage. With a resolving subdural hemorrhage, the flow of cerebrospinal fluid from the arachnoid granulations to the vasculature can be obstructed, leading to a communicating hydrocephalus (answer A), with a non-communicating hydrocephalus being due to an obstruction within the ventricular system in the brain. The image is not consistent with meningitis and contusions of the superior surface of the cerebral hemispheres, without underlying fractures, would be unlikely.

Answer 36: C (three or more contiguous ribs fractured in two or more locations)

A flail chest can occur when three or more ribs are fractured in two or more locations (answer C). Being aware of a flail chest as a possible mechanism of death in a decedent with blunt force injuries can be useful to know, especially when a decedent has few injuries and the mechanism of death is not otherwise clear.

Answer 37: C (vertebral artery laceration)

A blow to the chin or neck can lead to a vertebral artery laceration and even possibly a ponto-medullary laceration (answer C). Intracerebral hemorrhages can occur following trauma but are most often due to expansion of a contusion, and would not cause death so quickly. Similarly, a subdural hemorrhage would not cause death so quickly. Although an atlanto-occipital dislocation is not impossible, it would most likely be less likely than a vertebral artery laceration.

Answer 38: D (kinetic energy transfer and damage from gases)

The projectile passed superior to the level of the fragmented bone; however, the projectile passed very close to the bone and the bone would have fallen within the distribution of the temporary cavity. While a fall on the back of the head can result in fractures of the orbital plates, they would not be expected to be this extensive. There is no evidence of repair to indicate a previous injury.

Answer 39: A (red discoloration of the knees)

The lesions of the gastric mucosa are consistent with Wischnewski spots. Wischnewski spots are commonly associated with hypothermia. Another feature associated with hypothermia is frost erythema, which is red discoloration of the knees (answer A). While metastatic melanoma to the gastric mucosa is possible, this would be much less common of an autopsy finding. Erosions of the esophageal mucosa can occur in hypothermia (ie, acute esophageal necrosis, or black esophagus), but is a much less commonly seen finding.

APPENDIX B: SELF-ASSESSMENT ANSWERS   639

Answer 40: A (hypertension)

The intracerebral hemorrhage is centered on the left basal ganglia, which is one of three characteristic locations for an intracerebral hemorrhage due to hypertension (answer A). The remaining three choices could all potentially lead to an intracerebral hemorrhage; however, each is much less likely than a hypertensive hemorrhage.

Answer 41: A (bone marrow embolus)

In the vessel is a fragment of bone marrow (answer A), which can occur following resuscitation. While bone marrow and fat embolus can occur in the same setting, a fat embolus would not be so cellular. Although hematopoietic cells are present, so is adipose tissue, which would not be consistent with leukemia. While embolization of a fragment of a myelolipoma could potentially occur, it would be a very rare event.

Answer 42: C (intravenous drug use)

The polarizable material adjacent to the blood vessel is consistent with intravenous drug use. With ethylene glycol ingestion, polarizable oxalic acid crystals will be found in the kidney. While *Aspergillus niger* can produce oxalic acid, the crystals stay localized to the site of the infection, or can rarely enter the bloodstream and deposit in the kidneys. Hypercalcemia can lead to metastatic calcification, which can involve the lung; however, the calcification would not polarize.

Answer 43: D (non-human thoracic vertebrae)

The spinous processes are longer than on human vertebrae, and the facets for the rib heads identify the vertebrae as thoracic instead of cervical vertebrae.

Answer 44: B (anti-freeze)

The kidney has oxalic acid crystals, which form from the metabolism of ethylene glycol by alcohol dehydrogenase, and which is found in anti-freeze (answer B). Acetaminophen is not associated with crystals in the kidney and is most commonly associated with liver damage. Mercury can damage the kidney, but the findings are non-specific and do not include crystal formation.[1]

Answer 45: C (seizure disorder)

In the segment of Ammon's horn in the image, there are essentially no neurons, which would be consistent with mesial temporal sclerosis, which is associated with seizure disorder (answer C). While Alzheimer disease can cause tangles and plaques in the hippocampus and neuron death occurs, with ghost tangles identified; given the marked loss of neurons, the diagnosis of Alzheimer disease would be less likely. Diffuse Lewy body dementia can involve the entorhinal cortex; however, as with Alzheimer disease, the extreme loss of neurons would be less likely. Hippocampal asymmetry is associated with sudden death in children; however, the marked loss of neurons in the hippocampus is not a characteristic feature.[2-4]

Answer 46: C (colloid cyst)

The mass is smooth, which is consistent with a cyst (answer C) and located in the third ventricle, where it can obstruct the flow of cerebrospinal fluid. While it is possible for a berry aneurysm to extend from the circle of Willis into the cerebral parenchyma and potentially into a ventricle, there is no connection with the vasculature at the base of the brain in the image. A papilloma would not likely have such a smooth surface, and would appear as fronds.

Answer 47: A (CA1)

The image illustrates red neuron change, which, in adults, can be found in the hippocampus, the depths of the sulci, and the cerebellum (both dentate nucleus and Purkinje cells) as the earliest locations for the change. The CA1 sector of the hippocampus is most sensitive to hypoxic-ischemic injury of the four sectors in Ammon's horn.[5]

Answer 48: A (anomalous origin of right coronary artery from left sinus of Valsalva and subendocardial hemorrhage)

The right coronary artery arises from the left sinus of Valsalva and underlying the aortic valve is subendocardial hemorrhage. While a reperfused infarct cannot be completely excluded, subendocardial hemorrhage is a much more common finding at autopsy.

Answer 49: D (diabetes mellitus type 2)

The image illustrates amyloidosis of the pancreatic islet, which can be confirmed with a Congo Red stain. Amyloidosis of the pancreatic islets occurs associated with diabetes mellitus type 2 (answer D). Multiple myeloma is also associated with amyloidosis, but, if the islets are involved, the most likely cause is type 2 diabetes mellitus.

Answer 50: B (anatomic variant)

The cranium has a metopic suture, which is a suture line between the left and right frontal bones. While this suture completely fuses in most individuals, in some individuals a suture remains. It is not normal anatomy and can be described as an anatomic variant (answer B) but has no significance. An anomalous suture can always potentially be confused as a fracture or even as a natural disease process.

Answer 51: C (subdural hemorrhage)

The CT scan reveals a subdural hemorrhage (answer C). While most forensic pathologist offices only have access to radiographic equipment, some have CT scanners. In some locations, local hospitals may be willing to perform a CT scan for a medical examiner's office. In addition, clinical imaging studies are often available to the forensic pathologist. If interpretation of a CT scan is necessary to the evaluation of case, if appropriate, consultation with a radiologist may be useful (photograph courtesy of Herbert Tate).

References

1. Albers A, Gies U, Raatschen HJ, Klintschar M. Another umbrella murder?: a rare case of Minamata disease. *Forensic Sci Med Pathol*. 2020;16(3):504-509.
2. Hefti MM, Cryan JB, Haas EA, et al. Hippocampal malformation associated with sudden death in early childhood: a neuropathologic study—Part 2 of the investigations of The San Diego SUDC Research Project. *Forensic Sci Med Pathol*. 2016;12(1):14-25.
3. Rodriguez ML, McMillan K, Crandall LA, et al. Hippocampal asymmetry and sudden unexpected death in infancy: a case report. *Forensic Sci Med Pathol*. 2012;8(4):441-446.
4. Kinney HC, Armstrong DL, Chadwick AE, et al. Sudden death in toddlers associated with developmental abnormalities of the hippocampus: a report of five cases. *Pediatr Dev Pathol*. 2007;10(3):208-223.
5. Krupska O, Kowalczyk T, Beręsewicz-Haller M, et al. Hippocampal sector-specific metabolic profiles reflect endogenous strategy for ischemia-reperfusion insult resistance. *Mol Neurobiol*. 2021;58(4):1621-1633.

APPENDIX C: WRITING THE AUTOPSY REPORT

INTRODUCTION

While there is not one way in which an autopsy report must be written and while the format for writing an autopsy report will vary based upon office policies and the forensic pathologist's preferences, this chapter will provide some suggestions for completion of the autopsy report. The autopsy report is the formal record of the autopsy procedure and represents the forensic pathologist's work. Even if the best possible autopsy is performed by the forensic pathologist, if a poorly written autopsy report is the final result, the interpretation of the forensic pathologist's work will likely not be favorable. Unfortunately, written guides in the available literature as to how to write an autopsy report are sparse.[1]

> **PEARLS & PITFALLS**
>
> Dictating or otherwise recording the autopsy report the day of the autopsy is best, while the findings are still fresh in the forensic pathologist's mind. Supplementing written notes with memory is easier on the day of the autopsy than later.

CHECKLIST of sections to include in the autopsy report
- ☐ Summary of the scene investigation
- ☐ Summary of pathologic diagnoses
- ☐ Opinion regarding cause and manner of death
- ☐ Statement of autopsy date, time and location, and authorization for the autopsy
- ☐ Description of clothing and personal effects
- ☐ List of medical devices/findings associated with medical intervention
- ☐ Description of identifying features (including scars and tattoos)
- ☐ Description of injuries
- ☐ External examination of the body, including physical characteristics and post-mortem changes
- ☐ Internal examination of the body, including organ weights
- ☐ List of evidence collected
- ☐ List of histologic sections
- ☐ Description of microscopic findings
- ☐ List of additional studies performed (eg, blood cultures)

> **PEARLS & PITFALLS**
>
> Summarizing the pathologic findings at the beginning of the autopsy report can assist with a subsequent quick review when asked a question as well as with courtroom testimony. For example, a short listing of the entrance, injuries, exit, pathway, and other features of a gunshot wound in the summary section allows for quick and easy review.

PEARLS & PITFALLS

Other than in the summary of pathologic diagnoses, the body of the autopsy report itself should not include actual diagnoses. One reason for this is that the reader of the autopsy report has only the written word to formulate their own diagnoses. If the forensic pathologist writing the report indicates that the liver contains a cavernous hemangioma, the reader is dependent upon the ability of the forensic pathologist performing the autopsy to correctly identify a cavernous hemangioma. If instead the writer of the autopsy report describes the gross appearance of the mass in the liver (eg, a well-circumscribed dark red mass with a spongy texture), the reader can formulate their own diagnosis based upon the gross appearance. In actuality, using absolutely no diagnoses in the autopsy report is difficult and often ponderous, but the concept is important to follow as much as possible.

FAQ: Is a separate injuries section required?

Answer: While the injuries and the effects of the injuries can be described in the body of the report, both in the external examination and internal examination sections, including all of this information in a separate section can better allow the reader to assimilate the information because having the injuries scattered through the various portions of the external and internal examination can be difficult for the reader to follow.

FAQ: In an internal examination, what needs to be listed?

Answer: The record of the internal examination can vary from a brief list of weights of the organs and positive findings (eg, presence or absence of gallbladder and appendix, and list of natural disease present) to a detailed description of the normal appearance of the organs. One advantage of a detailed listing of normal findings is that the pathologist later will know what they did at the time of the autopsy. For example, if the tongue is not routinely removed at autopsy, and the autopsy report does not describe a normal tongue, at some point in the future, if asked if they removed the tongue, the pathologist will not likely know.

FAQ: Is it allowable to use a pre-formatted (ie, canned) autopsy report?

Answer: Yes, using a pre-formatted autopsy report can allow for speedier transcription of the autopsy report by either the pathologist themself or a transcriptionist. However, the pathologist must always be careful that normal findings are not left in place when the autopsy actually disclosed abnormal findings.

PEARLS & PITFALLS

When completing the autopsy report, it is best to review the autopsy photographs at the same time. Doing so will allow the forensic pathologist to identify errors made when dictating or typing the autopsy report draft, and to include details that may have been left out of the autopsy report draft. In this regard, detailed photography of the body (eg, the conjunctivae, the upper and lower lips reflected, the hands), different views of the body (eg, sides of the head, sides of the trunk), and more liberal photographs of the body as it was received as well as of internal findings, both natural disease and traumatic injuries, will help the forensic pathologist best re-visit the body while completing the final autopsy report. In short, the more photos a forensic pathologist has to review when completing their report, the better.

NEAR MISS

Near Miss #1: While essentially never of importance in determining the cause and manner of death, whether the penis is circumcised or not and whether the appendix and gallbladder are present or not is most often known by the family, and if the forensic pathologist records this information incorrectly, the family may doubt the remainder of their report. Instead of circumcised or not circumcised, the foreskin length can be described as short or long, and instead of absent, the appendix could be described as "not identified." Confirmation with medical records can assist but non-specific wording for details unimportant to the cause and/or manner of death can prevent future suspicions. Of course, if the body is not identified, better confirmation of the presence or absence of the appendix can be a potentially important detail.

Reference

1. Adams VI. *Guidelines for reports by autopsy pathologists.* Humana Press; 2008.

APPENDIX D: BIAS

INTRODUCTION

Bias can affect a forensic pathologist's ability to interpret patterns in the scene investigation or at autopsy and, in doing so, cause them to arrive at the incorrect determination of cause and/or manner of death or incorrectly interpret features about the cause and manner of death. Numerous forms of bias exist, with Croskerry describing 50 forms of bias that affect medicine.[1] While the term "bias" can be used in a narrow fashion indicating a negative social context (eg, bias against a certain groups of individuals), the concept of bias is much more broad and relates to how forensic pathologists acquire the information necessary to make their determinations, and bias may affect how they make those determinations. Being aware of the various forms of bias would help a forensic pathologist avoid or at least diminish the effect such biases may have on their determinations.

SPECIFIC FORMS OF BIAS

ALLITERATIVE BIAS

Description: This bias occurs when one forensic pathologist's determination is influenced by another forensic pathologist's determination on the same case.[2] The **bandwagon effect** is similar in that a forensic pathologist may make a determination just because numerous other forensic pathologists are doing the same thing.[1]

AMBIGUITY EFFECT

Description: This bias occurs when a physician avoids or ignores certain possibilities because of uncertainty.[1] In forensic pathology, this bias may be manifested by not ordering certain tests because of their cost or unavailability, or because of a lack of knowledge regarding how to interpret them.

ANCHORING BIAS

Description: This bias occurs when a forensic pathologist makes a determination early in the investigation or autopsy and fails to modify that determination as additional contrary information is discovered.[1-3]

AVAILABILITY BIAS

Description: This form of bias occurs when a forensic pathologist determines that a finding is more likely than another just because they remember it better.[1,2] Similar is the **mere exposure effect** in which a forensic pathologist prefers something just because of their familiarity with it.[1]

BELIEF BIAS

Description: This bias occurs when a forensic pathologist allows their personal belief to guide their determination.[1]

CONFIRMATION BIAS

Description: This bias occurs when a forensic pathologist looks for evidence to support their determination but does not look for or ignores evidence that refutes their determination.[1,3] A variation is the **sunken cost bias** in which the forensic pathologist is so invested in a particular diagnosis as a manifestation of their ego that they will not consider another diagnosis.[1]

CONTRAST EFFECT

Description: This bias occurs when one finding is diminished in its importance because of its contrast to another more significant finding.[1] For a forensic pathologist, an autopsy can present quite striking findings (eg, complete destruction of the cranium due to a contact gunshot wound with a rifle; however, faint linear scars on the ventral surface of the forearm may offer additional support for the manner of death determination as suicide). Similarly, a forensic pathologist may choose to concentrate on one striking autopsy finding and be less thorough in the remainder of their examination and thus potentially miss other important, less striking findings.

DIAGNOSIS MOMENTUM

Description: This form of bias occurs when a patient is determined to possibly have a certain disease process; however, with subsequent versions of the medical record that disease process is carried forward and the "possibly" disclaimer is lost, and the patient is instead labeled as having the disease, although a definitive diagnosis may never have been made.[1] For example, a patient who presents with shortness of breath on an emergency room visit may be labeled as "possible asthma"; however, during subsequent clinic visits, that "possible asthma" can become "asthma" through recording the medical record. Awareness of this bias can assist forensic pathologists in developing the medical profile of the decedent, as the family's diagnosis or ER physician's diagnosis may require a more extensive review before accepting.

EXPECTATION BIAS

Description: This bias occurs when researchers interpret, unconsciously manipulate, and report their data according to their expectations for the research.[1] As forensic pathologists often utilize medical journal articles when making their determinations, awareness of this bias can help prevent using faulty research.

FALSE CONSENSUS BIAS

Description: This bias occurs when a forensic pathologist overestimates how often other forensic pathologists would agree with them.[3] Similar is the **self-serving bias** in which a forensic pathologist overestimates their past successes and under-estimates their past failures.[1]

FRAMING EFFECT

Description: This bias occurs because of how a patient is presented to a physician (ie, in a positive or negative fashion, or as a benign or serious condition).[1,3,4] For forensic pathologists, the scene investigation and associated history of how the decedent was found dead, or how they came to die, is important in determining manner of death, and also, in some cases, the cause of death; however, this same information can lead to bias (eg, overcalling traumatic injuries in an infant because of history of alleged maltreatment of that infant).

GAMBLER'S FALLACY

Description: This bias occurs when a physician, who has had numerous patients with the same diagnosis present in a row, determines that the next person, with the same symptomatology cannot have the same diagnosis as all the others.[1]

GENDER BIAS/ASCERTAINMENT BIAS

Description: Gender bias occurs when a physician assigns a higher probability of a disease to a male or female, when no such higher probability has been determined by studies.[1]

Although the name of this bias is "gender bias," it would more aptly be named "sex bias" as gender is a social construct whereas sex is biological, with male and female being the two biologic sexes. **Ascertainment bias** occurs when a decision is based upon a prior expectation regarding certain characteristics about an individual.[1] Forensic pathologists autopsy a wide range of individuals from male to female, rich to destitute, and individuals with all forms of ancestral backgrounds, work backgrounds, and recreational activities. To incorrectly assign a higher probability of a disease or condition to any group without proven confirmation of that link is a manifestation of this form of bias.

HAWTHORNE EFFECT

Description: This bias occurs when individuals behave differently when someone is watching them. While this bias may not affect a forensic pathologist's determinations, it could certainly affect their workplace and reputation.[1]

HINDSIGHT BIAS

Description: This bias occurs because a person, knowing the outcome, misinterprets the past event.[1] At autopsy, a forensic pathologist is always looking at the final outcome and attempting to determine the past events. To a forensic pathologist, this bias is somewhat the opposite of the framing effect. In the framing effect, a forensic pathologist's knowledge of the scene investigation may bias their interpretation of the autopsy findings, and in hindsight bias, the forensic pathologist's knowledge of the autopsy findings may bias their interpretation of the events that led to the individual's demise.

ILLUSORY CORRELATION

Description: This bias occurs when a forensic pathologist links two conditions (cause and effect) just because they are juxtaposed in time.[1] **Attentional bias** is similar and occurs when a forensic pathologist links two conditions just because they are found together. Attentional bias has likely led to the publication of innumerable case reports, each because two conditions were found together.

INFORMATION BIAS

Description: This bias occurs when a forensic pathologist accumulates more information than necessary to support their determination. While this bias may not cause errors in a determination, it would impede the ability of a forensic pathologist to finish their workload in a timely fashion.[1]

NEED FOR CLOSURE BIAS

Description: This bias occurs when a forensic pathologist rushes their determination to appease family or law enforcement instead of taking the time necessary to finalize their determination.[1]

OUTCOME BIAS

Description: This bias is used to describe when a physician will opt for choices that favor a good outcome instead of a bad outcome, but can allow the worse disease to be missed.[1] This bias relates to forensic pathologists making decisions based upon how they feel law enforcement or the family will react to their decision, favoring those determinations that are less likely to be controversial.

OVERCONFIDENCE BIAS

Description: This bias occurs when a forensic pathologist places too much faith in their intuition or acts on incomplete information instead of carefully collecting enough evidence to support their determination.[1] The **visceral bias** is similar in that positive and negative feelings regarding a decedent may affect the forensic pathologist's determinations (eg, negative feelings toward a decomposed body may lead to a less than adequate autopsy evaluation).[1] The **blind spot bias** is also similar in that a forensic pathologist feels they are not as susceptible to bias as other individuals because of their perceived more effective self-awareness compared to others.[1,3]

PREMATURE CLOSURE

Description: This bias occurs when a forensic pathologist prematurely makes a determination without completely verifying that determination.[1,2] The **multiple alternative bias** is similar and occurs when a forensic pathologist for various reasons arbitrarily narrows a differential diagnosis just by excluding some conditions without actually ruling them out.[1] The **unpacking principle** is also similar and occurs when a forensic pathologist does not obtain all relevant information prior to making a determination.[1]

REACTANCE BIAS

Description: This bias occurs when a forensic pathologist finds their autonomy threatened such as being challenged in court, or being challenged by a non-forensic pathologist as to their findings or interpretation, and allowing that interaction to alter their determination.[1]

SEARCH SATISFICING BIAS

Description: This form of bias occurs when a forensic pathologist stops carefully looking for conditions after a cause of death or an important diagnosis is discovered. This bias can allow for other conditions of less importance to be missed; however, these additional diagnoses may also be important in other contexts (eg, identifying a heritable form of cancer or heart disease in an individual who died as the result of a gunshot wound inflicted by another person).[1,3]

SEMMELWEIS REFLEX

Description: This form of bias occurs when a forensic pathologist will not accept new evidence that contradicts an older established concept.[1] Another way to word this bias is **status quo bias**.[3]

SUTTON'S SLIP

Description: This form of bias occurs when a forensic pathologist does not consider conditions other than what is most obvious (eg, in a young individual with an oral foam cone, that the forensic pathologist does not consider a natural disease process instead of just a drug overdose would be an example of this form of bias).[1]

VERTICAL LINE FAILURE

Description: This form of bias occurs when an individual performs routine repetitive tasks, which can lead to inflexibility.[1] While each autopsy is potentially unique, general categories of autopsy (eg, a suspected drug overdose, a gunshot wound homicide) can be performed in a repetitive fashion and could promote this form of bias. To combat this bias, Croskerry suggests the simple question, "What else might this be?"[1]

ZEBRA RETREAT

Description: This bias occurs when a forensic pathologist fails to consider a rare diagnosis even though the likelihood of that rare diagnosis being present is great.[1] Similar is **representative restraint bias**, where, when a manifestation looks typical for a disease process or injury that another disease process or injury producing an atypical manifestation is not considered.[1] Somewhat the opposite of representative restraint bias is **aggregate bias**, where physicians do not think that clinical practice guidelines (ie, derived from aggregated data) do not apply to their patient,[1] which leads to ordering of more tests than necessary.[1]

References

1. Pat Croskerry. *50 Cognitive and Affective Biases in Medicine. Critical Thinking Program.* Dalhousie University; Accessed February 12, 2023. https://sjrhem.ca/wp-content/uploads/2015/11/CriticaThinking-Listof50-biases.pdf
2. Flemming DJ, White C, Fox E, Fanburg-Smith J, Cochran E. Diagnostic errors in musculoskeletal oncology and possible mitigation strategies. *Skeletal Radiol.* 2023;52(3):493-503.
3. Hammond MEH, Stehlik J, Drakos SG, Kfoury AG. Bias in medicine: lessons learned and mitigation strategies. *JACC Basic Transl Sci.* 2021;6(1):78-85.
4. Ogdie AR, Reilly JB, Pang WG, et al. Seen through their eyes: residents' reflections on the cognitive and contextual components of diagnostic errors in medicine. *Acad Med.* 2012;87(10):1361-1367.

APPENDIX E: RARE BUT IMPORTANT TO CONSIDER

INTRODUCTION

In forensic pathology, the autopsy is important for identifying both the cause and manner of death; however, a standard autopsy might not perform the dissections or microscopic examinations necessary to identify certain conditions. In addition, some conditions would require genetic testing, other ancillary testing, or a high index of suspicion based upon the known clinical history and lack of a competing cause of death. Although not a complete list, the following discussion should offer guidance to help identify some of these rare but important to consider diagnoses.

NERVOUS SYSTEM CONDITIONS

SUDDEN DEATH ASSOCIATED WITH SCHIZOPHRENIA

Autopsy findings: While decedents with schizophrenia can die related to the presence of cardiac disease such as coronary artery atherosclerosis or due to the effects of anti-psychotic medication on the QT interval, patients with schizophrenia also have an independent risk for sudden death.[1-3] Wang et al found that individuals with a higher number of psychiatric episodes had a higher risk for sudden death.[4] This predisposition to sudden cardiac death in schizophrenics may be genetic in origin.[5] With sudden death associated with schizophrenia, the autopsy would not identify any significant findings.

MYASTHENIA GRAVIS

Autopsy findings: Myasthenia gravis has been associated with vasculitis and myocarditis. The myocarditis can involve the cardiac conduction tissue, which can be a risk factor for a lethal cardiac dysrhythmia.[6]

Association with sudden death: Other than the risk for myocarditis, acute myasthenia gravis has been associated with acute respiratory muscle weakness requiring ventilator support, which could potentially lead to death. In addition to myocarditis, myasthenia gravis has been associated with various cardiac abnormalities including conduction disorders and congestive heart failure.[7,8] Testing for serum anti-acetylcholine receptor antibodies may assist with the diagnosis.[7]

WERNICKE-KORSAKOFF SYNDROME

Autopsy findings: In the acute phase, the mammillary bodies will be hemorrhagic and microscopic examination can reveal edema, petechial hemorrhages, and prominent capillaries due to hyperplasia and swelling of the endothelial cells[9] (Figure 1A and B). In the chronic phase, the mammillary bodies will be shrunken and brown-yellow discolored, with microscopic examination revealing loss of both neurons and myelinated fibers, as well as activated microglia, gliosis, and possible hemosiderin deposition[9,10] (Figure 1C). While the mammillary bodies are the most common area of the brain to be involved, other areas such as the thalamus, hypothalamus, and the periaqueductal gray matter can also have lesions.[10]

Associations: Wernicke encephalopathy has a 15% to 20% mortality rate, and patients can be found hypothermic and comatose[11]; thus, the condition could be associated with sudden death. While Wernicke encephalopathy is most commonly associated with chronic alcoholism, numerous other conditions can cause the disease, including various medical treatments (prolonged intravenous feeding and hemodialysis), gastrointestinal disorders

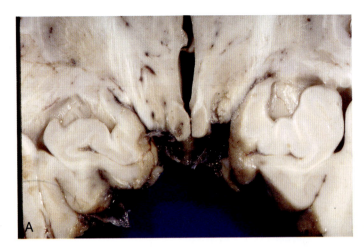
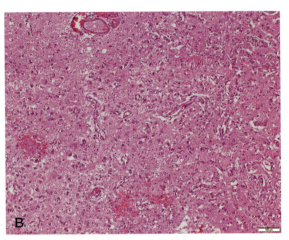
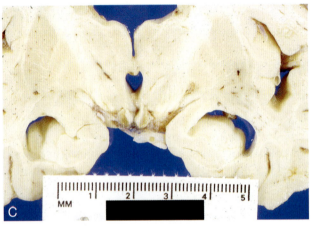

Figure 1. Wernicke-Korsakoff syndrome. In the acute stage, there will be hemorrhage of the mammillary bodies (**A**) and microscopic examination reveals petechiae, edema, and prominent vasculature (**B**), (Hematoxylin and eosin, high power). In the chronic stage or in decedents who have been treated, the mammillary bodies will be shrunken and brown discolored (**C**).

(enteritis and malabsorption), malignancy, anorexia nervosa, thyrotoxicosis, uremia, and human immunodeficiency virus infection.[10] If the mammillary bodies are not sectioned, the diagnosis will easily be missed at autopsy.

ENDOCRINE SYSTEM CONDITIONS

LYMPHOCYTIC HYPOPHYSITIS

Autopsy findings: Lymphocytic hypophysitis is inflammation of the pituitary gland that is most frequently of autoimmune origin.[12] The disease process can cause headache and hormone deficiencies, involve either the anterior or the posterior pituitary or both, and can potentially lead to death, likely through electrolyte abnormalities.[12]

Association with sudden death: Lymphocytic hypophysitis has been associated with sudden death.[13,14] The disease most commonly occurs in women, during pregnancy, or in the postpartum period.[15] If the pituitary gland is not examined microscopically, the diagnosis will be missed.

THYROGLOSSAL DUCT CYST

Autopsy findings: A cyst that develops at the base of the tongue from remnants of the thyroglossal duct.

Association with sudden death: A thyroglossal duct cyst can lead to airway compromise, which occurs mostly in children but also in adults and can be a cause of death.[16,17] If the tongue is not removed and examined, the diagnosis will be missed.

PARATHYROID GLAND HYPERPLASIA/ADENOMA

Autopsy findings: With dissection, the parathyroid glands can easily be identified and assessed for hyperplasia or an adenoma (Figure 2); however, frequently, an actual dissection of the parathyroid glands is not performed by the forensic pathologist at autopsy.

Association with sudden death: While the elevated calcium concentration produced by the adenoma or hyperplasia will shorten the QT interval, the resultant hypokalemia can lengthen the QT interval.[18] Individuals with primary hyperparathyroidism are at risk for cardiac dysrhythmia, which could be a potential cause of death, especially if combined with other conditions or drug therapy that could contribute to hypokalemia.

CARDIOVASCULAR SYSTEM CONDITIONS

MESOTHELIOMA OF THE ATRIOVENTRICULAR NODE

Autopsy findings: The tumor is potentially derived from endodermal or ultimobranchial heterotopia that become trapped in the region of the atrioventricular node, which represents an area of embryonic fusion.[19,20] The tumor is composed of cysts lined with non-ciliated cuboidal cells, solid nests of cells, and ducts.[19] The nuclei have a bland appearance and mitotic figures are not present. The tumor has been associated with congenital heart disease, including ventricular septal defect, ovarian and breasts cysts, and thyroglossal duct cysts.[19]

Association with sudden death: Mesotheliomas of the atrioventricular node are associated with sudden death.[19,21] If the atrioventricular nodal region is not examined microscopically, the cause of death will be missed.

WOLFF-PARKINSON-WHITE SYNDROME

Autopsy findings: While Pollanen reports no anatomical findings in Wolff-Parkinson-White (WPW) syndrome, there is an accessory bundle of conduction tissue which could possibly be identified.[22-24] Ideally, the diagnosis requires a documented cardiac dysrhythmia prior to death, with a subsequent electrocardiographic diagnosis.[25]

Association with sudden death: WPW is associated with sudden death; however, the risk is relatively low. The incidence of a life threatening event in WPW is 0.8 to 1.9 events per 1,000 person-years.[26]

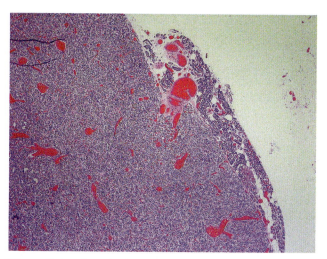

Figure 2. Parathyroid adenoma. On the right side of the image is a thin rim of normal gland, with interspersed adipose tissue, with the adenoma in the majority of the section (Hematoxylin and eosin, low power).

LONG QT SYNDROME AND TORSADE DE POINTES

Association with sudden death: A long QT interval can lead to the development of a polymorphic ventricular tachycardia (torsade de pointes), which can lead to sudden death.[27] Long QT syndrome (LQTS) can be either congenital or acquired. Congenital long QT syndrome is due to abnormalities in sodium or potassium ion channel genes, including SCN5A, KCNH2, KCNQ1, KCNE2, KCNE1, and KCNJ2.[28] The use of synthetic cathinones is associated with a greater risk of sudden death in individuals with KCNQ1 mutations.[29] NOS1AP and KCNQ1 are associated with drowning, with up to 30% of swimming-related drownings having a genetic abnormality.[30,31] Acquired LQTS and subsequent torsade de pointes can be associated with electrolyte abnormalities (hypokalemia, hypomagnesemia, hypocalcemia, and hypothyroidism), antiarrhythmic drugs (eg, amiodarone, procainamide), antibiotics (eg, erythromycin, macrolides, fluoroquinolones) antipsychotics (eg, haloperidol and olanzapine), liquid protein diets, and cisapride.[27,32] Anti-Ro/SSA-antibodies can also prolong the QT interval and could be associated with sudden death.[33] The autopsy of an individual who dies as the result of long QT syndrome will have no findings; however, if a congenital long QT syndrome is suspected, an appropriate sample should be maintained following autopsy.[34] This sample can include blood in a purple top tube (EDTA), heart frozen at −80 °C, or DNA extracted from paraffin-embedded tissue.[35,36]

> **PEARLS & PITFALLS**
>
> www.crediblemeds.org is an excellent resource for listing of drugs associated with prolongation of the QT interval.

> **PEARLS & PITFALLS**
>
> Two other conditions that can cause sudden cardiac death and would require genetic analysis for the diagnosis are Brugada syndrome and catecholaminergic polymorphic ventricular tachycardia (CPVT).[36]

INFECTIOUS CONDITIONS

WEST NILE VIRUS MYELITIS

Autopsy findings: An infection with West Nile virus can cause a fatal encephalitis and the inflammatory change may be most prevalent in the brainstem.[37] However, West Nile virus can also cause a myelitis.[38,39] If the myelitis is the prominent manifestation of the viral infection and causes death, unless the spinal cord is removed and examined microscopically, the diagnosis will be missed.

NAEGLERIA FOWLERI MENINGITIS

Antemortem history: *Naegleria fowleri* meningitis is most frequently associated with a history of swimming in warm stagnant water.[40] *Naegleria fowleri* has also been identified in tap water, including in the United States, and infections can occur from the use of a nasal irrigation device.[41,42]

Autopsy findings: *Naegleria fowleri* causes a hemorrhagic and necrotizing meningo-encephalitis often at the base of the brain.[40] If the meningitis is attributed to a bacterial infection and microscopic sections are not examined, or if the amoebae are missed in the review of the microscopic sections (Figure 3), the correct cause of death will not be identified.

RABIES

Autopsy findings: Microscopic examination of the brain can reveal Negri bodies (Figure 4).

HANTAVIRUS

Autopsy findings: Gross examination will reveal prominent pleural effusions (Figure 5A). Microscopic examination of the lungs can reveal marked interstitial and alveolar pulmonary

APPENDIX E: RARE BUT IMPORTANT TO CONSIDER

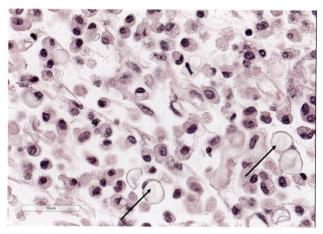

Figure 3. Amoebic encephalitis. Interspersed among the macrophages are amoebae (arrows), (Hematoxylin and eosin, high power).

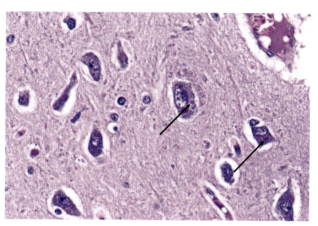

Figure 4. Rabies encephalitis. The neurons contain Negri bodies (arrows), (Hematoxylin and eosin, high power).

edema, with a mononuclear interstitial infiltrate[43] (Figure 5B). The virus can be confirmed with ELISA and PCR testing.[44,45]

ROCKY MOUNTAIN SPOTTED FEVER

Autopsy findings: The histologic features of the skin rash are a lymphohistiocytic capillaritis and venulitis associated with edema, extravasation of red blood cells, and edema.[46] Other findings in a fatal case can include severe vasculitis associated with interstitial nephritis and multifocal tubular necrosis, pericholangitis with bile stasis, microglial nodules in the brain, multifocal rhabdomyonecrosis, interstitial pneumonitis, and myocarditis.[47,48] Autopsy diagnosis of Rocky Mountain spotted fever can be done with PCR analysis for *Rickettsia rickettsii*.[49]

MISCELLANEOUS CONDITIONS

SNAKE BITE

Autopsy findings: Puncture marks from the snake's fangs will be present. While two puncture marks is most common, between one and four puncture marks can be seen.[50] If two puncture marks are present, it is good to record the distance between the two marks as this measurement can help allow for identification of the snake responsible for the bite.[50] At the site of the puncture marks will be edema, inflammation, hemorrhage, and necrosis.[50] Other

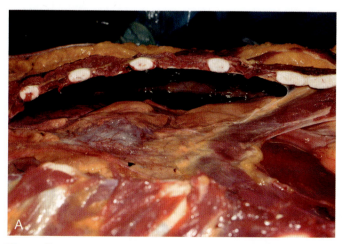 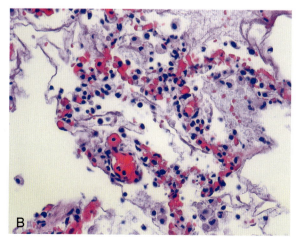

Figure 5. Hantavirus infection. The pleural cavities contain a watery pleural effusion (**A**). Microscopic examination revealed a lymphohistiocytic infiltrate (**B**), (Hematoxylin and eosin, high power).

autopsy findings are non-specific and can include visceral congestion or edema, petechial hemorrhages, myocardial hemorrhages, diffuse alveolar damage, and microthrombi.

SEROTONIN SYNDROME

Antemortem features: Patients with serotonin syndrome can have hyperthermia, mental status changes, autonomic instability, and abnormal muscle tone including rigidity.[51]

Associated with: Drugs that reduce metabolism of serotonin (eg, monoamine oxidase inhibitors), increase production of serotonin (eg, L-tryptophan), or inhibit serotonin uptake (eg, fluoxetine, meperidine, dextromethorphan, fenfluramine, and clomipramine) are associated with serotonin syndrome.[51] In addition, the use of illicit substances by patients on psychotropic medication could precipitate serotonin syndrome. For example, Khan et al described serotonin syndrome precipitated by cocaine and fentanyl.[52]

Complications of serotonin syndrome: Complications include rhabdomyolysis, renal failure, disseminated intravascular coagulation, seizures, and cardiac dysrhythmias.

ALLERGIC REACTION-ANAPHYLACTIC SHOCK

Autopsy findings: In a large series of deaths due to anaphylaxis, Bury et al identified angioedema of the upper airways (Figure 6A and B) and pulmonary edema in around 50% of decedents, and pulmonary congestion in around 25% of decedents; however, autopsy findings can also be completely absent in an individual who died from an anaphylactic reaction.[53,54]

Method for diagnosis: Serum tryptase is an excellent biomarker for anaphylactic shock (although other biomarkers such as chymase and histamine have been investigated). Increased immunoglobulin E (IgE) levels and identification of the specific IgE can also assist with the diagnosis.[55] Testing for the specific IgE (eg, IgE vs Hymenoptera venom) can be used to provide additional evidence supporting anaphylaxis as the cause of death.[56,57]

While the main method for identifying postmortem anaphylaxis is testing for tryptase, Garland et al and Busaro et al discuss considerations for interpreting such testing.[58,59] Other than just anaphylactic shock, elevated tryptase concentrations have been found in SIDS, hyperthermia, heroin deaths, and some heart conditions.[55] Randall and Butts report a series of cases of non-anaphylaxis related deaths associated with an elevated tryptase and caution that the diagnosis should be based upon the context of the case and not just testing for serum tryptase.[60] While there is a report identifying an elevated serum tryptase in decomposed bodies, another report indicates that both increased tryptase concentrations and decreased tryptase concentrations with an increasing postmortem interval have been reported.[55,61]

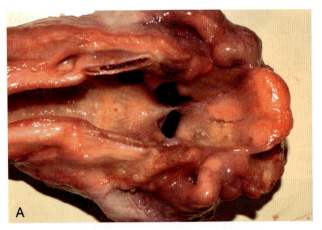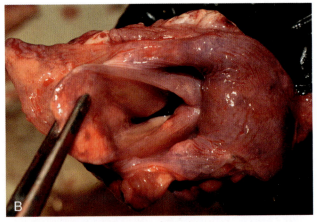

Figure 6. Laryngeal edema. Laryngeal edema will appear as a mucoid thickening of the soft tissue (**A** and **B**). In a decedent with no other explanation for laryngeal edema, testing for serum tryptase and, if known, the specific immunoglobulin E, can assist with the diagnosis of an anaphylactic reaction.

> **PEARLS & PITFALLS**
>
> If an anaphylactic death is suspected, after obtaining blood, centrifuge the blood tubes and remove the serum so as to prevent postmortem hemolysis from affecting the sample. If postmortem blood is not available, pericardial fluid may also work.[55]

> **PEARLS & PITFALLS**
>
> Diagnosing anaphylaxis requires an index of suspicion as the autopsy findings can be very subtle. While anaphylaxis is commonly associated with various drugs, insect and animal stings, and food allergies,[53,62,63] one important consideration is that during oral sex, an individual who has just eaten a substance can expose another person to that substance. McKibbin et al report fatal anaphylaxis in a male with a peanut allergy who received oral sex from another male who had just consumed peanut butter.[64]

ACUTE STRESS

Association with sudden death: Baltzer et al and Lou et al indicate that acute stress can cause death, if the patient is previously sensitized such as through drugs (eg, cocaine) and/or a psychiatric condition.[65,66] The authors propose that excited delirium syndrome, malignant catatonia, capture myopathy, and takotsubo cardiomyopathy are variants of the same pathophysiological phenomenon.

TOXINS AND POISONS

Autopsy considerations: The range of possible toxins and poisons that could be encountered at autopsy is significant. Unfortunately, most are not identified through routine toxicologic testing. The identification of such substances will require good scene investigation and consideration at autopsy, with additional specimens retained for testing, including hair and fingernails.

References

1. Vaiman EE, Shnayder NA, Zhuravlev NM, et al. Genetic biomarkers of antipsychotic-induced prolongation of the QT interval in patients with schizophrenia. *Int J Mol Sci.* 2022;23(24):15786.
2. He L, Yu Y, Zhang L, et al. A real-world study of risk factors for QTc prolongation in schizophrenia patients receiving atypical antipsychotics. *J Clin Psychopharmacol.* 2022;42(1):71-74.
3. Vohra J. Sudden cardiac death in schizophrenia: a review. *Heart Lung Circ.* 2020;29(10):1427-1432.
4. Wang S, He M, Andersen J, et al. Sudden unexplained death in schizophrenia patients: an autopsy-based comparative study from China. *Asian J Psychiatr.* 2023;79:103314.
5. Christiansen SL, Andersen JD, Themudo GE, et al. Genetic investigations of 100 inherited cardiac disease-related genes in deceased individuals with schizophrenia. *Int J Legal Med.* 2021;135(4):1395-1405.
6. Cohle SD, Lie JT. Myasthenia gravis-associated systemic vasculitis and myocarditis with involvement of the cardiac conducting tissue. *Cardiovasc Pathol.* 1996;5(3):159-162.
7. Payus AO, Leow Wen Hsiang J, Leong JQ, Ibrahim A, Raymond AA. Myasthenic crisis as the first presentation of myasthenia gravis: a case report. *Am J Case Rep.* 2021;22:e928419.
8. Călin C, Savu O, Dumitru D, et al. Cardiac involvement in myasthenia gravis—is there a specific pattern? *Rom J Intern Med.* 2009;47(2):179-189.
9. Gray F, Duyckaerts C, DeGirolami U. *Escourolle and Poirier's Manual of Basic Neuropathology.* 5th ed. Oxford University Press; 2014.
10. Hata Y, Takeuchi Y, Kinoshita K, Nishida N. An autopsy case of acute and nonalcoholic thiamine-deficient encephalopathy. *Eur Neurol.* 2014;71(5-6):230-232.

11. Lindberg MC, Oyler RA. Wernicke's encephalopathy. *Am Fam Physician*. 1990;41(4):1205-1209.
12. Gubbi S, Hannah-Shmouni F, Verbalis JG, Koch CA. Hypophysitis: an update on the novel forms, diagnosis and management of disorders of pituitary inflammation. *Best Pract Res Clin Endocrinol Metab*. 2019;33(6):101371.
13. Gonzalez-Cuyar LF, Tavora F, Shaw K, Castellani RJ, Dejong JL. Sudden unexpected death in lymphocytic hypophysitis. *Am J Forensic Med Pathol*. 2009;30(1):61-63.
14. Blisard KS, Pfalzgraf RR, Balko MG. Sudden death due to lymphoplasmacytic hypophysitis. *Am J Forensic Med Pathol*. 1992;13(3):207-210.
15. Brandes JC, Cerletty JM. Pregnancy in lymphocytic hypophysitis: case report and review. *Wis Med J*. 1989;88(11):29-32.
16. Sauvageau A, Belley-Côté EP, Racette S. Fatal asphyxia by a thyroglossal duct cyst in an adult. *J Clin Forensic Med*. 2006;13(6-8):349-352.
17. Hanzlick RL. Lingual thyroglossal duct cyst causing death in a four-week-old infant. *J Forensic Sci*. 1984;29(1):345-348.
18. Muzurović E, Medenica S, Kalezić M, et al. Primary hyperparathyroidism associated with acquired long QT interval and ventricular tachycardia. *Endocrinol Diabetes Metab Case Rep*. 2021;2021:21-0016.
19. Luc JGY, Phan K, Tchantchaleishvili V. Cystic tumor of the atrioventricular node: a review of the literature. *J Thorac Dis*. 2017;9(9):3313-3318.
20. Monma N, Satodate R, Tashiro A, Segawa I. Origin of so-called mesothelioma of the atrioventricular node. An immunohistochemical study. *Arch Pathol Lab Med*. 1991;115(10):1026-1029.
21. Bharati S, Bicoff JP, Fridman JL, Lev M, Rosen KM. Sudden death caused by benign tumor of the atrioventricular node. *Arch Intern Med*. 1976;136(2):224-228.
22. Pollanen MS. Forensic pathology and the miscarriage of justice. *Forensic Sci Med Pathol*. 2012;8(3):285-289.
23. Raharjo SB, Putro AH, Santoso A, et al. Simple electrocardiography algorithm for localizing accessory pathway in patients with Wolff-Parkinson-White syndrome. *Acta Cardiol*. 2022;77(8):729-733.
24. Wiedermann CJ, Becker AE, Hopferwieser T, Mühlberger V, Knapp E. Sudden death in a young competitive athlete with Wolff-Parkinson-White syndrome. *Eur Heart J*. 1987;8(6):651-655.
25. Qiu M, Lv B, Lin W, Ma J, Dong H. Sudden cardiac death due to the Wolff-Parkinson-White syndrome: a case report with genetic analysis. *Medicine (Baltimore)*. 2018;97(51):e13248.
26. Janson CM, Millenson ME, Okunowo O, et al. Incidence of life-threatening events in children with Wolff-Parkinson-White syndrome: analysis of a large claims database. *Heart Rhythm*. 2022;19(4):642-647.
27. Roden DM. A practical approach to torsade de pointes. *Clin Cardiol*. 1997;20(3):285-290.
28. Marcondes L, Crawford J, Earle N, et al. Long QT molecular autopsy in sudden unexplained death in the young (1-40 years old): lessons learnt from an eight year experience in New Zealand. *PLoS One*. 2018;13(4):e0196078.
29. Nagasawa S, Saitoh H, Kasahara S, et al. Relationship between KCNQ1 (LQT1) and KCNH2 (LQT2) gene mutations and sudden death during illegal drug use. *Sci Rep*. 2018;8(1):8443.
30. Tzimas I, Zingraf JC, Bajanowski T, Poetsch M. The role of known variants of KCNQ1, KCNH2, KCNE1, SCN5A, and NOS1AP in water-related deaths. *Int J Legal Med*. 2016;130(6):1575-1579.
31. Tester DJ, Medeiros-Domingo A, Will ML, Ackerman MJ. Unexplained drownings and the cardiac channelopathies: a molecular autopsy series. *Mayo Clin Proc*. 2011;86(10):941-947.
32. Al-Akchar M, Siddique MS. *Long QT Syndrome*. May 15, 2022. In: *StatPearls* [Internet]. StatPearls Publishing; 2022.
33. Lazzerini PE, Laghi-Pasini F, Boutjdir M, Capecchi PL. Anti-Ro/SSA antibodies and the autoimmune long-QT syndrome. *Front Med*. 2021;8:730161.
34. Basso C, Carturan E, Pilichou K, Rizzo S, Corrado D, Thiene G. Sudden cardiac death with normal heart: molecular autopsy. *Cardiovasc Pathol*. 2010;19(6):321-325.
35. Di Paolo M, Luchini D, Bloise R, Priori SG. Postmortem molecular analysis in victims of sudden unexplained death. *Am J Forensic Med Pathol*. 2004;25(2):182-184.
36. Michaud K, Fellmann F, Abriel H, Beckmann JS, Mangin P, Elger BS. Molecular autopsy in sudden cardiac death and its implication for families: discussion of the practical, legal and ethical aspects of the multidisciplinary collaboration. *Swiss Med Wkly*. 2009;139(49-50):712-728.

37. Sampson BA, Armbrustmacher V. West Nile encephalitis: the neuropathology of four fatalities. *Ann N Y Acad Sci*. 2001;951:172-178.
38. Jani C, Walker A, Al Omari O, et al. Acute transverse myelitis in West Nile Virus, a rare neurological presentation. *IDCases*. 2021;24:e01104.
39. Hiatt B, DesJardin L, Carter T, Gingrich R, Thompson C, de Magalhaes-Silverman M. A fatal case of West Nile virus infection in a bone marrow transplant recipient. *Clin Infect Dis*. 2003;37(9):e129-e131.
40. Gyori E. December 2002: 19-year old male with febrile illness after jet ski accident. *Brain Pathol*. 2003;13(2):237-239.
41. Cope JR, Ratard RC, Hill VR, et al. The first association of a primary amebic meningoencephalitis death with culturable *Naegleria fowleri* in tap water from a US treated public drinking water system. *Clin Infect Dis*. 2015;60(8):e36-e42.
42. Yoder JS, Straif-Bourgeois S, Roy SL, et al. Primary amebic meningoencephalitis deaths associated with sinus irrigation using contaminated tap water. *Clin Infect Dis*. 2012;55(9):e79-e85.
43. Guzmán GP, Tapia EO, Villaseca HM, et al. Hallazgos morfológicos en casos fatales de síndrome cardiopulmonar por hantavirus. Estudio de 7 autopsias [Morphological findings in fatal cases of hantavirus cardiopulmonary syndrome. Report of 7 autopsies]. *Rev Chilena Infectol*. 2010;27(5):398-405.
44. Figueiredo LT, Moreli ML, Almeida VS, et al. Hantavirus pulmonary syndrome (HPS) in Guariba, SP, Brazil. Report of 2 cases. *Rev Inst Med Trop Sao Paulo*. 1999;41(2):131-137.
45. Nuovo GJ, Simsir A, Steigbigel RT, Kuschner M. Analysis of fatal pulmonary hantaviral infection in New York by reverse transcriptase in situ polymerase chain reaction. *Am J Pathol*. 1996;148(3):685-692.
46. Kao GF, Evancho CD, Ioffe O, Lowitt MH, Dumler JS. Cutaneous histopathology of Rocky Mountain spotted fever. *J Cutan Pathol*. 1997;24(10):604-610.
47. Green WR, Walker DH, Cain BG. Fatal viscerotropic Rocky Mountain spotted fever. Report of a case diagnosed by immunofluorescence. *Am J Med*. 1978;64(3):523-528.
48. Marin-Garcia J, Gooch WM,III, Coury DL. Cardiac manifestations of Rocky Mountain spotted fever. *Pediatrics*. 1981;67(3):358-361.
49. Tribaldos M, Zaldivar Y, Bermudez S, et al. Rocky Mountain spotted fever in Panama: a cluster description. *J Infect Dev Ctries*. 2011;5(10):737-741.
50. Feola A, Marella GL, Carfora A, Della Pietra B, Zangani P, Campobasso CP. Snakebite envenoming a challenging diagnosis for the forensic pathologist: a systematic review. *Toxins*. 2020;12(11):699.
51. Palmiere C, Mangin P. Hyperthermia and postmortem biochemical investigations. *Int J Legal Med*. 2013;127(1):93-102.
52. Khan A, Lahmar A, Asif H, Haseeb M, Rai K. Serotonin syndrome precipitated by the use of cocaine and fentanyl. *Cureus*. 2022;14(3):e22805.
53. Bury D, Langlois N, Byard RW. Animal-related fatalities—part II: characteristic autopsy findings and variable causes of death associated with envenomation, poisoning, anaphylaxis, asphyxiation, and sepsis. *J Forensic Sci*. 2012;57(2):375-380.
54. Unkrig S, Hagemeier L, Madea B. Postmortem diagnostics of assumed food anaphylaxis in an unexpected death. *Forensic Sci Int*. 2010;198(1-3):e1-e4.
55. Heldring N, Kahn L, Zilg B. Fatal anaphylactic shock: a review of postmortem biomarkers and diagnostics. *Forensic Sci Int*. 2021;323:110814.
56. Riches KJ, Gillis D, James RA. An autopsy approach to bee sting-related deaths. *Pathology*. 2002;34(3):257-262.
57. Prahlow JA, Barnard JJ. Fatal anaphylaxis due to fire ant stings. *Am J Forensic Med Pathol*. 1998;19(2):137-142.
58. Garland J, Ondruschka B, Da Broi U, Palmiere C, Tse R. Post mortem tryptase: a review of literature on its use, sampling and interpretation in the investigation of fatal anaphylaxis. *Forensic Sci Int*. 2020;314:110415.
59. Busardò FP, Marinelli E, Zaami S. Is the diagnosis of anaphylaxis reliable in forensics? The role of β-tryptase and its correct interpretation. *Leg Med (Tokyo)*. 2016;23:86-88.
60. Randall B, Butts J, Halsey JF. Elevated postmortem tryptase in the absence of anaphylaxis. *J Forensic Sci*. 1995;40(2):208-211.

61. Radheshi E, Reggiani Bonetti L, Confortini A, Silingardi E, Palmiere C. Postmortem diagnosis of anaphylaxis in presence of decompositional changes. *J Forensic Leg Med.* 2016;38:97-100.
62. Byard RW. Death by food. *Forensic Sci Med Pathol.* 2018;14(3):395-401.
63. Martínez-Fernandez P, Vallejo-de-Torres G, Sánchez-de-León-Robles MS, et al. Medical and pathologic characteristics of fatal anaphylaxis: a Spanish nationwide 17-year series. *Forensic Sci Med Pathol.* 2019;15(3):369-381.
64. McKibbin LR, Siu SK, Roberts HT, Shkrum M, Jeimy S. Fatal anaphylaxis due to peanut exposure from oral intercourse. *Allergy Asthma Clin Immunol.* 2021;17(1):110.
65. Baltzer Nielsen S, Stanislaus S, Saunamäki K, Grøndahl C, Banner J, Jørgensen MB. Can acute stress be fatal? A systematic cross-disciplinary review. *Stress.* 2019;22(3):286-294.
66. Lou J, Chen H, Huang S, Chen P, Yu Y, Chen F. Update on risk factors and biomarkers of sudden unexplained cardiac death. *J Forensic Leg Med.* 2022;87:102332.

APPENDIX F: SUMMARY

The main purpose of the autopsy in forensic pathology is to determine the cause and manner of death. Secondary purposes include documentation of the cause of death, identification of the decedent if necessary, determination of time of death if possible, and identification of features in a traumatic injury that may help identify the source of injury (eg, the weapon type). To accomplish these tasks, the forensic pathologist must utilize information from the scene investigation (to include examination of the body at the scene, witness accounts, and medical record review), the autopsy (to include the external, internal, and microscopic examinations), radiography, toxicologic analysis, and other ancillary testing (to include cultures and other microbiologic testing and vitreous electrolyte testing). The overall combination of these various types of information available to the forensic pathologist forms a pattern, which must be interpreted correctly to determine the cause and manner of death. Unfortunately, in forensic pathology, patterns often overlap, with particular pathologic findings not being specific to any one etiology and unique situations (ie, a situation not completely described in the available literature) being quite common. Therefore, understanding how to identify the pattern, understanding how to search for more findings that will allow for better distinction of that pattern, and understanding how to document that pattern so that other people can make their own independent determinations are all vital parts of being a forensic pathologist.

Forensic pathologists must always remember that while the autopsy is a useful tool, it is only one tool to help determine the cause and manner of death, and, with some causes of death, the autopsy alone is inadequate. Pollanen listed causes of death with no or potentially no anatomical findings: epilepsy, Wolff-Parkinson-White syndrome, long QT syndrome (including torsade de pointes), anaphylaxis, excited delirium, smothering, positional asphyxia, asphyxiant gas, commotio cordis, and intoxications.[1] Pollanen also listed causes of death with minimal findings: drowning, electrocution, environmental hypothermia, heat stroke, air embolism, septicemia, fatty acid oxidant disorders, fat embolism, and chronic alcoholism.[1] Each of these conditions has been discussed in this book, and the context of when to search for each, and how, potentially, to identify each. Within that list of conditions described by Pollanen,[1] epilepsy, excited delirium, smothering, positional asphyxia, commotio cordis, drowning, hypothermia and hyperthermia, and chronic alcoholism are all essentially diagnoses of exclusion. In these types of the deaths, the purpose of the autopsy is to rule out a competing cause of death. Each of the above diagnoses would then require information from the death scene investigation combined with appropriate medical history to make the final diagnosis.

The breadth of conditions that a forensic pathologist will encounter in their career as well as the morphologic spectrum of findings associated with each condition is tremendous. Three important types of resources are available to help evaluate these cases. First of all, a good reference library is useful. This reference library at a minimum often includes texts on general forensic pathology,[2-5] specific forensic pathology topics (including gunshot wounds and neck trauma),[6,7] neuropathology,[8-10] cardiac pathology,[11] pulmonary pathology,[12] liver and kidney pathology,[13,14] pediatric pathology,[15,16] general autopsy pathology,[17,18] toxicology,[19-21] anthropology,[22-25] child abuse,[26] anatomy,[27] histology,[28] general pathology,[29] general forensic science,[30] and even clinical textbooks regarding surgery, pediatrics, obstetrics, emergency medicine, wilderness medicine, and dermatology.[31] Old references are not worthless by any means. In 1963, Rezek and Millard clearly described the challenges faced with diagnosing an asphyxial death and the non-specific changes that are often misinterpreted as an asphyxial death.[17] In addition to textbooks, other references are available. The National Association of Medical Examiners' "Classification of manners of death" is a useful reference, providing specific scenarios and the recommended manner of death determination.[32] In addition to textbooks, the utilization of medical journals, which can easily be found through www.PubMed.gov, or other search engines, is also important as new information is always coming to light and our understanding of the various traumatic and non-traumatic conditions encountered at autopsy changes. And, once again, old articles have useful information. Dr. Moritz's "Classic mistakes in forensic pathology" is timeless and always worthwhile to read.[33] The final resource for a forensic pathologist is their fellow forensic pathologist. Discussing cases between colleagues can often help in understanding a challenging case by providing a different perspective.

As described throughout this book, in forensic pathology, pattern interpretation is a vital component of the process; however, correct interpretation of the pattern requires understanding that an isolated autopsy finding (eg, petechiae of the conjunctivae) can most often have more than one cause, and interpreting the pattern most often requires a combination of autopsy and scene investigation findings, supplemented with toxicologic and other analyses. While pattern interpretation is important, of equal importance is learning how to search for the pattern as well as how to adequately document that pattern. In doing so, the forensic pathologist can identify the cause and manner of death as well as be able to defend that determination to families, to law enforcement, and in both criminal and civil courts.

References

1. Pollanen MS. Forensic pathology and the miscarriage of justice. *Forensic Sci Med Pathol.* 2012;8(3):285-289.
2. Spitz WU, Diaz FJ. *Spitz and Fisher's Medicolegal Investigation of Death.* 5th ed. Charles C. Thomas; 2020.
3. DiMaio VJ, DiMaio D. *Forensic Pathology.* 3rd ed. CRC Press; 2022.
4. Fisher RS, Petty CS. *Forensic Pathology: A Handbook for Pathologists.* National Institute of Law Enforcement and Criminal Justice, Law Enforcement Assistance Administration, US Department of Justice; 1977.
5. Dolinak D, Matshes E, Lew E. *Forensic Pathology: Principles and Practice.* Elsevier Academic Press; 2005.
6. DiMaio VJM. *Gunshot Wounds.* 2nd ed. CRC Press; 1999.
7. Vanezis P. *Pathology of Neck Injury.* Butterworts; 1989.
8. Dolinak D, Matshes E. *Medicolegal Neuropathology: A Color Atlas.* CRC Press; 2002.
9. Ellison D, Love S, Chimelli L, et al. *Neuropathology: A Reference Text of CNS Pathology.* 2nd ed. Mosby; 2004.
10. Gray F, Duyckaerts C, DeGirolami U. *Escourolle and Poirier's Manual of Basic Neuropathology.* 5th ed. Oxford University Press; 2014.
11. Buja LM, Butany J. *Cardiovascular Pathology.* 4th ed. Elsevier; 2016.
12. Mukhopadhyay S. *Non-neoplastic Pulmonary Pathology: An Algorithmic Approach to Histologic Findings in the Lung.* Cambridge University Press; 2016.
13. Scheuer PJ, Lefkowitch JH. *Liver Biopsy Interpretation.* 6th ed. Saunders; 2000.
14. Kern WF, Silva FG, Laszik ZG, et al. *Atlas of Renal Pathology.* WB Saunders Company; 1999.
15. Gilbert-Barness E, Debich-Spicer DE. *Handbook of Pediatric Autopsy Pathology.* Humana Press; 2005.
16. Bundock EA, Corey TS. *Unexplained Pediatric Deaths.* Academic Forensic Pathology International; 2019.
17. Rezek PR, Millard M. *Autopsy Pathology: A Guide for Pathologists and Clinicians.* Charles C. Thomas; 1963.
18. Ludwig J. *Handbook of Autopsy Practice.* 3rd ed. Humana Press; 2002.
19. Baselt RC. *Disposition of Toxic Drugs and Chemicals in Man.* 8th ed. Biomedical Publications; 2008.
20. Dolinak D. *Forensic Toxicology: A Physiologic Perspective.* Academic Forensic Pathology; 2013.
21. Drummer OH. *The Forensic Pharmacology of Drugs of Abuse.* Arnold; 2001.
22. Haglund WD, Sorg MH. *Advances in Forensic Taphonomy.* CRC Press; 2002.
23. Haglund WD, Sorg MH. *Forensic Taphonomy: The Postmortem Fate of Human Remains.* CRC Press; 1997.
24. France DL. *Human and Nonhuman Bone Identification: A Color Atlas.* CRC Press; 2009.

25. Iscan MY, Steyn M. *The Human Skeleton in Forensic Medicine*. 3rd ed. Charles C. Thomas; 2013.
26. Kleinman PK. *Diagnostic Imaging of Child Abuse*. 2nd ed. Mosby; 1998.
27. Clemente CD. *Anatomy: A Regional Atlas of the Human Body*. 3rd ed. Urban and Schwarzenberg; 1987.
28. Sternberg SS, ed. *Histology for Pathologists*. Lippincott-Raven Publishers; 1996.
29. Kumar V, Abbas AK, Aster JC, et al. *Robbins and Kumar Basic Pathology*. 11th ed. Elsevier; 2023.
30. Geberth VJ. *Practical Homicide Investigation: Checklist and Field Guide*. 2nd ed. CRC Press; 2014.
31. Ackerman AB, Kerl H, Sanchez J, et al. *A Clinical Atlas of 101 Common Skin Diseases With Histopathologic Correlation*. Ardor Scribendi; 2000.
32. Hanzlick R, Hunsaker JC, Davis GJ. *A Guide for Manner of Death Classification*. National Association of Medical Examiners; 2002.
33. Moritz AR. Classical mistakes in forensic pathology. *Am J Clin Pathol*. 1956;26(12):1383-1397.

INDEX

Note: Page numbers followed by "f" indicate figures and "t" indicates tables.

A

Abdominal aortic aneurysm, 106–107
Abrasions
    brush-burn type, 206, 208f
    face, 219, 220f
    marginal, 306f, 308, 308f
    mechanism, 206
    muzzle, 307f, 323
    patterned, 206, 209f–210f, 409f
    postmortem, 216, 218f
    stretch, 587, 588f
    unburned gunpowder, 636–637
Abusive head trauma, 382, 382f, 394, 403
    brain swelling, 404–405
    central venous pressure, 404–405
    dysphagic choking, 405
    encephalopathy, 404
    hypermobile Ehlers-Danlos syndrome, 406
    hypoxia, 404–405
    paroxysmal coughing, 405
    retinal hemorrhage, 404
    sagittal sinus thrombus, 405
    subdural hemorrhage, 404
    Valsalva retinopathy, 404
    versus cerebral aneurysms, 392
Accidental injury, 393–395, 395f–398f
Acetaminophen toxicity, 444, 446f
Acute cholecystitis, 135, 135f
Acute endometritis-myometritis, 156
Acute esophageal necrosis. *See* Black esophagus
Acute fatty liver, of pregnancy, 156
Acute pancreatitis
    autopsy, 136
    pearls and pitfalls, 137
    risk factors for, 136
Acute pyelonephritis
    autopsy, 140, 140f
    sudden death association, 141
Acute stress, 657
Acute tubular necrosis (ATN), 565
Adipocere, 52, 53f
Aggregate bias, 648
Aging of pulmonary thromboemboli, 486, 488f–489f
Aging of skeleton
    auricular surface, 540
    cranial suture closure, 540, 542f
    determination of, 539, 541f
    pubic symphysis, 540, 542f
    rib ends, 540, 542f
Air embolism
    circumstances, 490
    examination for, 599
    identification of, 490

Algor mortis, 42–43, 43t
Allergic reaction-anaphylactic shock, 656–657, 656f
Alliterative bias, 645
ALTE. *See* Apparent life-threatening event (ALTE)
Alzheimer disease, 629, 639
    autopsy findings, 90, 91f
    diagnosis of, 76
Ambiguity effect, 645
Ammon's horn, CA1, 630, 639–640
Ammunition
    birdshot, 293, 294f, 300f
    buckshot, 293, 294f
    frangible, 293, 296f
    high-powered rifle, 293, 294f
    with plastic nose, 298, 300f
    slugs, 293, 294f
Amniotic fluid embolism, 156
    circumstances, 492
    clinical signs of, 492
    identification of, 492, 492f
Amphetamine derivatives, 503
Amyloidosis, 631, 640
Anaphylactic shock, 565
Ancestry
    determination of, 543
    morphologic analysis for, 543, 544f–546f
Anchoring bias, 645
Aneurysms
    cerebral, 392
    incidence of, 391
    location of, 391
    presentation of, 391
    ruptured berry, 613, 635
    size of, 392
4-Anilino-N-phenethylpiperidine (4-ANPP), 454
Animal activity, 63, 63f–65f, 266f
Anterior neck, dissection of, 597–598, 597f
Anthropology, 534
    age
        auricular surface, 540
        cranial suture closure, 540, 542f
        determination of, 539, 541f
        pubic symphysis, 540, 542f
        rib ends, 540, 542f
    ancestry
        determination of, 543
        morphologic analysis for, 543, 544f–546f
    biological profile, 536
    near misses, 549, 549f
    non-human *vs.* human, 534, 535f–536f
        bear paw, 534, 537f
        bones, identification of, 534, 537f

        femur with saw marks, 536, 538f
        location, 536, 538f
    sex
        cranial features of, 539, 540f
        determination of, 536
        pelvic features of, 538–539
        skeletal features of, 538, 539f
    stature, 543
    variants and natural disease
        cranium, reconstruction of, 548, 548f
        hyperostosis frontalis, 546, 547f
        metopic suture, 546, 547f
        ossified thyroid and cricoid cartilage, 546, 547f
        prominent parietal foramen, 546, 547f
        removal and defleshing, of skeletal, 548, 548f
        Wormian bone, 546, 547f
Anti-freeze, 447, 628, 639
Anus, removal of, 604, 604f
Aortic dissection
    autopsy, 105, 106f
    documentation, 105, 107f
Aortic stenosis
    autopsy, 108, 108f
    sudden death association, 108
Apparent life-threatening event (ALTE), 403
Arnold-Chiari malformations, 569
Ascertainment bias, 646–647
Aspergillus niger, 447
Asphyxia
    autoerotic, 468, 469f
    autopsy, 175
    carbon monoxide poisoning, 193–195, 194f–195f
    checklist, 174
    drowning, 195–197, 197f
    lungs, oxygen failure to, 178–180, 179f
        choking, 180–181, 180f
        entrapment, 183
        mechanical asphyxia, 181–183, 181f–182f
        positional asphyxia, 181–183, 181f–182f
        smothering, traumatic asphyxia combined with, 183
        traumatic asphyxia, 181–183, 181f–182f, 184f
        vitiated atmosphere/suffocating gases, 183
    mechanisms of, 174
    near misses, 197–201, 198f–201f
    neck, external compression of
        hanging, 184–189, 185f–190f
        strangulation, 190–193, 190f–193f
    pearls and pitfalls, 175, 177, 178

665

666 INDEX

Asphyxial homicide, 468–471, 469f–473f
Asphyxial suicide, 468–471, 469f–473f
Asphyxiation, 430
Aspiration pneumonia
   autopsy, 125, 126f
   mimics, 126
Asthma, 18f, 633, 646
   autopsy, 127, 128f
Atrioventricular nodal artery dysplasia
   autopsy, 121, 121f
   sudden death association, 121
Atrioventricular node, dissection of, 600–601, 602f
Attentional bias, 647
Atypical gunshot wound, 327–332, 330f–332f
Autoerotic asphyxia, 468, 469f
Automobile accidents. *See* Motor vehicle accidents
Autopsy
   abdominal aortic aneurysm, 106–107
   acute cholecystitis, 135, 135f
   acute pancreatitis, 136
   acute pyelonephritis, 140, 140f
   allergic reaction-anaphylactic shock, 656
   Alzheimer disease, 90, 91f
   anaphylactic shock, 565
   anti-freeze, 628, 639
   aortic dissection, 105, 106f
   aortic stenosis, 108, 108f
   asphyxial death, 510–511
   aspiration pneumonia, 125, 126f
   asthma, 127, 128f
   atrioventricular nodal artery dysplasia, 121, 121f
   Barrett esophagus, 148
   bicuspid aortic valve, 108–109, 109f
   black esophagus, 149, 149f
   bone marrow embolus, 627, 639
   carbon monoxide poisoning, 193, 194f
   cardiogenic shock, 564–565
   cardiomyopathies, 116–117, 116f
   cavernous hemangioma, 138
   cerebral edema, 567–568, 568f–570f
   cerebral infarcts, 78–79, 80f–81f
   checklist for, 7
   cholesterol crystal embolism, 494, 494f
   chorioamnionitis, 559, 560f
   chronic rheumatic mitral valvulitis, 110, 110f
   chronic traumatic encephalopathy (CTE), 88–89
   colloid cyst, 92, 629, 639
   coronary artery aneurysm, 107, 108f
   coronary artery anomalies, 118
   coronary artery atherosclerosis, 93, 94f–95f, 95
   coronary artery dissection, 105, 107f
   cusp, endocardial fibrosis subjacent to, 620, 637
   death certification, 24
   death, manner of, 9
   decomposition, 619, 637
   dehydration, 412, 502
   diabetes mellitus type 2, 631, 640
   diffuse fatty liver, 129–130, 130f–131f
   diffuse Lewy body disease, 90–91
   documentation, 10
   drug overdose, 444–447
   elder abuse, 526, 527f
   elevated intracranial pressure, 622, 637
   emphysema, 126, 127f
   encephalitis, 91, 92f
   endocarditis, 111, 112f
   esophageal inlet patch, 147, 147f
   excited delirium syndrome, 519
   fatal dog attack, 435, 436f
   fat emboli, 491
   firearm injury, 305, 305f, 320
   Fitz-Hugh-Curtis syndrome, 135, 135f
   fly eggs, 610, 634
   food/medication, ingested, 609, 633
   globus pallidus/basal ganglia necrosis, 86, 87f
   green colon, 152, 152f
   hantavirus infection, 654–655, 655f
   Hashimoto thyroiditis, 144
   heart, 630, 640
   hemolytic uremic syndrome (HUS), 153, 154f
   hemorrhage, 382, 383f
      discoloration, of upper eyelids, 617, 636
   histologic examination
      brain, 478–479, 479f
      death, causes of, 476, 477f
      frequency of, 476–477
      pearls and pitfalls, 477–478, 479f
      traumatic injuries, 477
   hospital permit validity, 7
   hospital *vs.* forensic, 6, 6t–7t
   human teeth, 552
   hyperglycemia, 503
   hypertension, 626, 639
   hypertensive heart disease, 93
   hyperthermia, 424–425, 425f
   hyponatremia, 503
   hypothermia, 426–428
      frost erythema, 429–430
      gross and microscopic, 426, 427f–428f
      pancreatic adenoid cells, vacuolation of, 430
      proximal convoluted tubular epithelial cells, 430
      Wischnewski spots, 429
   hypovolemic shock
      blood loss, 564
      causes of, 564
      mechanism, 564
   incompetent diaphragm sella, 82
   interatrial septum, lipomatous hypertrophy of, 119–120, 119f
   intestinal diverticula, 150
   intracerebral hemorrhage, 76, 77f–78f
   intravenous drug use, 627, 639
   ischemic colitis, 150, 151f
   ketoacidosis, 504
   keyhole-type entrance gunshot wound, 612, 634
   lacunar infarct, 81
   liver, cirrhosis of, 132
   lymphocytic hypophysitis, 652
   malnourishment, 412
   meconium aspiration, 561, 561f
   meningitis, 84, 84f–85f
   Mesothelioma of the atrioventricular node, 653
   motor vehicle accidents, 584, 589, 611, 634
   multiple sclerosis, 88
   myasthenia gravis, 651
   myocarditis, 114, 114f
   myxomatous mitral valve, 109–110, 109f
   Naegleria fowleri meningitis, 654, 655f
   natural disease
      central nervous system, 76
      obesity, 75–76
   near misses, 479–480, 480f, 570, 570f
   nephrosclerosis, 139, 140f
   neurogenic shock, 565
   non-ischemic left ventricular scar, 120, 120f
   organ removal at, 8
   osmotic demyelination syndrome, 86, 87f
   parathyroid adenoma, 653
   parathyroid gland hyperplasia, 653
   pearls and pitfalls, 8–9
   peptic ulcer, 150, 150f
   pericarditis, 113, 113f
   pheochromocytoma, 144
   pituitary gland, infarction of, 142, 144f
   placenta, 559
      abruption, 560, 560f
   pneumonia, 123, 124f
   postmortem clot, 609, 634
   pulmonary thromboembolus, 618, 636
   rabies, 654, 655f
   red discoloration of the knees, 626, 638
   report, writing, 641–643
      checklist, 641
      internal examination, 642
      near miss, 643
      pre-formatted, 642
      separate injuries section, 642
   resuscitation, 621, 637
   Rocky Mountain spotted fever, 655
   ruptured berry aneurysm, 613, 635
   schizophrenia, 651
   seizure disorder, 89, 90f, 629, 639
   septic embolism, 493, 493f
   septic shock, 565
   with shock, 565, 566f–567f
   snake bite, 655–656
   snow immersion, 430
   splenic capsule, fibrosis of, 154–155, 154f
   subarachnoid hemorrhage, 82
   suicide, 471
   three or more contiguous ribs fractured, in two or more locations, 624, 638
   thrombotic thrombocytopenic purpura (TTP), 153
   thyroglossal duct cyst, 652
   tin foil with charred area, 612, 634
   toxins and poisons, 657
   treatment-related, 574–580
   vertebral artery laceration, 625, 638
   Wernicke-Korsakoff syndrome, 651
   West Nile virus myelitis, 654
   Wolff-Parkinson-White (WPW) syndrome, 653
Availability bias, 645
Avulsion fracture, 263

B

Back, dissection of, 599–600, 600f
Bandwagon effect, 645
Barotrauma, 433

Barrett esophagus
   autopsy, 148
   pearls and pitfalls, 148, 148f
Basal ganglia necrosis, 86, 87f
Basilar fracture, 225, 225f–226f
Bed-sharing, sudden unexpected infant death, 512
Belief bias, 645
Bell mania, 519
Bevel, exit gunshot wound in, 312, 314f
Bias, 645
   alliterative, 645
   anchoring, 645
   ascertainment, 646–647
   availability, 645
   belief, 645
   closure, 647
   confirmation, 645–646
   expectation, 646
   false consensus, 646
   gender, 646–647
   hindsight, 647
   information, 647
   outcome, 647
   overconfidence, 647–648
   reactance, 648
   search satisficing, 648
Bicuspid aortic valve
   autopsy, 108–109, 109f
   sudden death association, 109
Biologic profile, 543
Birdshot, 293, 294f, 300f
Bite mark, 290f
   analysis, 435
   evaluation of, 552
Black esophagus
   associations, 149
   autopsy, 149, 149f
Black thyroid, 145, 146f
Black widow bite, 437
Blind spot bias, 648
Bloating, 57, 57f–58f
Blood urea nitrogen (BUN), 502
Blunt force injuries, 348f
   abrasions, 206, 208, 208f–209f, 210f, 216, 217f
   contusions, 209, 211, 211f,–212f, 216, 217f
   documentation of, 216–217, 249–250
   extremities, 255
   fractures, 214
   head, 219, 220f–221f
   lacerations, 211, 213, 213f
   near misses, 268–269, 268f–269f
   neck, 250–251, 250f–251f
   pattern interpretation of, 214–215, 214f
   subgaleal hemorrhage, 219, 221–222, 221f
   trunk, 252–255, 254f
Body, physical findings on
   challenges, 36–37
   method, 36
Bone/cartilage, sharp force injuries, 286–287
   bony defects, 284–285, 285f
   class characteristics, identifying, 286
   pearls and pitfalls, 284, 286, 287–288, 287f–288f
Bone marrow embolus, 490, 491f, 627, 639
Bone trauma, timing of, 264–267
Brain autopsy, 478–479, 479f

Brain swelling, 404–405
Bronchopneumonia, 447
Brugada syndrome, 654
Bruising, 408–411, 408f–411f
Buckshot, 293, 294f, 333f
Bullet embolism, 493, 493f
Burns, 411
Butterfly fracture, 261–262, 262f

C

Carbon dioxide, poisoning of, 616, 636
Carbon monoxide, poisoning of
   autopsy, 193, 194f
   description, 193
   pearls and pitfalls, 195
Carboxyhemoglobin (COHb), 366–368
Cardiac conduction system, lesions of, 120–121
Cardiac myxoma, 494
Cardiogenic shock, 564–565
Cardiomyopathies, 447
   autopsy, 116–117, 116f
   cardiac dilation, 117
   mimics of, 117, 117f
   pearls and pitfalls, 118
   sudden death association, 117
Cardiopulmonary resuscitation (CPR), 398–400, 400f, 576
   bone marrow embolus, 627, 639
Cardiovascular system
   long QT syndrome (LQTS), 654
   Mesothelioma of the atrioventricular node, 653
   natural disease of, 92
   pearls and pitfalls, 92
   torsade de pointes, 654
   Wolff-Parkinson-White (WPW) syndrome, 653
Cards, identification
   challenges, 37
   method, 37
Catecholaminergic polymorphic ventricular tachycardia (CPvT), 654
Cavernous hemangioma
   autopsy, 138
   sudden death association, 138
Central venous pressure, 404–405
Centrilobular necrosis, of liver, 614, 635
Cerebellum, red neurons in, 568, 570f
Cerebral aneurysm, 392
Cerebral edema, 382, 383f, 445, 446f, 503. *See also* Herniation
   autopsy, 567–568, 568f–570f
Cerebral infarcts
   autopsy, 78–79, 80f–81f
   pearls and pitfalls, 79, 81f
Cervical vertebral column, dissection of, 598
Charcot-Leyden crystals, 633
Cheek, abrasions of, 412, 412f
Chest
   close range gunshot wound of, 308, 309f
   compression of, 576
   flail, 218, 254f, 586–587
   Tardieu spots, 49f
Child abuse
   abusive head trauma, 382, 382f, 403
   brain swelling, 404–405

   central venous pressure, 404–405
   dysphagic choking, 405
   encephalopathy, 404
   hypermobile Ehlers-Danlos syndrome, 406
   hypoxia, 404–405
   paroxysmal coughing, 405
   retinal hemorrhage, 404
   sagittal sinus thrombus, 405
   subdural hemorrhage, 404
   Valsalva retinopathy, 404
   accidental injury, 393–395, 395f–398f
   aneurysms
      incidence of, 391
      location of, 391
      presentation of, 391
      size of, 392
   axonal spheroids in, 382, 382f
   bruising and lacerations, 408–411, 408f–411f
   burns, 411
   coagulation disorders, 392–393
   congenital heart disease, 389
   dehydration, 412
   diastatic fracture, 382, 383f
   forehead, close-range gunshot wound of, 380, 380f
   fractures, 406–407, 407f
   galactosemia, 389
   glutaric aciduria type I, 389
   hypernatremia, 392
   inflicted head injury in, 382, 382f
   inflicted head trauma
      versus apparent life-threatening event (ALTE), 403
      versus falls, 401–402
      with rib fractures, 395–400, 399f–401f
   leukemia, 389
   malnourishment, 412
   meningitis, 389
   near misses, 412–416, 412f–416f
   neurosurgical complications, 391
   peritonitis, 380, 380f
   retinal hemorrhages
      backlit sectioned eyes, 387, 387f
      differential diagnosis of, 389, 390t
      distribution of, 387, 388f
      importance, 386
      location, 387–388
      microscopic images of, 387, 388f
      photographically documenting, 387, 387f
   retinoschisis, 389, 389f
   shaken baby syndrome, 380–381
   subdural hemorrhage
      differential diagnosis of, 389, 390t
      space-occupying, 383, 386f
      thin-film, 383, 384f–385f
   suspicious infant death, 381
   traumatic labor, 391
Choking
   autopsy, 180–181
   description, 180, 180f
   pearls and pitfalls, 181
Cholesterol crystal embolism, 494, 494f
Chop wound
   description, 281, 282f
   pearls and pitfalls, 281, 282f–283f

Chorioamnionitis
    autopsy, 559, 560f
    potential mimics, 560
Chronic alcoholism, 456, 624, 638
Chronic rheumatic mitral valvulitis
    autopsy, 110, 110f
    potential mimic, 110, 110f
Chronic traumatic encephalopathy (CTE)
    autopsy, 88–89
    pearls and pitfalls, 89
Circumstantial identification, 30
Closed scissors, 610, 634
Closure bias, 647
Coagulation disorders, 392–393
Cocaine, 447
Codeine, 449
Colloid cyst, 92, 629, 639
Comminuted fracture, 227, 227f, 261
Communicating hydrocephalus, 624, 638
Complete fractures, 259–261
Complex fractures, 224, 224f
Complex skull fracture, 406, 407f
Computed tomography (CT), 313, 433
Conducted electrical weapons, 520–521
Confirmation bias, 645–646
Congenital heart disease, 389
Congested conjunctivae, 178f
Conjunctival edema, 444, 445f
Conjunctival petechiae, 579
Contact entrance gunshot wound, 620, 637
Contrast effect, 646
Contre-coup contusions, 240–241, 241f–244f
Contusions, 209, 211, 211f, 212f, 216, 217f
    contre-coup, 240–241, 241f–244f
    coup, 240, 241f
    fracture, 242
    gliding, 246, 247f–248f
    herniation, 242, 244f–245f
    intermediary, 246, 246f
    pearls and pitfalls, 249
Copper-jacketed projectile, 343, 343f
Coral snake injury
    clinical features of, 436
    pathologic features of, 436
Corneal clouding, 54
Coronary artery aneurysm
    associations, 107
    autopsy, 107, 108f
Coronary artery anomalies
    anomalous origin of
        autopsy, 118
        sudden death association, 118
    tunneling/bridging of
        autopsy, 119, 119f
        sudden death association, 119
Coronary artery atherosclerosis
    acute myocardial infarct
        complications of, 102–103, 103f
        gross and microscopic aging of, 96–101, 99f–101f
        pearls and pitfalls, 101, 102f
    autopsy, 93, 94f–95f, 95
    death certificate, 104–105
    documentation of, 96
    sudden death association, 96
Coronary artery dissection
    associations, 105

autopsy, 105, 107f
    pearls and pitfalls, 105
Coup contusions, 240, 241f
CPR. See Cardiopulmonary resuscitation (CPR)
Cranial fractures, 413f
    basilar fracture, 225, 225f–226f
    comminuted fracture, 227, 227f
    depressed fracture, 224, 224f–225f
    diastatic fracture, 227–228, 228f
    linear fracture, 223–224, 223f
    pearls and pitfalls, 226, 227f
    ring fracture, 225, 225f
    stellate/complex fracture, 224, 224f
Cranial injury, farming accident, 310, 311f
Craniocerebral trauma, 394
Craniocerebrocervical trauma, 394
Cranium, exit gunshot wound in, 312, 314f
Crohn disease, 609, 633
Cytochrome P450 (CYP) enzymes, 450

D

DAI. See Diffuse axonal injury (DAI)
Death. See also specific types
    cause of, 22, 24, 476, 477f
    determination time, 62, 63f
    manner of, 9, 23, 25
    mechanism of, 23
Death certification, 25–26
    autopsy, 24
    cause of, 365
    death, cause of, 22, 24
    death, manner of, 23, 25
    death, mechanism of, 23
    gunshot wound for, 323
    near miss, 26
    pearls and pitfalls, 23, 25–26
Death scene investigation
    basics of, 12–14
    checklist, 13–14
    discovery history and terminal events documentation, 17–18, 17f
    importance of, 14
    near misses, 18–19
    pearls and pitfalls, 15, 17–18
    photography, 14
    postmortem changes, documentation of, 15, 16f
Decomposition, 619, 637
    adipocere, 52, 53f
    corneal clouding, 54
    factors affecting, 51
    hemolysis, 54
    marbling, 54
    mummification and postmortem drying, 54, 55f
    pearls and pitfalls, 54, 55, 56, 56f, 57f
    postmortem blisters, 53, 53f
    postmortem bullae, 53, 53f
    skin, green discoloration of, 52, 52f–53f
    skin slippage, 56, 56f
    stages of, 59t
    swelling/bloating, 57, 57f–58f
    tache noire, 59, 59f
Decubitus ulcers, 529f
    causes, 528
    classification of, 529
    complications of, 530

pearls and pitfalls, 530
    risk factors for, 528
Deep vein thrombus, 495, 495f
Defensive-type injuries, 466, 467f
Dehydration, 44, 412
    autopsy, 424, 502
Delirious mania, 519
Dental examination, 553
    requirements, 35
    time frame, 35
Depressed fracture, 224, 224f–225f
Dermal melanosis, 410f
Diabetes mellitus (DM), 142, 143f, 631, 640
Diabetic ketoacidosis, 617, 636
Diagnosis momentum, 646
Diaper rash, 415f
Diastatic fracture, 227–228, 228f
Diffuse axonal injury (DAI), 382
Diffuse fatty liver
    autopsy, 129–130, 130f–131f
    death, cause of, 130
    potential mimics, 131, 132f
Diffuse injury, 386
Diffuse Lewy body disease, 90–91
Disseminated intravascular coagulation (DIC), 153, 153f
Distal femoral fracture, in infant, 416f
DNA analysis
    requirements, 34, 34f
    time frame, 35
Documentation, 339f
    aortic dissection, 105
    autopsy, 10
    blunt force injuries, 216–217, 249–250
    coronary artery atherosclerosis, 96
    discovery history, 17–18, 17f
    postmortem changes, 15, 16f
    stab wound, 274, 275f–277f
    terminal events, 17–18, 17f
Dog attacks, 434–435, 435f–436f
Dog mauling, 435, 435f
Doll re-enactment, 508, 509f
Dorsal root ganglia, 396f
    hemorrhage in, 397f, 413f
Double-edged knife, 610, 634
Drowning
    autopsy, 194f–195f, 195
    description, 195
    diagnosis, 196
    freshwater vs. salt water, 197
    pearls and pitfalls, 195–197
    suicide by, 439f
    water immersion, 196
Drug overdose, 444
    acetaminophen toxicity, 444, 446f
    autopsy, 444–447
    baggie, in stomach, 445, 447f
    cerebral edema, 445, 446f
    death, cause of, 444, 452
    death, manner of, 452
    external findings of, 444, 445f
    foreign material, in lung, 447, 448f
    oronasal foam cones, 444, 445f
    oxalic acid, in kidney, 447, 448f
    track marks, 444, 446f
Drugs, metabolites of, 454, 454t
Dust cleaners, 453
Dysphagic choking, 405

E

Ear, gunshot wound of, 352f–353f
Ectopic pregnancy, 157, 158f
Edema, conjunctival, 444, 445f
Elder abuse, 526
   decubitus ulcers, 529f
      causes, 528
      classification of, 529
      complications of, 530
      pearls and pitfalls, 530
      risk factors for, 528
   forms of, 526
   near misses, 530–531, 530f
   risk factors for, 526
      autopsy, 526, 527f
   senile ecchymoses, 528, 528f
Electrocution, 434, 439f
   gross appearance, 434, 434f
   microscopic appearance, 434, 435f
Embalming artifacts, 65–66, 66f–67f
Embolism, 484
   air
      circumstances, 490
      identification of, 490
   amniotic fluid
      circumstances, 492
      clinical signs of, 492
      identification of, 492, 492f
   bullet, 493
   cholesterol crystal, 494, 494f
   fat
      circumstances, 490
      clinical signs of, 490
      identification of, 490, 491f
      pearls and pitfalls, 491
   near misses, 496, 496f–497f
   other forms of, 494–495, 495f
   pulmonary thromboembolus
      aging of, 486, 488f–489f
      circumstances, 484
      complications of, 484–486, 486f–488f
      identification of, 484, 485f–486f
   septic, 493, 493f
Emphysema
   autopsy, 126, 127f
   pearls and pitfalls, 127–128
Encephalitis
   autopsy, 91, 92f
   pearls and pitfalls, 91
Encephalopathy, 404
Endocarditis
   associations of, 111, 113f
   autopsy, 111, 112f
Endocrine system
   lymphocytic hypophysitis, 652
   natural disease of, 142
   parathyroid adenoma, 653, 653f
   parathyroid gland hyperplasia, 653
   thyroglossal duct cyst, 652
Entrance gunshot wounds, 301, 301f
   damaged head with, 336f
   decomposed body, 327f
   decomposition preclude identification of, 322
   determination of, 312
   features, 316
   for handguns/rifles, 306, 306f–311f, 308–310
   head, 309, 310f
   marginal abrasion, 325f
   muzzle abrasion, 316, 323f
   shotguns and relative range of fire, 332–336, 333f–336f
   soot deposition on skin, 316, 320f–321f
   surgical intervention, 309
Entrapment
   autopsy, 183
   description, 183
Environmental deaths, 424
   animal attack, 437
   dog attacks, 434–435, 435f–436f
   electrocution, 434, 434f–435f
   high-altitude cerebral edema, 437
   high-altitude pulmonary edema, 437
   hyperthermia, 424
      autopsy, 424–425, 425f
      exogenous, 425
      heat stroke, 424
      infant/child, left inside a car, 426
   hypothermia, 426
      autopsy, 426–428
      certification of death, 429
   near misses, 438–439, 438f–439f
   scuba diving-related deaths
      barotrauma, 433
      causes of, 432–433
      gas embolism, 433
   snake bite, 436
   snow immersion, 430
   spider bite, 437
   water, bodies found in, 430
      cardiovascular disease, 431
      environmental and human factors, 431
      postmortem artifacts, 432, 432f–433f
Epidural hemorrhage, 228–230, 229f
Esophageal inlet patch
   autopsy, 147, 147f
   potential mimics, 148
Esophagus, examination of, 602, 603f
Ethanol, 454–456
Ethylene glycol, ingestion of, 447
Excited delirium syndrome, 519
   autopsy, 519
   checklist of, 519
   diagnosis of, 520
   features of, 519
Exclusionary identification, 30
Exit gunshot wounds, 614, 635
   decomposed body, 327f
   decomposition preclude identification of, 322
   determination of, 312
   features, 316
   with gunpowder, 306, 307f
   handguns/rifles, 310, 312–313, 312f–319f, 316
   head, 309, 310f
   misconception, 309
   shotguns and relative range of fire, 332–336, 333f–336f
   surgical intervention, 309
Expectation bias, 646
Explosion-related deaths, 374
External injuries, resuscitation attempts, 575, 575f
Extra-cerebral hemorrhage
   epidural hemorrhage, 228–230, 229f
   subarachnoid hemorrhage, 235–239, 237f–239f
   subdural hemorrhage, 230–234, 232f–233f, 232t, 234t, 235f
Eyes, 178f, 206f
   close range gunshot wound of, 310, 311f
   dissection of, 596–597
   on light stand, 387f
   retinoschisis, 389
   tan plastic cap on, 66f

F

Falls, 401–402
False consensus bias, 646
Fat embolism
   circumstances, 490
   clinical signs of, 490
   identification of, 490, 491f
   pearls and pitfalls, 491
Female genitalia
   contusion of, 415f
   en bloc removal of, 604, 604f
Femur, gunshot wound, 313, 315f
Fentanyl, 449, 452
Fingerprints
   pearls and pitfalls, 34
   requirements, 33
   time frame, 33
Firearm injuries
   entrance and exit wounds, 332–336, 333f–336f
   evaluation of, 292
   external examination, 299
      autopsy, 305, 305f
      close range gunshot wound, 302, 302f
      entrance wound, 301, 301f
      gunshot residue testing, 304–305
      head, 302, 302f–304f
      intra-oral shotgun wound, 303, 304f
      self-inflicted shotgun wound, 302, 302f
   gunshot wounds, 306
      death determination, manner of, 344–346, 344f–347f
      death, mechanism of, 340–342, 341f–342f
      entrance wounds, 306, 306f–311f, 308–310
      exit wounds, 310, 312–313, 312f–319f, 316
      range of fire, 316–323, 320f–323f, 324t, 325f–327f
      special types of, 325–332, 328f–332f
   internal examination
      cranium, endocranial surface of, 340, 340f
      documentation of, 338, 339f
      hand, 337, 338f
      head, 337, 337f
      microscopic examination, for soot, 339, 339f
      orbital plates fracture, 337, 338f
      temporary cavity, 337
      wrist, 337, 338f
   near misses, 346–351, 348f–353f

Firearm injuries (*Continued*)
  projectiles, composition of, 342–343, 343f–344f
  radiography, 299f
    0.25 ACP Winchester Expanding Point ammunition, 293, 295f
    birdshot, 293, 294f, 300f
    buckshot, 293, 294f
    copper and lead, 293, 293f, 298
    frangible ammunition, 293, 296f
    Glaser round, 293, 295f
    gunshot wound of neck, 298, 301f
    in head, 296, 297f
    hemothorax, 292, 293f
    high-powered rifle ammunition, 293, 294f
    intra-oral gunshot wound, 296, 298f
    Liberty Ammunition Civil Defense round, 293, 297f
    lower extremity, 297, 299f
    plastic nose, ammunition with, 298, 300f
    pneumothorax, 292, 293f
    purposes of, 292
    shotgun at close range, 298, 300f
    shotgun slug, 293, 294f
    snakeshot, 293, 295f
Fire deaths, 361f
  autopsy, 368–369, 369f–371f
  carboxyhemoglobin (COHb), 366–368
  checklist, 361
  death certification, cause of, 365
  explosion-related deaths, 374
  flash fire description, 367, 367f
  heat-related fractures, 371–373, 372f–373f
  near misses, 375, 375f–378f
  orthopedic hardware, 360, 360f
  pearls and pitfalls, 361, 362f, 365, 366f, 373–374, 374f
  thermal injury, 365, 365f
Fitz-Hugh-Curtis syndrome, autopsy, 135, 135f
Flail chest, 586–587, 587f
Flash fire, 367, 367f
Fly eggs, 610, 634
Foot, gunshot wound of, 310, 311f
Fordisc™ program, 543
Forensic pathology, pattern interpretation in, 1–3
Fournier gangrene, 141
Fractures, 214, 255–257. See also specific types
  antemortem fractures, 265
  avulsion, 263
  butterfly, 261–262, 262f
  classification, 257–258, 258t
  comminuted, 261
  complete, 259–261
  contusions, 242
  greenstick, 259
  incomplete, 258
  longitudinal, 261
  oblique, 260
  perimortem injuries, 265–267
  postmortem fractures, 265, 268f
  segmental, 262, 263f
  specific types, 257–258
  spiral, 261
  terminology, 257–258
  torus/buckle, 259
  transverse, 259–260
Framing effect, 646
Frangible ammunition, 293, 296f
Frenulum, laceration of, 411, 411f
Frost erythema, 429–430
Funisitis, 559, 560f

G

Galactosemia, 389
Gambler's fallacy, 646
Gas embolism, 433
Gastrointestinal hemorrhage, 146f
Gastrointestinal system, natural disease of, 145, 146f
Gender bias, 646–647
Glaser round, 293, 295f, 298
Glasgow Coma Scale, 394
Gliding contusions, 246, 247f–248f
Globus pallidus, 86–88, 87f
Glutaric aciduria type I, 389
Graze wound, 326, 328f
Green colon, 152, 152f
  autopsy, 152, 152f
  pearls and pitfalls, 152
  potential mimic, 152
Greenstick fractures, 259
Gunshot residue testing, 304–305
Gunshot wounds
  chest with aspiration of blood, 615, 635
  close range, 302, 302f
  death
    certificate, 323
    determination manner, 344–346, 344f–347f
    mechanism of, 340–342, 341f–342f
  description in report, 322–323
  documenting, 346
  entrance, 306, 306f–311f, 308–310
  exit, 310, 312–313, 312f–319f, 316
  fire, range of, 316–323, 320f–323f, 324t, 325f–327f
  homicide vs. suicide, 465–466
  with intervening object, 623, 638
  keyhole-type entrance, 612, 634
  kinetic energy transfer and damage from gases, 625, 638
  neck, 298, 301f
  scientific terminology, 323
  special types, 325
    graze, 326, 328f
    re-entrance wound/atypical, 327–332, 330f–332f
    shored exit, 326, 328f
    superficial perforating, 327, 330f
    tangential, 326–327, 329f
  terminology used for, 324t
  unburned gunpowder, abrasions from, 619, 636–637

H

Handgun wounds, 292
  ammunition, 293
  cause of death for, 336
  entrance wounds, 306, 306f–311f, 308–310
  exit wounds, 310, 312–313, 312f–319f, 316
  small-caliber, 292
Hands, 46f, 215f
  defensive type injuries of, 288f, 345f
  gunshot wound of, 337, 338f
  mummification of, 55f
  rust colored deposit on, 347f
Hanging
  autopsy, 184–185, 185f–187f
  description, 184
  pearls and pitfalls, 188–189, 188f–189f
Hantavirus infection, 654–655, 655f
Hashimoto thyroiditis
  autopsy, 144
  sudden death association, 144
Hawthorne effect, 647
Head, firearm injuries
  contusions, in gunshot wound, 337, 337f
  entrance wounds of, 309, 310f
  exit wounds of, 310, 313f
  external examination, 302, 302f–304f
  radiography, 296, 297f
Heart
  acute myocardial infarct, 103f
  incidental and microscopic findings in
    basophilic degeneration, 122, 122f
    contraction band necrosis, 122, 122f
    lymphocytes, clusters of, 121
    sarcoidosis of, 101f
Heat-related fractures, 371–373, 372f–373f
Heat stroke, 424–425. See also Hyperthermia
HELLP syndrome, 157, 157f
Hemangioma, of skin, 411f
Hematolymphoid system, natural disease of, 153
Hemolysis, 54
Hemolytic uremic syndrome (HUS), 153, 154f
Hemorrhages, 382, 383f
  in dorsal root ganglia, 397f
  intracranial, 392
  Menkes disease, 390
  optic nerve sheath, 389, 389f
  preretinal, 388
  retinal
    backlit sectioned eyes, 387, 387f
    differential diagnosis of, 389, 390t
    distribution of, 387, 388f
    importance, 386
    location, 387–388
    microscopic images of, 387, 388f
    photographically documenting, 387, 387f
  subarachnoid, 383, 385f, 597
  subdural, 391f
    differential diagnosis of, 389, 390t
    space-occupying, 383, 386f
    thin-film, 383, 384f–385f
  subendocardial, 424, 425f
  subgaleal, 383
  subretinal, 388
Hemothorax, 292, 293f, 608, 633
Hepatobiliary system, natural disease of, 129
Herniation
  of cerebellar tonsils, 568
  with cerebral edema, 568, 569f
  complications of, 568, 570f

contusions, 242, 244f–245f
transtentorial, 568
Heroin, 453
Hesitation marks, 466, 467f
High-altitude cerebral edema, 437
High-altitude pulmonary edema, 437
High-voltage electrocution,
434, 434f
Hindsight bias, 647
Hit-and-run, 585, 585f
Homicides, 344f
child abuse, 403
vs. suicides
asphyxial, 468–471, 469f–473f
gunshot wounds, 465–466
sharp force injuries, 466–468, 467f
weapon, 345
Hospital autopsy permit validity, 7
Human dentition, 552
Hyperglycemia, 503
Hyperinflated lungs, 607, 633
Hypermobile Ehlers-Danlos syndrome, 406
Hypernatremia, 392
Hypertension, 626, 639
Hypertensive heart disease
autopsy, 93
death, cause of, 93
pearls and pitfalls, 93
sudden death association, 93
Hyperthermia, 424
autopsy, 424–425, 425f
exogenous, 425
heat stroke, 424
infant/child, left inside a car, 426
Hypoglycemia, 504
Hyponatremia
autopsy, 503
causes of, 503
clinical features of, 503
Hypothermia, 1, 426, 438f, 626, 638
autopsy, 426–428
frost erythema, 429–430
gross and microscopic, 426,
427f–428f
pancreatic adenoid cells, vacuolation of,
430
proximal convoluted tubular epithelial
cells, 430
Wischnewski spots, 429
certification of death, 429
scene investigative features in, 428
Hypovolemic shock
blood loss, 564
causes of, 564
mechanism, 564
Hypoxia, 404–405
Hypoxic ischemic encephalopathy,
568, 570f

I

Identification
body, physical findings on
challenges, 36–37
method, 36
cards
challenges, 37
method, 37
circumstantial identification, 30

dental examination
requirements, 35
time frame, 35
DNA analysis
requirements, 34, 34f
time frame, 35
exclusionary identification, 30
fingerprints
pearls and pitfalls, 34
requirements, 33
time frame, 33
near miss, 39–40, 39f
non-scientific methods of, 36
other methods, 38
pearls and pitfalls, 37
personal effects, 38
positive identification, 30–33
presumptive identification, 30
scientific identification, other forms of, 35,
35f–36f
scientific methods to, 33
tentative identification, 30
visual identification, 36
challenges, 36
method, 36
Illicit substances, 454
Illusory correlation, 647
Immunoglobulin E (IgE), 656
Incidental liver masses, 138, 139f
Incidental renal masses
adenoma, 141
adrenal gland rest, 141
renal cell carcinoma, 141
renomedullary interstitial cell tumor, 141, 142f
Incised wound
description, 279–280, 280f
pearls and pitfalls, 280–281
Incomplete fractures, 258
In-custody deaths
checklist for, 518
conducted electrical weapons, 520–521
death, manner of, 521
electronic control devices, 520–521
excited delirium syndrome, 519
autopsy, 519
checklist of, 519
diagnosis of, 520
features of, 519
pearls and pitfalls, 518
prone restraint cardiac arrest, 520
restraint asphyxia, 520
types of, 518
Infectious conditions
hantavirus, 654–655, 655f
Naegleria fowleri meningitis, 654, 655f
rabies, 654, 655f
Rocky Mountain spotted fever, 655
West Nile virus myelitis, 654
Inflicted head injury, in infants, 382
Inflicted head trauma, 394
versus apparent life-threatening event
(ALTE), 403
versus falls, 401–402
with rib fractures, 395–400, 399f–401f
Information bias, 647
Interatrial septum, lipomatous hypertrophy of
autopsy, 119–120, 119f
sudden death association, 120

Intermediary contusions, 246, 246f
Internal injuries, resuscitation attempts, 576,
576f–578f
Intestinal diverticula, 150
Intracerebral hemorrhage, 626, 639
autopsy, 76, 77f–78f
with endocarditis, 415f
etiologies of, 78, 79f
pearls and pitfalls, 76
Intracranial hemorrhage, 392
Intra-oral handgun wound, 303, 304f
Intra-thoracic petechiae, 511, 512f
Intravenous drug use, 627, 639
Intubation, 576, 576f
ulcers, 577f
Ischemic colitis
autopsy, 150, 151f
potential mimic, 150, 151f
Isopropyl alcohol, 504

K

Ketoacidosis, 1, 504–505
Ketones, 504
Keyhole defects, 313, 319f
Keyhole-type entrance gunshot wound,
612, 634
Kidney, oxalic acid in, 447, 448f

L

Labor, traumatic, 391
Lacerations, 211, 213, 213f, 408–411,
408f–411f
of liver, 580, 580f
occipital region, of scalp, 616, 636
vertebral artery, 625, 638
Lacunar infarct, 81
Lead projectile, 343, 343f–344f
Leukemia, 389
Linear fracture, 223–224, 223f
Linear skull fracture, 406, 407f
Liver
centrilobular necrosis of, 614, 635
cirrhosis of
autopsy, 132
bleeding, risk factor for, 134
complications of, 133–134, 133f
pearls and pitfalls, 132, 133f, 134, 135f
potential mimics, 132
sudden cardiac death, 134
laceration of, 580, 580f
Lividity, 49–51
other uses of, 50
pearls and pitfalls, 50
Tardieu spots, 49, 49f–50f
Livor mortis, 46–48, 46f–47f, 49t
Longitudinal fracture, 261
Long QT syndrome (LQTS), 519, 654
Lower extremities, dissection of, 585, 586f,
600
Lungs
body position, 608, 633
foreign material in, 447, 448f
hyperinflated, 607, 633
incidental microscopic findings in
corpora amylacea, 128, 129f
lentils, 128, 129f
pulmonary chemodectoma, 128, 129f
Lymphocytic hypophysitis, 652

M

Macerated infant brain, underwater removal of, 603
Magnetic resonance imaging (MRI), 313, 433
Mallory-Weiss laceration, 147f
Malnourishment, 412
Marbling, 54
Marginal abrasion, 313, 321, 325f
Mass disasters, 556
Mechanical asphyxia
    autopsy, 183, 184f
    description, 181, 182f
Meconium, 449
    aspiration, 561, 561f
Mendosal sutures, 413f
Meningitis, 389
    autopsy, 84, 84f–85f
    pearls and pitfalls, 84–85
    potential mimics, 85, 86f
Menkes disease, 390
Mere exposure effect, 645
Mesothelioma of the atrioventricular node, 653
Methadone overdose, 445, 446f
Methamphetamine, 238, 453
    pulmonary hypertension, 447
    toxicity, 618, 636
Middle ears, dissection of, 596, 596f
Motor vehicle accidents, 584
    atlanto-occipital fracture/dislocation, 587, 588f
    basilar skull fracture, 586, 587f
    checklist for, 584
    delayed death, 592
        splenic laceration, 592, 592f
    flail chest, 586–587, 587f
    hit-and-run, 585, 585f
    internal injuries, confirmation of, 589, 591f
    lower extremities, dissection of, 585, 586f
    near misses, 592, 592f
    scene investigation of, 584, 585f
    seatbelt injuries, 589, 590f
    stretch abrasions/lacerations, 587–592, 591f–592f
        gross description, 587, 588f
    transection of the aorta, 586, 586f
Multiple alternative bias, 648
Multiple gunshot wounds, 336, 338f
Multiple injuries, in suicides, 471f
Multiple remote rib fractures, 406, 407f
Multiple sclerosis, 623, 638
    autopsy, 88
    pearls and pitfalls, 88
Mummification, 54, 55f
Musculoskeletal system, natural disease of, 155
Muzzle abrasion, 306, 307f, 325f, 622, 638
    at entrance wound, 316, 323f
Myasthenia gravis, 651
Myelolipoma, 145, 145f
Myocarditis
    autopsy, 114, 114f
    death, cause of, 115
    mimics of, 115, 115f
    pearls and pitfalls, 115

Myxomatous mitral valve
    autopsy, 109–110, 109f
    potential mimics, 110
    sudden death association, 110

N

Naegleria fowleri meningitis, 654, 655f
Nasogastric tube, misplacement of, 574, 574f
National Oceanic and Atmospheric Administration website, 426
Natural disease
    cardiovascular system, 92
    central nervous system, 76
    endocrine system, 142
    hepatobiliary system, 129
    near misses, 158–160, 158f–162f
    respiratory system, 123
Neck, 250–251, 250f–251f
    blunt force injuries, 250–251, 250f–251f
    green discoloration of, 53f
    hanging, 184–185, 185f–187f
    noose furrow, 189
    strangulation, 190–191
    Tardieu spots, 49f
Nephrosclerosis, 139, 140f
Nervous system
    myasthenia gravis, 651
    schizophrenia, 651
    Wernicke-Korsakoff syndrome, 651–652, 652f
Neurogenic shock, 565
Neurosurgical complications, 391
Non-alcoholic fatty liver disease (NAFLD), 130
Non-human thoracic vertebrae, 628, 639
Non-ischemic left ventricular scar
    autopsy, 120, 120f
    sudden death association, 120
Non-scientific methods of identification, 36

O

Oblique fracture, 260
Odontology
    bite mark, 552
    forensic, 552–553
    human dentition, 552
    postmortem, 552
Opioid-type drug overdose, 445
Optic nerves
    dissection of, 596–597, 596f
    sheath hemorrhage, 389, 389f
Oral tears, 349f
Orbital plates, fracture of, 337, 338f
Oronasal foam cones, 444, 445f
Osmotic demyelination syndrome
    association, 86
    autopsy, 86, 87f
    potential mimics, 86
Outcome bias, 647
Overconfidence bias, 647–648
Oxalic acid, in kidney, 447, 448f
Oxycodone, 449

P

Pancreatic hemorrhage, 427
Papillary fibroelastoma, 494

Parathyroid adenoma, 653, 653f
Parathyroid glands
    dissection of, 601, 602f
    hyperplasia, 653
Parenchymal cleft of brain, 398f
Parenchymal contusions of brain, 395, 398f
Paroxysmal coughing, 405
Patterned abrasion, 409f
Peptic ulcer, 150, 150f
Pericarditis
    autopsy, 113, 113f
    etiologies of, 113
Peri-oral tears, 349f
Peripartum cardiomyopathy, 156–157
Peritonitis, 380, 380f
Petechial hemorrhages, 175, 176f
Phenice criteria, 538
Pheochromocytoma, 144, 145f
    autopsy, 144
Pituitary gland, infarction of
    association, 142
    autopsy, 142, 144f
Pit viper injury
    clinical features of, 436
    pathologic features of, 436
Placenta
    abruption, 560, 560f
    accreta, 156
    examination of, 559, 559f
    increta, 156
    percreta, 156
Pneumonia, 609, 634
    aspiration pneumonia. *See* Aspiration pneumonia
    autopsy, 123, 124f
    pearls and pitfalls, 123
    potential mimics of, 123, 125f
Pneumothorax, 292, 293f, 433
    examination for, 598–599, 599f
Polymicrobial cultures, 500
Positive identification, 30–33
Positive postmortem culture, 500
Posterior neck, dissection of, 597–598, 598f
Posterior rib fracture, 398, 399f
Postmortem changes
    animal activity, 63, 63f–65f
    decomposition, 51
        adipocere, 52, 53f
        corneal clouding, 54
        factors affecting, 51
        hemolysis, 54
        marbling, 54
        mummification and postmortem drying, 54, 55f
        pearls and pitfalls, 54, 55, 56, 56f, 57f
        postmortem blisters, 53, 53f
        postmortem bullae, 53, 53f
        skin, green discoloration of, 52, 52f–53f
        skin slippage, 56, 56f
        stages of, 59t
        swelling/bloating, 57, 57f–58f
        tache noire, 59, 59f
    documentation of, 15, 16f
    embalming artifacts, 65–66, 66f–67f
    identification of, 42
    lividity, 49–51
        other uses of, 50

pearls and pitfalls, 50
Tardieu spots, 49, 49f–50f
near misses, 67–68
postmortem entomology, 61, 61f–62f
  death determination, time of, 62, 63f
  pearls and pitfalls, 62
scene indicators, 60, 60f–61f
time/early death
  algor mortis, 42–43, 43t
  livor mortis, 46–48, 46f–47f, 49t
  pearls and pitfalls, 42–43
  postmortem vitreous potassium measurements, 44
  rigor mortis, 44, 44f
  supravitality, 44
Postmortem clots, 494, 495f, 609, 634
Postmortem drying, 54, 55f
Postmortem entomology, 61, 61f–62f
  death determination, time of, 62, 63f
  pearls and pitfalls, 62
Postmortem fractures, 265, 268f
Postmortem microbiology, 500
Postmortem redistribution, 451–452
Postmortem toxicology
  alcohol, 455
  cavity blood, 449
  chronic alcoholism, 456
  drug overdose, 444
    acetaminophen, 444, 446f
    autopsy, 444–447
    baggie, in stomach, 445, 447f
    cause of death, 444, 452
    cerebral edema, 445, 446f
    external findings of, 444, 445f
    foreign material, in lung, 447, 448f
    manner of death, 452
    oronasal foam cones, 444, 445f
    oxalic acid, in kidney, 447, 448f
    track marks, 444, 446f
  drugs
    metabolites of, 454, 454t
    oral hygiene associated with, 444, 446f
  ethanol, 454–456
  interpretation of, 450
  obtaining specimens for, 447–449
  pearls and pitfalls, 449–450
  postmortem drug concentrations, 451
  postmortem redistribution and importance, 451–452
  specific drugs, 453
Postmortem urine drug screen, 449
Postmortem vitreous potassium measurements, 44
Post-splenectomy patients, 500
Powder tattooing, 318, 321, 322f
Pre-eclampsia/eclampsia, 157
Pre-formatted autopsy report, 642
Pregnancy-related deaths, 155–156
Preretinal hemorrhages, 388
Prescription medications, 444
Presumptive identification, 30
Prone restraint cardiac arrest, 520
Pseudo-stippling, 321
  on skin, 326f
Psoriasis, 612, 634
Pulmonary barotrauma, 432

Pulmonary fat emboli, 491
Pulmonary hypertension, methamphetamine, 447
Pulmonary thromboembolus, 608, 618, 633, 636
  aging of, 486, 488f–489f
  circumstances, 484
  complications of, 484–486, 486f–488f
  identification of, 484, 485f–486f
  lower extremity dissections, 495
  right ventricle, inflammation of, 496, 497f

R
Rabies encephalitis, 654, 655f
Radiography, 74
  antemortem, 39f
  dental examination, 35
  firearm injuries, 292–293, 299f, 350f–352f
    0.25 ACP Winchester Expanding Point ammunition, 293, 295f
    birdshot, 293, 294f, 300f
    buckshot, 293, 294f
    copper and lead, 293, 293f, 298
    frangible ammunition, 293, 296f
    Glaser round, 293, 295f
    gunshot wound of neck, 298, 301f
    in head, 296, 297f
    hemothorax, 292, 293f
    high-powered rifle ammunition, 293, 294f
    intra-oral gunshot wound, 296, 298f
    Liberty Ammunition Civil Defense round, 293, 297f
    lower extremity, 297, 299f
    plastic nose, ammunition with, 298, 300f
    pneumothorax, 292, 293f
    purposes of, 292
    shotgun at close range, 298, 300f
    shotgun slug, 293, 294f
    snakeshot, 293, 295f
  neck, 250f
  stab wound, 282f
  vertebral arteries, 597f
Ratshot, 293, 295f
Reactance bias, 648
Recluse bite, 437
Re-entrance wound, 327–332, 330f–332f
Representative restraint bias, 648
Respiratory system, natural disease of, 123
Restraint asphyxia, 520
Resuscitation, 574, 621, 637
  conjunctival petechiae, 579
  external injuries, 575, 575f
  internal complications of, 577f–578f
  internal injuries, 576, 576f–578f
  retinal hemorrhages, 579
Retinal hemorrhages, 392, 404
  accidental injury, 393
  apparent life-threatening event (ALTE), 403
  backlit sectioned eyes, 387, 387f
  differential diagnosis of, 389, 390t
  distribution of, 387, 388f
  dysphagic choking, 405
  importance, 386
  location, 387–388
  microscopic images of, 387, 388f
  paroxysmal coughing, 405

photographically documenting, 387, 387f
resuscitation, 579
sagittal sinus thrombus, 405
Retinoschisis, 389, 389f
Rib fractures, 395
  cardiopulmonary resuscitation (CPR), 398–400, 400f
  location of, 396
  microscopic examination of, 400, 401f
  posterior, 398, 399f
Rickettsia rickettsii, 655
Rifle wounds, 292
  cause of death for, 336
  entrance, 306, 306f–311f, 308–310
  exit, 310, 312–313, 312f–319f, 316
  high-powered, 293, 294f, 303f
Rigor mortis, 44, 44f
Ring fracture, 225, 225f
Rocky Mountain spotted fever, 655
Ruptured berry aneurysm, 613, 635

S
Saddle pulmonary thromboembolus, 485, 486f
Sagittal sinus thrombus, 405
Scalloped shotgun wound entrance, 334f
Scene indicators for time of death, 60, 60f–61f
Scientific identification, 35, 35f–36f
Scrotum, gunshot wound of, 310, 311f
Scuba diving-related deaths
  barotrauma, 433
  causes of, 432–433
  gas embolism, 433
Search satisficing bias, 648
Seatbelt injuries, 589, 590f
Segmental fracture, 262, 263f
Seizure disorder, 439, 439f, 629, 639
  autopsy, 89, 90f
  pearls and pitfalls, 89–90
  sudden death association, 89
Self-serving bias, 646
Semmelweis reflex, 648
Senile ecchymoses, 215f, 528, 528f, 530f
Septic embolism, 493, 493f
Septic shock, 565
Serotonin syndrome, 656
Sex
  cranial features of, 539, 540f
  determination of, 536
  pelvic features of, 538–539
  skeletal features of, 538, 539f
Sexual trauma, 380
Shaken baby syndrome, 380–381, 394
Sharp force injuries, 466–468, 467f
  bone and cartilage, 286–287
    bony defects, 284–285, 285f
    class characteristics, identifying, 286
    pearls and pitfalls, 284, 286, 287–288, 287f–288f
  chop wound
    description, 281, 282f
    pearls and pitfalls, 281, 282f–283f
  incised wound
    description, 279–280, 280f
    pearls and pitfalls, 280–281
  near misses, 288, 288f–290f
  stab wound
    depth, determination of, 278, 278f

Sharp force injuries (*Continued*)
    description, 274, 274f, 278
    documentation of, 274, 275f
    multiple stab wounds, 279, 279f
    pearls and pitfalls, 275, 276f–277f, 277, 278, 279
Shored exit wounds, 313, 317f–318f, 326, 328f
Shotgun wounds, 292
    ammunition, 293
    death, cause of, 336
    entrance and exit wounds for, 332–336, 333f–336f
    head, 302, 302f–304f
    intra-oral wound, 303, 304f
    pellets, wadding, and shot sleeve, 344f
    self-inflicted wound, 302, 302f
    wound range, 333
SIDS. *See* Sudden infant death syndrome (SIDS)
Single-edged knife, 610, 634
Sinoatrial node, dissection of, 600–601, 601f
SIRS. *See* Systemic inflammatory response syndrome (SIRS)
Skin
    green discoloration of, 52, 52f–53f
    slippage, 56, 56f
    tenting, 412, 412f
Slugs, 293, 294f
Smothering
    autopsy, 180
    description, 178, 179f
Snake bite, 436, 655–656
Snakeshot, 293, 295f
Snow immersion, 430
Space-occupying subdural hemorrhage, 383, 386f
Spider bite, 437
Spinal cord, quick removal of, 603
Spinal nerves, 396f
Spiral fracture, 261
Splenic capsule, fibrosis of
    autopsy, 154–155, 154f
Splenic laceration, 592, 592f
Stab wound
    depth, determination of, 278, 278f
    description, 274, 274f, 278
    documentation of, 274, 275f
    multiple stab wounds, 279, 279f
    pearls and pitfalls, 275, 276f–277f, 277, 278, 279
Staphylococcus aureus, 500
Stature, 543
Stellate fracture, 224, 224f
Stillbirths, 558
    chorioamnionitis
        autopsy, 559, 560f
        potential mimics, 560
    distinguishing live birth from, 558
    meconium aspiration, 561, 561f
    near miss, 561, 561f
    organs in, 559
    placenta, examination of, 559, 559f
    placental abruption, 560, 560f
    stillborn fetus, 558, 559f
    stillborn infant, 558
Stippling, 318, 321, 322f
Strangulation
    autopsy, 191, 192f–193f
    description, 190
    pearls and pitfalls, 190–193, 191f, 193f
Streptococcus pneumoniae, 500
Streptococcus pyogenes, 500
Stretch-type injuries, of femoral region, 587, 588f
Subarachnoid hemorrhage, 235–239, 237f–239f, 382–383, 383f, 385f, 597
    contre-coup contusions associated with, 243f
    natural causes of
        autopsy, 82
        etiologies of, 82, 83f
        pearls and pitfalls, 83–84
        potential mimics of, 83, 84f
Subdural hemorrhage, 230–234, 232f–233f, 232t, 234t, 235f, 404, 413f, 449, 632, 640
    differential diagnosis of, 389, 390t
    herniated and hemorrhagic right uncus, 615, 635
    sagittal sinus thrombus, 405
    space-occupying, 383, 386f
    subarachnoid space, benign enlargement of, 405
    thin-film, 383, 384f–385f
Subendocardial hemorrhage, 424, 425f
Subgaleal hemorrhage, 219, 221–222, 221f, 383
Subretinal hemorrhages, 388
Sudden infant death syndrome (SIDS), 403, 510
Sudden unexpected infant death, 508
    asphyxial death at autopsy, 510–511
    bed-sharing, 512
    histologic sections, 508–509, 510f
    intra-thoracic petechiae, 511, 512f
    investigation of, 508, 509f
    microbiology studies, 512–513
    near miss, 513
    vs. sudden unexplained infant death (SUID), 513
    virological studies, 513
Sudden unexpected infant death investigation (SUIDI), 381, 508
Sudden unexplained infant death (SUID), 510, 513
Sugar spleen. *See* Splenic capsule, fibrosis of
Suicide(s), 344f, 464
    by drowning, 438, 439f
    vs. homicide
        asphyxial, 468–471, 469f–473f
        gunshot wounds, 465–466
        sharp force injuries, 466–468, 467f
    manner of death, 345, 464–465
    near misses, 473
    notes, 464, 465f
SUID. *See* Sudden unexplained infant death (SUID)
SUIDI. *See* Sudden unexpected infant death investigation (SUIDI)
Sunken cost bias, 645
Superficial perforating wound, 327, 330f
Supravitality, 44
Suspected inflicted head injury, 607, 633
Suspicious infant death, 381
Sutton's slip, 648
Swelling, 57, 57f–58f
Systemic inflammatory response syndrome (SIRS), 565

T
Tache noire, 59, 59f
Tangential wound, 326–327, 329f
Tardieu spots, 49, 49f–50f
Tentative identification, 30
Terson syndrome, 392
Thermal injury, 365, 365f
Thin-film subdural hemorrhage, 383, 384f–385f, 414f
Thoracotomy artifact, 579f
Thrombotic thrombocytopenic purpura (TTP), 153
Thymic involution, 509, 510f
Thyroglossal duct cyst, 652
Thyroid cartilage, 2
    maceration of, 604
Torsade de pointes, 654
Torus/buckle fractures, 259
Track marks, 444, 446f, 612, 634
Tramadol, 449
Transtentorial herniation, 568
Transverse fracture, 259–260
Traumatic asphyxia, smothering
    autopsy, 183
    description, 183
Treatment-related autopsy, 574
    medical devices, 574, 574f
    near misses, 579–580, 579f–580f
    resuscitation
        external injuries, 575, 575f
        internal injuries, 576, 576f–578f
Trunk, 252–255, 254f
    blunt force injuries, 252–255, 254f
    exit wounds of, 310, 313f

U
Ulcers, decubitus. *See* Decubitus ulcers

V
Valsalva retinopathy, 404
Ventriculostomy tubes, 578f
Vertebral arteries
    dissection of, 597, 597f
    laceration, 625, 638
Vertical line failure, 648
Vicks vapoInhaler™, 453
Visceral bias, 647
Visual identification, 36
    challenges, 36
    method, 36

Vitiated atmosphere/suffocating gases
   autopsy, 183
   description, 183
Vitreous electrolyte analysis, 502
   hyperglycemia, 503
   hyponatremia
      autopsy, 503
      causes of, 503
      clinical features of, 503
   ketoacidosis, 504–505
   patterns, 502–503, 502t

Vitreous urea nitrogen (VUN), 502
von Willebrand disease (vWD), 392

W

Wadding lodged, in body, 333, 334f
Water, bodies found in, 430
   cardiovascular disease, 431
   environmental and human factors, 431
   postmortem artifacts, 432, 432f–433f
Wernicke-Korsakoff syndrome, 651–652, 652f

West Nile virus myelitis, 654
Widmark equation, 453
Wischnewski spots, 429, 429f, 626, 638
   elder abuse, 530f, 531
Wolff-Parkinson-White (WPW) syndrome, 653
Wrist, gunshot wound of, 337, 338f

Z

Zebra retreat, 648
Zip guns, 292